Bioinspired Materials for Medical Applications

Related titles

Biomaterials for Cancer Therapeutics: Diagnosis, Prevention and Therapy
(ISBN 978-0-85709-664-7)

Biomimetic Biomaterials
(ISBN 978-0-85709-416-2)

Biomaterials Science 3e,
(ISBN 978-0-12-374626-9)

Woodhead Publishing Series in Biomaterials: Number 121

Bioinspired Materials for Medical Applications

Edited By

Lígia Rodrigues and ***Manuel Mota***

University of Minho, Braga, Portugal

ELSEVIER

AMSTERDAM • BOSTON • CAMBRIDGE • HEIDELBERG
LONDON • NEW YORK • OXFORD • PARIS • SAN DIEGO
SAN FRANCISCO • SINGAPORE • SYDNEY • TOKYO
Woodhead Publishing is an imprint of Elsevier

WP WOODHEAD PUBLISHING

Woodhead Publishing is an imprint of Elsevier
The Officers' Mess Business Centre, Royston Road, Duxford, CB22 4QH, United Kingdom
50 Hampshire Street, 5th Floor, Cambridge, MA 02139, United States
The Boulevard, Langford Lane, Kidlington, OX5 1GB, United Kingdom

Library of Congress Cataloging-in-Publication Data
A catalog record for this book is available from the Library of Congress

British Library Cataloguing-in-Publication Data
A catalogue record for this book is available from the British Library

ISBN: 978-0-08-100741-9 (print)
ISBN: 978-0-08-100746-4 (online)

Publisher: Matthew Deans
Acquisition Editor: Laura Overend
Editorial Project Manager: Lucy Beg
Production Project Manager: Poulouse Joseph
Designer: Maria Inês Cruz

Typeset by SPi Global, India

Contents

Contributors

N.F. Azevedo University of Porto, Porto, Portugal

C.C. Barrias i3S – Instituto de Investigação e Inovação em Saúde, University of Porto, Porto, Portugal

V.F. Cardoso University of Minho, Braga, Portugal; University of Minho, Guimarães, Portugal

S. Catarino University of Minho, Guimarães, Portugal

A.F. Cruz University of Coimbra, Coimbra, Portugal

J.F. da Silva Domingues Institute of Pharmacology and Structural Biology, CNRS UMR 5089, Toulouse Cedex, France

L.G. Dias Polytechnic Institute of Bragança, ESA, Bragança, Portugal; University of Trás-os-Montes e Alto Douro, CQ-VR, Vila Real, Portugal

J. Durão i3S – Instituto de Investigação e Inovação em Saúde, University of Porto, Porto, Portugal

D. Ferreira University of Minho, Centre of Biological Engineering, Braga, Portugal

G.P. Chaves Filho Universidade Federal do Rio Grande do Norte, Natal, Brazil

N.A. Fonseca University of Coimbra, Coimbra, Portugal; TREAT U, Coimbra, Portugal

L. Gales i3S – Instituto de Investigação e Inovação em Saúde, University of Porto, Porto, Portugal

M. Gama University of Minho, Braga, Portugal

S. Gorgieva University of Maribor, Maribor, Slovenia

A.C. Gregório University of Coimbra, Coimbra, Portugal

N.M. Guimarães University of Porto, Porto, Portugal

V.P. Hytönen University of Tampere, Tampere, Finland

S. Lanceros-Mendez University of Minho, Braga, Portugal; BC Materials, Technology and Scientific Park of Bizkaia, Derio, Spain; KERBASQUE, Basque Foundation for Science, Bilbao, Spain

V. Leiro i3S – Instituto de Investigação e Inovação em Saúde, University of Porto, Porto, Portugal

J. Leppiniemi University of Tampere, Tampere, Finland

R. Lima University of Minho, Guimarães, Portugal; Faculty of Engineering of the University of Porto, Porto, Portugal

R.M. Lopes University of Coimbra, Coimbra, Portugal

R. Machado University of Minho, Braga, Portugal

I.M. Martins University of Minho, Centre of Biological Engineering, Braga, Portugal

S.G. Meirinho University of Minho, Centre of Biological Engineering, Braga, Portugal

G. Minas University of Minho, Guimarães, Portugal

S.M.G. Moreira Universidade Federal do Rio Grande do Norte, Natal, Brazil

L. Moreira University of Porto, Porto, Portugal

J.N. Moreira University of Coimbra, Coimbra, Portugal

P.M. Moreno i3S – Instituto de Investigação e Inovação em Saúde, University of Porto, Porto, Portugal

V. Moura University of Coimbra, Coimbra, Portugal; TREAT U, Coimbra, Portugal

M. Oliveira University of Minho, Braga, Portugal

A.P. Pêgo i3S – Instituto de Investigação e Inovação em Saúde, University of Porto, Porto, Portugal

A.C. Peixoto University of Minho, Braga, Portugal

I. Pereira University of Minho, Braga, Portugal

A.M. Peres Polytechnic Institute of Bragança, ESA, Bragança, Portugal; University of Porto, LSRE-LCM, Porto, Portugal

C. Ribeiro University of Minho, Braga, Portugal

C. Rodrigues University of Minho, Braga, Portugal

A. Rodrigues University of Minho, Braga, Portugal

L.R. Rodrigues University of Minho, Centre of Biological Engineering, Braga, Portugal

J.L. Rodrigues University of Minho, Centre of Biological Engineering, Braga, Portugal

B. Sarmento i3S – Instituto de Investigação e Inovação em Saúde, University of Porto, Porto, Portugal; CESPU – Instituto de Investigação e Formação Avançada em Ciências e Tecnologias da Saúde, Instituto Superior de Ciências da Saúde-Norte, Gandra, Portugal

V. Sencadas University of Wollongong, Wollongong, NSW, Australia

A.F. Silva University of Minho, Braga, Portugal

S. Simões University of Coimbra, Coimbra, Portugal

J.J.T.M. Swartjes University of Groningen, Groningen, The Netherlands; Current address: Ecole Polytechnique Fédérale de Lausanne (EPFL), Institut des Matériaux and Institut des Sciences et Ingénierie Chimiques, Laboratoire des Polymères Bâtiment MXD Station 12 CH-1015 Lausanne, Switzerland

Â. Valério-Fernandes University of Coimbra, Coimbra, Portugal

T.G. Van Kooten University of Groningen, Groningen, The Netherlands

A.C.A. Veloso University of Minho, Centre of Biological Engineering, Braga, Portugal; Instituto Politécnico de Coimbra, ISEC, DEQB, Coimbra, Portugal

Woodhead Publishing Series in Biomaterials

1 **Sterilisation of tissues using ionising radiations**
Edited by J. F. Kennedy, G. O. Phillips and P. A. Williams

2 **Surfaces and interfaces for biomaterials**
Edited by P. Vadgama

3 **Molecular interfacial phenomena of polymers and biopolymers**
Edited by C. Chen

4 **Biomaterials, artificial organs and tissue engineering**
Edited by L. Hench and J. Jones

5 **Medical modelling**
R. Bibb

6 **Artificial cells, cell engineering and therapy**
Edited by S. Prakash

7 **Biomedical polymers**
Edited by M. Jenkins

8 **Tissue engineering using ceramics and polymers**
Edited by A. R. Boccaccini and J. Gough

9 **Bioceramics and their clinical applications**
Edited by T. Kokubo

10 **Dental biomaterials**
Edited by R. V. Curtis and T. F. Watson

11 **Joint replacement technology**
Edited by P. A. Revell

12 **Natural-based polymers for biomedical applications**
Edited by R. L. Reiss et al

13 **Degradation rate of bioresorbable materials**
Edited by F. J. Buchanan

14 **Orthopaedic bone cements**
Edited by S. Deb

15 **Shape memory alloys for biomedical applications**
Edited by T. Yoneyama and S. Miyazaki

16 **Cellular response to biomaterials**
Edited by L. Di Silvio

17 **Biomaterials for treating skin loss**
Edited by D. P. Orgill and C. Blanco

18 **Biomaterials and tissue engineering in urology**
Edited by J. Denstedt and A. Atala

19 **Materials science for dentistry**
B. W. Darvell

20 **Bone repair biomaterials**
Edited by J. A. Planell, S. M. Best, D. Lacroix and A. Merolli

21 **Biomedical composites**
Edited by L. Ambrosio

22 **Drug–device combination products**
Edited by A. Lewis

23 **Biomaterials and regenerative medicine in ophthalmology**
Edited by T. V. Chirila

24 **Regenerative medicine and biomaterials for the repair of connective tissues**
Edited by C. Archer and J. Ralphs

25 **Metals for biomedical devices**
Edited by M. Niinomi

26 **Biointegration of medical implant materials: Science and design**
Edited by C. P. Sharma

27 **Biomaterials and devices for the circulatory system**
Edited by T. Gourlay and R. Black

28 **Surface modification of biomaterials: Methods analysis and applications**
Edited by R. Williams

29 **Biomaterials for artificial organs**
Edited by M. Lysaght and T. Webster

30 **Injectable biomaterials: Science and applications**
Edited by B. Vernon

31 **Biomedical hydrogels: Biochemistry, manufacture and medical applications**
Edited by S. Rimmer

32 **Preprosthetic and maxillofacial surgery: Biomaterials, bone grafting and tissue engineering**
Edited by J. Ferri and E. Hunziker

33 **Bioactive materials in medicine: Design and applications**
Edited by X. Zhao, J. M. Courtney and H. Qian

34 **Advanced wound repair therapies**
Edited by D. Farrar

35 **Electrospinning for tissue regeneration**
Edited by L. Bosworth and S. Downes

36 **Bioactive glasses: Materials, properties and applications**
Edited by H. O. Ylänen

37 **Coatings for biomedical applications**
Edited by M. Driver

38 **Progenitor and stem cell technologies and therapies**
Edited by A. Atala

39 **Biomaterials for spinal surgery**
Edited by L. Ambrosio and E. Tanner

40 **Minimized cardiopulmonary bypass techniques and technologies**
Edited by T. Gourlay and S. Gunaydin

41 **Wear of orthopaedic implants and artificial joints**
Edited by S. Affatato

42 **Biomaterials in plastic surgery: Breast implants**
Edited by W. Peters, H. Brandon, K. L. Jerina, C. Wolf and V. L. Young

43 **MEMS for biomedical applications**
Edited by S. Bhansali and A. Vasudev

44 **Durability and reliability of medical polymers**
Edited by M. Jenkins and A. Stamboulis

45 **Biosensors for medical applications**
Edited by S. Higson

46 **Sterilisation of biomaterials and medical devices**
Edited by S. Lerouge and A. Simmons
47 **The hip resurfacing handbook: A practical guide to the use and management of modern hip resurfacings**
Edited by K. De Smet, P. Campbell and C. Van Der Straeten
48 **Developments in tissue engineered and regenerative medicine products**
J. Basu and J. W. Ludlow
49 **Nanomedicine: Technologies and applications**
Edited by T. J. Webster
50 **Biocompatibility and performance of medical devices**
Edited by J-P. Boutrand
51 **Medical robotics: Minimally invasive surgery**
Edited by P. Gomes
52 **Implantable sensor systems for medical applications**
Edited by A. Inmann and D. Hodgins
53 **Non-metallic biomaterials for tooth repair and replacement**
Edited by P. Vallittu
54 **Joining and assembly of medical materials and devices**
Edited by Y. (Norman) Zhou and M. D. Breyen
55 **Diamond-based materials for biomedical applications**
Edited by R. Narayan
56 **Nanomaterials in tissue engineering: Fabrication and applications**
Edited by A. K. Gaharwar, S. Sant, M. J. Hancock and S. A. Hacking
57 **Biomimetic biomaterials: Structure and applications**
Edited by A. J. Ruys
58 **Standardisation in cell and tissue engineering: Methods and protocols**
Edited by V. Salih
59 **Inhaler devices: Fundamentals, design and drug delivery**
Edited by P. Prokopovich
60 **Bio-tribocorrosion in biomaterials and medical implants**
Edited by Y. Yan
61 **Microfluidic devices for biomedical applications**
Edited by X-J. James Li and Y. Zhou
62 **Decontamination in hospitals and healthcare**
Edited by J. T. Walker
63 **Biomedical imaging: Applications and advances**
Edited by P. Morris
64 **Characterization of biomaterials**
Edited by M. Jaffe, W. Hammond, P. Tolias and T. Arinzeh
65 **Biomaterials and medical tribology**
Edited by J. Paolo Davim
66 **Biomaterials for cancer therapeutics: Diagnosis, prevention and therapy**
Edited by K. Park
67 **New functional biomaterials for medicine and healthcare**
E. P. Ivanova, K. Bazaka and R. J. Crawford
68 **Porous silicon for biomedical applications**
Edited by H. A. Santos
69 **A practical approach to spinal trauma**
Edited by H. N. Bajaj and S. Katoch
70 **Rapid prototyping of biomaterials: Principles and applications**
Edited by R. Narayan

71 **Cardiac regeneration and repair Volume 1: Pathology and therapies**
Edited by R-K. Li and R. D. Weisel
72 **Cardiac regeneration and repair Volume 2: Biomaterials and tissue engineering**
Edited by R-K. Li and R. D. Weisel
73 **Semiconducting silicon nanowires for biomedical applications**
Edited by J. L. Coffer
74 **Silk biomaterials for tissue engineering and regenerative medicine**
Edited by S. Kundu
75 **Biomaterials for bone regeneration: Novel techniques and applications**
Edited by P. Dubruel and S. Van Vlierberghe
76 **Biomedical foams for tissue engineering applications**
Edited by P. Netti
77 **Precious metals for biomedical applications**
Edited by N. Baltzer and T. Copponnex
78 **Bone substitute biomaterials**
Edited by K. Mallick
79 **Regulatory affairs for biomaterials and medical devices**
Edited by S. F. Amato and R. Ezzell
80 **Joint replacement technology Second edition**
Edited by P. A. Revell
81 **Computational modelling of biomechanics and biotribology in the musculoskeletal system: Biomaterials and tissues**
Edited by Z. Jin
82 **Biophotonics for medical applications**
Edited by I. Meglinski
83 **Modelling degradation of bioresorbable polymeric medical devices**
Edited by J. Pan
84 **Perspectives in total hip arthroplasty: Advances in biomaterials and their tribological interactions**
S. Affatato
85 **Tissue engineering using ceramics and polymers Second edition**
Edited by A. R. Boccaccini and P. X. Ma
86 **Biomaterials and medical-device associated infections**
Edited by L. Barnes and I. R. Cooper
87 **Surgical techniques in total knee arthroplasty (TKA) and alternative procedures**
Edited by S. Affatato
88 **Lanthanide oxide nanoparticles for molecular imaging and therapeutics**
G. H. Lee
89 **Surface modification of magnesium and its alloys for biomedical applications Volume 1: Biological interactions, mechanical properties and testing**
Edited by T .S. N. Sankara Narayanan, I. S. Park and M. H. Lee
90 **Surface modification of magnesium and its alloys for biomedical applications Volume 2: Modification and coating techniques**
Edited by T .S. N. Sankara Narayanan, I. S. Park and M. H. Lee
91 **Medical modelling: the application of advanced design and rapid prototyping techniques in medicine Second Edition**
Edited by R. Bibb, D. Eggbeer and A. Paterson
92 **Switchable and responsive surfaces and materials for biomedical applications**
Edited by Z. Zhang

93 **Biomedical textiles for orthopaedic and surgical applications: fundamentals, applications and tissue engineering**
Edited by T. Blair
94 **Surface coating and modification of metallic biomaterials**
Edited by C. Wen
95 **Hydroxyapatite (HAP) for biomedical applications**
Edited by M. Mucalo
96 **Implantable neuroprostheses for restoring function**
Edited by K. Kilgore
97 **Shape memory polymers for biomedical applications**
Edited by L. Yahia
98 **Regenerative engineering of musculoskeletal tissues and interfaces**
Edited by S. P. Nukavarapu, J. W. Freeman and C. T. Laurencin
99 **Advanced cardiac imaging**
Edited by K. Nieman, O. Gaemperli, P. Lancellotti and S. Plein
100 **Functional Marine Biomaterials: Properties and Applications**
Edited by S. K. Kim
101 **Shoulder and elbow trauma and its complications: Volume 1: The Shoulder**
Edited by R. M. Greiwe
102 **Nanotechnology-Enhanced Orthopedic Materials: Fabrications, Applications and Future Trends**
Edited by L. Yang
103 **Medical devices: Regulations, standards and practices**
Edited by S. Ramakrishna, L. Tian, C. Wang, S. L. and T. Wee Eong
104 **Biomineralisation and biomaterials: fundamentals and applications**
Edited by C. Aparicio and M. Ginebra
105 **Shoulder and elbow trauma and its complications: Volume 2: The Elbow**
Edited by R. M. Greiwe
106 **Characterisation and Design of Tissue Scaffolds**
Edited by P. Tomlins
107 **Biosynthetic Polymers for Medical Applications**
Edited by L. Poole-Warren, P. Martens and R. Green
108 **Advances in Polyurethane Biomaterials**
Edited by S. L. Cooper
109 **Nanocomposites for Musculoskeletal Tissue Regeneration**
Edited by H. Liu
110 **Thin Film Coatings for Biomaterials and Biomedical Applications**
Edited by H. J. Griesser
111 **Laser surface modification of biomaterials**
Edited by R. Vilar
112 **Biomaterials and regenerative medicine in ophthalmology Second edition**
Edited by T. V. Chirila and D. Harkin
113 **Extracellular Matrix-derived Medical Implants in Clinical Medicine**
Edited by D. Mooradian
114 **Wound Healing Biomaterials: Volume 1: Therapies and Regeneration**
Edited by M. S. Ågren
115 **Wound Healing Biomaterials: Volume 2: Functional biomaterials**
Edited by M. S. Ågren

116 **Materials for the Direct Restoration of Teeth**
J. Nicholson and B. Czarnecka
117 **Science and principles of biodegradable and bioresorbable medical polymers**
Edited by X. Zhang
118 **Medical Biosensors for Point of Care (POC) Applications**
Edited by R. Narayan
119 **Biocompatibility of Dental Biomaterials**
Edited by R. Shelton
120 **Bioresorbable Polymers for Biomedical Applications: From Fundamentals to Translational Medicine**
Edited by G. Perale
121 **Bioinspired materials for medical applications**
Edited by L. Rodrigues and M. Mota
122 **Chitosan based biomaterials Volume 1, Fundamentals**
Edited by J. A. Jennings and J. D. Bumgardner
123 **Chitosan based biomaterials Volume 2, Tissue Engineering and Therapeutics**
Edited by J. A. Jennings and J. D. Bumgardner
124 **Material-tissue interfacial phenomena**
Edited by P. Spencer
125 **Mechanical testing of orthopaedic implants**
Edited by E. Friis
126 **Management of periprosthetic joint infections (PJIs)**
Edited by A. J. Arts and J. A. P. Guerts
127 **Bone response to dental implant materials**
Edited by A. Piattelli
128 **Orthodontic Applications of Biomaterials: A Clinical Guide**
Edited by T. Eliades & W. A. Brantley
129 **Biofilms and implantable medical devices: Infection and control**
Edited by Y. Deng & W. Lv

Preamble

The relation between mankind and the surrounding environment began as soon as the first man stood upright. The development of tools commenced soon after. Wherever man has lived, tools have been found that were made from materials of biological origin.

Bones, animal skins, animal hair, horns, shells, wood, plant fibers, plant leaves, straw, for all of them man found a use and discovered novel applications.

The transformation of these collected biomaterials also began very early in man's development. Fire was used to harden wooden spears; animal hair and plant fibers were transformed into clothes or used to make baskets.

Much later, around 7500 BC, man discovered the possibility of extracting new materials from the earth, such as mud, which could be transformed by blending it with straw and sun drying. Later, c.5000 BC, bricks started to be made in kilns, giving rise to one of the strongest and cheapest building materials.

Modified kilns were used to extract metals from rocks and the hegemony of organic materials began to fade over the following centuries.

This situation changed dramatically in the 19th century, when several scientists became interested by in strange properties of several natural substances.

Around 1834, Hancock in Great Britain and Goodyear in the United States successfully improved the structural properties of latex rubber by adding sulfur.

In addition, cellulose was isolated from plant material in 1838 by the French chemist Anselme Payen, who determined its chemical formula. Soon, several materials derived from cellulose were made, namely, nitrocellulose, celluloid, cellulose acetate, cotton powder. The starch composition was shown to be identical to that of cellulose, the same being the case for glycogen.

One aspect remained, however, without explanation, that is, if starch and glycogen have exactly the same chemical composition, then why are starch and glycogen so different from cellulose as far as behavior and function are concerned? The answer to this enigma was given by Hermann Staudinger in 1920, who published work that opened up a new world for organic chemistry (Staudinger, 1920). Not only did he proved that rubber and other biomolecules, such as starch, glycogen, cellulose and proteins, which he named macromolecules, are long chains of repeating molecular units linked by covalent bonds, but also he showed that different ways of covalent bonding were responsible for different properties, even when the global chemical composition was the same. He also coined the term polymers. During his career he developed several methods to determine the molecular weight of polymers. As a result of this groundbreaking work, Staudinger won the Nobel Prize of Chemistry in 1953.

We can say that Staudinger's work was inspired by the biomaterials he worked with: cellulose, starch, glycogen, and rubber. If so, we can accept that the first bioinspired materials were the synthetic polymers that are so widely used nowadays.

The developments in molecular biology opened up further doors within this area. More and more macromolecules were discovered that were linked to very specific functions inside cells. Another landmark was setup when Watson and Crick disclosed the complex structure of DNA and how it could explain the mechanism of hereditary conservation of characteristics from parents to children (Watson and Crick, 1953). DNA is not a single polymer chain as many polymers are. DNA is a double-stranded molecule with hydrogen bonds between nitrogen bases, these bases being placed in a strict matching mechanism.

The accuracy of Watson and Crick's description of how the DNA double helix unfolds to replicate and self-assemble afterwards provided another exciting tool for bioinspired materials, namely a way of controlling self-assemblage. The possibility of controlling the assembling and disassembling cycles of DNA molecules became a reality with the introduction of the polymerase chain reaction (PCR) as a way to synthesize novel DNA molecules. With a very small amount of DNA, we are now able to replicate it billions of times in a machine called a thermocycler and use the synthetic DNA to transform living cells or to produce completely different materials. Kary Mullis won the Nobel Prize of Chemistry in 1993 for the invention of PCR.

The combination of new methods for DNA sequencing and PCR gave rise to astounding breakthroughs; one of the most striking examples being the in vitro/in silico (ie, by exocellular means combined with powerful computational methodologies) synthesis of an artificial bacterium, *Mycoplasma mycoides* JCVI-syn1.0, by the Craig Venter's group. As the authors stated:

> *We report the design, synthesis, and assembly of the 1.08-mega-base pair* Mycoplasma mycoides *JCVI-syn1.0 genome starting from digitized genome sequence information and its transplantation into a* M. capricolum *recipient cell to create new* M. mycoides *cells that are controlled only by the synthetic chromosome. The only DNA in the cells is the designed synthetic DNA sequence, including "watermark" sequences and other designed gene deletions and polymorphisms, and mutations acquired during the building process. The new cells have expected phenotypic properties and are capable of continuous self-replication.*
>
> *(Gibson et al., 2010)*

The frontier of synthetic biology was wide open. An exciting new field was offered to researchers.

On the other hand, researchers from the area of materials were moving fast. A number of new methodologies to characterize macromolecules were developed in the last decade. Advanced techniques address molecular weight determination, molecular and structural characterization by spectroscopic techniques, morphology and structural characterization by microscopy and diffraction, thermal analysis, in addition to techniques such as atomic force microscopy, and circular dichroism, XPS, micro-FTIR, MALDI-TOFF, NMR, micro-CT, among others.

However, new problems arose when bioinspired materials started to be assayed to tackle real-world issues. We can say that, in most cases of materials science, macromolecules have a primary orientation axis. In turn, in the real world of tissue engineering, macromolecules are not oriented in the same direction, since we have many different macromolecules coexisting and interacting. As a matter of fact, each organic tissue has its own preference, but in the vast majority of cases, organs in general present different cell-layer arrangements depending not only on their function (eg, lung, heart, bone, liver, kidney, among others) but also on their location in the human body (eg, skin, brain, eye).

Take an apparently simple example. Skin is a multilayered tissue, the outermost layer being the epidermis, which is indeed composed of four distinct layers: the one directly in contact with the outside world is called the stratum corneum, and going inside the body, we have the stratum granulosum, the stratum spinosum and the stratum basale. We now know that skin barrier capacity is controlled by lipids filling the extracellular space of the skin's surface layer—the stratum corneum.

Then comes the dermis, which is mainly connective tissue harboring a great number of cells, mainly fibroblasts, but also a number of organelles of different kinds—hair follicles, oil glands, sweat glands, nerves, etc., where the outer layer (ectoderm) is rather different from the medium layer (mesoderm) and from the innermost layer (endoderm). In other words, organs are far from being homogeneous.

In general terms, when you have a tissue you will have a simplified 2D organization, whereas when you are working with an organ you will have a multilayered 3D organization, as is the case of the skin where the ectodermis, endodermis and mesodermis will be present, or a quite intricate and even a rather corrugated structure, as in the case of the bones, lung, or brain.

For these reasons we are still far from being able to create artificial organs from scratch. The best way to produce tissues will be, for quite a while, the use of stem cells. The reason is simple. Stem cells have inscribed in their genome all the information needed to synthesize the right tissues and to coordinate the self-assemblage, on the one hand, and the 3D organization on the other.

Nevertheless, bioinspired materials are already under very active investigation and are proving their usefulness in many fields.

This is why we present this book, which is organized in distinct topics.

The first topic is composed by six chapters that present a general overview and discuss sensitive subjects such as *Design and preparation of biomimetic and bioinspired materials*, *Preparative methods and devices of bioinspired materials in drug-delivery systems*, *Metamorphic biomaterials*, *Molecular signaling mechanisms of host–materials interactions*, *Multifunctional biomaterials and their bioinspired systems for bioactive molecules delivery*, and the *Perspectives of bioinspired materials in regenerative medicine*.

The second topic is devoted to methodologies, tackling subjects such as *Advanced techniques for characterizing bioinspired materials* and *Imaging strategies for bioinspired materials*.

The third topic deals with biomaterials that are already on the market or are on the verge of being purchased in view of the clinical phases they are undergoing. In this topic we can find five chapters on *Injectable hydrogels as a delivery system for bone regeneration*, *Therapeutic proteins in bioactive materials for wound healing*, *Smart devices: micro and nanosensors*, *Smart devices: Lab-on-a-chip*, and *Electronic tongues and aptasensors*.

Finally, a set of three chapters discuss the challenges and the opportunities that recent advances in biology can offer to bioinspired materials. This is the case of *Advances on nucleic acid delivery with nonviral vectors*, *Artificial virus particles*, and *Synthetic Biology strategies towards the development of new bioinspired technologies for medical applications*.

Notwithstanding the impossible task of covering all of the exciting themes around this subject, there is still the need to point out future developments, including:

1. The feature of identification and spontaneous assembly present in several biomolecules might be explored to the benefit of a number of bioinspired materials. Spontaneous assembly involves two stages, namely the identification of the target and the attachment to the target at a special site that may be called the docking site. Spontaneous attachment has been recognized for many years, because this is what explains, for instance, the activity of antibodies, which identify and attach to antigens, or the activity of phages. The news is that we now know which are the molecules directly involved in a particular attachment mechanism, and we also know there are sticky molecules of various kinds. The first to be discovered were the nucleic acids, as we saw with the work of Watson and Crick. But soon after, many nucleic acid-binding proteins were described. Following these came the description of carbohydrate-binding molecules, called lectins. Although we have been aware of lectins since the 19th century, they have been increasingly used in the affinity separation of sugar mixtures. Lectins display a high affinity for sugar moieties and, as a result, they stick to a pure carbohydrate or to the carbohydrate part of a glycoprotein or a glycolipid. They are used in the most common assay to identify the different blood types by simple agglutination. Nowadays, injectable hydrogels are being used for bone regeneration. Many of the injectable hydrogels are composed of carbohydrate parts, as is the case of hyaluronic acid, an anionic, nonsulfated glycosaminoglycan, or of hydroxypropyl-methylcellulose. We may speculate that the decoration of these hydrogels with lectins might prevent a fast biodegradation or dampen the immune response.
2. Recently, specifically around 1999, the discovery of sillafins brought to light the role of these peptides in the templating process of exquisite diatom silica skeletons. The same happened with sponges, organisms that have also a silicious skeleton, though they are quite different from diatoms. In both cases, the involvement of proteins in the control of the silification process was unveiled. For example, sillafin-R5, a 19-aminoacid cationic peptide very rich in lysine and serine residues is able to induce precipitation of silica in seconds, at room temperature and at pH 5 or more. On the other hand, the spiculas from sponges are formed via the enzyme sylicatein involving a different mechanism. What is interesting is the potential utilization of the biosilica for bone regeneration. Indeed, both silaffins and silicatein have potential utilization in stimulating the growth of osteocytes (Gough et al., 2004). This is another aspect that needs to be more deeply explored in the future. Additionally, the flexibility brought about by the control of silica templating at a micro and nano scale opens up new possibilities in the design of smart devices, micro- and nanosensors and lab-on-a-chip (Rai and Perry, 2010; Miles et al., 2012; Otzen, 2012).

3. If, as expected, the number of surgical implants increases exponentially, then there will be an opportunity for the development of small, inexpensive and portable devices, able to monitor the postsurgical recovery process.
4. The fast development of the new tools discovered in the recent years for genome editing, as well as emergent approaches to assemble DNA parts will certainly foster the development of new bioinspired materials for medical applications.

As editors of this book, we have tried to organize it in an order that raises the readers' interest, by making it as easy to understanding as possible. This is why we have a comprehensive list of terms, abbreviations and acronyms for each chapter. The chapter sequence was also set out in such a way that similar subjects are assembled.

We hope that, by putting together a set of different fields, pertaining, all of them, to the domain of bioinspired materials, several novel ideas will spark and give a new thrust to this exciting subject. If so, we think we have done our job, by contributing to efforts to make the life of millions of people suffering every day from many health issues less painful, providing relief, if not a cure, with the help of novel, durable, biocompatible biomaterials applicable in less invasive ways. Enjoy your reading.

The Editors
Lígia Rodrigues and Manuel Mota

References

Gibson, D.G., Glass, J.I., Lartigue, C., Noskov, V.N., Chuang, R.Y., Algire, M.A., et al., 2010. Creation of a bacterial cell controlled by a chemically synthesized genome. Science 329 (5987), 52–56.

Gough, J.E., Notingher, I., Hench, L.L., 2004. Osteoblast attachment and mineralized nodule formation on rough and smooth 45S5 bioactive glass monoliths. J. Biomed. Mater. Res. A 68 (4), 640–650.

Miles, D., Wilcox, R., Aggeli, A., 2012. Self-assembling peptides as a new class of medical device for regenerative medicine. In: Castillo, J., Sasso, L., Svendsen Winnie, E. (Eds.), Self-Assembled Peptide Nanostructures: Advances and Applications in NanoBiotechnology. CRC Press, Boca Raton, FL.

Otzen, D., 2012. The role of proteins in biosilicification. Scientifica 2012, 1–22. http://dx.doi.org/10.6064/2012/867562, Article ID 867562.

Rai, A., Perry, C.C., 2010. Facile fabrication of uniform silica films with tunable physical properties using silicatein protein from sponges. Langmuir 26 (6), 4152–4159.

Staudinger, H., 1920. Über polymerisation. Ber. Deut. Chem. Ges. 53 (6), 1073–1085.

Watson, J.D., Crick, F.H.C., 1953. A structure for deoxyribose nucleic acid. Nature 171, 737–738.

Design and preparation of biomimetic and bioinspired materials

1

V. Leiro, P.M. Moreno*, B. Sarmento*,†, J. Durão*, L. Gales*, A.P. Pêgo*, C.C. Barrias**

*i3S – Instituto de Investigação e Inovação em Saúde, University of Porto, Porto, Portugal, †CESPU – Instituto de Investigação e Formação Avançada em Ciências e Tecnologias da Saúde, Instituto Superior de Ciências da Saúde-Norte, Gandra, Portugal

1.1 General introduction

1.1.1 Drug delivery—The need for new solutions for an old challenge

For a long time drug-delivery systems have been investigated and explored as a strategy to improve the efficacy and safety of therapeutic agents. The quest is to find "the magic cannon"—a carrier-system that transports the drug of interest to a specific target. Different approaches have been proposed, with many already in the clinic, to improve drug solubility, increase drug half-life, control the drug release profile and attain tissue/cell targeting. These have differently contributed to the enhancement of the pharmacokinetics and pharmacodynamics of many drugs, with demonstrated improvements in terms of efficacy, reduction of side effects, and even reduction of the number of the required administrations. Success stories include the PEGylated (where PEG stands for poly(ethylene glycol)) liposomal formulations for the delivery of doxorubicin (DOX) (Doxil/Caelyx) (Allena and Cullisb, 2013) or protein-bound paclitaxel for the treatment of ovarian and breast cancer (Liang et al., 2015), respectively.

Nevertheless, many clinical problems are still unanswered. With the increase of life expectancy, the prevalence of age-related diseases, like neurodegenerative diseases, osteoarticular diseases, and even cancer, is also increasing. Efficient drug-delivery systems to the central nervous system (CNS) have been expected for a long time. The challenge, still to be answered, has been to beat the blood–brain barrier (BBB), blood–cerebrospinal fluid barrier, blood–retinal barrier and, the blood–CNS tumor barrier. Some progress has been achieved (Chena and Liub, 2012). Targeting a specific cell population has also not been a trivial issue. While tethering antibodies to a drug or the surface of a particulate delivery system has been an advanced solution, the use of such an approach has been very limited so far. Escaping immune-surveillance and attaining efficient specificity have been hurdles that have been difficult to overcome. Even in the case of solutions already in the clinics unexpected side effects have come up, as in the previously referred to case of Doxil/Caelyx (Chang and Yeh, 2012). Consequently, the field of drug delivery is still eager to find new and/or improved systems that can solve the caveats of the current existing solutions.

Bioinspired Materials for Medical Applications. http://dx.doi.org/10.1016/B978-0-08-100741-9.00001-2

1.1.2 Biomimetic and bioinspired materials

As our understanding of cell biology, as well as of tissue homeostasis and pathology improves, the interest in biomimetic and bioinspired materials is growing. Here, this class of biomaterials is defined as a material that recapitulates key features of natural materials and/or biological structures. They can be of natural origin, as in the case of naturally derived sugars, be based on natural occurring monomer units, as in the case of nucleic acid (NA)-based molecules, or fully synthetic.

Due to their similarities with biologically relevant structures, either at the chemical, physical, or morphological level, biomimetic and bioinspired materials are expected to outperform many of the currently available materials. At the chemical level one can take advantage of the similarity of biological constituents to attain chemical specificity, reduce cytotoxicity, or tune biodegradability. Self-assembly features have also been explored at large, mimicking the membranes of cytoplasmic vesicles, as in the case of liposomes, and forming cross-linked hydrogels resembling our natural "drug reservoir"—the extracellular matrix (ECM), as in the case of engineered protein-, peptide-, or polysaccharide-based hydrogels (Barros et al., 2015).

Vector size and structure can also be key to the success of an advanced solution. To illustrate the advantage of the use of a bioinspired material in this case one can highlight the use of NA technology and NAs as vector-building blocks, which has allowed precise control of intermolecular interactions, and finally the design of NA cages that combine therapeutic functions with vectorizing features. In this context, synthetically derived biopolymers have particularly raised a lot of attention, due to several advantageous features. In contrast with the simpler and stochastic structure of purely synthetic polymers commonly used in the field (e.g., poly(lactic-*co*-glycolic acid)), synthetically derived biopolymers can be engineered to attain a complex and reproducible structure.

Furthermore, by being synthesized using solid-phase synthesis or recombinant technology (eventually combined with genetic engineering), they are monodisperse in nature. Finally, these are inherently recognized by enzymes, and consequently biodegradable. In parallel, dendrimers, a new class of fully synthetic macromolecules, have also been proposed as promising carriers for drug delivery due to not only their monodispersion and controllable nanosize but also their unique structural characteristics (globular, well-defined, and very branched structure). While fully synthetic, they mimic many of defined features of biological molecules.

In the last few years these materials have been explored as drug-delivery systems, with different degrees of developmental success. Here we discuss the design and preparation of five of the most promising classes of bioinspired and biomimetic materials for this application.

1.2 Lipid-based systems

1.2.1 Structure and properties of lipids

Lipids are a large class of materials that includes fatty acids, glycerides, phospholipids, sphingolipids, waxes, and sterols. These compounds are usually insoluble in water, or amphiphilic, and are identified by their fatty-acid composition, melting point, hydrophilic–lipophilic balance, and solubility in organic solvents. Lipid-based systems have gained much interest in the recent years for drug-delivery purposes mainly due to their ability to improve the solubility and bioavailability of drugs with poor water solubility.

However, lipid-based systems have also demonstrated superior efficacy for hydrophilic drugs, tailoring the release profile of the active payloads in a biofunctional manner.

The most significant dosage forms are liposomes, solid lipid nanoparticles (SLN), nanostructured lipid carriers (NLC), and self-emulsifying drug-delivery systems (SEDDS).

1.2.2 Design of lipid-based delivery systems

1.2.2.1 Liposomes

Liposomes are spherical vesicles composed of bilayers of phospholipids, cholesterol, and/or other lipids (Mishra et al., 2010). Lecithin, phosphatidylglycerol, phosphatidylinositol, phosphatidylethanolamine, and phosphatidylserine are the mainly used phospholipids (Cryan, 2005). They can be classified according to their lamellarity as uni, oligo, and multilamellar, or by size as small, intermediate, and large. Due to its structure, they allow the incorporation of hydrophilic drugs in the aqueous core, and lipophilic drugs within the lipid bilayer (Fig. 1.1; Martins et al., 2007). Possessing higher core, unilamellar liposomes are preferred for encapsulation of hydrophilic drugs, while multilamellar liposomes are especially used to encapsulate hydrophobic drugs due to the higher lipid content (Immordino et al., 2006). Depending on the number and composition of the bilayers and the presence of coating, it is possible to obtain systems with modified release characteristics (Grenha et al., 2008; Faraji and Wipf, 2009). Besides the marketed formulations, liposomes have been suggested for administration of several drugs, including peptides and therapeutic proteins, as well as for gene therapy (Cryan, 2005). Stealth liposomes like Doxil/Caelyx, Novantrone, or Lipoplatin are commercially available examples of second-generation liposomes, surface-decorated with PEG moieties, resulting in improvement of blood circulation time and the therapeutic efficacy of many drugs through the avoidance of opsonization, that is, removal by immune cells, and escape from reticuloendothelial system (Immordino et al., 2006).

1.2.2.2 SLNs and NLC

Lipid nanoparticles generally comprise two types of structures, SLN and NLC (Fig. 1.1B and C; Martins et al., 2007; Müller et al., 2007). They comprise a solid lipid matrix, usually highly purified triacylglycerols, complex acylglycerol mixtures, and even waxes, at room and body temperatures, dispersed in aqueous solution and stabilized with a layer of emulsifier agent, usually phospholipids (Faraji and Wipf, 2009). Lipid nanoparticles emerged as an alternative to liposomes because of the superior stability in biological fluids. They are colloidal carriers made of nontoxic (Muller et al., 1996), biodegradable and well-tolerated solid lipids dispersed either in water or in an aqueous surfactant solution. The lipid composition can delay degradation by hindering the anchorage of enzyme complexes (Olbrich and Muller, 1999), justifying their potential for controlled drug delivery. Additional advantages of SLN are their particulate nature, ability to incorporate both hydrophilic and hydrophobic drugs, the avoidance of organic solvents in the production procedures and the possibility to produce highly concentrated lipid suspensions, lower cytotoxicity, and scale-up feasibility (Joshi and Müller, 2009).

Hydrophobic anticancer drugs such as camptothecin (Martins et al., 2013), antirheumatics such as methotrexate (Albuquerque et al., 2015), or immunosuppressants as cyclosporine (Sandri et al., 2010) have been encapsulated into SLN for modulating their in vivo biodistribution and target drugs for their local of action. SLNs are also able to encapsulate biopharmaceutical drugs with high aqueous solubility, retaining their structure after encapsulation and even freeze-drying (Soares et al., 2013). Therapeutic proteins (Fonte et al., 2011) or genetic material (Jin et al., 2011) are currently formulated into solid lipid matrix, resulting in biocompatible and environment-friendly conditions to stabilize those biologicals.

A second generation of lipid nanoparticles is the so-called NLC (Muller et al., 2002). These particles are prepared not from a solid lipid but from a blend of solid and liquid (oils) lipids, which must be solid at least at 40°C. The main difference between SLN and NLC is that the latter are formulated by nano-structuring the lipid matrix to increase drug loading and prevent drug expulsion. Using spatially different lipids leads to larger distances between the fatty acid chains of the acylglycerols and general imperfections in the crystal, providing more room to accommodate drugs. The highest drug loads could be achieved by mixing solid lipids with small amounts of liquid lipids. Many drugs show a higher solubility in oils than in solid lipids, thus they can be dissolved in the oil and still be protected from degradation by the surrounding solid lipids.

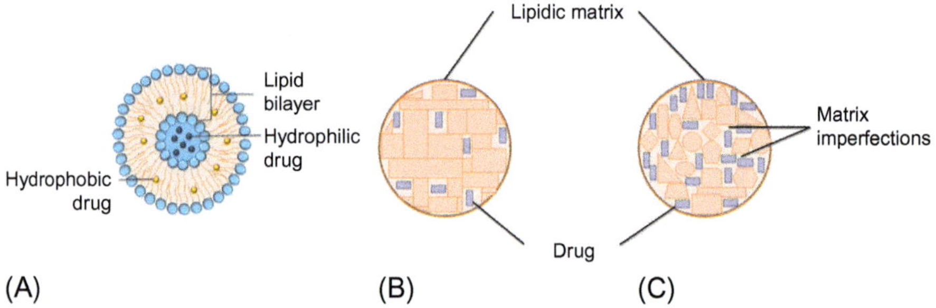

Fig. 1.1 Schematic representation of a liposome (A), a SLN (B), and a NLC (C).

1.2.2.3 Self-emulsifying drug-delivery systems

SEDDS are isotropic mixtures of lipid, surfactant, cosurfactant and, sometimes, cosolvents, and drug substance that can spontaneously form fine oil-in-water microemulsions under mild agitation following dilution with an aqueous phase (Neslihan Gursoy and Benita, 2004). On dilution in an aqueous phase they form fine stable oil-in-water (o/w) emulsions or fine lipid droplets, which is characteristic of these systems.

Compared with classical emulsions, SEDDS are physically more stable and easier to manufacture, being ready-to-use formulations to entrap lipophilic drugs with dissolution rate–limited absorption. Consequently, these systems may offer an improvement in the rate and extent of absorption, tailor pharmacokinetic profiles, and result in more reproducible blood–time profiles.

SEDDS are particularly applicable for orally administered drugs, in soft or hard gelatin capsules that disintegrate in the gastrointestinal fluids (Sandri et al., 2010). Drugs with dissolution and bioavailability issues as fenofibrate (Soares et al., 2013), celecoxib (Fonte et al., 2011), or cyclosporine (Jin et al., 2011) have been formulated into SEDDS with success improvement of the oral controlled release of those drugs.

1.3 Glycan-based systems

1.3.1 Structure and properties of glycans

Carbohydrates, sometimes called "sugars," are an important class of biomolecules found abundantly in nature. Monosaccharides, the simplest sugars, are the basic structural units of carbohydrates. These units have three to nine carbons and a characteristic carbonyl group, which can be either an aldehyde, in aldoses, or a ketone, in ketoses. Monosaccharides exist primarily in cyclic form, and can be linked together via "α" or "β" glycosidic bonds, forming linear or branched chains of oligosaccharides (2–20 units), with the general formula $(CH_2O)_n$. Chains with more than 20 monosaccharide residues are referred to as polysaccharides. The generic term "glycan" is often used to refer to any oligo- and polysaccharide, either free or covalently linked to other molecules, such as proteins or lipids, in the form of glycoconjugates.

The field of glycobiology has been developing at a great pace over the past decades. Although carbohydrates were primarily considered mainly as storage and structural materials, it is nowadays clear that they exhibit a plurality of biological activities (Varki et al., 2009; Stick, 2001; Raman et al., 2005). This is in large part associated with their great diversity, for which several factors contribute. There is a wide array of monosaccharides. The ones commonly found in animal glycans include: (i) neutral sugars—pentoses and hexoses; (ii) hexosamines—hexoses with a free or N-acetylated amino group; (iii) deoxyhexoses—hexoses without an hydroxyl group at position 6; (iv) uronic acids—hexoses with a negatively charged carboxyl group; and (v) sialic acids—family of 9-carbon acidic sugars (Varki et al., 2009; Stick, 2001; Raman et al., 2005). Apart from the already mentioned modifications, hydroxyl groups of monosaccharides can also be chemically modified by methylation and esterification (phosphate, acyl, and sulfate esters). Moreover, the presence of asymmetrical (chiral) carbons in monosaccharides gives rise to different isomeric forms, with distinct biochemical properties. To form higher-order structures, monosaccharides can be linked together in many different ways, because of the various possible isomers that can be formed between two units. The glycosidic linkage can involve alternative stereoisomers (α or β) at the anomeric carbon of the former unit, and the various hydroxyl groups at the subsequent unit allow several possibilities of isomerization (Varki et al., 2009; Stick, 2001; Raman et al., 2005). The common occurrence of branching also contributes to the structural diversity of glycans (Varki et al., 2009; Stick, 2001; Raman et al., 2005). This way, depending on the type of glycosidic linkage, sugar chains of identical composition can assume very different conformations and bioactivities. A classic example is that of starch and cellulose, which are both homopolymers of glucose found in plants, where they play storage and structural roles, respectively. While α1–4 linkages and branching in starch results in helical chains and a more disorganized three-dimensional (3D) structure, β1–4 linkages in cellulose result in a straight chain 3D structure, strengthen by interchain hydrogen bonds (Varki et al., 2009; Stick, 2001; Raman et al., 2005). These structural differences account for their quite distinct biochemical properties and biological function.

The major classes of animal glycans include glycosaminoglycans (GAGs) that, with the exception of hyaluronic acid, occur as proteoglycans and other conjugates such as glycoproteins and glycolipids. Glycans can mediate a wide range of biological processes by virtue of their physical properties, such as charge, molecular conformation, mass or gel-forming ability, and their biochemical function is determined by their nanoscale organization (Varki et al., 2009; Stick, 2001; Raman et al., 2005; Fernández-Tejada et al., 2015; Miller et al., 2014).

On the other hand, many of the more specific functions of glycans implicate recognition by glycan-binding proteins (GBPs), such as lectins and GAG-binding proteins (Varki et al., 2009; Stick, 2001). In nature, all cells and many macromolecules carry a set of covalently linked glycans. The presence of glycans at the cell surface and in the ECM, place them in optimal position for mediating a variety of processes underlying cell–cell, cell–matrix, and cell–molecule interactions, not only within an organism, but also between different organisms. Inspired by their biological roles, different biomimetic materials have been designed using native, modified, and synthetic glycans as building blocks.

1.3.2 Design of glycan-based delivery systems

Glycan-based biomaterials, from more simple oligosaccharides to more complex polysaccharides, can be engineered with unique properties and defined structures, being particularly appealing for the design of advanced drug-delivery systems (Fernández-Tejada et al., 2015; Miller et al., 2014; Lenci et al., 2016; Chen et al., 2014). In these applications, glycans from animal, nonanimal, and synthetic origins have been used, often chemically modified to achieve specific and consistent physicochemical properties and bioactivity (Fernández-Tejada et al., 2015; Miller et al., 2014; Lenci et al., 2016; Chen et al., 2014). To meet different needs, glycan-based biomaterials have been processed into various shapes, including micelles, nano/microparticles, hydrogels, nano/micro-fibers, and porous 3D scaffolds (Miller et al., 2014; Lenci et al., 2016; Chen et al., 2014; Zhang et al., 2013; Singh et al., 2014; Azevedo and Pashkuleva, 2015; Boddohi and Kipper, 2010).

The design of glycan-based drug-delivery systems exploits different properties of this highly diverse family of natural compounds. Depending on the type of carbohydrate, some key properties may include (Miller et al., 2014; Lenci et al., 2016; Chen et al., 2014; Zhang et al., 2013; Singh et al., 2014; Azevedo and Pashkuleva, 2015; Boddohi and Kipper, 2010): (i) gel-forming ability, commonly used in the development of matrix-type drug carriers; (ii) hydrophilic nature, which can be explored to enhance the circulatory half-lives of different types of drugs; (iii) polyelectrolyte nature, to promote bottom-up nano-assembly and/or complexation between glycans and drugs of opposite charge via electrostatic interactions; (iv) bioadhesiveness, frequently exploited as a means to increase drug retention at certain locations, namely at mucosal surfaces; and (v) affinity for GBPs, commonly employed in the design of targeted carriers, such as glycan-decorated particles.

There are also sugar-based compounds with very particular properties. This is the case of cyclodextrins, a family of cyclic oligosaccharides made up of glucose monomers bound together in a ring. Given the unique nature imparted by their structure, where the interior is considerably less hydrophilic than the exterior, cyclodextrins are able to form host–guest complexes with hydrophobic molecules, enhancing their solubility, physical chemical stability, and bioavailability (Fig. 1.2; Rodell et al., 2015; Dan et al., 2015). As such, these compounds have recently found a large number of applications in the drug-delivery field (Rodell et al., 2015; Dan et al., 2015).

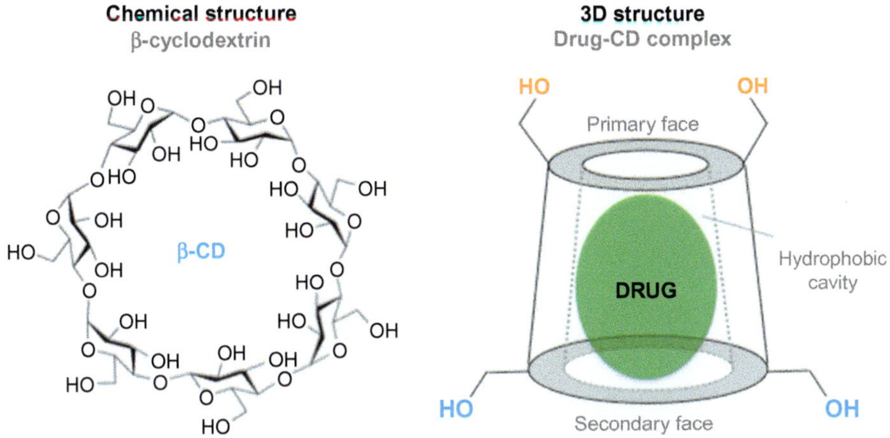

Fig. 1.2 *Left:* Chemical structure of β-cyclodextrin (seven glucose units). *Right:* Schematic representation (3D structure) of a cyclodextrin encasing a hydrophobic drug.

Hydrogel-based matrix-type drug carriers have been gaining increasing popularity as ECM mimics for regenerative medicine and tissue engineering. In the ECM, gel-forming glycans provide hydration, structural stability, and selective permeability (Azevedo and Pashkuleva, 2015; Hynes, 2009; Hudalla and Murphy, 2011). They are also involved in specific, noncovalent binding of several endogenous molecules, such as growth factors, regulating their bioavailability and bioactivity, namely by assisting in the establishment of gradients (Azevedo and Pashkuleva, 2015; Hynes, 2009; Hudalla and Murphy, 2011). Several polysaccharides, including alginate, chitosan, pectin, and hyaluronic acid, among many others, are able to form highly hydrated 3D networks under mild conditions, being extensively used as matrix-type reservoirs for numerous biomolecules. Hydrogels can be prepared from unmodified or bio-functionalized polysaccharides, and can range from nearly bioinert networks to bioactive "smart" or "cell-instructive/responsive" matrices, which more closely recapitulate the complex nature of native ECMs (Hudalla and Murphy, 2011; Neves et al., 2015; Fonseca et al., 2014; Maia et al., 2014; Zhao et al., 2015; Giammanco et al., 2015; Chan et al., 2009; Daniel-da-Silva et al., 2011). Different drug-immobilization strategies have been described. While simple matrix-entrapment generally results in poorly controllable diffusion-driven drug release, electrostatic and Van der Waals interactions or covalent immobilization via labile linkers may provide additional levels of control over release kinetics. Moreover, the use of environmentally sensitive hydrogels offers a means to spatially and/or temporally control drug release, which occurs in response to specific physiological triggers, such as pH, temperature, ionic strength, enzymatic activity, or external stimuli such as magnetic or electric fields (Fonseca et al., 2014; Zhao et al., 2015; Giammanco et al., 2015; Chan et al., 2009; Daniel-da-Silva et al., 2011). Multicomponent hydrogels, such as interpenetrating polymeric networks (IPNs) and semi-IPNs, which may show physicochemical properties remarkably different from those of their macromolecular constituents, have also emerged as a promising alternative for drug delivery (Matricardi et al., 2013).

While the widespread utility of carbohydrates has been undeniably demonstrated, covering all the relevant aspects of their applications in drug delivery in a single thematic issue is recognizably difficult. Therefore this section is intended to provide only a brief overview of the field, being illustrative rather than all-inclusive.

1.4 Peptide-based systems

1.4.1 Structure and properties of peptides

Peptides offer several advantages as building blocks for the design of drug-delivery systems. They are endogenous molecules, which reduces the risk of adverse effects; are composed of nonpolar, polar, or charged amino acids, allowing a certain level of prediction of the self-assembly properties through the meticulous selection of the peptide sequence; may range from short to long and more flexible chains enabling the construction of structural diverse arrangements, from solid crystals to soft disordered materials; and are relatively easy to synthesize and in some cases (short peptides) are commercially available at reasonable prices. Moreover, the remarkable physicochemical properties of peptides enable them to originate responsive materials to stimulus such as temperature, pH, or the presence of specific molecules.

1.4.2 Design of peptide-based delivery systems

Short peptides have been vastly used in the preparation of both crystalline and of soft materials. Diphenylalanine emerged as probably the most versatile (Yan et al., 2010), with application in nanoelectronics (Reches and Gazit, 2003), tissue engineering (Jayawarna et al., 2006; Mahler et al., 2006), or as a model to investigate the molecular mechanisms of protein aggregation in amyloidogenisis (Adler-Abramovich et al., 2012). Several hydrophobic dipeptides, including diphenylalanine, are able to generate microporous crystals formed by hydrogen bond-induced head-to-tail assembly of dipeptides into helical arrangements (Görbitz, 2007).

The crystal frameworks typically contain 1D channels with a diameter of 3–10 Å (Fig. 1.3). They were tested as adsorbents (Afonso et al., 2012) of several gases such as Xe (Soldatov et al., 2004), CO_2 (Durão and Gales, 2013), CH_4, H_2 (Comotti et al., 2009), Ar (Afonso et al., 2014), N_2, and O_2 (Afonso et al., 2010) and may find interesting biomedical application in the delivery of gasotransmitter molecules. Dipeptides were also incorporated in hybrid metal–organic materials (Adler-Abramovich et al., 2012; Emami et al., 2014; Rabone et al., 2010) showing interesting adsorption properties. Oligopeptides may self-assemble into several different architectures with perhaps even higher biomedical interest than microporous crystals, such as tubes, rods, fibrils, spheres, vesicles, and gels (Gazit, 2007; Koley and Pramanik, 2012).

Nanovesicular structures have been intensely investigated for the delivery of hydrophobic drugs (Koley et al., 2012; Zhao et al., 2010). Also 3D cultures of nerve cells, endothelial cells, and chondrocytes (Mahler et al., 2006; Holmes et al., 2000; Genové et al., 2005; Zhang, 2003) were already successfully conducted in highly hydrated short-peptides-based scaffolds, like, for example, from the simple amphiphilic building blocks consisting of dipeptides linked to fluorenylmethoxycarbonyl (Fmoc, broadly used as a protecting group in peptide chemistry). The incorporation of small organic moieties or of unnatural amino acids has been frequently used to regulate the physicochemical properties and to increase the proteolytic and thermal stability of these peptides (Koley and Pramanik, 2011; Maity et al., 2011). The properties of the final material are also governed by the experimental conditions during the self-assembly. For instance, Greenfield et al. (2010) have studied a peptide amphiphile (PA) hydrogel produced by two different triggers, HCl and $CaCl_2$, resulting in gels with similar structure but remarkably different viscoelastic properties. Whereas $CaCl_2$ produced a stronger gel with tighter inter- and intrafibril crosslinks, HCl induced a more flexible structure capable of rapidly recovering its shape after deformation.

It is still a major challenge to design a novel peptide-based material with predetermined properties. Several design strategies are being refined, mainly involving either the production of PAs or the application of the knowledge gained from protein secondary structural motifs, such as α-helix and β-sheet. Although a greater number of studies have concentrated on peptides folding into β-sheets, possibly as a result of the high research activity on amyloid-like structures, α-helical folding has recently been receiving increasing attention. This fact could be linked to the well-defined set of rules that have been established for the assembly of α-helices that can lead to a rational molecular design.

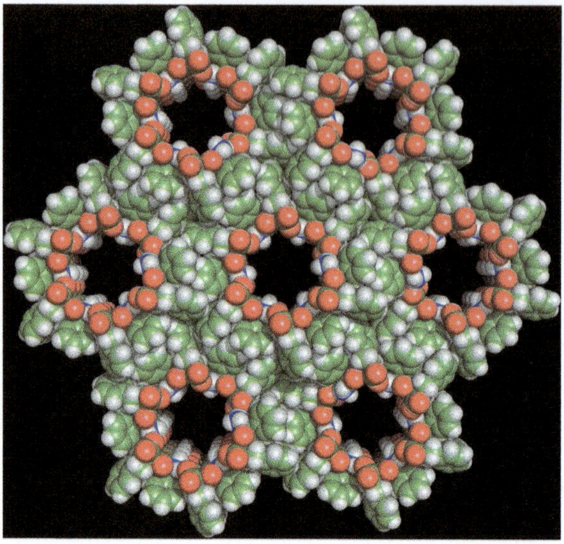

Fig. 1.3 Example of one dipeptide crystal (leucine–serine) displaying 1D nanochannel.

1.4.2.1 α-Helix

α-Helix is a key secondary structure of natural proteins that consists of a peptide chain coiled into a right-handed spiral conformation and stabilized by hydrogen bonds between the N–H and the C=O groups in the backbone. Methionine, alanine, leucine, glutamate, and lysine have special propensity to be part of α-helix structures while proline and glycine have poor helix-forming propensities. A particularly abundant α-helix-based structural motif is the coiled coil, in which the α-helix is frequently characterized by a seven residue repeating unit of alternating hydrophobic and hydrophilic residues, often denoted as $(abcdefg)_n$ (Fig. 1.4; Banwell et al., 2009; Woolfson, 2010; Woolfson and Ryadnov, 2006; Wagner et al., 2005; Zimenkov et al., 2004; Burkhard et al., 2001; Parry et al., 2008). Coiled coils have been used for drug delivery isolated or incorporated in liposomes and for the design of supramolecular materials. Coiled coils display an inner hydrophobic core that can be explored to carry hydrophobic drugs. Eriksson et al. (2009) studied the potential of loading cisplatin, a hydrophobic chemotherapeutic drug, into a right-handed coiled coil (RHCC). RHCC containing the drug was able to bind and enter cells in vitro. Naturally occurring coiled coils, such as the leucine zipper, led to the recognition of sequence requirements for the assembly of these structures. A generally accepted rule for coiled coil formation is the positioning of hydrophobic (H) and polar (P) residues in the following order $(HPPHPPP)_n$. A two-stranded coiled coil is formed through interhelical hydrophobic interactions of residues in positions a and d, which form the core of this motif.

The peripheral residues of the coiled coil arrangement are likely to be involved in interfibril interactions. Single point mutations may originate very different materials.

For example, Zimenkov et al. reported that the heptad with a histidine residue onto position d assembles in response to pH (Zimenkov et al., 2006). In another study, it was shown that positions b, c, and f have an influence on fibril thickness, with positively charged residues generating long and narrow nanofibers of approximately 4 nm thickness (Dong et al., 2008). Moreover, temperature responsive materials were already designed (Banwell et al., 2009) by interchanging amino acids at this same peripheral region; in one case they incorporated alanine to promote hydrophobic interactions between fibrils and in another by glutamine to foster hydrogen bonding. In both cases physical hydrogels were obtained, with the particularity that glutamine-based gels were formed at low temperature whereas alanine-based gels were achieved at high temperature.

Thermoresponsive coiled-coil peptides were also inserted in liposome membranes to allow greater control over the release of enclosed compounds in response to temperature (Al-Ahmady et al., 2012). In a recent work by More et al. engineered a supercharged coiled coil structure bearing several arginine residues that was successfully complexed with plasmid DNA and encapsulated it in a liposome for gene therapy (More et al., 2014).

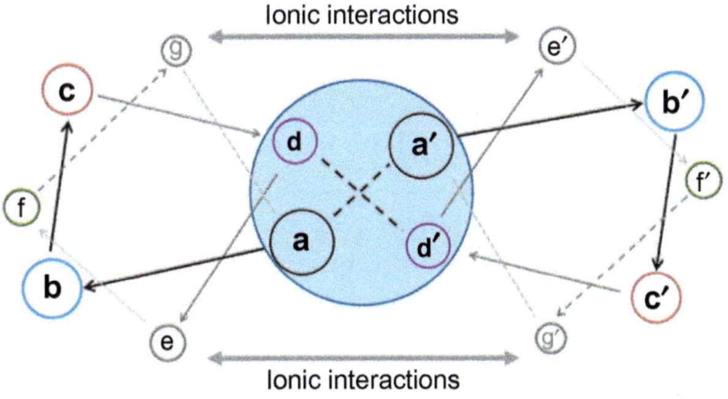

Fig. 1.4 Representation of coiled coil viewed from the top. Hydrophobic interactions take place within the core residues (a and d) whereas ionic interactions occur between proximal residues (e and g).

1.4.2.2 β-Sheet

β-Sheet is the other form of secondary structure present in proteins and consists of β-strands connected laterally by backbone hydrogen bonds and arranged in a parallel or antiparallel fashion. Much like the α-helix, β-sheets can be made amphiphilic to facilitate the creation of design guidelines. Since in β-sheets, the side chains alternately stick out of the plan in opposite directions, the HPHPHP pattern forms β-sheets with a hydrophilic side and a hydrophobic side, which spontaneously self-assemble. One of such assemblies (RADA16, where R stands for arginine, A for alanine, and D for aspartic acid) is now marketed, primarily for research purposes, under the commercial name PuraMatrix. Several studies have employed these hydrogels for cell culture, demonstrating its potential for tissue engineering applications (Genové et al., 2005; Zhang et al., 1995; Gelain et al., 2006).

It was also shown that RADA16 is suitable for the slow delivery of proteins (Koutsopoulos et al., 2009); the releasing kinetics is dependent on the size and charge of the macromolecules but it is also a function of the peptide density in the gel. By introducing a phenylalanine residue on the RADA16 sequence, Zhao et al. intentionally created a motif for interaction with hydrophobic drugs (Zhao et al., 2010). This group investigated two peptide sequences, RADAFI and RADAFII, the hydrogels were shown to entrap molecules containing the phenyl group, apparently by π–π interaction, providing another ground evidence of the potential of these materials for drug delivery. An ingenious design was reported by Schneider et al. (2002) who synthesized a peptide, MAX1, that adopts a β-hairpin secondary structure in response to pH switch, when pH is below the pK_a of the constituting lysines, they become charged causing repulsion between them and subsequently unfolding. This was accomplished by introducing a tetrapeptide (V^DPPT, where V^D stands for the D-form of valine, P for proline, and T for threonine), which favors a type II′ turn structure, in the middle of lysines intercalated with valines residues, known to have a great propensity for β-sheet generation. This sequence does not contain negatively charged residues, as opposed to the abovementioned β-sheet hydrogels.

1.4.2.3 Peptide amphiphiles

PAs are double character molecules whose self-assembling mechanism resembles that of phospholipids in cell membranes. To design a PA, a hydrophobic structural domain—usually in the form of a polymer or alkyl chain, or less frequently, a sequence of nonpolar amino acids—is linked to hydrophilic peptides.

When placed in aqueous environment such amphipathic character molecules tend to assemble into supramolecular architectures such as spherical or cylindrical micelles. The ability to encapsulate hydrophilic molecules has already been shown by van Hell et al. (2007) who reported the design of several PAs, which self-assemble into vesicles. In addition to providing a capable carrier environment, these systems also present the advantage of allowing a fine control of the properties of the assembly surface by judicious selection of composing amino acids. Liang et al. (2014) have shown this versatility by incorporating lysines in the design of a PA molecule to confer pH-responsiveness. The PAs self-assembled into micelle, entrapping DOX, an antineoplastic drug that is released when placed in acidic conditions due to electrostatic repulsions between the protonated lysine molecules. Other successful drug carriers based on PAs have been created (Bulut et al., 2011; Kim et al., 2009; Matson et al., 2012; Webber et al., 2012) and a compilation of carriers based on peptide self-assembly is provided on Table 1.1.

Table 1.1 List of peptide-based carriers

Peptide sequence/carrier	Secondary structure	Guest/drug	References
Polypeptide chain fragment from protein tetrabrachion (*Staphylothermus marinus*)	α-Helix/coiled coil	Cisplatin	Eriksson et al. (2009), Stetefeld et al. (2000)
MRGSHHHHHHGSGRLRPQMLREL QRTNAALRDVRELLRQQVKEITRL KNTVRRSRASGKLN	α-Helix/coiled coil	DNA	More et al. (2014)
$(IAALEKE)_2$ IAALEKG	α-Helix/coiled coil	Methotrexate	Apostolovic et al. (2011)
$[VSSLESK]_2$VSKLESKKSKLESKVS KLESKVSSLESK]-NH_2	α-Helix/coiled coil	Doxorubicin	Al-Ahmady et al. (2012)
RADA16=$(RADA)_4$	β-Sheet	Phenol red, bromophenol pyranine, 4-PSA, CBBG	Nagai et al. (2006)
RADAFI ([CH_3CONH]-RADARAD**F**$(RADA)_2$-[$CONH_2$]) RADAFII ([CH_3CONH]-RAD**F**$(RADA)_3$-[$CONH_2$])	β-Sheet	L-Phenylalanine	Zhao et al. (2010)
RADA16 RADA16-DGE: Ac-$(RADA)_4$GGDGEA-$CONH_2$ RADA16-PFS:Ac-$(RADA)_4$GGPFSSTKT-$CONH_2$	β-Sheet	Human recombinant BDNF, βFGF, and VEGF121	Gelain et al. (2006)
RADA16	β-Sheet	Lysozyme, trypsin inhibitor, BSA, and IgG	Koutsopoulos et al. (2009)
ac-(RADA)4-$CONH_2$ ac-(KLDL)3-$CONH_2$	β-Sheet	IgG	Koutsopoulos and Zhang (2012)

Continued

Table 1.1 Continued

Peptide sequence/carrier	Secondary structure	Guest/drug	References
MAX1: $(VK)_4V^DPPT\text{-}(KV)_4$ MAX8: $(VK)_4V^DPPTKVEVKVKV$	β-Hairpin	FITC–dextran of different sizes	Branco et al. (2009)
MAX8	β-Hairpin	Curcumin	Altunbas et al. (2011)
PSFCFKFEP	β-Sheet, β-turn	Pyrene	Ruan et al. (2009)
Ac-AAVVLLLWE2-COOH Ac-AAVVLLLWE7-COOH	Peptide amphiphile	Calcein	van Hell et al. (2007)
$(V)_6$KKGRGDS	Peptide amphiphile	Doxorubicin	Liang et al. (2014)
CH3(CH2)14CONHGTAGLIGQRGDS-COOH	Peptide amphiphile	Cisplatin	Kim et al. (2009)
C16-$V_2A_2E_2$	Peptide amphiphile	Dexamethasone	Webber et al. (2012)
C12-VVAGK-Am	Peptide amphiphile	Bcl-2 antisense oligodeoxynucleotide	Bulut et al. (2011)
C16-V2A2E2K(Hydrazide) C16-V2A2K(Hyd)E2 C16-V2K(Hyd)A2E2 C16-K(Hyd)V2A2E2	Peptide amphiphile	Prodan	Matson et al. (2012)

Adapted from Durão, J., Gales, L., 2015. Peptide self-assembly for therapeutic applications. Curr. Org. Chem. 19, 1874–1881.

1.4.2.4 Peptides as functional motifs

It is important to mention that, in view of the several physiological roles played by peptides, peptide-based materials not only constitute a structural platform, but also can convey specific biological activities. The implementation of such functional motifs may have applications in drug delivery by allowing the targeted transport of the vehicle to the specific cell, tissue, or organ in need of therapeutic action (Ruoslahti, 2012). This field of peptide application it too vast to be covered in the present chapter (Ruoslahti, 2012; Majumdar and Siahaan, 2012; Wang et al., 2014). Among the relevant examples of employed peptide motifs are the RGD (where R stands for arginine, G for glycine, and D for aspartic acid) peptide, which targets $\alpha_{\nu}B_{3}$ integrin (Xiong et al., 2002), a protein overexpressed in many tumors and the laminin-derived sequence. Another class of peptides that holds great biomedical interest is the cell penetrating peptides as they may facilitate the transport of various biologically active molecules inside living cells (Wang et al., 2014).

1.5 NAs-based systems

1.5.1 Structure and properties of NAs

The field of DNA nanotechnology, which arose from the seminal work of Nadrian Seeman (Kallenbach et al., 1983), has, during the last decade, progressed to a stage where it is starting to provide new tools for the construction of innovative smart drug delivery vehicles. These particularly stand out from the classical carriers such as liposomes (Allen and Cullis, 2013) and polymers (Liechty et al., 2010) due to special characteristics enabling the quantitative loading of drugs, stoichiometric and precise geometric placement of targeting entities as well as intelligent control of drug delivery.

1.5.1.1 Principles governing NAs-based nanostructure assembly

Perhaps the foundational principles for the comprehension of structural DNA technology can be listed as: (i) sequence specific hybridization rules governed by Watson–Crick base pairing (Watson and Crick, 1953); (ii) connection of independent DNA species through "sticky-ended" cohesive interactions, for the formation of single molecule entities (Cohen et al., 1973; Qiu et al., 1997); and (iii) the realization of stable NAs junctions (Kallenbach et al., 1983; Winfree et al., 1998) and application of sequence symmetry minimization (Seeman, 1982; Seeman, 1990).

Following some or all of these principles has led to the construction of a variety of NAs-based structures. These can be made purely out of NAs with an exquisite control over the structures' geometrical properties, or from NAs–hybrid material conjugates such as inorganic material–DNA hybrids (Rosi et al., 2006; Brown et al., 2013) and DNA-polymer/lipid hybrid conjugates (Talom et al., 2011; Liu et al., 2010), which, although with somewhat decreased structural control, can provide extra functionalities. In this section we will focus mostly on NAs-based systems assembled through the principles of structural DNA technology.

1.5.1.2 Pure NAs nanostructures

Pure NAs 3D nanostructure construction has suffered several evolutionary steps. It initially started with the construction of the 4-way junction tile which, by subsequent self-assembly through sticky end connections, and after several successive catenation and purification steps, yielded the first DNA cube (Fig. 1.5(1); Kallenbach et al., 1983; Chen and Seeman, 1991). This initial nanostructure did not possess the necessary rigidity to produce a well-defined structure geometry with the self-assembly process suffering from low yields. The necessary increase in rigidity allowing the production of well-defined DNA structures came with the introduction of the double-crossover motif (Fig. 1.5(2); Fu and Seeman, 1993; Li et al., 1996) and its derivatives (e.g., triple crossover also designated TX motif (LaBean et al., 2000), paranemic crossover also designated PX motif (Zhang et al., 2002)). Other important DNA motifs are represented by the 4×4 cross-tile (Yan et al., 2003) which, through subsequent use of the "sequence symmetry" concept made possible the achievement of large and high yield 2D assemblies (Yan et al., 2003), and the 3-point star motif (He et al., 2005). Both tiles subsequently gave rise to the development of 3D structures (Fig. 1.5(3); He et al., 2008; He et al., 2010).

The above design principles were further advanced by the seminal contribution of Rothemund to the field of DNA nanotechnology, which was the introduction of the DNA origami method (Fig. 1.5(4); Rothemund, 2006). This technology allowed the folding of a DNA scaffold strand into virtually any desired shape through the hybridization of single-stranded oligonucleotide "staple strands." Although initially, DNA origami produced essentially planar structures it soon evolved into complex 3D assemblies (Andersen et al., 2009; Douglas et al., 2009), with intricate curvatures (Han et al., 2011). The high pace of technical evolution in the field has also recently led to the production of large complex structures without the need of a scaffold strand, using for that purpose only single stranded oligonucleotides, designated by short single stranded tiles (SSTs) (Yin et al., 2008; Wei et al., 2012). The SST itself gave rise to the concept of single-stranded "bricks" for the creation of a 3D "molecular canvas" where each single-stranded DNA (ssDNA, DNA brick) function as a LEGO-like brick and allows the assembly of arbitrary 3D shapes (Ke et al., 2012).

Apart from the abovementioned general principle of relying on DNA crossovers for the construction of rigid nano-objects, another method also contributes for the structural rigidity necessary for achieving stable tridimensional architectures. Hence, using the triangulation, and compression and tension (tensegrity) concepts, where flexible DNA branches work as vertices connecting stiff double stranded regions, enables the construction of stable 3D wireframe and tensegrity structures (Simmel et al., 2014). One example of a DNA structure using triangulation to achieve rigidity is the DNA tetrahedron, first introduced by the group of Turberfield (Goodman et al., 2005). The tetrahedron could be built by hybridization of 4 ssDNA strands of around 60 nucleotides each, with 20 bp composing each edge.

Other seemingly simple concepts nonetheless also have been successively applied for the construction of several different DNA nanostructures. The group of Sleiman has generated different DNA polyhedra using a small set of ssDNA building blocks where cyclization plays a decisive role by providing the structural integrity needed for achieving three-dimensionality. In this approach, the cyclic single-stranded blocks work as faces or sides of the intended 3D structure (Fig. 1.5(5); Aldaye and Sleiman, 2007; McLaughlin et al., 2011).

Apart from DNA, RNA is also being used for the construction of nanostructures. The interest in RNA derives in part from being a molecule capable of performing multiple biological functions, some directly deriving from its naturally occurring and diverse structural assemblies. Some of the naturally occurring

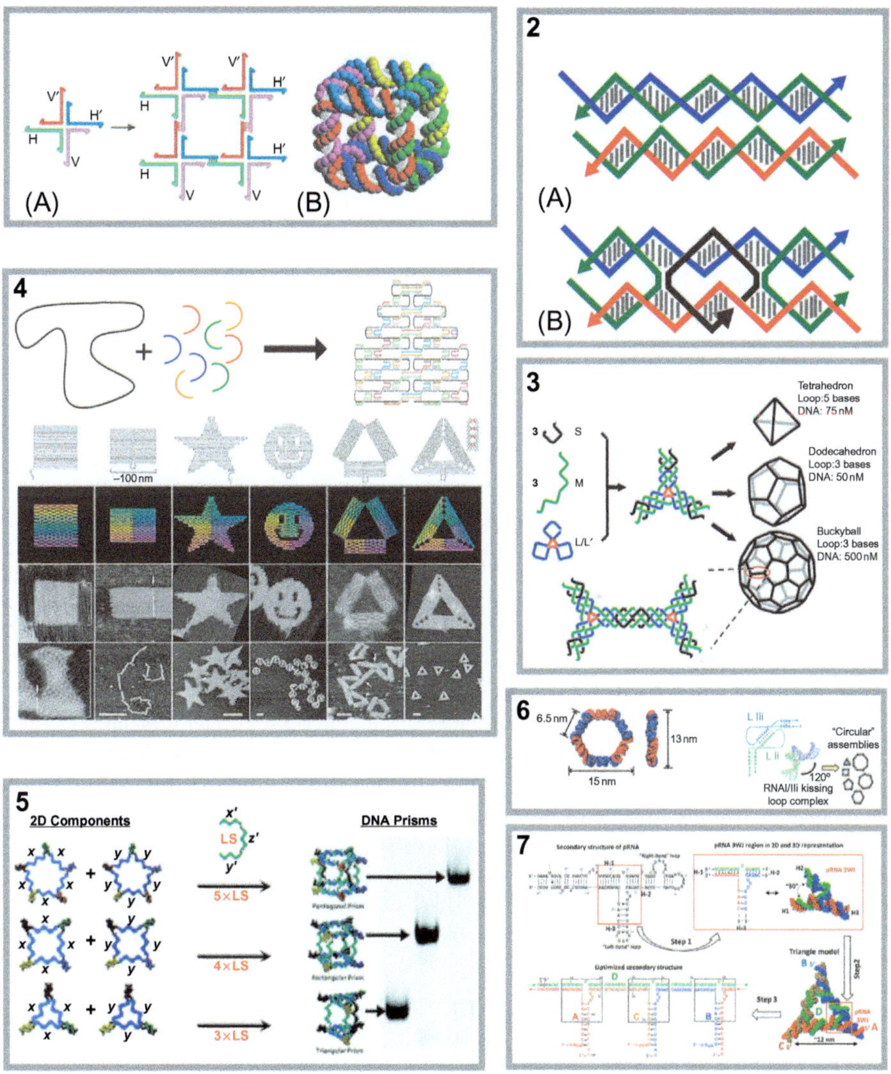

Fig. 1.5 See caption on next page.

RNA structural motifs are directly used as building blocks "tecto RNAs" for the construction of stable nano-assemblies. As such, three different 90 degree-angle motifs, coming from the participating RNA in the translational machinery (right-angle motif, 3-way junction motif (3WJ-motif), and tRNA-motif) have been used for the assembly of square-shaped RNA nanoparticles (Severcan et al., 2009). Additionally, the RNAI/RNAII inverse (RNAI/IIi) kissing complex, with loop–loop interactions that form a bend of approximately 120 degrees between adjacent helices, was utilized to form a hexagonal RNA nanoring (Fig. 1.5(6); Grabow et al., 2011). Another natural RNA motif, the pRNA, included in the DNA-packaging motor of bacterial virus phi29, also has been used for the assembly of ring structures through Watson–Crick interactions between individual pRNA loops (Shu et al., 2003). Moreover, the 3WJ that characterizes the pRNA secondary structure was additionally used for the production of RNA triangle nanoparticles (Fig. 1.5(7); Khisamutdinov et al., 2014). Finally, the assembly

Fig. 1.5 Examples of DNA nanostructure principles and designs. (1) (A) A 4-way immobile DNA junction as envisioned by Seeman and its use in the formation of a self-assembling array; (B) a cube-like structure formed by the interlocking of six cyclic single-stranded DNA. (Reprinted with permission from Seeman, N.C., 2003. DNA in a material world. Nature. 421(6921), 427–431, Copyright © 2003, Nature Publishing Group.) (2) (A) Two parallel DNA double helix; (B) conversion of the parallel helix into a DNA double cross over motif as a result of two reciprocal exchanges between antiparallel DNA strands. (Image adapted from Mao, C., 2004. The emergence of complexity: lessons from DNA. PLoS Biol. 2(12), e431.) (3) Asymmetric 3-point-star motif (made with three strands) used for assembly of three different polyhedra. (Adapted with permission from He, Y., Ye, T., Su, M., Zhang, C., Ribbe, A.E., Jiang, W., et al., 2008. Hierarchical self-assembly of DNA into symmetric supramolecular polyhedra. Nature. 452(7184), 198–201, Copyright © 2008, Nature publishing Group.) (4) DNA origami—a DNA scaffold strand is folded into desired shapes through the binding of several "staple" oligonucleotides. (Adapted with permission from Rothemund, P.W.K., 2006. Folding DNA to create nanoscale shapes and patterns. Nature. 440(7082), 297–302, Copyright 2006, Nature Publishing Group.) (5) Building DNA 3D nanostructures through the use of a multistrand approach with initial assembly of cyclic DNA motifs. (Reprinted with permission from McLaughlin, C.K., Hamblin, G.D., Aldaye, F.A., Yang, H., Sleiman, H.F., 2011. A facile, modular and high yield method to assemble three-dimensional DNA structures. Chem. Commun. 47(31), 8925–8927, Copyright © 2011, Royal Society of Chemistry.) (6) The pRNA 3WJ motif used for the construction of a 2D triangular nanoparticle. (Adapted with permission from Khisamutdinov, E.F., Jasinski, D.L., Guo, P., 2014. RNA as a boiling-resistant anionic polymer material to build robust structures with defined shape and stoichiometry. ACS Nano. 8(5), 4771–4781, Copyright © 2014 American Chemical Society.) (7) RNA nanorings assembled through the 120 degrees loop–loop interactions as found in the RNAI/RNAII inverse (RNAI/IIi) kissing complex. (Adapted with permission from Grabow, W.W., Zakrevsky, P., Afonin, K.A., Chworos, A., Shapiro, B.A., Jaeger, L., 2011. Self-assembling RNA nanorings based on RNAI/II inverse kissing complexes. Nano Lett. 11(2), 878–887, Copyright © 2011, American Chemical Society.)

of a 3D RNA nanocube has also been described using a minimum of six RNA strands (Afonin et al., 2010).

1.5.2 Design of NAs-based delivery systems

1.5.2.1 Delivery by branched or 2D—NAs structures

One of the first examples using NAs-based nanoparticles for oligonucleotide delivery comes from the group of Peixuan Guo, through the use of the abovementioned pRNA motif (Shu et al., 2003). The pRNA motif was modified to include either a small interfering RNA (siRNA) or targeting moieties such as the CD4 RNA aptamer or folate. These were then assembled into dimers or trimmers creating nanoparticles of 20–40 nm in size, which were then shown to enter cells by receptor mediated uptake and silence genes in vitro, albeit using an optimized buffer during cell incubation (Khaled et al., 2005). Still, the work showed the potential of using pure NAs-based nanosystems (in this case a 2D system), without the aid of transfection reagents, for oligonucleotide delivery.

Shapiro and Jaeger functionalized RNA nanorings (Grabow et al., 2011) (mentioned in the previous section) with siRNAs and different types of aptamers (both for visualization and cell targeting), as well as fluorescent proteins (e.g., phycoerythrin labeled streptavidin (STV)) and tested for siRNA efficiency in vitro and in vivo in a tumor xenograft mouse model. The properties of this multifunctional RNA nanoparticle were highlighted by showing increased siRNA efficiency over regular double-stranded siRNA counterparts, ability of cell targeting through aptamer recognition, and fluorescent imaging detection of the nanoparticles (Afonin et al., 2014).

Perhaps the simplest NAs-based nanosystem is the one based on the structurally flexible 3WJ DNA motif. This motif, designated by Y-DNA was initially shown to give rise to dendrimer-like DNA structures by ligation of several complementary Y-DNA units (Li et al., 2004). The Y-DNA was later used as a structure to carry immunostimulatory CpG motifs (specific DNA oligonucleotide sequences characterized by the presence of the dinucleotide CG) (Weiner et al., 1997) by inclusion into the Y-DNA sequence. The Y-DNA was shown to stimulate an enhanced uptake by macrophage-like cell lines and generated significantly higher levels of cytokines compared with double- stranded oligonucleotide, albeit showing a decreased resistance to degradation (Nishikawa et al., 2008). This concept was further expanded to CpG carrying dendrimer- like DNA through ligation of Y-DNA monomers with 5′-cohesive ends, were CpG motifs are present at the external layers of the dendrimer structure (Rattanakiat et al., 2009). In addition, different types of branched DNA structures equivalent to 3-, 4-, 5-, 6-, and even 8-way DNA junctions (respectively designated by tripodna, tetrapodna, pentapodna, hexapodna, octapodna) were also tested for CpG delivery (Fig. 1.6(1)). An increase in immunostimulation was observed with increasing number of branches, although at the expense of serum stability, thus suggesting a relation between structural complexity and toll-like receptor 9 recognition/activation (Mohri et al., 2012).

1.5.2.2 Delivery by wireframe and origami DNA structures

A particularly interesting and revealing experiment made by Turberfield demonstrated for the first time the possibility for the DNA tetrahedron, a structure made entirely of pure NAs, to be taken up by cells. In addition, it was observed, by fluorescence resonance energy transfer analysis, that the DNA tetrahedron could maintain integrity over a period of 48 h inside cells, illustrating that DNA structural rigidity could play an important role in improving DNA degradation resistance (Walsh et al., 2011). The ability to be taken up by cells and the resistance to extra and intracellular degradation are central features for a drug-delivery system and in fact of special importance for negatively charged systems made of DNA, as the negative charge diminishes the ability to interact with cellular membranes and DNA is normally a material naturally sensitive to nuclease degradation.

Nonetheless, several examples employing DNA nanostructures have provided insights into their utility as delivery systems.

The abovementioned DNA tetrahedron was used by Li et al. (2011) who modified the structure to carry one CpG motif at each vertex. The tetrahedron was shown to be taken up by RAW264.7 cells without any transfection reagents, residing mainly in intracellular vesicles. It was additionally shown to maintain integrity for 4 h in 50% fetal bovine serum (FBS) in contrast to double-stranded DNA (dsDNA) that was almost completely degraded already after 2 h. It was finally shown to induce greater immunostimulation than control CpG oligonucleotide, especially when the tetrahedron was fully modified with four CpG motifs.

CpG motifs were also used to decorate a hollow DNA origami tube (carrying up to 62 CpG sequences). The high stimulatory activity when incubated with mouse splenocytes was especially attributed to the construct's compactness, size (80 nm length; 20 nm diameter), and stability, being able to maintain a high degree of integrity for up to 6 h in FBS containing medium, which also resulted in higher cell uptake (Schüller et al., 2011). Also, importantly, in contrast to transfection of CpG ON with lipofectamine, origami structures did not show any appreciable toxicity to splenocytes.

Besides CpG ON cargoes, DNA nanostructures have been also utilized to deliver other NAs-based drugs such as antisense oligonucleotides.

The abovementioned tetrahedron has been explored for the delivery of a ssDNA antisense sequence, for inducing RNase H mediated mRNA cleavage. This was achieved by designing one of the strands participating in the tetrahedron formation to contain an extra 20 nucleotide antisense sequence, which formed a bulged out loop able to hybridize to the specific intracellular mRNA. These structures needed mixing with lipofectamine (transfection reagent) for increased cellular uptake, but nonetheless, once inside the cell were able to promote targeted mRNA downregulation (Keum et al., 2011). Later, the same group also introduced into the tetrahedron an aptamer sequence, AS1411 (Soundararajan et al., 2008), against the nucleolin receptor expressed at the surface of cancer cells. To introduce the aptamer sequences they used a previously developed strategy (mentioned later) (Lee et al., 2012) consisting in DNA overhangs protruding from the structure, which act as anchor points and allow hybridization of the extended aptamer sequences. The aptamers enhanced cellular uptake of the DNA nanostructures without any transfection reagents and in parallel could elicit tumor growth inhibition (Charoenphol and Bermudez, 2014).

An important study by Lee et al. showed, for the first time, the in vivo use of the tetrahedron as a carrier of siRNA sequences for tumor delivery (Fig. 1.6(2); Lee et al., 2012). In this study each edge of the tetrahedron contained a protruding overhang DNA sequence to which an extended siRNA sequence could hybridize. The siRNAs sequences were further modified with folic acid (FA) in such a way that in the final nanostructure siRNA–FA molecules were placed at defined geometrical orientations. The structure was shown to have a hydrodynamic size of around 29 nm. After i.v. delivery in a xenograft tumor mouse model, the nanostructures were seen to specifically accumulate in the tumor and downregulate luciferase from implanted Luc-modified KB cancer cell line.

A DNA nanotube carrier, assembled through the dimerization of the symmetric 3-point-star motif (mentioned previously), was also used as a scaffold for the attachment of siRNAs through overhang sequence complementarity. The DNA nanotube had a dimension of 6 nm in diameter and 13 nm in length and could bear six siRNA sequences. In this study, in vitro cell uptake of the nanotubes was aided by a transfection reagent showing, nonetheless, a higher downregulation efficiency of mTOR in pulmonary arterial smooth muscle cells when compared to regular double stranded siRNAs (You et al., 2015).

Single-stranded antisense oligonucleotides (ssAON) were also introduced in 3D DNA prisms. One of the main differences from the abovementioned tetrahedron studies was that the ssAON strands were an integral part of the DNA structure framework. After cell uptake, aided by complexation with a transfection reagent, it was shown that the antisense activity was higher than an ssAON and approximately equal to a double-stranded antisense oligonucleotide control (Fakhoury et al., 2014). Overall, the study highlights the possibility to integrate different NAs therapeutics into a DNA nanostructure framework, which could increase their resistance to degradation potentially leading to prolonged therapeutic effects. Additionally, it could also provide more possibilities for further functionalization of the DNA structures through hybridization.

Apart from NA therapeutics delivery, other types of molecules could also be employed with NAs-based nanostructure vectors.

Erben et al. could demonstrate in 2006 the encapsulation of a single-molecule protein inside a DNA tetrahedron. To achieve this, they first conjugated cytochrome *c* with one of the four oligonucleotides that assemble into the tetrahedron. The central cavity of the tetrahedron was estimated to hold a sphere with radius of 2.6 nm, corresponding to proteins up to 60 kDa, which was enough to accommodate the 12.4 kDa cytochrome *c* protein. Depending on the attachment point of the protein along the oligonucleotide, the protein could be introduced facing inward or outwards the tetrahedron. With such strategy one could control the accessibility to the protein once in the intracellular environment. Liu et al. used a similar strategy for encapsulation of STV in CpG bearing DNA tetrahedrons

(Fig. 1.6(3); Liu et al., 2012). Their structure was based on the 3-point-star motif developed by the group of Chengde Mao (He et al., 2008, 2010) with additional overhang sequences containing the CpG motifs. STV, used as model antigen, was loaded into the tetrahedron during the structure assembly process, with a final purification step to isolate STV containing tetrahedrons. The tetrahedron was shown to maintain a good integrity level after an incubation of up to 5 h in 50% FBS. The full STV–tetrahedron–CpG system was used for mice immunization and, when compared to a mixture of antigen and CpG molecules, was shown to induce a strong and long-lasting antibody response against the antigen without stimulating a reaction to the DNA nanostructure itself.

Chang et al. (2011) utilized five DNA strands to assemble a 5-point-star motif with 5′ overhangs in order to further assemble it in a DNA icosahedron 3D structure. Using six DNA strands they further developed a 6-point-star motif with sticky ends, which further assembled into a MUC1 aptamer-containing DNA icosahedron. This nanostructure was then loaded with DOX through its DNA intercalation property and shown to be specifically taken up by MCF7 cells, producing higher cytotoxic effects than free DOX.

Also several origami structures were used for the delivery of DOX. Hogbergs group tested two different origami tubes with the first type consisting of a straight nanotube structure (S-Tube) and the second exhibiting a twisted structure (T-Tube) (Zhao et al., 2012). The T-Tube showed higher loading efficiency of DOX in comparison to S-Tube, a slower release profile, and induced a higher toxicity towards different cancer cell lines in relation to free DOX and S-Tube loaded DOX. The reasons for the increased activity were attributed to enhanced cell uptake of DOX by the origami scaffold and inhibition of lysosomal acidification induced by the origami structure, which led to a redistribution of the drug to the target sites even overcoming DOX-resistant cancer cell lines.

Similarly, two different origami structures, a 2D triangular structure and a 3D tubular structure, were shown to incorporate around twofold more DOX than unstructured dsDNA inducing enhanced cytotoxicity in DOX-resistant cancer cell lines, in contrast to free DOX (Fig. 1.6(4); Jiang et al., 2012).

A very interesting demonstration of the possibilities of DNA nanostructures as intelligent delivery vectors comes from the study by Douglas et al. where a DNA origami strategy was used to construct a hexagonal barrel DNA structure with dimensions of 35 nm × 35 nm × 45 nm (Douglas et al., 2012). The structure was designed in a way that the barrel is divided longitudinally in two domains connected at the rear by single-stranded scaffold hinges and at the front by DNA aptamer staple sequences that work as an open/close mechanism through binding of the specific aptamer ligands. The structure can be loaded with different cargoes, such as antibodies, which can then only interact with cells once the robot is activated (opened) in the presence of specific cellular membrane cues. Hence, this structure allows specific delivery of molecular payloads for cell targeting.

Below we present a table summarizing this section and highlighting the uses of NAs structures as delivery systems (Table 1.2).

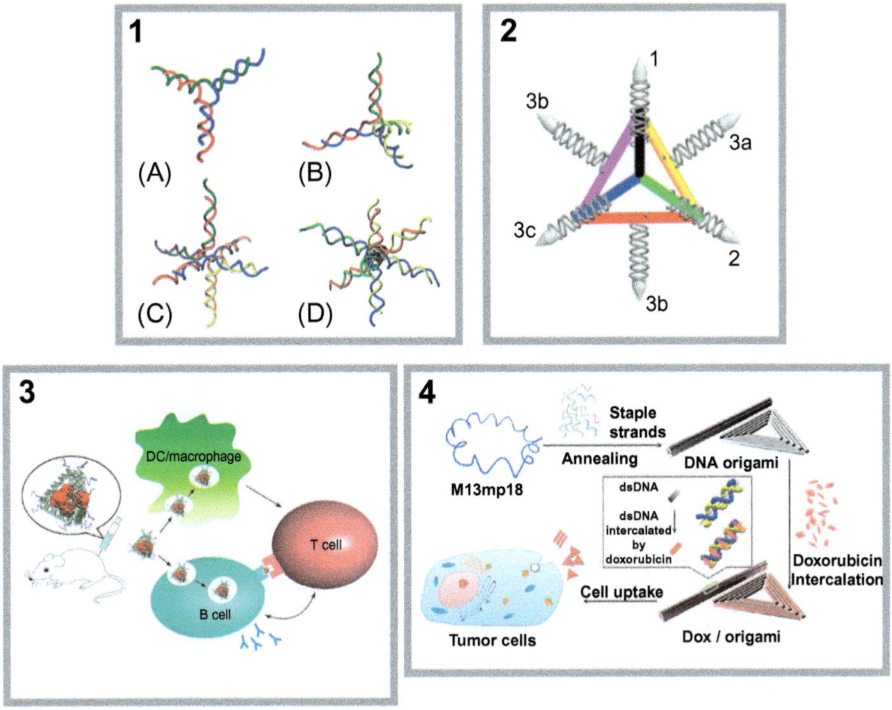

Fig. 1.6 Examples of nucleic acids-based nanostructures used as drug delivery systems. (1) Schematic representation of polypodna formed by 3-, 4-, 6-, 8-way DNA junction motifs, respectively designated by tripodna (A), tetrapodna (B), hexapodna (C), octapodna. (Reprinted with permission from Mohri, K., Nishikawa, M., Takahashi, N., Shiomi, T., Matsuoka, N., Ogawa, K., et al., 2012. Design and development of nanosized DNA assemblies in polypod-like structures as efficient vehicles for immunostimulatory CpG motifs to immune cells. ACS Nano. 6(7), 5931–5940, Copyright © 2012 American Chemical Society.) (2) Schematic representation of the DNA tetrahedron carrying a maximum of six siRNA molecules and six folate molecules as cancer targeting moieties for targeted delivery. (Adapted with permission from Lee, H., Lytton-Jean, A.K.R., Chen, Y., Love, K.T., Park, A.I., Karagiannis, E.D., et al., 2012. Molecularly self-assembled nucleic acid nanoparticles for targeted in vivo siRNA delivery. Nat. Nanotechnol. 7(6), 389–393, Copyright © 2012, Nature Publishing Group.) (3) Representation of DNA tetrahedron structure, assembled from the 3-point-star DNA motif, carrying CpG oligonucleotides and encapsulating streptavidin demonstrating a scaffolded adjuvant–antigen vaccine complex. (Reprinted with permission from Liu, X., Xu, Y., Yu, T., Clifford, C., Liu, Y., Yan, H., et al., 2012. A DNA nanostructure platform for directed assembly of synthetic vaccines. Nano Lett. 12(8), 4254–4259, Copyright © 2012, American Chemical Society.) (4) Two DNA origami structures (Tube and Triangle) are loaded with Doxorubicin and act as delivery systems for cancer cells. (Reprinted with permission from Jiang, Q., Song, C., Nangreave, J., Liu, X., Lin, L., Qiu, D., et al., 2012. DNA origami as a carrier for circumvention of drug resistance. J. Am. Chem. Soc. 134(32), 13396–13403, Copyright © 2012, American Chemical Society.)

Table 1.2 Summary of nucleic acids-based structures as delivery systems

Structure	Cargo	Targeting ligands	Delivery	References
Dimers and trimmers of pRNA motif	siRNA	CD4 RNA aptamer; folate	In vitro (cancer cell lines)—free uptake	Khaled et al. (2005)
RNA nanorings (RNAI/IIi) kissing complex	siRNA/PE-STV	EGFR-specific J18 aptamer	(i) In vitro (human breast cancer cells: MDA-MB-231)—transfection mediated (ii) Cell binding through aptamer interaction (human epidermoid carcinoma cells: A431) (iii) Intratumoral injection in xenograft mouse model	Afonin et al. (2014)
Y-shape DNA; polypodna; dendrimeric polypodna	CpG ODN	–	In vitro (RAW264.7 macrophage cell line)—free uptake	Nishikawa et al. (2008), Rattanakiat et al. (2009), Mohri et al. (2012), Mohri et al. (2015)
DNA tetrahedron (four strand assembly)	CpG ODN	–	In vitro (RAW264.7 macrophage cell line)—free uptake	Li et al. (2011)
DNA origami tube	CpG ODN	–	Isolated mouse splenocytes—free uptake	Schüller et al. (2011)
DNA tetrahedron (four strand assembly)	ssAON	–	In vitro (HeLa, C2C12, MCF7)—transfection mediated	Keum et al. (2011)
DNA tetrahedron (four strand assembly)	Aptamer AS1411	AS1411 aptamer	In vitro (HeLa)—free uptake	Charoenphol and Bermudez (2014)

DNA tetrahedron (six strand assembly)	siRNA	Folate	(i) In vitro (HeLa, KB)—free uptake; (ii) I.v. and intratumoral injection in xenograft mouse model	Lee et al. (2012)
DNA nanotube (3-point-star motif)	siRNA	–	In vitro (pulmonary arterial smooth muscle cells) transfection mediated	You et al. (2015)
3D DNA prism (12 strand assembly)	ssAON	–	In vitro (HeLa)—transfection mediated	Fakhoury et al. (2014)
DNA tetrahedron (3-point-star motif)	CpG	–	(i) In vitro (RAW264.7; primary DC) (ii) Subcutaneous immunization in mice	Liu et al. (2012)
DNA icosahedron (6-point-star motif)	DOX	MUC1 aptamer	In vitro (MCF7)—free uptake	Chang et al. (2011)
DNA origami—straight tube (S-Tube) and twisted tube (T-Tube)	DOX	–	In vitro (breast cancer cell lines—MDA-MB-231, MDA-MB-468, and MCF-7)—free uptake	Zhao et al. (2012)
DNA origami—2D triangle and 3D tube	DOX	–	In vitro (MCF 7; doxorubicin-resistant MCF 7)—free uptake	Jiang et al. (2012)
DNA origami—hexagonal barrel with open/close mechanism	Antibody	Aptamers: platelet-derived growth factor (PDGF); sTE17; sgc8c	In vitro cell surface tagging of different cancer cell lines	Douglas et al. (2012)

1.6 Dendrimer-based systems

1.6.1 Structure and properties of dendrimers

Currently, the biomimetic and bioinspired strategy has become a predominant guide for the design and development of novel macromolecular-based materials. Since the demand increases, a higher control over their structure, properties, and development is being pursued. In this context, dendritic structures (Fig. 1.7) arose as one of the most promising innovative nanocarriers in nanomedicine. They are the result of great advances and innovations in organic chemistry and polymer science, exhibiting significant improved physicochemical properties comparing to traditional linear polymers. Because of this, they are also coined as "polymers of the 21st century."

Dendritic architectures emerged from a new class of very branched polymers "cascade molecules", firstly synthesized by Voegtle et al. in 1978 (Buhleier et al., 1978). Later, Denkewalter, Tomalia, Newkome, Frechet, and coworkers further increased the complexity level of these branched molecules, giving rise to larger dendritic structures, then renamed as "dendrimers" (Denkewalter et al., 1981; Tomalia et al., 1985; Newkome et al., 1985; Hawker and Frechet, 1990). The word *dendrimer* arises from the Greek *dendron* ("tree" or "branch") and *meros* ("part"), and refers to the distinctive organization of branched units. Dendrimers consist of: (a) a central core with two or more reactive groups, (b) repeated units covalently attached to the central core and organized in layers called "generations" (G), and (c) high number of terminal functional groups on their surface (Fig. 1.7).

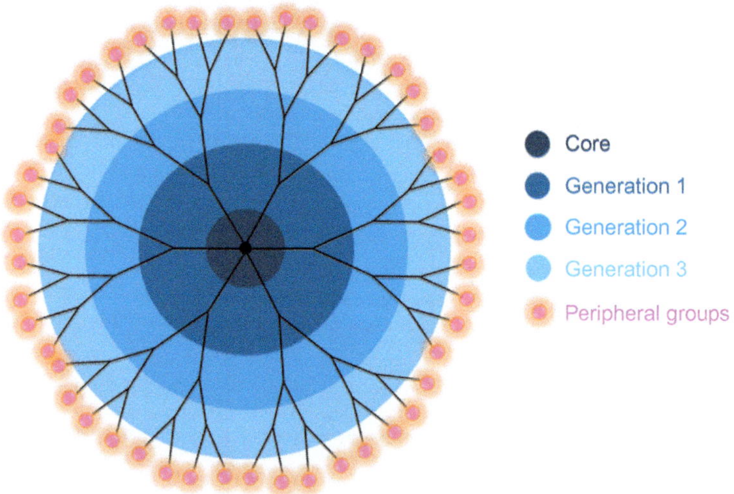

Fig. 1.7 Schematic representation of a dendrimer with three generations and terminal functional groups.

The first synthesized dendrimers were poly(amide amine) (PAMAM) (Tomalia et al., 1985), poly(propylene imine) (PPI) (Buhleier et al., 1978) and poly(lysine)-based dendrimers (PLL) (Rao and Tam, 1994). They are the most commonly used dendrimers and all are commercially available nowadays. These and other dendrimers have something very special to offer in many biomedical applications due to their unique structural characteristics: a globular, well-defined, and very branched structure, as well as their monodispersion and controllable nanosize. Moreover, the abundance of terminal functional groups allows the tethering of different ligands and/or drugs in a specific and controllable manner, simulating the multivalency present in different biological systems. This bioinspired multivalency is the greater virtue of dendrimers: the enhanced effect that stems from presenting lots of several bioactive molecules at the same time and place. Additionally, dendrimers can also cargo a molecule of interest by forming nanosized structures stabilized by noncovalent interactions.

Although the internal dendrimer structure also plays a significant role (Caminade et al., 2015), the characteristics of their surface groups predominantly will determine their physicochemical properties, and therefore also their biological activity (toxicity and pharmacokinetics) and biocompatibility (Duncan and Izzo, 2005; Kaminskas et al., 2011a). For example, cationic dendrimers will more readily interact with the negatively charged surface of the cell membranes but also have been found to be more cytotoxic than anionic or neutral ones (Duncan and Izzo, 2005). Surface decoration of amino positive terminated dendrimers exhibited improved pharmacokinetics and lower toxicity profiles as compared with plain amine-terminated dendrimers (Kaminskas et al., 2011a; Malik et al., 2000). In this regard, the most common approach for masking the dendrimers charge and improving their solubility and biocompatibility, while increasing their circulation time in the blood stream, is to tether chains of PEG) to the dendritic backbone (Thakur et al., 2015). This strategy was also carried out in the case of *DEP docetaxel dendrimer*, which is in Phase 1 clinical trials for the treatment of a wide range of solid tumors. Other dendrimers have also reached clinical trials: VivaGel, an antimicrobial agent G4 poly(L-lysine)-based dendrimer, is in Phase 3 trials; and Gadomer-17, a PLL-based dendrimer, is in Phase 2 trials for its use as dendritic contrast agent (CA) for diagnosis in magnetic resonance imaging (MRI).

1.6.2 Design of dendrimer-based delivery systems

1.6.2.1 Design, preparation and types of dendrimers

The tunable chemistry of dendrimers allows a precise "chemical makeup" through designing of critical nanoscale parameters: size, shape, surface, and internal chemistry, flexibility/rigidity, and architecture.

The synthetic routes through which dendrimers are synthesized allow this accurate design and are mainly two reverse approaches: divergent (Buhleier et al., 1978; Tomalia et al., 1985; Newkome et al., 1985) or convergent (Hawker and Frechet, 1990). The divergent synthesis, introduced by Tomalia, Newkome, and Voegtle, involves the growth of the dendrimers from the core towards the periphery, layer-by-layer, in an "inside-outward" approach. The core molecule reacts with monomeric molecules giving the first-generation dendrimer (G1). This reacts with more monomers to give G2. Then, the process is repeated until the desired generation and size dendrimer is formed. In the convergent approach, established by Fréchet et al. (Hawker and Frechet, 1990), the growth is from the terminal groups towards focal points in an inward layer-by-layer process, yielding individual dendrons. Finally, the obtained several dendrons are attached with a multifunctional core.

The divergent methodology is susceptible to defective monomer assembly due to the higher number of reactions performed at the same time, and thus, usually requires purification after each step (Mintzer and Grinstaff, 2010). The probability of byproduct formation increases with generation, rendering lower purification rates. On the contrary, in convergent synthesis only a limited number of groups are active per reaction, reducing the probability of structural defects (Mintzer and Grinstaff, 2010). The main drawback is its low ability to produce dendrimers of higher generations due to the steric hindrance between dendrons in the last step, although an adequate choice of core size and multivalency can reduce steric hindrances (Mintzer and Grinstaff, 2010).

To overcome these drawbacks, new user- and environmentally friendly synthetic approaches have been reported, including "click chemistry" (Arseneault et al., 2015), Lego chemistry (Maraval et al., 2003), and accelerated (Walter and Malkoch, 2012) and orthogonal synthesis strategies (Brauge et al., 2001), which resulted in higher reaction efficiency and step number reduction.

In general, all these strategies yield products with well-defined structures and monodisperse sizes, which is quite attractive not only for synthesis reproducibility but also for reducing experimental variability in the applications (Mintzer and Grinstaff, 2010).

The development and optimization of these highly efficient and rapid synthetic methodologies in combination with the design of novel orthogonal building blocks have allowed the synthesis of an ample range of dendritic compounds. Besides the already introduced PAMAM, PPI, and PLL, today there is a wide range of different dendritic families (Fig. 1.8) with potential applications in biomedical and pharmaceutical areas (Tomalia et al., 2012).

For these bio-applications, biocompatible dendrimers are crucial. Thus, the surface modification [with emphasis on the already mentioned PEGylation (Thakur et al., 2015), as well as acetylation (Kolhatkar et al., 2007; Zhuo et al., 1999), glycosylation (Shaunak et al., 2004), and amino-acid functionalization (Kim et al., 2006)] is a common strategy for improving biocompatibility in dendrimers. Moreover, some authors have synthesized dendrimers with biocompatible units with the human body, such as natural metabolites: succinic acid (Carnahan and Grinstaff, 2001) and adipic acid (Carnahan and Grinstaff, 2006) "biodendrimers"; glycerol (Tschiche et al., 2014); amino acids (Kui et al., 2011); and oligo PEG chains (Dhanikula and Hildgen, 2006).

Despite these improvements on the dendrimers design for biomedical applications, the nondegradability, under physiological conditions, of the most currently used dendrimers can result in cytotoxicity induced by the accumulation of nondegradable synthetic materials inside cells or in tissues (Malik et al., 2000; Jain et al., 2010). To overcome these possible hurdles, a number of teams have been focusing on the design of biodegradable dendritic structures (Leiro et al., 2015), mainly polyester-based architectures (Fig. 1.8). Moreover, the development of biodegradable dendrimers is also put forward in the context of the design of "smart" controlled delivery systems in which one aims at triggering and/or sustaining the release of a therapeutic agent via the control of the degradation profile of its vector.

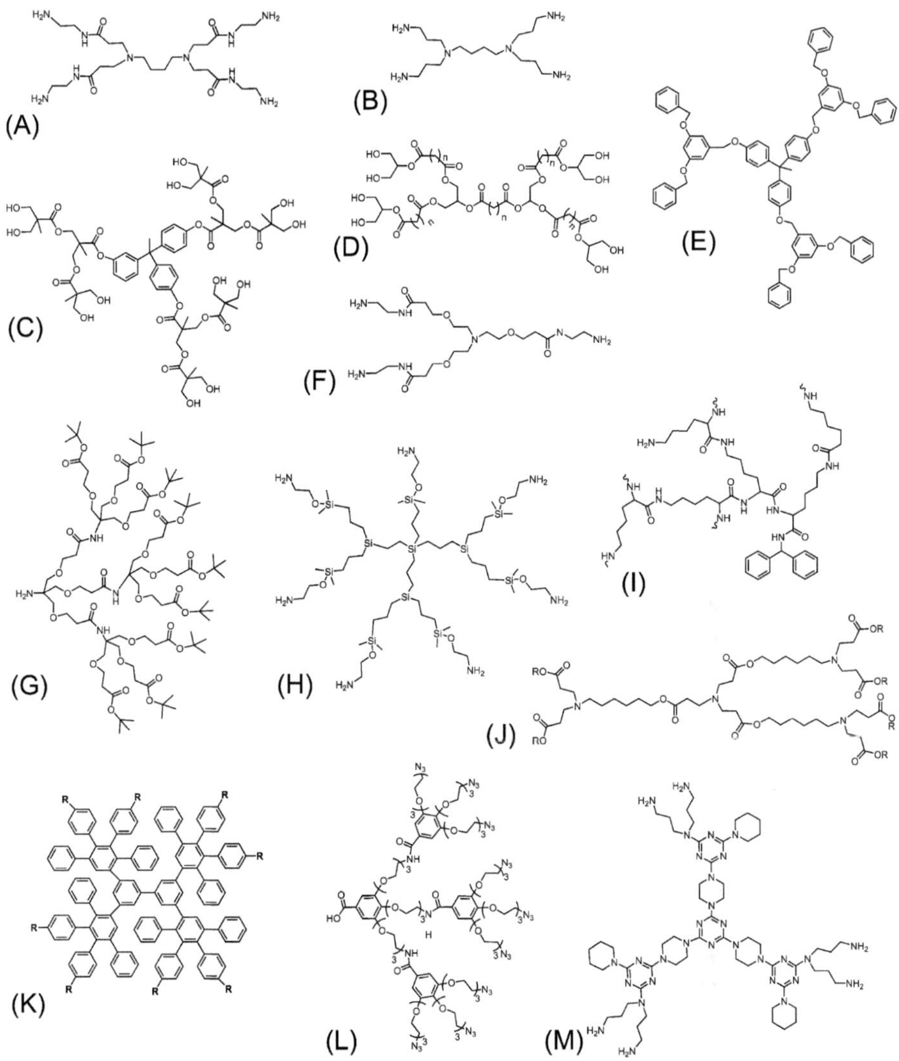

Fig. 1.8 Partial structure of some representative dendritic families: (A) PAMAM, (B) PPI, (C) polyester, (D) succinic and/or adipic-based ("biodendrimers"), (E) polyether, (F) poly(ether amine), (G) amino-poly(ether ester), (H) carbosilane, (I) PLL, (J) poly (ester amine), (K) polyphenylene, (L) gallic acid triethylene glycol (GATG), and (M) s-triazine dendrimers.

However, the progress of biodegradable dendritic compounds with suitable physicochemical and pharmacodynamic properties is challenging due to undesired and/or premature degradation during synthesis, purification, and subsequent functionalization and processing steps (van der Poll et al., 2010). In fact, these obstacles may explain the still reduced number of reports where biodegradable dendrimers are applied for a particular function in biomedicine (Leiro et al., 2015).

Also, it is worth mentioning that, although most of reported dendrimers are monofunctional systems, the more and more sophisticated synthetic methodologies have allowed the synthesis of some heterofunctional dendrimers, mainly bifunctionals, with two (or more) terminal functional groups (Navath et al., 2010; de Jong et al., 2015).

1.6.2.2 Applications of dendrimers as drug delivery systems

Dendrimers are being used as promising carriers of chemical drugs (Medina and El-Sayed, 2009; Caminade and Turrin, 2014) and therapeutic NAs (Dufes et al., 2005; Biswas and Torchilin, 2013), as well as macromolecular CAs (Langereis et al., 2007; Qiao and Shi, 2015). Here, there is a crucial application to be stressed: their function as carriers to deliver bioactives to the CNS. The deficient BBB permeability leads to a poor access of theranostic agents into CNS, which limits the efficacy of noninvasive treatment and diagnosis for CNS diseases. Thus, to cross the brain parenchyma has become one of the most significant challenges in the development of CNS theranostics. In this context, dendrimers present very attractive features to mediate bioactives delivery to the brain, since their adaptable solubility, monodispersion, and nanosize allow the tight control and tuning of the size of the resulting dendritic nanoparticle, here targeted to be lower than 100 nm (Sukrut and Christine, 2014).

Dendrimers in chemical drug delivery: Dendrimers serve as appropriate host of guest chemical drugs: (i) by entrapping in the interior cavities or (ii) by attaching to offer a dendrimer–drug conjugate. Indeed, due to the easy multifunctionalization, target molecules can be attached to dendrimers in both cases with the aim of improving their cell-specificity (Kesharwani and Lyer, 2015). (i) *Drug encapsulation*. Drugs can be accommodated inside dendrimers ("dendritic box") (Jansen et al., 1994) through noncovalent interactions (hydrogen bonding (Dhanikula and Hildgen, 2007), hydrophobic (Dhanikula and Hildgen, 2007; Morgan et al., 2003) and/or electrostatic interactions (Cheng et al., 2007; Sadekar et al., 2013). In most cases, dendrimers allow the increase of the solubilization of the often poorly water-soluble bioactives (Gupta et al., 2007; Shadrack et al., 2015) (anticancer, antiviral, antibacterial, antitubercular, and antimalarial drugs). (ii) D*rugs conjugation*. The high density of functional groups on dendrimers provides an unprecedented chance for ionic-coordination (Malik et al., 1999; Haririan et al., 2010) or covalent attachment of drugs. In the last case, they can be attached to the dendrimers through different linkages (ester (Malik et al., 2000; Bi et al., 2007), hydrazone (Lee et al., 2006; Kaminskas et al., 2011b), carbamate (Lee et al., 2006), amide (Zhuo et al., 1999; Qi et al., 2015), disulfide (Navath et al., 2008), oximes (Seo et al., 2014), among others).

This strategy provides better control in terms of kinetics of drug release (avoiding a premature release) (Patri et al., 2005), through cleavage, chemical (pH, redox) or enzymatic, of the bonds linking the drugs (Gingras et al., 2007); and allows to engineer stimuli-sensitive targeted drug-delivery systems. However, some cons include the more complex conjugate design and the direct contact of the drugs with enzymes and body fluids. In this regard, the encapsulated drug into the dendrimer remains more protected. Still, a lower number of bioactives can be encapsulated and the guest molecules can rapidly diffuse out of the dendrimer (Patri et al., 2005). As briefly seen, both strategies have their own pros and cons (Kaminskas et al., 2012), thus, some researchers have evaluated the combination of both approaches simultaneously (Patri et al., 2005). Because dendrimers can render drugs more water soluble, bioavailable, and biocompatible, different routes of administration, besides intravenous (Malik et al., 1999; Gajbhiye and Jain, 2011), have been successfully proved: oral (Sadekar et al., 2013; Goldberg et al., 2011), transdermal (Chauhan et al., 2003), ocular (Shaunak et al., 2004; Spataro et al., 2010), and pulmonary (Dong et al., 2011).

Dendrimers in NA deliver: Dendrimers represent another attractive nonviral vehicle in the gene therapy field (Dufes et al., 2005; Biswas and Torchilin, 2013). In their cationic form, they are able to complex and protect NAs through electrostatic interactions, originating dendriplexes (Shcharbin et al., 2014), and contribute to overcoming the different extra- and intracellular barriers encountered in order to efficiently deliver exogenous and therapeutic NAs into cells with minimal toxicity. Moreover, the possibility of precise chemical multidecoration allows the design of an almost unlimited number of molecules, as well as the conjugation of several ligands and target molecules tailored to attain an efficient and site-specific NA delivery (Yang et al., 2015).

Even though several groups reported the success of dendrimers as NA carriers (Luo et al., 2002; Santos et al., 2010; de la Fuente et al., 2012), the nonbiodegradability of the used dendritic structures in this field remains a drawback yet to be solved (Duncan and Izzo, 2005; Mintzer and Grinstaff, 2010; Jain et al., 2010). Biodegradability besides preventing cytotoxicity (Malik et al., 1999, 2000; Jain et al., 2010) can contribute to a better release of the transported NA (Barnard et al., 2014), rendering higher transfection efficiencies.

Dendrimers as macromolecular CAs: A particular case of drug–dendrimer conjugation is the covalent linkage of diagnosis agents for their use as macromolecular CAs in techniques such as X-ray (Peng and Shi, 2013) and MRI for medical diagnostics (Langereis et al., 2007; Qiao and Shi, 2015). Briefly, the objective is to synthesize large molecular weight CAs to enhance the image contrast, stability, water solubility, biocompatibility, and pharmacokinetic behavior, while decreasing toxicity and the dose of currently available small CAs. Some researchers have explored organometallic (Bi and Sn) complexes of dendrimers and dendritic nanoparticles with heavy isotopes of iodine as X-ray CAs (Yordanov et al., 2002; Fu et al., 2006). In the MRI case, the most widely used CAs are small molecules based on paramagnetic gadolinium(III) chelates (Gd(III)–DTPA (DTPA = diethylenetriaminepentaacetic acid, Magnevist) and Gd(III)–DOTA (Dotarem)) (Langereis et al., 2007). Due to their multivalency, dendrimers represent one of the most appealing platforms to carry multiple CAs moieties (Langereis et al., 2007; Wiener et al., 1994; Misselwitz et al., 2001; Kobayashi and Brechbiel, 2003; Parrott et al., 2009), as well as to graft target molecules, offering a unique opportunity to enhance site-specific image contrast (Langereis et al., 2007; Swanson et al., 2008; Ye et al., 2013). Moreover, some authors have proposed the use of degradable dendrimers as macromolecular CAs for overcoming long-term Gd(III) tissue accumulation (Ye et al., 2012).

1.7 Concluding remarks and future perspectives

In conclusion, the use of biomimetic and bioinspired materials as drug-delivery systems is exponentially increasing, supported by progress in our understanding of the mechanisms of diseases, cell biology, and drug mechanism of action. This has allowed the design of more efficient and targeted drug-vector systems and exploration of alternative routes of administration taking advantage of our more in-depth knowledge of pathological states (e.g., the enhanced permeability and retention effect, in the case of vascularized tumors).

Technological advances in the field of recombinant proteins, solid-phase synthesis, and polymer chemistry (e.g., "click chemistry") have also contributed greatly to progress in this area as previously reviewed. Bioinformatics and mathematical modeling have also been instrumental in the field, contributing to the in silico testing of many of the proposed systems, advancing mechanisms of action, and permitting a better design of the drug vectors. Further developments in these fields, combined with advances in genomics, proteomics, and the emerging field of glycomics, will certainly broaden the spectrum of smarter drug delivery systems.

Nonetheless, many of the proposed drug-delivery system systems, although they have successfully conquered a number of hurdles in vitro and/or in preclinical animal models, have failed to reach the bedside. So it is our belief that research being conducted in this field will greatly profit from progress being made in many other areas, such as tissue engineering, with important contributions to the design of more reliable tissue models for use as screening platforms, stem cell technology (in particular induced pluripotent stem cell technology), (quantitative) bioimaging (both in vitro, including high throughput screening, and in vivo), and bioinformatics.

References

Adler-Abramovich, L., Vaks, L., Carny, O., Trudler, D., Magno, A., Caflisch, A., et al., 2012. Phenylalanine assembly into toxic fibrils suggests amyloid etiology in phenylketonuria. Nat. Chem. Biol. 8, 701–706.

Afonin, K.A., Bindewald, E., Yaghoubian, A.J., Voss, N., Jacovetty, E., Shapiro, B.A., et al., 2010. In vitro assembly of cubic RNA-based scaffolds designed in silico. Nat. Nanotechnol. 5 (9), 676–682.

Afonin, K.A., Viard, M., Koyfman, A.Y., Martins, A.N., Kasprzak, W.K., Panigaj, M., et al., 2014. Multifunctional RNA nanoparticles. Nano Lett. 14 (10), 5662–5671.

Afonso, R.V., Durão, J., Mendes, A., Damas, A.M., Gales, L., 2010. Dipeptide crystals as excellent permselective materials: sequential exclusion of argon, nitrogen, and oxygen. Angew. Chem. Int. Ed. Engl. 49, 3034–3036.

Afonso, R., Mendes, A., Gales, L., 2012. Peptide-based solids: porosity and zeolitic behavior. J. Mater. Chem. 22, 1709–1723.

Afonso, R., Mendes, A., Gales, L., 2014. Hydrophobic dipeptide crystals: a promising Ag-free class of ultramicroporous materials showing argon/oxygen adsorption selectivity. Phys. Chem. Chem. Phys. 16, 19386–19393.

Al-Ahmady, Z.S., Al-Jamal, W.T., Bossche, J.V., Bui, T.T., Drake, A.F., Mason, A.J., et al., 2012. Lipid-peptide vesicle nanoscale hybrids for triggered drug release by mild hyperthermia in vitro and in vivo. ACS Nano 6, 9335–9346.

Albuquerque, J., Moura, C.C., Sarmento, B., Reis, S., 2015. Solid lipid nanoparticles: a potential multifunctional approach towards rheumatoid arthritis theranostics. Molecules 20 (6), 11103–11118.

Aldaye, F.A., Sleiman, H.F., 2007. Modular access to structurally switchable 3D discrete DNA assemblies. J. Am. Chem. Soc. 129 (44), 13376–13377.

Allen, T.M., Cullis, P.R., 2013. Liposomal drug delivery systems: from concept to clinical applications. Adv. Drug Deliv. Rev. 65 (1), 36–48.

Allena, T.M., Cullisb, P.R., 2013. Liposomal drug delivery systems: from concept to clinical applications. Adv. Drug Deliv. Rev. 65 (1), 36–48.

Altunbas, A., Lee, S.J., Rajasekaran, S.A., Schneider, J.P., Pochan, D.J., 2011. Encapsulation of curcumin in self-assembling peptide hydrogels as injectable drug delivery vehicles. Biomaterials 32, 5906–5914.

Andersen, E.S., Dong, M., Nielsen, M.M., Jahn, K., Subramani, R., Mamdouh, W., et al., 2009. Self-assembly of a nanoscale DNA box with a controllable lid. Nature 459 (7243), 73–76.

Apostolovic, B., Deacon, S.P.E., Duncan, R., Klok, H.-A., 2011. Cell uptake and trafficking behavior of non-covalent, coiled-coil based polymer-drug conjugates. Macromol. Rapid Commun. 32, 11–18.

Arseneault, M., Wafer, C., Morin, J.F., 2015. Recent advances in click chemistry applied to dendrimer synthesis. Molecules 20 (5), 9263–9294.

Azevedo, H.S., Pashkuleva, I., 2015. Biomimetic supramolecular designs for the controlled release of growth factors in bone regeneration. Adv. Drug Deliv. Rev. 94, 63–76.

Banwell, E.F., Abelardo, E.S., Adams, D.J., Birchall, M.A., Corrigan, A., Donald, A.M., et al., 2009. Rational design and application of responsive [alpha]-helical peptide hydrogels. Nat. Mater. 8, 596–600.

Barnard, A., Posocco, P., Fermeglia, M., Tschiche, A., Calderon, M., Pricl, S., et al., 2014. Double-degradable responsive self-assembled multivalent arrays—temporary nanoscale recognition between dendrons and DNA. Org. Biomol. Chem. 12 (3), 446–455.

Barros, D., Amaral, I.F., Pêgo, A.P., 2015. Biomimetic synthetic self-assembled hydrogels for cell transplantation. Curr. Top. Med. Chem. 15 (13), 1209–1226.

Bi, X., Shi, X., Majoros, I.J., Shukla, R., Baker, J.R., 2007. Multifunctional poly(amidoamine) dendrimer-taxol conjugates: synthesis, characterization and stability. J. Comput. Theor. Nanosci. 4 (6), 1179–1187.

Biswas, S., Torchilin, V.P., 2013. Dendrimers for siRNA delivery. Pharmaceuticals 6 (2), 161–183.

Boddohi, S., Kipper, M.J., 2010. Engineering nanoassemblies of polysaccharides. Adv. Mater. 22, 2998–3016.

Branco, M.C., Pochan, D.J., Wagner, N.J., Schneider, J.P., 2009. Macromolecular diffusion and release from self-assembled β-hairpin peptide hydrogels. Biomaterials 30, 1339–1347.

Brauge, L., Magro, G., Caminade, A.M., Majoral, J.P., 2001. First divergent strategy using two AB(2) unprotected monomers for the rapid synthesis of dendrimers. J. Am. Chem. Soc. 123 (27), 6698–6699.

Brown, P.K., Qureshi, A.T., Moll, A.N., Hayes, D.J., Monroe, W.T., 2013. Silver nanoscale antisense drug delivery system for photoactivated gene silencing. ACS Nano 7 (4), 2948–2959.

Buhleier, E., Wehner, W., Vogtle, F., 1978. "Cascade"- and "non-skid-chain-like" syntheses of molecular cavity topologies. Synthesis 2, 155–158.

Bulut, S., Erkal, T.S., Toksoz, S., Tekinay, A.B., Tekinay, T., Guler, M.O., 2011. Slow release and delivery of antisense oligonucleotide drug by self-assembled peptide amphiphile nanofibers. Biomacromolecules 12, 3007–3014.

Burkhard, P., Stetefeld, J., Strelkov, S.V., 2001. Coiled coils: a highly versatile protein folding motif. Trends Cell Biol. 11, 82–88.

Caminade, A.M., Turrin, C.O., 2014. Dendrimers for drug delivery. J. Mater. Chem. B 2 (26), 4055–4066.

Caminade, A.M., Fruchon, S., Turrin, C.O., Poupot, M., Ouali, A., Maraval, A., et al., 2015. The key role of the scaffold on the efficiency of dendrimer nanodrugs. Nat. Commun. 6, 7722.

Carnahan, M.A., Grinstaff, M.W., 2001. Synthesis and characterization of poly(glycerol-succinic acid) dendrimers. Macromolecules 34 (22), 7648–7655.

Carnahan, M.A., Grinstaff, M.W., 2006. Synthesis of generational polyester dendrimers derived from glycerol and succinic or adipic acid. Macromolecules 39 (2), 609–616.

Chan, A.W., Whitney, R.A., Neufeld, R.J., 2009. Semisynthesis of a controlled stimuli-responsive alginate hydrogel. Biomacromolecules 10 (3), 609–616.

Chang, H.-I., Yeh, M.-K., 2012. Clinical development of liposome-based drugs: formulation, characterization, and therapeutic efficacy. Int. J. Nanomedicine 7, 49–60.

Chang, M., Yang, C.-S., Huang, D.-M., 2011. Aptamer-conjugated DNA icosahedral nanoparticles as a carrier of doxorubicin for cancer therapy. ACS Nano 5 (8), 6156–6163.

Charoenphol, P., Bermudez, H., 2014. Aptamer-targeted DNA nanostructures for therapeutic delivery. Mol. Pharm. 11 (5), 1721–1725.

Chauhan, A.S., Sridevi, S., Chalasani, K.B., Jain, A.K., Jain, S.K., Jain, N.K., et al., 2003. Dendrimer-mediated transdermal delivery: enhanced bioavailability of indomethacin. J. Control. Release 90 (3), 335–343.

Chen, J.H., Seeman, N.C., 1991. Synthesis from DNA of a molecule with the connectivity of a cube. Nature 350 (6319), 631–633.

Chen, X., Ramström, O., Yan, M., 2014. Glyconanomaterials: emerging applications in biomedical research. Nano Res. 7 (10), 1381–1403.

Chena, Y., Liub, L., 2012. Modern methods for delivery of drugs across the blood-brain barrier. Adv. Drug Deliv. Rev. 64 (7), 640–665.

Cheng, Y.Y., Man, N., Xu, T.W., Fu, R.Q., Wang, X.Y., Wang, X.M., et al., 2007. Transdermal delivery of nonsteroidal anti-inflammatory drugs mediated by polyamidoamine (PAMAM) dendrimers. J. Pharm. Sci. 96 (3), 595–602.

Cohen, S.N., Chang, A.C., Boyer, H.W., Helling, R.B., 1973. Construction of biologically functional bacterial plasmids in vitro. Proc. Natl. Acad. Sci. U. S. A. 70 (11), 3240–3244.

Comotti, A., Bracco, S., Distefano, G., Sozzani, P., 2009. Methane, carbon dioxide and hydrogen storage in nanoporous dipeptide-based materials. Chem. Commun. 284–286.

Cryan, S., 2005. Carrier-based strategies for targeting protein and peptide drugs to the lungs. AAPS J. 7, E20–E41.

Dan, Z., Cao, H., He, X., Zeng, L., Zou, L., Shen, Q., Zhang, Z., 2015. Biological stimuli-responsive cyclodextrin-based host–guest nanosystems for cancer therapy. Int. J. Pharm. 483, 63–68.

Daniel-da-Silva, A.L., Ferreira, L., Gil, A.M., Trindade, T., 2011. Synthesis and swelling behavior of temperature responsive k-carrageenan nanogels. J. Colloid Interface Sci. 355 (2), 512–517.

de Jong, E.R., Deloch, N., Knoll, W., Turrin, C.O., Majoral, J.P., Caminade, A.M., et al., 2015. Synthesis and characterization of bifunctional dendrimers: preliminary use for the coating of gold surfaces and the proliferation of human osteoblasts (HOB). New J. Chem. 39 (9), 7194–7205.

de la Fuente, M., Raviña, M., Sousa-Herves, A., Correa, J., Riguera, R., Fernandez-Megia, E., et al., 2012. Exploring the efficiency of gallic acid-based dendrimers and their block copolymers with PEG as gene carriers. Nanomedicine 7 (11), 1667–1681.

Denkewalter, R.G., Kolc, J., Lukasavage, W.J., inventors; Google Patents, assignee, 1981. Surface modifying agents, metal chelating agents, substrates for drugs. Patent U.S. 4289872.

Dhanikula, R.S., Hildgen, P., 2006. Synthesis and evaluation of novel dendrimers with a hydrophilic interior as nanocarriers for drug delivery. Bioconjug. Chem. 17 (1), 29–41.

Dhanikula, R.S., Hildgen, P., 2007. Influence of molecular architecture of polyether-*co*-polyester dendrimers on the encapsulation and release of methotrexate. Biomaterials 28 (20), 3140–3152.

Dong, H., Paramonov, S.E., Hartgerink, J.D., 2008. Self-assembly of α-helical coiled coil nanofibers. J. Am. Chem. Soc. 130, 13691–13695.

Dong, Z.Q., Hamid, K.A., Gao, Y., Lin, Y.L., Katsumi, H., Sakane, T., et al., 2011. Polyamidoamine dendrimers can improve the pulmonary absorption of insulin and calcitonin in rats. J. Pharm. Sci. 100 (5), 1866–1878.

Douglas, S.M., Dietz, H., Liedl, T., Högberg, B., Graf, F., Shih, W.M., 2009. Self-assembly of DNA into nanoscale three-dimensional shapes. Nature 459 (7245), 414–418.

Douglas, S.M., Bachelet, I., Church, G.M., 2012. A logic-gated nanorobot for targeted transport of molecular payloads. Science 335 (6070), 831–834.

Dufes, C., Uchegbu, I., Schatzlein, A., 2005. Dendrimers in gene delivery. Adv. Drug Deliv. Rev. 57 (15), 2177–2202.

Duncan, R., Izzo, L., 2005. Dendrimer biocompatibility and toxicity. Adv. Drug Deliv. Rev. 57 (15), 2215–2237.

Durão, J., Gales, L., 2013. Guest diffusion in dipeptide crystals. CrystEngComm 15, 1532–1535.

Emami, S., Paz, F.A.A., Mendes, A., Gales, L., 2014. Toward the construction of 3D dipeptide-metal frameworks. Cryst. Growth Des. 14, 4777–4780.

Eriksson, M., Hassan, S., Larsson, R., Linder, S., Ramqvist, T., Lövborg, H., Vikinge, T., Figgemeier, E., Müller, J., Stetefeld, J., Dalianis, T., Ozbek, S., 2009. Utilization of a right-handed coiled-coil protein from archaebacterium *Staphylothermus marinus* as a carrier for cisplatin. Anticancer Res. 29, 11–18.

Fakhoury, J.J., McLaughlin, C.K., Edwardson, T.W., Conway, J.W., Sleiman, H.F., 2014. Development and characterization of gene silencing DNA cages. Biomacromolecules 15 (1), 276–282.

Faraji, A., Wipf, P., 2009. Nanoparticles in cellular drug delivery. Bioorg. Med. Chem. 17 (8), 2950–2962.

Fernández-Tejada, A., Cañada, F.J., Jiménez-Barbero, J., 2015. Recent developments in synthetic carbohydrate-based diagnostics, vaccines, and therapeutics. Chemistry 21 (30), 10616–10628.

Fonseca, K.B., Granja, P.L., Barrias, C.C., 2014. Engineering proteolytically-degradable artificial extracellular matrices. Prog. Polym. Sci. 39, 2010–2029.

Fonte, P., Nogueira, T., Gehm, C., Ferreira, D., Sarmento, B., 2011. Chitosan-coated solid lipid nanoparticles enhance the oral absorption of insulin. Drug Deliv. Transl. Res. 1 (4), 299–308.

Fu, T.J., Seeman, N.C., 1993. DNA double-crossover molecules. Biochemistry 32 (13), 3211–3220.

Fu, Y.J., Nitecki, D.E., Maltby, D., Simon, G.H., Berejnoi, K., Raatschen, H.J., et al., 2006. Dendritic iodinated contrast agents with PEG-cores for CT imaging: synthesis and preliminary characterization. Bioconjug. Chem. 17 (4), 1043–1056.

Gajbhiye, V., Jain, N.K., 2011. The treatment of glioblastoma xenografts by surfactant conjugated dendritic nanoconjugates. Biomaterials 32 (26), 6213–6225.

Gazit, E., 2007. Self-assembled peptide nanostructures: the design of molecular building blocks and their technological utilization. Chem. Soc. Rev. 36, 1263–1269.

Gelain, F., Bottai, D., Vescovi, A., Zhang, S., 2006. Designer self-assembling peptide nanofiber scaffolds for adult mouse neural stem cell 3-dimensional cultures. PLoS One 1.

Genové, E., Shen, C., Zhang, S., Semino, C.E., 2005. The effect of functionalized self-assembling peptide scaffolds on human aortic endothelial cell function. Biomaterials 26, 3341–3351.

Giammanco, G.E., Sosnofsky, C.T., Ostrowski, A.D., 2015. Light-responsive iron(III)-polysaccharide coordination hydrogels for controlled delivery. ACS Appl. Mater. Interfaces 7 (5), 3068–3076.

Gingras, M., Raimundo, J.M., Chabre, Y.M., 2007. Cleavable dendrimers. Angew. Chem. Int. Ed. 46 (7), 1010–1017.

Goldberg, D.S., Vijayalakshmi, N., Swaan, P.W., Ghandehari, H., 2011. G3.5 PAMAM dendrimers enhance transepithelial transport of SN38 while minimizing gastrointestinal toxicity. J. Control. Release 150 (3), 318–325.

Goodman, R.P., Schaap, I.A.T., Tardin, C.F., Erben, C.M., Berry, R.M., Schmidt, C.F., et al., 2005. Rapid chiral assembly of rigid DNA building blocks for molecular nanofabrication. Science 310 (5754), 1661–1665.

Görbitz, C.H., 2007. Microporous organic materials from hydrophobic dipeptides. Chem. Eur. J. 13, 1022–1031.

Grabow, W.W., Zakrevsky, P., Afonin, K.A., Chworos, A., Shapiro, B.A., Jaeger, L., 2011. Self-assembling RNA nanorings based on RNAI/II inverse kissing complexes. Nano Lett. 11 (2), 878–887.

Greenfield, M.A., Hoffman, J.R., De La Cruz, M.O., Stupp, S.I., 2010. Tunable mechanics of peptide nanofiber gels. Langmuir 26, 3641–3647.

Grenha, A., Remuñán-López, C., Carvalho, E.L., Seijo, B., 2008. Microspheres containing lipid/chitosan nanoparticles complexes for pulmonary delivery of therapeutic proteins. Eur. J. Pharm. Biopharm. 69 (1), 83–93.

Gupta, U., Agashe, H.B., Jain, N.K., 2007. Polypropylene imine dendrimer mediated solubility enhancement: effect of pH and functional groups of hydrophobes. J. Pharm. Pharm. Sci. 10 (3), 358–367.

Han, D., Pal, S., Nangreave, J., Deng, Z., Liu, Y., Yan, H., 2011. DNA origami with complex curvatures in three-dimensional space. Science 332 (6027), 342–346.

Haririan, I., Alavidjeh, M.S., Khorramizadeh, M.R., Ardestani, M.S., Ghane, Z.Z., Namazi, H., 2010. Anionic linear-globular dendrimer-cis-platinum (II) conjugates promote cytotoxicity in vitro against different cancer cell lines. Int. J. Nanomedicine 5, 63–75.

Hawker, C.J., Frechet, J.M.J., 1990. Preparation of polymers with controlled molecular architecture. A new convergent approach to dendritic macromolecules. J. Am. Chem. Soc. 112 (21), 7638–7647.

He, Y., Chen, Y., Liu, H., Ribbe, A.E., Mao, C., 2005. Self-assembly of hexagonal DNA two-dimensional (2D) arrays. J. Am. Chem. Soc. 127 (35), 12202–12203.

He, Y., Ye, T., Su, M., Zhang, C., Ribbe, A.E., Jiang, W., et al., 2008. Hierarchical self-assembly of DNA into symmetric supramolecular polyhedra. Nature 452 (7184), 198–201.

He, Y., Su, M., Fang, P.-A., Zhang, C., Ribbe, A.E., Jiang, W., et al., 2010. On the chirality of self-assembled DNA octahedra. Angew. Chem. Int. Ed. Engl. 49 (4), 748–751.

Holmes, T.C., De Lacalle, S., Su, X., Liu, G., Rich, A., Zhang, S., 2000. Extensive neurite outgrowth and active synapse formation on self- assembling peptide scaffolds. Proc. Natl. Acad. Sci. U. S. A. 97, 6728–6733.

Hudalla, G.A., Murphy, W.L., 2011. Biomaterials that regulate growth factor activity via bioinspired interactions. Adv. Funct. Mater. 21 (10), 1754–1768.
Hynes, R.O., 2009. The extracellular matrix: not just pretty fibrils. Science 326, 1216–1219.
Immordino, M.L., Dosio, F., Cattel, L., 2006. Stealth liposomes: review of the basic science, rationale, and clinical applications, existing and potential. Int. J. Nanomedicine 1 (3), 297–315.
Jain, K., Kesharwani, P., Gupta, U., Jain, N.K., 2010. Dendrimer toxicity: let's meet the challenge. Int. J. Pharm. 394 (1-2), 122–142.
Jansen, J.F.G.A., Debrabandervandenberg, E.M.M., Meijer, E.W., 1994. Encapsulation of guest molecules into a dendritic box. Science 266 (5188), 1226–1229.
Jayawarna, V., Ali, M., Jowitt, T.A., Miller, A.F., Saiani, A., Gough, J.E., et al., 2006. Nanostructured hydrogels for three-dimensional cell culture through self-assembly of fluorenylmethoxycarbonyl-dipeptides. Adv. Mater. 18, 611–614.
Jiang, Q., Song, C., Nangreave, J., Liu, X., Lin, L., Qiu, D., et al., 2012. DNA origami as a carrier for circumvention of drug resistance. J. Am. Chem. Soc. 134 (32), 13396–13403.
Jin, J., Bae, K.H., Yang, H., Lee, S.J., Kim, H., Kim, Y., Joo, K.M., Seo, S.W., Park, T.G., Nam, D.H., 2011. In vivo specific delivery of c-Met siRNA to glioblastoma using cationic solid lipid nanoparticles. Bioconjug. Chem. 22 (12), 2568–2572.
Joshi, M.D., Müller, R.H., 2009. Lipid nanoparticles for parenteral delivery of actives. Eur. J. Pharm. Biopharm. 71 (2), 161–172.
Kallenbach, N.R., Ma, R.-I., Seeman, N.C., 1983. An immobile nucleic acid junction constructed from oligonucleotides. Nature 305 (5937), 829–831.
Kaminskas, L.M., Boyd, B.J., Porter, C.J., 2011a. Dendrimer pharmacokinetics: the effect of size, structure and surface characteristics on ADME properties. Nanomedicine (London) 6 (6), 1063–1084.
Kaminskas, L.M., Kelly, B.D., McLeod, V.M., Sberna, G., Owen, D.J., Boyd, B.J., et al., 2011b. Characterisation and tumour targeting of PEGylated polylysine dendrimers bearing doxorubicin via a pH labile linker. J. Control. Release 152 (2), 241–248.
Kaminskas, L.M., McLeod, V.M., Porter, C.J.H., Boyd, B.J., 2012. Association of chemotherapeutic drugs with dendrimer nanocarriers: an assessment of the merits of covalent conjugation compared to noncovalent encapsulation. Mol. Pharm. 9 (3), 355–373.
Ke, Y., Ong, L.L., Shih, W.M., Yin, P., 2012. Three-dimensional structures self-assembled from DNA bricks. Science 338 (6111), 1177–1183.
Kesharwani, P., Lyer, A.K., 2015. Recent advances in dendrimer-based nanovectors for tumor-targeted drug and gene delivery. Drug Discov. Today 20 (5), 536–547.
Keum, J.-W., Ahn, J.-H., Bermudez, H., 2011. Design, assembly, and activity of antisense DNA nanostructures. Small 7 (24), 3529–3535.
Khaled, A., Guo, S., Li, F., Guo, P., 2005. Controllable self-assembly of nanoparticles for specific delivery of multiple therapeutic molecules to cancer cells using RNA nanotechnology. Nano Lett. 5 (9), 1797–1808.
Khisamutdinov, E.F., Jasinski, D.L., Guo, P., 2014. RNA as a boiling-resistant anionic polymer material to build robust structures with defined shape and stoichiometry. ACS Nano 8 (5), 4771–4781.
Kim, J.B., Choi, J.S., Nam, K., Lee, M., Park, J.S., Lee, J.K., 2006. Enhanced transfection of primary cortical cultures using arginine-grafted PAMAM dendrimer, PAMAM-Arg. J. Control. Release 114 (1), 110–117.
Kim, J.-K., Anderson, J., Jun, H.-W., Repka, M.A., Jo, S., 2009. Self-assembling peptide amphiphile-based nanofiber gel for bioresponsive cisplatin delivery. Mol. Pharm. 6, 978–985.
Kobayashi, H., Brechbiel, M.W., 2003. Dendrimer-based macromolecular MRI contrast agents: characteristics and application. Mol. Imaging 2 (1), 1–10.

Koley, P., Pramanik, A., 2011. Nanostructures from single amino acid-based molecules: stability, fibrillation, encapsulation, and fabrication of silver nanoparticles. Adv. Funct. Mater. 21, 4126–4136.

Koley, P., Pramanik, A., 2012. Multilayer vesicles, tubes, various porous structures and organo gels through the solvent-assisted self-assembly of two modified tripeptides and their different applications. Soft Matter 8, 5364–5374.

Koley, P., Gayen, A., Drew, M.G.B., Mukhopadhyay, C., Pramanik, A., 2012. Design and self-assembly of a leucine-enkephalin analogue in different nanostructures: application of nanovesicles. Small 8, 984–990.

Kolhatkar, R.B., Kitchens, K.M., Swaan, P.W., Ghandehari, H., 2007. Surface acetylation of polyamidoamine (PAMAM) dendrimers decreases cytotoxicity while maintaining membrane permeability. Bioconjug. Chem. 18 (6), 2054–2060.

Koutsopoulos, S., Zhang, S., 2012. Two-layered injectable self-assembling peptide scaffold hydrogels for long-term sustained release of human antibodies. J. Control. Release 160, 451–458.

Koutsopoulos, S., Unsworth, L.D., Nagai, Y., Zhang, S., 2009. Controlled release of functional proteins through designer self-assembling peptide nanofiber hydrogel scaffold. Proc. Natl. Acad. Sci. U. S. A. 106, 4623–4628.

Kui, L., Caixia, L., Gang, W., Yu, N., Bin, H., Yao, W., et al., 2011. Peptide dendrimers as efficient and biocompatible gene delivery vectors: synthesis and in vitro characterization. J. Control. Release 155 (1), 77–87.

LaBean, T.H., Yan, H., Kopatsch, J., Liu, F., Winfree, E., Reif, J.H., et al., 2000. Construction, analysis, ligation, and self-assembly of DNA triple crossover complexes. J. Am. Chem. Soc. 122 (9), 1848–1860.

Langereis, S., Dirksen, A., Hackeng, T.M., van Genderen, M.H.P., Meijer, E.W., 2007. Dendrimers and magnetic resonance imaging. New J. Chem. 31 (7), 1152–1160.

Lee, C.C., Gillies, E.R., Fox, M.E., Guillaudeu, S.J., Fréchet, J.M.J., Dy, E.E., et al., 2006. A single dose of doxorubicin-functionalized bow-tie dendrimer cures mice bearing C-26 colon carcinomas. Proc. Natl. Acad. Sci. U. S. A. 103 (45), 16649–16654.

Lee, H., Lytton-Jean, A.K.R., Chen, Y., Love, K.T., Park, A.I., Karagiannis, E.D., et al., 2012. Molecularly self-assembled nucleic acid nanoparticles for targeted in vivo siRNA delivery. Nat. Nanotechnol. 7 (6), 389–393.

Leiro, V., Garcia, J.P., Tomas, H., Pego, A.P., 2015. The present and the future of degradable dendrimers and derivatives in theranostics. Bioconjug. Chem. 26 (7), 1182–1197.

Lenci, E., Menchi, G., Trabocchi, A., 2016. Carbohydrates in diversity-oriented synthesis: challenges and opportunities. Org. Biomol. Chem. 14 (3), 808–825.

Li, X., Yang, X., Qi, J., Seeman, N.C., 1996. Antiparallel DNA double crossover molecules as components for nanoconstruction. J. Am. Chem. Soc. 118 (26), 6131–6140.

Li, Y., Tseng, Y.D., Kwon, S.Y., d'Espaux, L., Bunch, J.S., McEuen, P.L., et al., 2004. Controlled assembly of dendrimer-like DNA. Nat. Mater. 3 (1), 38–42.

Li, J., Pei, H., Zhu, B., Liang, L., Wei, M., He, Y., et al., 2011. Self-assembled multivalent DNA nanostructures for noninvasive intracellular delivery of immunostimulatory CpG oligonucleotides. ACS Nano 5 (11), 8783–8789.

Liang, J., Wu, W.-L., Xu, X.-D., Zhuo, R.-X., Zhang, X.-Z., 2014. pH Responsive micelle self-assembled from a new amphiphilic peptide as anti-tumor drug carrier. Colloids Surf. B: Biointerfaces 114, 398–403.

Liang, C., Li, L., Fraser, C.D., Ko, A., Corzo, D., Enger, C., Patt, D., 2015. The treatment patterns, efficacy, and safety of nab (®)-paclitaxel for the treatment of metastatic breast cancer in the United States: results from health insurance claims analysis. BMC Cancer 15 (1), 1019.

Liechty, W.B., Kryscio, D.R., Slaughter, B.V., Peppas, N.A., 2010. Polymers for drug delivery systems. Annu. Rev. Chem. Biomol. Eng. 1, 149–173.
Liu, H., Zhu, Z., Kang, H., Wu, Y., Sefan, K., Tan, W., 2010. DNA-based micelles: synthesis, micellar properties and size-dependent cell permeability. Chemistry 16 (12), 3791–3797.
Liu, X., Xu, Y., Yu, T., Clifford, C., Liu, Y., Yan, H., et al., 2012. A DNA nanostructure platform for directed assembly of synthetic vaccines. Nano Lett. 12 (8), 4254–4259.
Luo, D., Haverstick, K., Belcheva, N., Han, E., Saltzman, W.M., 2002. Poly(ethylene glycol)-conjugated PAMAM dendrimer for biocompatible, high-efficiency DNA delivery. Macromolecules 35 (9), 3456–3462.
Mahler, A., Reches, M., Rechter, M., Cohen, S., Gazit, E., 2006. Rigid, self-assembled hydrogel composed of a modified aromatic dipeptide. Adv. Mater. 18, 1365–1370.
Maia, F.R., Barbosa, M., Gomes, D.B., Vale, N., Gomes, P., Granja, P.L., Barrias, C.C., 2014. Hydrogel depots for local co-delivery of osteoinductive peptides and mesenchymal stem cells. J. Control. Release 189, 158–168.
Maity, S., Jana, P., Maity, S.K., Haldar, D., 2011. Fabrication of hollow self-assembled peptide microvesicles and transition from sphere-to-rod structure. Langmuir 27, 3835–3841.
Majumdar, S., Siahaan, T.J., 2012. Peptide-mediated targeted drug delivery. Med. Res. Rev. 32, 637–658.
Malik, N., Evagorou, E.G., Duncan, R., 1999. Dendrimer-platinate: a novel approach to cancer chemotherapy. Anti-Cancer Drugs 10 (8), 767–776.
Malik, N., Wiwattanapatapee, R., Klopsch, R., Lorenz, K., Frey, H., Weener, J.W., et al., 2000. Dendrimers: relationship between structure and biocompatibility in vitro, and preliminary studies on the biodistribution of 125I-labelled polyamidoamine dendrimers in vivo. J. Control. Release 65 (1-2), 133–148.
Maraval, V., Pyzowski, J., Caminade, A.M., Majoral, J.P., 2003. "Lego" chemistry for the straightforward synthesis of dendrimers. J. Org. Chem. 68 (15), 6043–6046.
Martins, S., Sarmento, B., Ferreira, D.C., Souto, E.B., 2007. Lipid-based colloidal carriers for peptide and protein delivery—liposomes versus lipid nanoparticles. Int. J. Nanomedicine 2 (4), 595–607.
Martins, S.M., Sarmento, B., Nunes, C., Lúcio, M., Reis, S., Ferreira, D.C., 2013. Brain targeting effect of camptothecin-loaded solid lipid nanoparticles in rat after intravenous administration. Eur. J. Pharm. Biopharm. 85 (3 Pt A), 488–502.
Matricardi, P., Di Meo, C., Coviello, T., Hennink, W.E., Alhaique, F., 2013. Interpenetrating polymer networks polysaccharide hydrogels for drug delivery and tissue engineering. Adv. Drug Deliv. Rev. 65 (9), 1172–1187.
Matson, J.B., Newcomb, C.J., Bitton, R., Stupp, S.I., 2012. Nanostructure-templated control of drug release from peptide amphiphile nanofiber gels. Soft Matter 8, 3586–3595.
McLaughlin, C.K., Hamblin, G.D., Aldaye, F.A., Yang, H., Sleiman, H.F., 2011. A facile, modular and high yield method to assemble three-dimensional DNA structures. Chem. Commun. 47 (31), 8925–8927.
Medina, S.H., El-Sayed, M.E.H., 2009. Dendrimers as carriers for delivery of chemotherapeutic agents. Chem. Rev. 109 (7), 3141–3157.
Miller, T., Goude, M.C., McDevitt, T.C., Temenoff, J.S., 2014. Molecular engineering of glycosaminoglycan chemistry for biomolecule delivery. Acta Biomater. 10 (4), 1705–1719.
Mintzer, M.A., Grinstaff, M.W., 2010. Biomedical applications of dendrimers: a tutorial. Chem. Soc. Rev. 40 (1), 173–190.
Mishra, B., Patel, B., Tiwari, S., 2010. Colloidal nanocarriers: a review on formulation technology, types and applications toward targeted drug delivery. Nanomedicine 6, 9–24.

Misselwitz, B., Schmitt-Willich, H., Ebert, W., Frenzel, T., Weinmann, H.J., 2001. Pharmacokinetics of Gadomer-17, a new dendritic magnetic resonance contrast agent. MAGMA 12 (2-3), 128–134.

Mohri, K., Nishikawa, M., Takahashi, N., Shiomi, T., Matsuoka, N., Ogawa, K., et al., 2012. Design and development of nanosized DNA assemblies in polypod-like structures as efficient vehicles for immunostimulatory CpG motifs to immune cells. ACS Nano 6 (7), 5931–5940.

Mohri, K., Kusuki, E., Ohtsuki, S., Takahashi, N., Endo, M., Hidaka, K., et al., 2015. Self-assembling DNA dendrimer for effective delivery of immunostimulatory CpG DNA to immune cells. Biomacromolecules 16 (4), 1095–1101.

More, H.T., Frezzo, J.A., Dai, J., Yamano, S., Montclare, J.K., 2014. Gene delivery from supercharged coiled-coil protein and cationic lipid hybrid complex. Biomaterials 35, 7188–7193.

Morgan, M.T., Carnahan, M.A., Immoos, C.E., Ribeiro, A.A., Finkelstein, S., Lee, S.J., et al., 2003. Dendritic molecular capsules for hydrophobic compounds. J. Am. Chem. Soc. 125 (50), 15485–15489.

Muller, R.H., Maaβen, S., Weyhers, H., Specht, F., Lucks, J.S., 1996. Cytotoxicity of magnetite-loaded polylactide, polylactide/glycolide particles and solid lipid nanoparticles. Int. J. Pharm. 138 (1), 85–94.

Muller, R.H., Radtke, M., Wissing, S.A., 2002. Solid lipid nanoparticles (SLN) and nanostructured lipid carriers (NLC) in cosmetic and dermatological preparations. Adv. Drug Deliv. Rev. 54 (1), S131–S155.

Müller, R., Petersen, R.D., Hommoss, A., Pardeike, J., 2007. Nanostructured lipid carriers (NLC) in cosmetic dermal products. Adv. Drug Deliv. Rev. 59 (6), 522–530.

Nagai, Y., Unsworth, L.D., Koutsopoulos, S., Zhang, S., 2006. Slow release of molecules in self-assembling peptide nanofiber scaffold. J. Control. Release 115, 18–25.

Navath, R.S., Kurtoglu, Y.E., Wang, B., Kannan, S., Romero, R., Kannan, R.M., 2008. Dendrimer–drug conjugates for tailored intracellular drug release based on glutathione levels. Bioconjug. Chem. 19 (12), 2446–2455.

Navath, R.S., Menjoge, A.R., Wang, B., Romero, R., Kannan, S., Kannan, R.M., 2010. Amino acid-functionalized dendrimers with heterobifunctional chemoselective peripheral groups for drug delivery applications. Biomacromolecules 11 (6), 1544–1563.

Neslihan Gursoy, R., Benita, S., 2004. Self-emulsifying drug delivery systems (SEDDS) for improved oral delivery of lipophilic drugs. Biomed. Pharmacother. 58 (3), 173–182.

Neves, S.C., Gomes, D.B., Sousa, A., Bidarra, S., Petrini, P., Moroni, M., Barrias, C.C., Granja, P.L., 2015. Biofunctionalized pectin hydrogels as 3D cellular microenvironments. J. Mater. Chem. B 3, 2096–2108.

Newkome, G.R., Yao, Z.Q., Baker, G.R., Gupta, V.K., 1985. Micelles. Part 1. Cascade molecules: a new approach to micelles. A [27]-arboro. J. Org. Chem. 50, 2003–2004.

Nishikawa, M., Matono, M., Rattanakiat, S., Matsuoka, N., Takakura, Y., 2008. Enhanced immunostimulatory activity of oligodeoxynucleotides by Y-shape formation. Immunology 124 (2), 247–255.

Olbrich, C., Muller, R.H., 1999. Enzymatic degradation of SLN—effect of surfactant and surfactant mixtures. Int. J. Pharm. 80 (1), 31–39.

Parrott, M.C.B.S., Saab, C., Lemon, J.A., Parker, S., Valliant, J.F., Adronov, A., 2009. Synthesis, radiolabeling, and biological imaging of high-generation polyester dendrimers. J. Am. Chem. Soc. 131, 2906–2916.

Parry, D.A.D., Fraser, R.D.B., Squire, J.M., 2008. Fifty years of coiled-coils and α-helical bundles: a close relationship between sequence and structure. J. Struct. Biol. 163, 258–269.

Patri, A.K., Kukowska-Latallo, J.F., Baker, J.R., 2005. Targeted drug delivery with dendrimers: comparison of the release kinetics of covalently conjugated drug and non-covalent drug inclusion complex. Adv. Drug Deliv. Rev. 57 (15), 2203–2214.

Peng, C., Shi, X.Y., 2013. Dendrimer-based nanoscale CT contrast agents: preparation and biomedical applications. Yingxiang Kexue yu Guanghuaxue 31 (2), 81–90.

Qi, R., Majoros, I., Misra, A.C., Koch, A.E., Campbell, P., Marotte, H., et al., 2015. Folate receptor-targeted dendrimer-methotrexate conjugate for inflammatory arthritis. J. Biomed. Nanotechnol. 11 (8), 1431–1441.

Qiao, Z., Shi, X., 2015. Dendrimer-based molecular imaging contrast agents. Prog. Polym. Sci. 44, 1–27.

Qiu, H., Dewan, J.C., Seeman, N.C., 1997. A DNA decamer with a sticky end: the crystal structure of d-CGACGATCGT1. J. Mol. Biol. 267 (4), 881–898.

Rabone, J., Yue, Y.F., Chong, S.Y., Stylianou, K.C., Bacsa, J., Bradshaw, D., et al., 2010. An adaptable peptide-based porous material. Science 329, 1053–1057.

Raman, R., Raguram, S., Venkataraman, G., Paulson, J.C., Sasisekharan, R., 2005. Glycomics: an integrated systems approach to structure-function relationships of glycans. Nat. Methods 2, 817–824.

Rao, C., Tam, J.P., 1994. Synthesis of peptide dendrimer. J. Am. Chem. Soc. 16, 6975–6976.

Rattanakiat, S., Nishikawa, M., Funabashi, H., Luo, D., Takakura, Y., 2009. The assembly of a short linear natural cytosine-phosphate-guanine DNA into dendritic structures and its effect on immunostimulatory activity. Biomaterials 30 (29), 5701–5706.

Reches, M., Gazit, E., 2003. Casting metal nanowires within discrete self-assembled peptide nanotubes. Science 300, 625–627.

Rodell, C.B., Mealy, J.E., Burdick, J.A., 2015. Supramolecular guest-host interactions for the preparation of biomedical materials. Bioconjug. Chem. 26 (12), 2279–2289.

Rosi, N.L., Giljohann, D.A., Thaxton, C.S., Lytton-Jean, A.K.R., Han, M.S., Mirkin, C.A., 2006. Oligonucleotide-modified gold nanoparticles for intracellular gene regulation. Science 312 (5776), 1027–1030.

Rothemund, P.W.K., 2006. Folding DNA, to create nanoscale shapes and patterns. Nature 440 (7082), 297–302.

Ruan, L., Zhang, H., Luo, H., Liu, J., Tang, F., Shi, Y.-K., et al., 2009. Designed amphiphilic peptide forms stable nanoweb, slowly releases encapsulated hydrophobic drug, and accelerates animal hemostasis. Proc. Natl. Acad. Sci. U. S. A. 106, 5105–5110.

Ruoslahti, E., 2012. Peptides as targeting elements and tissue penetration devices for nanoparticles. Adv. Mater. 24, 3747–3756.

Sadekar, S., Thiagarajan, G., Bartlett, K., Hubbard, D., Ray, A., McGill, L.D., et al., 2013. Poly(amido amine) dendrimers as absorption enhancers for oral delivery of camptothecin. Int. J. Pharm. 456 (1), 175–185.

Sandri, G., Bonferoni, M.C., Gökçe, E.H., Ferrari, F., Rossi, S., Patrini, M., Caramella, C., 2010. Chitosan-associated SLN: in vitro and ex vivo characterization of cyclosporine A loaded ophthalmic systems. J. Microencapsul. 27 (8), 735–746.

Santos, J.L., Oliveira, H., Pandita, D., Rodrigues, J., Pêgo, A.P., Granja, P.L., et al., 2010. Functionalization of poly(amidoamine) dendrimers with hydrophobic chains for improved gene delivery in mesenchymal stem cells. J. Control. Release 144 (1), 55–64.

Schneider, J.P., Pochan, D.J., Ozbas, B., Rajagopal, K., Pakstis, L., Kretsinger, J., 2002. Responsive hydrogels from the intramolecular folding and self-assembly of a designed peptide. J. Am. Chem. Soc. 124, 15030–15037.

Schüller, V.J., Heidegger, S., Sandholzer, N., Nickels, P.C., Suhartha, N.A., Endres, S., et al., 2011. Cellular immunostimulation by CpG-sequence-coated DNA origami structures. ACS Nano 5 (12), 9696–9702.

Seeman, N.C., 1982. Nucleic acid junctions and lattices. J. Theor. Biol. 99 (2), 237–247.
Seeman, N.C., 1990. De novo design of sequences for nucleic acid structural engineering. J. Biomol. Struct. Dyn. 8 (3), 573–581.
Seo, J.W., Baek, H., Mahakian, L.M., Kusunose, J., Hamzah, J., Ruoslahti, E., et al., 2014. Cu-64-labeled LyP-1-dendrimer for PET-CT imaging of atherosclerotic plaque. Bioconjug. Chem. 25 (2), 231–239.
Severcan, I., Geary, C., Verzemnieks, E., Chworos, A., Jaeger, L., 2009. Square-shaped RNA particles from different RNA folds. Nano Lett. 9 (3), 1270–1277.
Shadrack, D.M., Mubofu, E.B., Nyandoro, S.S., 2015. Synthesis of polyamidoamine dendrimer for encapsulating tetramethylscutellarein for potential bioactivity enhancement. Int. J. Mol. Sci. 16 (11), 26363–26377.
Shaunak, S., Thomas, S., Gianasi, E., Godwin, A., Jones, E., Teo, I., et al., 2004. Polyvalent dendrimer glucosamine conjugates prevent scar tissue formation. Nat. Biotechnol. 22 (8), 977–984.
Shcharbin, D., Janaszewska, A., Klajnert-Maculewicz, B., Ziemba, B., Dzmitruk, V., Halets, I., et al., 2014. How to study dendrimers and dendriplexes III. Biodistribution, pharmacokinetics and toxicity in vivo. J. Control. Release 181, 40–52.
Shu, D., Huang, L.P., Hoeprich, S., Guo, P., 2003. Construction of phi29 DNA-packaging RNA monomers, dimers, and trimers with variable sizes and shapes as potential parts for nanodevices. J. Nanosci. Nanotechnol. 3 (4), 295–302.
Simmel, S.S., Nickels, P.C., Liedl, T., 2014. Wireframe and tensegrity DNA nanostructures. Acc. Chem. Res. 47 (6), 1691–1699.
Singh, D., Han, S.S., Shin, E.J., 2014. Polysaccharides as nanocarriers for therapeutic applications. J. Biomed. Nanotechnol. 10 (9), 2149–2172.
Soares, S., Fonte, P., Costa, A., Andrade, J., Seabra, V., Ferreira, D., Reis, S., Sarmento, B., 2013. Effect of freeze-drying, cryoprotectants and storage conditions on the stability of secondary structure of insulin-loaded solid lipid nanoparticles. Int. J. Pharm. 456 (2), 370–381.
Soldatov, D.V., Moudrakovski, I.L., Ripmeester, J.A., 2004. Dipeptides as microporous materials. Angew. Chem. Int. Ed. Engl. 43, 6308–6311.
Soundararajan, S., Chen, W., Spicer, E.K., Courtenay-Luck, N., Fernandes, D.J., 2008. The nucleolin targeting aptamer AS1411 destabilizes Bcl-2 messenger RNA in human breast cancer cells. Cancer Res. 68 (7), 2358–2365.
Spataro, G., Malecaze, F., Turrin, C.O., Soler, V., Duhayon, C., Elena, P.P., et al., 2010. Designing dendrimers for ocular drug delivery. Eur. J. Med. Chem. 45 (1), 326–334.
Stetefeld, J., Jenny, M., Schulthess, T., Landwehr, R., Engel, J., Kammerer, R.A., 2000. Crystal structure of a naturally occurring parallel right-handed coiled coil tetramer. Nat. Struct. Biol. 7, 772–776.
Stick, R.V., 2001. Carbohydrates: The Sweet Molecules of Life. Academic Press, New York, NY.
Sukrut, S., Christine, D., 2014. Applications of dendrimers for brain delivery and cancer therapy. Nanomedicine (London) 9 (15), 2403–2414.
Swanson, S.D., Kukowska-Latallo, J.F., Patri, A.K., Chen, C., Ge, S., Cao, Z., et al., 2008. Targeted gadolinium-loaded dendrimer nanoparticles for tumor-specific magnetic resonance contrast enhancement. Int. J. Nanomedicine 3 (2), 201–210.
Talom, R.M., Fuks, G., Kaps, L., Oberdisse, J., Cerclier, C., Gaillard, C., et al., 2011. DNA-polymer micelles as nanoparticles with recognition ability. Chemistry 17 (48), 13495–13501.
Thakur, S., Kesharwani, P., Tekade, R.K., Jain, N.K., 2015. Impact of pegylation on biopharmaceutical properties of dendrimers. Polymer 59, 67–92.
Tomalia, D.A., Baker, H., Dewald, J., Hall, M., Kallos, G., Martin, S., et al., 1985. A new class of polymers: starburst-dendritic macromolecules. Polym. J. 17 (1), 117–132.

Tomalia, D.A., Christensen, J.B., Boas, U., 2012. Dendrimers, Dendrons and Dendritic Polymers: Discovery, Applications, and the Future. Cambridge University Press, Cambridge.

Tschiche, A., Staedtler, A.M., Malhotra, S., Bauer, H., Bottcher, C., Sharbati, S., et al., 2014. Polyglycerol-based amphiphilic dendrons as potential siRNA carriers for in vivo applications. J. Mater. Chem. B 2 (15), 2153–2167.

van der Poll, D.G., Kieler-Ferguson, H.M., Floyd, W.C., Guillaudeu, S.J., Jerger, K., Szoka, F.C., et al., 2010. Design, synthesis, and biological evaluation of a robust, biodegradable dendrimer. Bioconjug. Chem. 21 (4), 764–773.

van Hell, A.J., Costa, C.I.C.A., Flesch, F.M., Sutter, M., Jiskoot, W., Crommelin, D.J.A., et al., 2007. Self-assembly of recombinant amphiphilic oligopeptides into vesicles. Biomacromolecules 8, 2753–2761.

Varki, A., Cummings, R.D., Esko, J.D., et al. (Eds.), 2009. Essentials of Glycobiology. second ed. Cold Spring Harbor Laboratory Press, Cold Spring Harbor, NY.

Wagner, D.E., Phillips, C.L., Ali, W.M., Nybakken, G.E., Crawford, E.D., Schwab, A.D., et al., 2005. Toward the development of peptide nanofilaments and nanoropes as smart materials. Proc. Natl. Acad. Sci. U. S. A. 102, 12656–12661.

Walsh, A.S., Yin, H., Erben, C.M., Wood, M.J.A., Turberfield, A.J., 2011. DNA cage delivery to mammalian cells. ACS Nano 5 (7), 5427–5432.

Walter, M.V., Malkoch, M., 2012. Simplifying the synthesis of dendrimers: accelerated approaches. Chem. Soc. Rev. 41 (13), 4593–4609.

Wang, F., Wang, Y., Zhang, X., Zhang, W., Guo, S., Jin, F., 2014. Recent progress of cell-penetrating peptides as new carriers for intracellular cargo delivery. J. Control. Release 174, 126–136.

Watson, J.D., Crick, F.H., 1953. Molecular structure of nucleic acids; a structure for deoxyribose nucleic acid. Nature 171 (4356), 737–738.

Webber, M.J., Matson, J.B., Tamboli, V.K., Stupp, S.I., 2012. Controlled release of dexamethasone from peptide nanofiber gels to modulate inflammatory response. Biomaterials 33, 6823–6832.

Wei, B., Dai, M., Yin, P., 2012. Complex shapes self-assembled from single-stranded DNA tiles. Nature 485 (7400), 623–626.

Weiner, G.J., Liu, H.M., Wooldridge, J.E., Dahle, C.E., Krieg, A.M., 1997. Immunostimulatory oligodeoxynucleotides containing the CpG motif are effective as immune adjuvants in tumor antigen immunization. Proc. Natl. Acad. Sci. U. S. A. 94 (20), 10833–10837.

Wiener, E., Brechbiel, M.W., Brothers, H., Magin, R.L., Gansow, O.A., Tomalia, D.A., et al., 1994. Dendrimer-based metal chelates: a new class of magnetic resonance imaging contrast agents. Magn. Reson. Med. 31 (1), 1–8.

Winfree, E., Liu, F., Wenzler, L.A., Seeman, N.C., 1998. Design and self-assembly of two-dimensional DNA crystals. Nature 394 (6693), 539–544.

Woolfson, D.N., 2010. Building fibrous biomaterials from α-helical and collagen-like coiled-coil peptides. Pept. Sci. 94, 118–127.

Woolfson, D.N., Ryadnov, M.G., 2006. Peptide-based fibrous biomaterials: some things old, new and borrowed. Curr. Opin. Chem. Biol. 10, 559–567.

Xiong, J.P., Stehle, T., Zhang, R., Joachimiak, A., Frech, M., Goodman, S.L., et al., 2002. Crystal structure of the extracellular segment of integrin αVβ3 in complex with an Arg-Gly-Asp ligand. Science 296, 151–155.

Yan, H., Park, S.H., Finkelstein, G., Reif, J.H., LaBean, T.H., 2003. DNA-templated self-assembly of protein arrays and highly conductive nanowires. Science 301 (5641), 1882–1884.

Yan, X., Zhu, P., Li, J., 2010. Self-assembly and application of diphenylalanine-based nanostructures. Chem. Soc. Rev. 39, 1877–1890.

Yang, J.P., Zhang, Q., Chang, H., Cheng, Y.Y., 2015. Surface-engineered dendrimers in gene delivery. Chem. Rev. 115 (11), 5274–5300.

Ye, M., Qian, Y., Shen, Y., Hu, H., Sui, M., Tang, J., 2012. Facile synthesis and in vivo evaluation of biodegradable dendritic MRI contrast agents. J. Mater. Chem. 22 (29), 14369–14377.

Ye, M., Qian, Y., Tang, J., Hu, H., Sui, M., Shen, Y., 2013. Targeted biodegradable dendritic MRI contrast agent for enhanced tumor imaging. J. Control. Release 169 (3), 239–245.

Yin, P., Hariadi, R.F., Sahu, S., Choi, H.M.T., Park, S.H., LaBean, T.H., et al., 2008. Programming DNA tube circumferences. Science 321 (5890), 824–826.

Yordanov, A.T., Lodder, A.L., Woller, E.K., Cloninger, M.J., Patronas, N., Milenic, D., et al., 2002. Novel iodinated dendritic nanoparticles for computed tomography (CT) imaging. Nano Lett. 2 (6), 595–599.

You, Z., Qian, H., Wang, C., He, B., Yan, J., Mao, C., et al., 2015. Regulation of vascular smooth muscle cell autophagy by DNA nanotube-conjugated mTOR siRNA. Biomaterials 67, 137–150.

Zhang, S., 2003. Fabrication of novel biomaterials through molecular self-assembly. Nat. Biotechnol. 21, 1171–1178.

Zhang, S., Holmes, T.C., DiPersio, C.M., Hynes, R.O., Su, X., Rich, A., 1995. Self-complementary oligopeptide matrices support mammalian cell attachment. Biomaterials 16, 1385–1393.

Zhang, X., Yan, H., Shen, Z., Seeman, N.C., 2002. Paranemic cohesion of topologically-closed DNA molecules. J. Am. Chem. Soc. 124 (44), 12940–12941.

Zhang, Nan, Wardwell, Patricia R., Bader, Rebecca A., 2013. Polysaccharide-based micelles for drug delivery. Pharmaceutics 5, 329–352.

Zhao, Y., Tanaka, M., Kinoshita, T., Higuchi, M., Tan, T., 2010. Nanofibrous scaffold from self-assembly of β-sheet peptides containing phenylalanine for controlled release. J. Control. Release 142, 354–360.

Zhao, Y.-X., Shaw, A., Zeng, X., Benson, E., Nyström, A.M., Högberg, B., 2012. DNA origami delivery system for cancer therapy with tunable release properties. ACS Nano 6 (10), 8684–8691.

Zhao, W., Odelius, K., Edlund, U., Zhao, C., Albertsson, A.C., 2015. In situ synthesis of magnetic field-responsive hemicellulose hydrogels for drug delivery. Biomacromolecules 16 (8), 2522–2528.

Zhuo, R.X., Du, B., Lu, Z.R., 1999. In vitro release of 5-fluorouracil with cyclic core dendritic polymer. J. Control. Release 57 (3), 249–257.

Zimenkov, Y., Conticello, V.P., Guo, L., Thiyagarajan, P., 2004. Rational design of a nanoscale helical scaffold derived from self-assembly of a dimeric coiled coil motif. Tetrahedron 60, 7237–7246.

Zimenkov, Y., Dublin, S.N., Ni, R., Tu, R.S., Breedveld, V., Apkarian, R.P., et al., 2006. Rational design of a reversible pH-responsive switch for peptide self-assembly. J. Am. Chem. Soc. 128, 6770–6771.

Preparative methods and devices of bioinspired materials in drug-delivery systems

2

S. Gorgieva
University of Maribor, Maribor, Slovenia

2.1 Biomimetics: An overview

Relying on the idea that no model is better in the development processes as nature is, the biomimetic concept looks to nature for inspiration in the accomplishment of interdisciplinary (art, architecture, engineering, medicine and technique) needs, while resolving relevant issues. Indeed, the fact that engineering cannot outperform the nature's perfection, which has been developed over the time and evolution, encourages the emergence of biomimetics as a practical, sustainable, time- and, often, cost-efficient principle that goes beyond the simple use of natural properties as the basis for the design of new products (Hwang et al., 2015). Also, the process of mimicking biological systems may proceed at different stages of technical innovation (from functional and morphological design, principle, strategy, amongst others), as well as at different length scales, thus making this concept highly versatile.

By using completely different mechanisms, living things have realized equal or superior functionalities to man-made equivalents. The super hydrophobicity of the lotus leaf due to its micro/nanostructure, the fluid dynamics featured by the sharkskin riblet, structural colours displayed by butterflies and jewel beetles, the highly adhesive properties of gecko's fingers, the antireflective structure of the moss eye, are amongst the most studied aspects of nature in the search for a new generation of biomimetic materials (Shimomura, 2010).

Recent research activities in medicine-related disciplines and specialties, such as biomedical engineering, robotics, neuromorphic engineering, biomaterials design and biofabrication, attest to the growing interest in the transformation of biological solutions into various technical endeavours (Larkin et al., 2014). The examples of the biomimetic-originated success stories in the biomedical field (Fig. 2.1) express the confidence in the transformative role of biology in interdisciplinary progress. The artificial cornea being processed on photographically patterned and nutrition-permeable, hydrogel-like material Duoptix, has demonstrated growth of corneal epithelial and fibroblast cells in a core-skirt keratoprothesis design (Jabbari, 2014). Owing to its specific composition, that is, two interpenetrating polymer networks from polyethylene glycol (PEG) and polyacrylic acid (PAA) molecules, this material can swell to a water content of 80%, which is about the same as in biological tissues, at the same time resisting surface protein accumulation and inflammation (Levy, 2006). The engineering and design of a fly-ear inspired, miniature, directional microphone, a recent

Bioinspired Materials for Medical Applications. http://dx.doi.org/10.1016/B978-0-08-100741-9.00002-4

innovation in hearing-aid technology that is able to locate sounds and eliminate background noise, is being developed by the University of Strathclyde and the MRC/CSO Institute for Hearing Research (IHR)-Scottish Section at the Glasgow Royal Infirmary. The synthesis of antimicrobial furanone-based coatings on medical devices is inspired by the behaviour of the marine macro alga *Delisea pulchra*, which protects itself from bacterial infection by exuding the biofilm-inhibiting natural furanones.

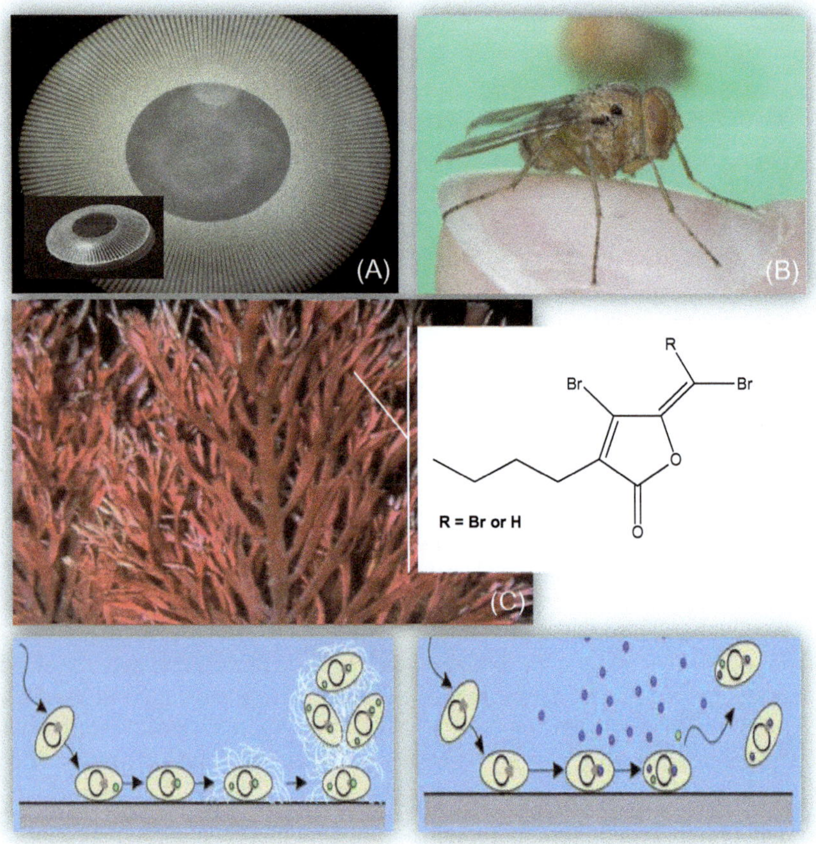

Fig. 2.1 Some of the biomimetic-originated successful stories in biomedicine: artificial cornea (A), insect ear-inspiration for miniature directional microphone (B) and furanones—the compounds excluded by *Delisea pulchra* for biofilms inhibition (C).
Adapted from Levy, D., 2006. An artificial cornea is in sight, thanks to biomimetic hydrogels. Stanford report. http://news.stanford.edu/news/2006/september13/cornea-091306.html (accessed 10.01.16.). (A), http://phys.org/news/2015-04-insects-aids.html (B) and http://www.medgadget.com/2006/06/biosignal_furan.html (C).

Within the field of robotics, different natural manipulators such as elephant trunks, octopus arms, squid tentacles and snakes have been considered as models for the development of high-performance (means of locomotion or grasping) robotic devices.

A very recent invention is the flexible manipulator for minimally invasive surgery application (Ranzani et al., 2015), designed to reach the surgical target while simultaneously interacting with biological structures. Soft, light-driven and fast-response robotics, using the polydimethylsiloxane-/graphene-based nanocomposites, have also recently been introduced (Jiang et al., 2014), and are foreseen as being used in implantable surgery robotics for clinical medicine or drug-delivery devices. The bionanorobotics systems are a subgroup employing various biological elements (proteins and DNA in particular) as motors, mechanical joints, transmission elements or sensors with capacity to apply forces and manipulate objects on a nanoscale for information transfer, amongst other things.

The biomimetic sensor technology is an emerging branch of sensor research being inspired by the incredible variety of sensors for navigation, spatial orientation, and prey and object detection (Stroble et al., 2009) developed by nature itself. Insights related to the high sensing abilities of insects such as beetles from the genus *Melanophila acuminate* with their highly mechanosensitive infrared sensors (Siebke et al., 2014), crickets with their extremely sensitive flow sensors (Izadi et al., 2007), honey bees with their unique flight patterns and behaviour, drosophilae (fruit flies), dragonflies, etc., all provide ideas for improvements in existing or even development of new technologies.

The motivation to pursue biomimicry in a diversity of innovations is also widely diverse. Importantly, these innovations are, in general, simple, cheap to manufacture and apply, and work much better than the existing technologies addressing the same issues. Several important investments for the development of innovative biomimicry solutions have been reported by institutions, such as Biomimicry Institute, Biomimicry Guild (USA), BIOKON (Germany), BIONIS (UK) and the Century Centre of Excellence (Japan) (Wu et al., 2007; Matsumoto et al., 2012), which additionally highlight the potential and promise of this scientific field.

2.2 Drug-delivery systems

The main goal of pharmacologists is to develop targeted drug-delivery systems that can be considered advantageous over the conventional systems due to an improved therapeutic efficiency, decreased toxicity, better biocompatibility, controlled drug release and reduction of side effects. This relatively old, yet highly appealing concept (dating from 1906 when Ehrlich first postulated the "magic bullet", Fahmy et al., 2005) is supposed to use different delivery "cargoes" and, besides carrying the drug, it must: (a) allow a high drug loading, (b) efficiently prevent the disintegration and clearance of the drug, (c) release the drug under particular triggers at the site of action and (d) be safe (Batrakova et al., 2011). The immobilized drug has to remain stable for a sufficient timeframe, especially while passing through different biological barriers (eg, mucociliary escalator, macrophage phagocytosis, clearance via lymphatic system and uptake by alveolar type II epithelial cells during pulmonary delivery, vascular endothelium, basement membrane in intravenous administration), as well as be retained for a given period at the targeted site in order to promote the desired action.

Therefore the drug-delivery systems should provide nonreactive matrixes for physical protection of the incorporated drug load from destructive factors (eg, oxygen, light, enzymes), be physically separated from other reactive components and be able to deliver the drug to the target site. These may be broadly categorized as polymer, lipid and surfactant-based systems (micro- and nanospheres, liposomes, nanoliposomes, vesicular phospholipid gels, archaeosomes and niosomes) or combinations thereof [micelles and nanoparticles (NPs)]. However, the main limitation of the current synthetic delivery systems is their cytotoxicity, as well as the permeability to a few large NPs, which makes them highly undesirable in biomedical applications (Ye et al., 2015).

NPs are multifunctional systems of a size similar to proteins and other macromolecular structures found inside living cells, which enables them to take advantage of the existing cellular machinery for drug delivery. When properly designed, NPs may confer a multitude of desired attributes to the drug being encapsulated, dispersed, adsorbed or conjugated to them, such as improved stability, (bio)distribution and pharmacokinetics, decreased toxicity due to the use of biocompatible nanomaterials, prolonged and tuneable circulation time, reduced reticuloendothelial uptake through minimization of plasma protein coating, opsonization and recognition, as well as superior protection from biological degradation in the blood or after cellular internalization, etc.

Up-to-date, various nanoplatforms (Fig. 2.2) have been explored for biological applications. These can be divided into the following categories: organic [liposomes, polymers (Jain et al., 2016), molecular conjugates, dendrimers, and carbon-based including fullerenes, carbon dots, nanodiamonds and nanofoams (Naahidi et al., 2013)], inorganic (quantum dots, silica and gold NPs) and a combination of the two—the hybrid particles [dendrimer-entrapped gold NPs (Sharma and Kakkar, 2015), lipid-polymer hybrid NPs (Mandal et al., 2013)], the latter providing superior performance due to their biomimetic (from lipids) and architectural advantage (from polymer).

Liposomes are amongst the most exploited type of drug nanocarriers. These are cell membrane-like composites made of an aqueous core surrounded by natural (phospholipid) or synthetic bilayers (Fig. 2.3). Due to their biocompatibility, non-immunogenicity, biodegradability, nonpyrogenicity, biological inertness and ability for the compartmentalization of both types (hydrophilic and hydrophobic) of drugs, liposomes are the most well-established nanoplatforms with a wide range of clinical applications (eg, ocular, pulmonary, cancer) and US Food and Drug Administration (FDA)-approved formulations [eg, Cytarabine, Daunorubicin, Amphotericin B, Doxorubicin (DOX)]. Successful liposome-based formulations in the market include AmBisome (for fungal infection), Doxil (for Kaposi's sarcoma) and Visudyne (for age-related macular degeneration and choroidal neovascularization), all exhibiting reduced invasiveness of the drug treatment (Ariga et al., 2014). Several liposome-based formulations, such as EndoTAG-1 (paclitaxel-loaded cationic liposomes), Lipoplatin (cisplatin-loaded long-circulating liposomes), Stimuvax (a cancer vaccine) and ThermoDox (DOX-loaded liposomes) also show promising therapeutic value in clinical studies. Epaxal (the hepatitis A virus vaccine) and Infelxal V (the influenza vaccine) are clinically approved virosomes, that is, liposome-based vaccines bearing viral surface antigens and synthetic lipids simulating the viral membrane for an enhanced and targeted vaccine delivery (Fan and Zhang, 2013).

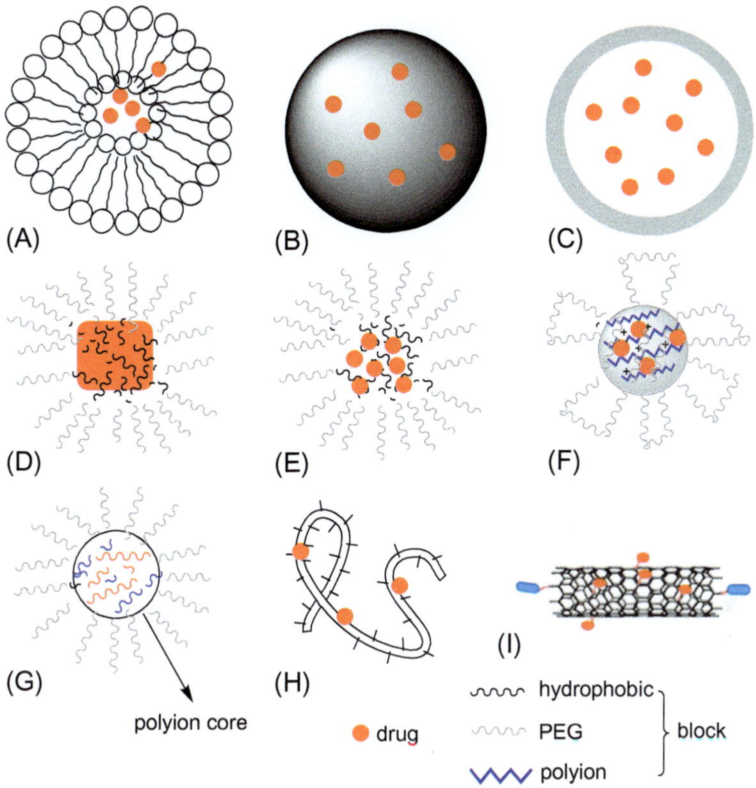

Fig. 2.2 Types of nanocarriers for drug delivery. (A) Liposomes; (B) polymer and lipid NPs; (C) nanospheres and nanocapsules; (D) nanosuspensions; (E) polymer micelles; (F) nanogels; (G) block ionomer complexes; (H) nanofibers and (I) nanotubes.
Adapted from Kabanov, A.V., Batrakova, E.V., 2008. Neuroimmune Pharmacology. Springer, Boston, MA. https://uncch.pure.elsevier.com/en/publications/polymer-nanomaterials (accessed 20.02.16.).

Due to their bilayer (phospho-) lipid membrane, the liposomes are often considered biomimetic products, even though the complexity of living cells membranes is hardly achievable by their simple structure. In order to approach that complexity, several preparation methods are used to tune the liposomes physicochemical and colloidal characteristics (mechanical agitation, solvent evaporation, solvent injection, detergent solubilization, etc.).

More stable and less permeable to small, water-soluble molecules from classical liposomes are polymersomes, the more recent generation of artificial vesicles. They are made of synthetic amphiphilic block copolymers, forming a polymeric shell that offers a protective barrier to proteins, peptides, DNA and RNA fragments against potential deleterious factors in the biological environment. These nanostructures with a size range of 50 nm–5 μm have relatively high multidrug loading capacity, membrane robustness and stealth properties, making them very attractive carriers for hydrophilic and hydrophobic drugs (Lee and Feijen, 2012), which, however, lack specific cellular interactions.

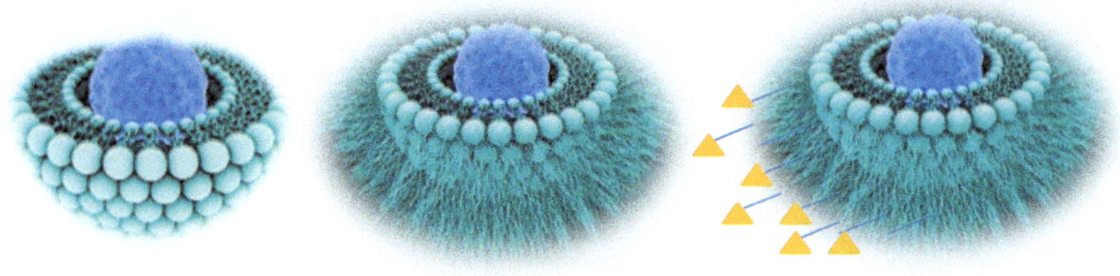

Fig. 2.3 Brief illustration of chronology in the liposomes development.

The large family of liposome-originated carriers is summarized in Table 2.1, which display the major advantages, putting them in the mainstream of modern drug-delivery systems.

Table 2.1 New generation liposomes and their features

Type	Main constituent	Advantage
Polymersomes	Amphiphilic block copolymers	High stability, high loading capacity
Archaeosomes	One or more lipids containing diether linkages	High stability at several conditions
Niosomes	Nonionic surfactant and cholesterol	Less prone to the action of bile salts
Novasomes	Monoester of polyoxyethylene fatty acids, cholesterol and free fatty acids. Two to seven bilayer shells	High loading capacity
Transfersomes	Lipid supramolecular aggregates	More flexible, hence enhancing transdermal delivery
Ethosomes	Phospholipids and alcohol in relatively high concentration	More disruptive in the skin lipid bilayer organization; improved transdermal delivery
Virosomes	Lipids surface modified with fusogenic viral envelope proteins	Intracellular delivery of antigens, drugs and DNA
Cryptosomes	Phospholipids and polaxamers or PEG	High stability
Emulsomes	Internal solid fat core surrounded by phospholipid bilayer	High encapsulation efficiency of hydrophobic drugs
Vesesomes	Multilamellar liposomes	Multidrug formulations are possible

Adapted from Melis Çağdaş, A.D.S., Sezer, S.B., 2014. Application of Nanotechnology in Drug Delivery. InTech, Rijeka. http://www.intechopen.com/books/application-of-nanotechnology-in-drug-delivery/liposomes-as-potential-drug-carrier-systems-for-drug-delivery (accessed 29.09.15.).

Bile salts are one of the agents that affect the liposome structure during intestinal digestion. These amphiphilic molecules synthesized in human liver are gaining increased attention from the pharmaceutical industry due to their ability to interact with, and even enhance the permeability of biological membranes, consequently improving the drug absorption (Stojančević et al., 2014). To act as drug-delivery carriers, they are prestructured in the form of mixed micelles (as in the human body, they self-associate with phospholipids, fatty acids and monoglycerides), bilosomes or form chemical conjugates with the drug molecules. Mixed micelles from randomly methylated β-cyclodextrin, chitosan (CS) and bile components (dehydrocholic acid or ursodeoxycholic acid and their sodium salts) significantly improve the adsorption of the poorly water soluble, nonsteroidal antiinflammatory drug oxaprosine (Maestrelli et al., 2011), while a combination of bile salt sodium taurocholate with spermine, a typical polyamine, was found to enhance the rebamibide adsorption (Mukaizawa et al., 2009).

Fuelled by many advances in nanotechnology and biotechnology, the last six decades have witnessed a rapid growth in the research and development of numerous novel dosage forms and complex delivery therapies (Park, 2014).

2.3 Modification of drug-delivery carriers

The current trend in personalized medicine is to base all clinical practice on the diagnosis and only afterwards treatment. In this respect, it is often required that NPs play a dual, therapeutic and diagnostic, or so-called theranostic role. The targeting abilities of particulate drug-delivery systems, as well as their prolonged circulation time and effective distribution of drug doses, may be efficiently tuned by suitable surface modifications, generally based on adsorption or covalent grafting processes.

The manipulation of NPs' surface may extend their multifunctionality while allowing:

i. Specificity and recognition via both passive and active drug targeting, through the attachment of specific ligands, such as antibodies, aptamers or peptides.
ii. Monitoring and diagnosis by linking to imaging agents, for example, dyes, quantum dots or through the use of magnetic NPs.
iii. Extension of blood circulation solubility, stability and biocompatibility (polymers and polypeptides coupling).
iv. Enhanced cellular penetration by coupling specific peptides, cationic polymers, cationic lipids and transferrin (Sharma and Kakkar, 2015).

The general purpose of surface modification of drug-delivery particulates is to provide a hydrophilic and stable steric barrier that will minimize plasma protein adsorption, opsonization and recognition. PEG-based coating is one of most popular and successful methods to obtain long-circulating biologically stable liposomes. Moreover, the in vivo circulation time of liposomes, as well as the reduction of their aggregation is obtained by grafting hydrophilic polymers onto the head groups of phospholipids, or through the addition of water-soluble polymers containing several hydrophobic groups. The PEG coating acts as an inhibitor of electrostatic interactions between the drug carriers and biological surfaces (protein matrix or cell membrane).

It has also been demonstrated that this coating improves safety and efficiency without loss of the biological function, while reducing the invasiveness of drug-treatment protocols by reducing the frequency of administration.

One example is the administration of insulin, where the immunogenicity, allergenicity and antigenicity, caused by insulin aggregation, were consequently eliminated (Hinds and Kim, 2002). Doxil is the liposomal DOX formulation available in the market, which is stable for more than 18 months in the liquid state due to drug-delivery system stabilization using PEG. Despite the well-known PEG chemistry and its successful use to modify liposome surfaces, its immunogenicity, together with hypersensitivity, unexpected changes in pharmacokinetic behaviour, toxic side products and an antagonism arising from the easy degradation of the polymer under mechanical stress (Knop et al., 2010) may seriously affect its targeting efficiency.

Alternatively, sterically protecting polymers are also being explored. The substitute candidate polymers should also be biocompatible, soluble, hydrophilic and highly flexible for drug delivery. Some of these polymers are synthetic polymers of the vinyl series, that is, polyvinyl pyrrolidone and polyacrylamide (PAA).

Other class of surface-modifying agents are poloxamers, the triblock [poly(ethylene oxide)–poly(propylene oxide)–poly(ethylene oxide) (PEO–PPO–PEO)] copolymer-based, nonionic, surface active agents, also known as Supronic, Pluronic or Tetronic. They provide multiple physicochemical, as well as biological functions to drug-delivery formulations. Poloxamers' action as solubilizers, emulsifiers and stabilizers is generally related to efficient thermo-reversible properties, concentration and/or temperature-dependent micelles versus gel-formation ability (Devi et al., 2013). Their frequent administration in drug-carrier synthesis generally relies on reported positive effects, such as reduction of protein-like molecules adsorption onto hydrophobic surfaces and consequent phagocytosis reduction (Shubhra et al., 2014), improved drug release in cases of periodontal intrapocket administration (Garala et al., 2013), decreased drug dissolution rate (Ur-Rehman et al., 2011), increased permeation across human stratum cornea, inhibition of lipoprotein lipase (Johnston, 2010), increased bioavailability of the drug for topical ocular delivery (Devi et al., 2013), etc. Their application in cancer therapy has also been explored (eg, DOX formulated with Pluronics demonstrating an increased drug accumulation in the brain in comparison with a Pluronic-free formulation) and recognized as a promising therapy platform for drug-resistant cancers (Batrakova et al., 2010).

In the case of magnetic nanocarriers, the surface modifications (Fig. 2.4) are commonly explored to diminish their toxicity, as well as to reduce opsonization, to prolong the plasma half-life and provide the specific tissue targeting. For toxicity reduction, several (co)polymeric formulations have been used, such as the PEO triblock copolymers (PEO–COOH–PEO) (Häfeli et al., 2009), polyvinyl alcohol, dimercaptosuccinic acid (Auffan et al., 2006), PEI-*g*-PEG (poly(ethyleneimine)-graft-poly(ethylene glycol)), PEG, CS, dextran, different surfactants and albumin (Seyda Bucak and Sezer, 2012). Although magnetic targeting is an efficient way to target drugs to the desired site (eg, tumours), in particular cases, specific targeting ligands, such as folic acid (folate), are used to improve the binding to specific receptors.

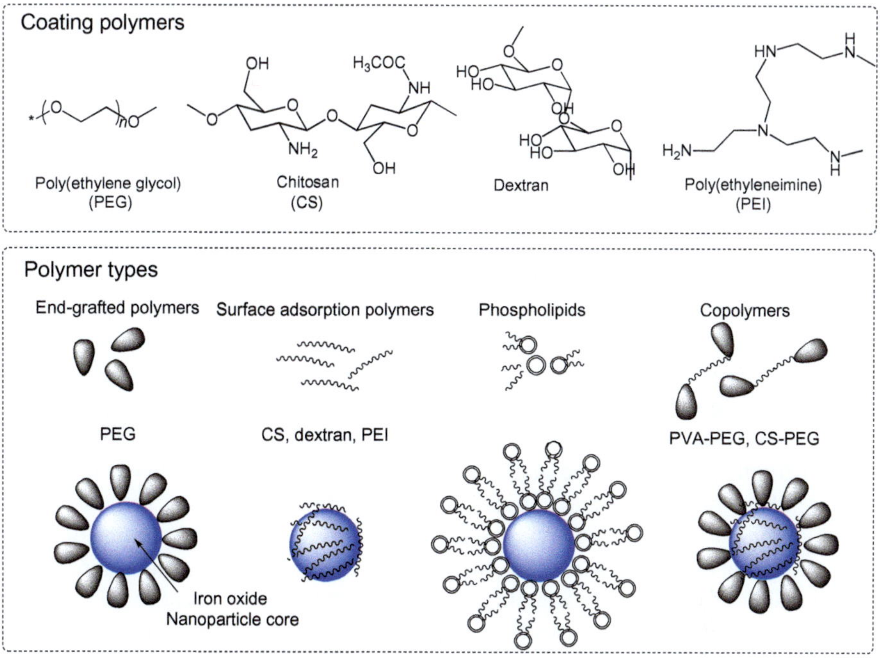

Fig. 2.4 Assembly of polymers onto the surface of magnetic nanoparticle (NP) cores. Adapted from Veiseh, O., Gunn, J.W., Zhang, M., 2010. Design and fabrication of magnetic nanoparticles for targeted drug delivery and imaging. Adv. Drug Deliv. Rev. 62 (3), 284–304. http://www.pubmedcentral.nih.gov/articlerender.fcgi?artid=2827645&tool=pmcentrez&rendertype=abstract (accessed 05.10.15.).

Aptamers are known as promising delivery devices for chemotherapy drugs (eg, DOX, docetaxel, daunorubicin and cisplatin), toxins (eg, gelonin and various photodynamic therapy agents) and a variety of small interfering RNAs (Zhang et al., 2011). Moreover, they may be only indirectly involved in the delivery process, that is, conjugated to NPs via synthetic modification route (Farokhzad et al., 2004; Zhu et al., 2014), and as such to provide enhanced affinity and specificity to target different proteins, phospholipids, iron channels, nucleic acids and even whole cells. These "smart ligands" are short, single-stranded and 3D-configured DNA or RNA oligonucleotides (Tan et al., 2011) and offer superior advantages in terms of small size, flexible structure, elective internalization and intratumour penetration, facile and inexpensive synthesis, low antigenic and immunogenic potential. Although the reported results of their use are very promising (Bruno, 2013), much remains to be done before aptamer-mediated drug delivery can successfully complete the clinical trials in progress.

Due to the high retention capacities, swelling and colloidal properties, clays and clay minerals have been proposed as useful materials to modify drug-delivery systems (Datta and Kaur, 2014). The interactions of ibuprofen (Zheng et al., 2007), nicotine, timolol and donepezil (Park et al., 2008), a well-known drug for Alzheimer's disease, with montmorillonite, saponite and laponite clays have been investigated for their effect on drug solubility and release kinetics.

2.4 Cells as a biomimetic model or drug-delivery vehicle

The rigorous regulations in clinical translation are not constantly met by the synthetic drug carriers, making the natural particulates preferable for multiple therapeutic payloads including DNA, vaccines, peptides and/or proteins, small molecules, which rely on the possession of highly optimized biological functions and features. With this motivation, a substantial effort has been undertaken towards understanding their key features as delivery vesicles, such as natural tropisms, self-markers, cell entry mechanisms, antigenic components and physicochemical properties. Ranging from mammalian cells to pathogens, in native, as well as biotechnology reengineered form, the various natural systems become materials of choice in recent drug-delivery research.

The endogenous nature and intrinsic biocompatibility of natural cells are areas of developing research in a new generation of drug-delivery systems in personalized medicine (Tan et al., 2015). Moreover, direct cell loading with therapeutic agents make the processing of these carriers facile and much simplified in respect to NPs synthesis. Up to now, different cell types have been investigated for their appropriateness as drug cargoes (briefly summarized in Table 2.2), such as erythrocytes [red blood cells (RBC)], (mesenchymal) stem cells (due to tumour-tropic properties) or immune cells (Corbo et al., 2014) (dendritic cells, monocytes, macrophages, neutrophils and lymphocytes), the latest being exploited as Trojan horses due to their high mobility, and migration ability across impermeable barriers such as blood–brain or blood–tumour barriers (Batrakova et al., 2011).

Use of cell membranes and extracellular vesicles (EL Andaloussi et al., 2013) as synthetically applied coatings to polymer particles is another approach for utilization of cells' biological features, which endows carriers with the same desirable biofunctions and targeting specificities as the parent cells, without further modifications. Inspired by the biology of white blood immune cells (leucocytes) and their "safeness" concerning immune reactions, the hybrid particles named leukolike vectors (LLVs) were recently produced (Parodi et al., 2013) in the form of injectable NPs containing a nanoporous silicon core with a camouflage shell from a purified leucocyte cell membrane. Due to an active recognition of tumour endothelium and high tumouritropic accumulation, the LLVs are foreseen as promising devices for chemotherapeutics delivery to cancer.

2.4.1 *Erythrocyte-inspired delivery systems*

The surface inertness towards serum proteins, as well as to reticuloendothelial cells makes the RBCs appropriate models for drug delivery with intravascular application (eg, delivery of antileukemic enzyme L-asparaginase, Agrawal et al., 2013). Owing to their long life-span, unique shape, mechanical properties and presence of a self-marker on their surface, they are also capable of circulating and delivering oxygen for

Table 2.2 Bio-inspired, bioengineered and biomimetic drug-delivery carriers

Categories	Key attributes	Applications	Current status	Challenges and/or limitations
Virus mimetics				
Bacterial ghosts	No cytoplasmic contents Intact surface properties Large drug-loading capacity Natural tropism to various tissues, including tumours Considerable safety and low production cost	Drug or DNA delivery Vaccine delivery	Preclinical	Potential immunogenicity owing to lipopolysaccharide Limited in vivo data
Viruses				
Virus-like particles	Self-assembled particles that are composed of viral capsids Easy to scale up at a low cost Preserve antigenicity Drug-loading capabilities Natural tropism and targeting ability with further modification	Drug or DNA delivery Vaccine delivery	FDA-approved vaccines [Gardasil (Merck) and Cervarix (GlaxoSMithKline)]	Potential immunogenicity when used for nonvaccine delivery
Eukaryotic cells				
Red blood cells (RBCs)	Prolonged circulation (~120 days) Large volume for drug encapsulation Ability to carry NPs and thrombolytics	Drug delivery Targeting the RES	Preclinical	Difficult to maintain integrity Limited targeting ability

Continued

Table 2.2 Continued

Categories	Key attributes	Applications	Current status	Challenges and/or limitations
Virus mimetics				
pH-sensitive nanogels	Capsid-like structure pH-sensitive reversible swelling is followed by drug release and endosomal escape	Targeting tumours	In vitro	Vulnerable to immune recognition In vivo validation needed
Cell mimetics				
Synthetic red blood cells	Ability to mimic shape and mechanical property of RBCs Drug-loading ability Oxygen-carrying ability	Drug delivery Compartment of artificial blood	Preclinical	Vulnerable to immune recognition Detailed in vivo validation needed
Compartmentalization				
Vesosomes	Liposomes within a liposome distinct inner compartments separated from the external membrane Sustained release profile	Drug delivery	Preclinical	Vulnerable to immune recognition In vivo validation needed

Reproduced from Yoo, J.-W., et al., 2011. Bio-inspired, bioengineered and biomimetic drug delivery carriers. Nat. Rev. Drug Discov. 10 (7), 521–535. http://dx.doi.org/10.1038/nrd3499, with permission of Nature Publishing Group (http://www.nature.com/nrd/journal/v10/n7/full/nrd3499.html).

a prolonged period of time, being preferable for encapsulation (via electroporation or by osmosis-driven swelling methodology) or binding (via electrostatic interactions, van der Waals and/or hydrophobic interactions). Due to the semipermeability of their membranes, diverse cargoes, such as antiretroviral agents, antibiotics and cardiovascular drugs, were loaded into the RBCs to avoid their rapid clearance and achieve the sustained release with improved biodistribution (Tan et al., 2015). Besides applicability as a whole, RBCs' membranes are also used as intertissue drug transport vehicles (antimicrobial peptide K-S3), as well as carriers of NPs with incorporated drugs. By membrane-camouflage polymeric carriers combine the mechano- and chemo-biological advantageous properties of natural RBCs and synthetic biomaterials (Hu et al., 2011).

2.4.2 Virus-like particles as drug-delivery vesicles

The translation of pathogenic invader (ie, bacteria and viruses) biological mechanisms is another biomimetic strategy being integrated into of the application of smart drug nanocarriers (Vauthier and Labarre, 2008). Up-to-date virus-like particles (VLPs) have been explored as NP vehicles for diverse biotechnological applications, such as vaccines, drug delivery, imaging agents, biocatalysts, amongst others. However, their instability, antigen fusion limitations, intrinsic immunogenicity generally limit their further development. To overcome these issues, an *Escherichia coli*-based cell-free protein synthesis was performed, which allowed the production of nonimmunogenic, hepatitis B core protein variants stabilized with artificial covalent di-sulphide bridges, capable of conforming in VLPs with desired properties (Lu et al., 2015).

2.5 Bioinspired preparation methodologies for drug-delivery systems

The use of multilayered particles is emerging as a powerful pharmaceutical platform for targeted, triggered and sustained drug delivery, exhibiting several advantages over single-layered particles (Saha and Loo, 2015), such as higher drug loading, improved drug stability and programmable (delayed or pulsatile) drug release schedules, avoiding the burst phenomena. The most common methodologies being used in the preparation of multilayer particles are emulsion solvent evaporation (Xiao et al., 2013), dip coating/layer-by-layer (LbL) assembling (Bhat et al., 2013), spray drying (Mladenovska et al., 2007; Bhalekar et al., 2013), ionic gelation (Anal et al., 2003), coaxial ultrasonic atomization (Si et al., 2012), polyelectrolyte complexation (Lankalapalli and Kolapalli, 2009) and supercritical fluids precipitation (Lima et al., 2012; Miladi et al., 2014). However, the production of layered carriers may be challenging whenever production procedures involve aggressive environments, such as organic solvents, extreme temperatures, mechanical stress and pressure, all being fairly unsuitable for encapsulation of cells, proteins or other unstable molecules. In addition, they may not provide loading of a functional amount of bioactive molecules.

To overcome such issues, several preparation methodologies with nature-inspired platforms have been developed and will be discussed in the following section.

2.5.1 Bioinspired nanoarchitectonics

Nanoarchitectonics evolved recently as a new technological system capable to produce architectures organized on multiple length scales, bearing closer resemblance to biological matrices. It comprises a number of methodologies that can be used to arrange nanoscale structural units into a required configuration, such as atom/molecules manipulation, chemical nanomanipulation, field-induced control for ordering/orientation and controlled self-assembly and organization (Ariga et al., 2014). Knowing that very complex functions are performed by simple biological molecules (ie, amino acids, saccharides and lipids) and are the consequence of the correct assembly of those components interacting on extremely small length scales (Kramer, 2011), gives reason to view nanoarchitectonics as a promising approach for the controlled design of drug-delivery carriers.

The artificial supramolecular systems are building-up from the spontaneously processed nanosized molecular assemblies, amongst which the most representative are self-assembled monolayers, Langmuir–Blodgett films and LbL assemblies. The latter (LbL) approach is most versatile due to the required mild conditions as well as the variety of materials that can be included in supramolecular assemblies (ranging from organic-, bio- and inorganic one) on flat substrates (Fig. 2.5A) and microscopic colloidal particles (Fig. 2.5B).

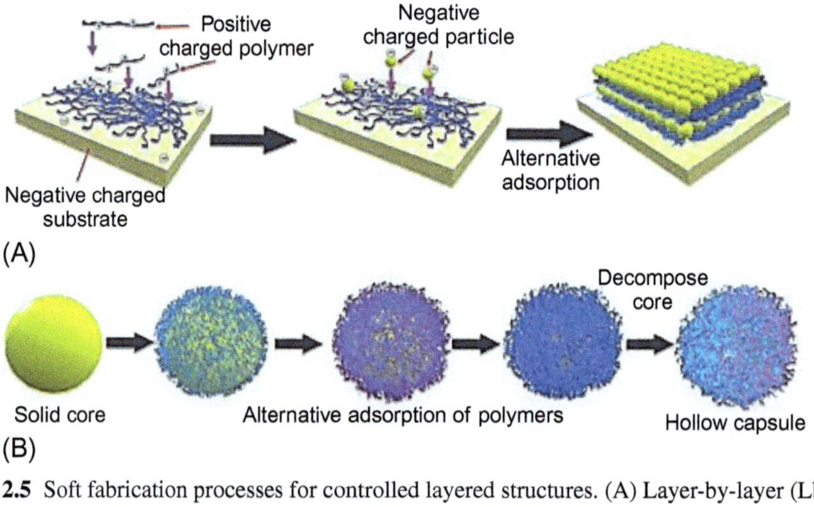

Fig. 2.5 Soft fabrication processes for controlled layered structures. (A) Layer-by-layer (LbL) assembly in flat film mode and (B) LbL assembly in colloidal mode.
Reproduced from Ariga, K., et al., 2012. Forming nanomaterials as layered functional structures toward materials nanoarchitectonics. NPG Asia Mater. 4 (5), e17. http://dx.doi.org/10.1038/am.2012.30, with permission of Nature Publishing Group (http://www.nature.com/am/index.html).

Dipping, spin coating and spraying are frequent application modalities in LbL assembling. The human serum albumin (HSA) nanotubes have been designed as viral traps by alternating LbL assembly HSA and oppositely charged poly(L-arginine) into a nanoporous polycarbonate membrane followed by depositions of poly(L-glutamic acid) and hepatitis B surface antibody and subsequent dissolution of template membrane (Komatsu et al., 2011). The same technique was used for preparation of mesoporous nanocompartment films composed of silica particles and hollow silica capsules, possessing stimuli-free auto-modulated stepwise release of drug molecules (Ji et al., 2008). Besides drug delivery from substrates, the LbL assemblies are also used as drug carriers. Some examples are alkylated hyaluronic acid assembled with poly(L-lysine) into hollow capsules for hydrophobic drugs entrapment (Cui et al., 2011), the nanocomplex of gold NPs, cystamine, small interfering RNA and hyaluronic acid for target-specific drug delivery for the systemic treatment of various liver diseases (Lee et al., 2011), or even for tumour hypoxia (Poon et al., 2011).

The self-(micro)emulsifying drug-delivery systems are isotropic mixtures of drug, oil, surfactants, solvents and co-solvents/surfactants (Rahman, 2013), which under mild agitation in the stomach/small intestine to form the oil-in-water (micro)emulsions that are indeed very similar to the bile salt micelles or high-/low-density lipoproteins. These formulations enhance the drug absorption by improving its solubility, maintaining the drug in solution throughout the gastrointestinal tract, inhibiting the P-glycoprotein-mediated drug efflux and preabsorptive metabolism by gut membrane-bound cytochrome enzymes, and promoting the lymphatic transport that delivers the drug to the systemic circulation (Patel et al., 2013).

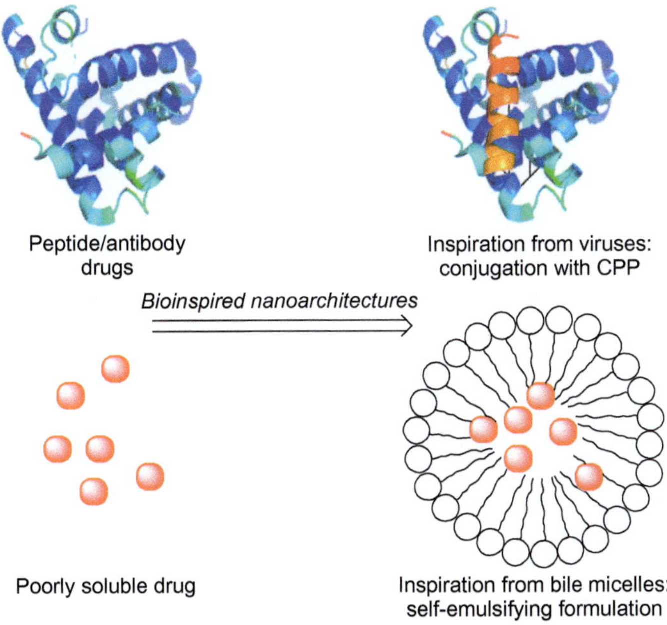

Fig. 2.6 Bioinspired nanoarchitectures for improving oral bioavailability of poorly absorbable drugs. *CPP*, cell-penetrating peptides.
Adapted from Ariga, K., et al., 2014. Bioinspired nanoarchitectonics as emerging drug delivery systems. New J. Chem. 38 (11), 5149–5163. http://xlink.rsc.org/?DOI=C4NJ00864B.

The process of physico/chemical conjugation of cell-penetrating peptides to large molecules, such as peptides and oligonucleotides, as well as its ability to promote permeation across biological membranes was first discovered during study of the HIV.

In order to introduce the "gating" properties on the channel inlets, the inorganic, mesoporous structures were modified with organic groups (Acosta et al., 2014). This allows drug storage and release upon certain stimuli, such as UV, temperature or pH changes. The release processes occurring in mesoporous drug-delivery systems are similar to the release of signal molecules and ions through membrane channels upon specific interactions at the cell surface. Therefore drug-delivery systems comprising gate-controlled mesoporous materials can be classified as bioinspired nanosystems (Fig. 2.6).

The bioinspired nanoarchitectonics design strategy was employed in the construction of n-type organic semiconductor naphthalene diimide (NDi) 2D sheets with tuneable shape, size and promising solid-state optical properties (Pandeeswar and Govindaraju, 2014). Different strength (due to directionality of intermolecular hydrogen bonding interactions), self-assembled 2D sheets were obtained by NDi pre-functionalization with amino acid-glycine derivatives (carboxylic acid, amide and ester).

2.5.2 Bioinspired processing of drug-delivery carriers

The formation of multicompartmentalized particles, offering simultaneous release of various bioactive agents with different kinetics, which can fulfil the therapeutic demands of multifactor disease and regenerative processes (Zou et al., 2012) relies on the bioinspired event consisting of the rolling of water droplets onto super hydrophobic surfaces with low surface free energy (like the lotus leaf). Up to 100% of encapsulation efficiency of different bioactive agents (drugs, enzymes, flavours or cells) on the polymers was achieved by employing a fast dispensing system and few cycle repetitions (Fig. 2.7), as well as suitable crosslinking routes for multilayered particles stabilization (Lima et al., 2013).

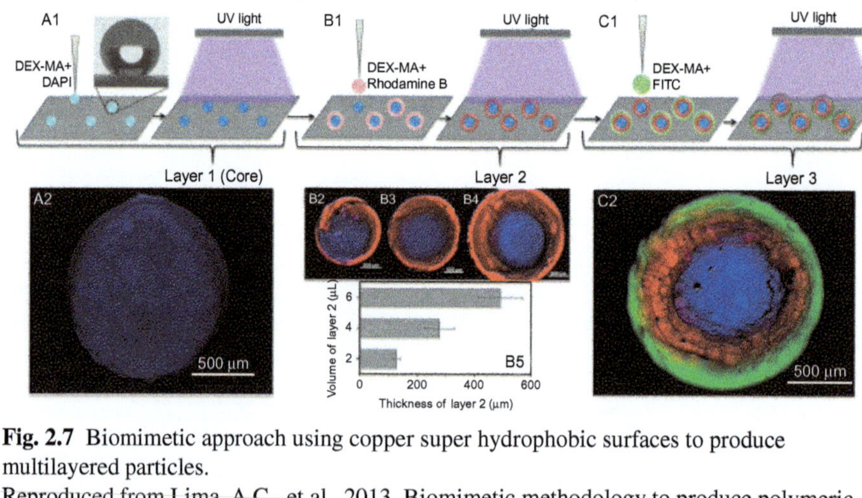

Fig. 2.7 Biomimetic approach using copper super hydrophobic surfaces to produce multilayered particles.
Reproduced from Lima, A.C., et al., 2013. Biomimetic methodology to produce polymeric multilayered particles for biotechnological and biomedical applications. Small, 9 (15), 2487–2492, with permission of John Wiley and Sons (http://onlinelibrary.wiley.com/journal/10.1002/(ISSN)1613-6829).

Besides topical and oral drug delivery, the resultant micro- to milimetre-sized particles are also suitable for other biomedical applications, like wound healing, tissue engineering scaffolds, cell reservoirs to implant inside damaged tissues and organ printing.

In vivo bio-mineralization, the main process involved in the formation of bone tissues, has been exploited in another facile, bottom-up, self-assembling method for processing nanostructured, calcium phosphate (CaP) NPs (Loomba and Sekhon, 2015) and CaP/polymer hybrids (eg, poly(ethylene glycol)-*b*-polylactide (PEG-PLA)/CaP nanocomposites, poly(acrylic acid-*b*-isoprene)/CaP hybrid nanocapsules, poly(*N*-isopropylacrylamide) (PNIPAAm)/CaP) (Fig. 2.8), the later possessing dual (pH- and thermal-) responsive control over the (drug) release process (Shi et al., 2012).

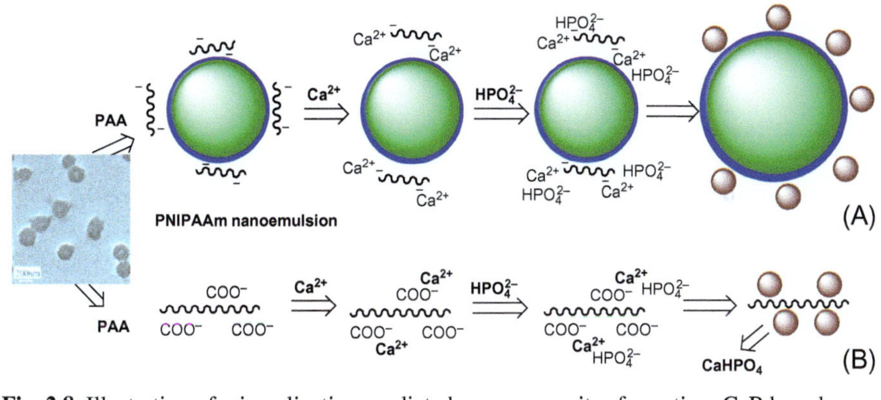

Fig. 2.8 Illustration of mineralization-mediated nanocomposites formation. CaP-based nanocrystalites nucleate on the outer surface of PNIPAAm microgels (A) and at near-surface regions of the PAA polymer nanostructures (B). *CaP*, calcium phosphate; *PNIPAAm*, poly(*N*-isopropylacrylamide); and *PAA*, polyacrylamide.
Adapted from Shi, J., et al., 2012. Biomimetic self-assembly of calcium phosphate templated by PNIPAAm nanogels for sustained smart drug delivery. Mater. Sci. Eng. C, 32 (5), 1299–1306. http://dx.doi.org/10.1016/j.msec.2012.04.008.

CaP-based NPs are popular as drug-delivery vehicles due to their high bioactivity, biocompatibility, chemical stability, nontoxicity, biodegradability and strong adsorption ability under physiological conditions, as well as their pH-dependent solubility profiles that allow tuning the drug release. The CaP/carboxymethyl-chitosan (CaP/CMC) (Wang et al., 2013) and the CaP/heparin/$CaCO_3$ hybrid NPs (Liang et al., 2013) were reported to provide a sustainable release of DOX, the latter being further improved by decorating the NPs with cationic amphipathic cell-penetrating peptide KALA (with the sequence WEAKLAKALAKALAKHLAKALAKALKACEA), and a self-assembling process, forming the drug-loaded CaP/CMC/KALA NPs. The CaP NPs were found to be useful for the local delivery of methazolamine (Chen et al., 2010) used to treat glaucoma, the amphiphilic gelatin-iron oxide core/calcium phosphate shell (AGIO/CaP-DOX) NPs for anticancer treatment (Li et al., 2013), and the PEGylated CaP NPs for oral delivery of insulin (Ramachandran et al., 2009).

Silica-based NPs used as drug-delivery systems have attracted considerable attention, given their ability to control drug loading, porosity, surface chemistry, degradability and "GRAS" (generally recognized as safe) status (Thakur and Thakur, 2015). The conventional, multistep preparation routes of silica NPs, require elevated temperature, high pressure, very high/low pH. However, control over the drug encapsulation and release is poor. Contrarily, a green route for silica synthesis has been reported (Sano et al., 2010) as being facile regarding time and energy consumption, providing control over the particles' size and porosity by simple adjustment of preparation conditions and addition of different additives (diethylenetriamine, tetraethylenepentamine, pentaethylenehexamine and polyallylamine hydrochloride (Steven et al., 2014). The inspiration was found in unicellular organisms, such as diatoms, which use specific structuring and templating biomolecules (small proteins and polyamines) to produce silica shells with hierarchically ordered nano- to micro-sized pores and remarkable mechanical and structural properties (Sun et al., 2004).

2.6 Conclusions/future perspectives

So far, the main research efforts have been conducted on the study and development of drug-delivery carriers, ranging from the traditional designs, up to the "modern", the nanotechnology-driven, and, most recently, the biomimetically inspired ones. By mimicking nature, scientists are attempting to (and partially succeeding) design and synthesize smart materials that are reactive and responsive towards biological tissues by releasing bioactive molecules in a manner preferably controlled by physiological or pathological stimuli and not by matrix-tailored physicochemical properties.

By going far beyond scientific curiosity and simply relying on the clinically successful "stories", the biomimetically oriented drug-delivery designs and formulations certainly should be considered as a reasonable approach that requires multiinterdisciplinary expertise (eg, polymer, science, pharmaceutics, biology, engineering). The substantial requirements for the proposed designs include a fundamental understanding of nanosized systems interactions with cell membranes and receptors, and their intracellular pathways, intracellular sorting mechanisms, and biodistribution between blood proteins and tissues.

The new (hybrid) materials, the ways of combining nano/microstructures, and the applications and alternative ways of production are yet to be integrated into a single Research & Development & Innovation (R&D&I) procedure for drug-delivery vesicles. The nanoarchitectonics' methodological set-up should certainly be foreseen as an integral part, being already recognized as advantageous over the existing technological approaches.

References

Acosta, C., et al., 2014. Polymer composites containing gated mesoporous materials for on-command controlled release. ACS Appl. Mater. Interfaces 6 (9), 6453–6460. http://www.ncbi.nlm.nih.gov/pubmed/24707920 (accessed 09.01.16.).

Agrawal, V., et al., 2013. Red blood cell-encapsulated L-asparaginase: potential therapy of patients with asparagine synthetase deficient acute myeloid leukemia. Protein Pept. Lett. 20 (4), 392–402. http://www.ncbi.nlm.nih.gov/pubmed/23016580 (accessed 22.02.16.).

Anal, A.K., et al., 2003. Chitosan-alginate multilayer beads for gastric passage and controlled intestinal release of protein. Drug Dev. Ind. Pharm. 29 (6), 713–724. http://www.ncbi.nlm.nih.gov/pubmed/12889789 (accessed 20.02.16.).

Ariga, K., et al., 2014. Bioinspired nanoarchitectonics as emerging drug delivery systems. New J. Chem. 38 (11), 5149–5163. http://xlink.rsc.org/?DOI=C4NJ00864B.

Auffan, M., et al., 2006. In vitro interactions between DMSA-coated maghemite nanoparticles and human fibroblasts: a physicochemical and cyto-genotoxical study. Environ. Sci. Technol. 40 (14), 4367–4373. http://www.ncbi.nlm.nih.gov/pubmed/16903272 (accessed 10.01.16.).

Batrakova, E.V., et al., 2010. Effects of pluronic and doxorubicin on drug uptake, cellular metabolism, apoptosis and tumor inhibition in animal models of MDR cancers. J. Control. Release 143 (3), 290–301. http://www.pubmedcentral.nih.gov/articlerender.fcgi?artid=3089980&tool=pmcentrez&rendertype=abstract (accessed 21.02.16.).

Batrakova, E.V., Gendelman, H.E., Kabanov, A.V., 2011. Cell-mediated drug delivery. Expert Opin. Drug Deliv. 8 (4), 415–433. http://www.pubmedcentral.nih.gov/articlerender.fcgi?artid=3062753&tool=pmcentrez&rendertype=abstract (accessed 07.01.16.).

Bhalekar, M., et al., 2013. Formulation and optimisation of sustained release spray-dried microspheres of glipizide using natural polysaccharide. PDA J. Pharm. Sci. Technol. 67 (2), 146–154. http://www.ncbi.nlm.nih.gov/pubmed/23569075 (accessed 20.02.16.).

Bhat, S.K., et al., 2013. Preparation, characterization and in-vitro release studies of enteric coated gelatin capsules containing guar gum microspheres for targeted delivery of 5-fluorouracil to colon. Der Pharma Chem. 5 (3), 221–231.

Bruno, J.G., 2013. A review of therapeutic aptamer conjugates with emphasis on new approaches. Pharmaceuticals 6 (3), 340–357.

Chen, R., et al., 2010. Methazolamide calcium phosphate nanoparticles in an ocular delivery system. Yakugaku Zasshi: J. Pharm. Soc. Jpn. 130 (3), 419–424. http://www.ncbi.nlm.nih.gov/pubmed/20190526 (accessed 10.01.16.).

Corbo, C., et al., 2014. Proteomic profiling of a biomimetic drug delivery platform. Curr. Drug Targets 15 (999), 1. http://www.eurekaselect.com/openurl/content.php?genre=article&doi=10.2174/1389450115666141109211413.

Cui, D., et al., 2011. Hydrophobic shell loading of biopolyelectrolyte capsules. Adv. Mater. (Deerfield Beach, FL) 23 (24), H200–H204. http://www.ncbi.nlm.nih.gov/pubmed/21590815 (accessed 03.02.16.).

Datta, M., Kaur, M., 2014. In vitro release of sodium diclofenac from poloxamer 188 modified montmorillonite as an oral drug delivery vehicle. Int. J. Pharm. Pharm. Sci. 6 (5), 100–110.

Devi, D.R., Sandhya, P., Hari, B.N.V., 2013. Poloxamer: a novel functional molecule for drug delivery and gene therapy. J. Pharm. Sci. Res. 5 (8), 159–165.

EL Andaloussi, S., et al., 2013. Extracellular vesicles: biology and emerging therapeutic opportunities. Nat. Rev. Drug Discov. 12 (5), 347–357. http://dx.doi.org/10.1038/nrd3978.

Fahmy, T.M., et al., 2005. Targeted for drug delivery. Mater. Today 8 (8), 18–26. http://www.sciencedirect.com/science/article/pii/S1369702105710336 (accessed 29.12.15.).

Fan, Y., Zhang, Q., 2013. Development of liposomal formulations: from concept to clinical investigations. Asian J. Pharm. Sci. 8 (2), 81–87. http://www.sciencedirect.com/science/article/pii/S1818087613000111 (accessed 18.10.15.).

Farokhzad, O.C., et al., 2004. Nanoparticle-aptamer bioconjugates: a new approach for targeting prostate cancer cells. Cancer Res. 64, 7668–7672.

Garala, K., et al., 2013. Formulation and evaluation of periodontal in situ gel. Int. J. Pharm. Invest. 3 (1), 29–41. http://www.pubmedcentral.nih.gov/articlerender.fcgi?artid=3687234&tool=pmcentrez&rendertype=abstract (accessed 04.03.16.).

Häfeli, U.O., et al., 2009. Cell uptake and in vitro toxicity of magnetic nanoparticles suitable for drug delivery. Mol. Pharm. 6 (5), 1417–1428. http://www.ncbi.nlm.nih.gov/pubmed/19445482 (accessed 10.01.16.).

Hinds, K.D., Kim, S.W., 2002. Effects of PEG conjugation on insulin properties. Adv. Drug Deliv. Rev. 54 (4), 505–530. http://www.ncbi.nlm.nih.gov/pubmed/12052712 (accessed 09.01.16.).

Hu, C.-M.J., Zhang, L., Aryal, S., Cheung, C., Fang, R.H., Zhang, L., 2011. Erythrocyte membrane-camouflaged polymeric nanoparticles as a biomimetic delivery platform. Proc. Nat. Acad. Sci. 108 (27), 10980–10985. http://dx.doi.org/10.1073/pnas.1106634108.

Hwang, J., et al., 2015. Biomimetics: forecasting the future of science, engineering, and medicine. Int. J. Nanomedicine 10, 5701–5713. http://www.pubmedcentral.nih.gov/articlerender.fcgi?artid=4572716&tool=pmcentrez&rendertype=abstract (accessed 05.01.16.).

Izadi, N., Jaganatharaja, R.K., Floris, J., Krijnen, G.J.M., 2007. Optimization of cricket-inspired, biomimetic artificial hair sensors for flow sensing. In: Proceedings of the Ninth International Symposium on Design, Test, Integration and Packaging of MEMS/MOEMS, 25–27 April 2007, Stresa, Italy, pp. 112–115.

Jabbari, E., 2014. Handbook of Biomimetics and Bioinspiration: Biologically-Driven Engineering of Materials, Processes, Devices, and Systems. World Scientific, New Jersey.

Jain, A., et al., 2016. Fabrication, characterization and cytotoxicity studies of ionically cross-linked docetaxel loaded chitosan nanoparticles. Carbohydr. Polym. 137 (2016), 65–74. http://linkinghub.elsevier.com/retrieve/pii/S0144861715009923.

Ji, Q., et al., 2008. Stimuli-free auto-modulated material release from mesoporous nanocompartment films. J. Am. Chem. Soc. 130 (8), 2376–2377. http://dx.doi.org/10.1021/ja076139s.

Jiang, W., et al., 2014. Photoresponsive soft-robotic platform: biomimetic fabrication and remote actuation. Adv. Funct. Mater. 24 (48), 7598–7604. http://dx.doi.org/10.1002/adfm.201402070.

Johnston, T.P., 2010. Poloxamer 407 as a general lipase inhibitor: its implications in lipid metabolism and atheroma formation in C57BL/6 mice. J. Pharm. Pharmacol. 62 (12), 1807–1812. http://www.ncbi.nlm.nih.gov/pubmed/21054409 (accessed 04.03.16.).

Knop, K., et al., 2010. Poly(ethylene glycol) in drug delivery: pros and cons as well as potential alternatives. Angew. Chem. 49 (36), 6288–6308. http://www.ncbi.nlm.nih.gov/pubmed/20648499 (accessed 04.11.15.) (in English).

Komatsu, T., et al., 2011. Virus trap in human serum albumin nanotube. J. Am. Chem. Soc. 133 (10), 3246–3248. http://dx.doi.org/10.1021/ja1096122.

Kramer, W., 2011. Transporters, Trojan horses and therapeutics: suitability of bile acid and peptide transporters for drug delivery. Biol. Chem. 392 (1–2), 77–94. http://www.ncbi.nlm.nih.gov/pubmed/21194371 (accessed 10.01.16.).

Lankalapalli, S., Kolapalli, V.R.M., 2009. Polyelectrolyte complexes: a review of their applicability in drug delivery technology. Indian J. Pharm. Sci. 71 (5), 481–487. http://www.pubmedcentral.nih.gov/articlerender.fcgi?artid=2866337&tool=pmcentrez&rendertype=abstract (accessed 20.02.16.).

Larkin, W., Etienne-Cummings, R., Van der Spiegel, J., 2014. Bioinspired imaging: discovery, emulation, and future prospects [scanning the issue]. Proc. IEEE 102 (10), 1404–1410. https://www.infona.pl//resource/bwmeta1.element.ieee-art-000006899785 (accessed 14.02.16.).

Lee, J.S., Feijen, J., 2012. Polymersomes for drug delivery: design, formation and characterization. J. Control. Release 161 (2), 473–483. http://linkinghub.elsevier.com/retrieve/pii/S0168365911009576.

Lee, M.-Y., et al., 2011. Target-specific gene silencing of layer-by-layer assembled gold-cysteamine/siRNA/PEI/HA nanocomplex. ACS Nano 5 (8), 6138–6147. http://www.ncbi.nlm.nih.gov/pubmed/21739990 (accessed 22.02.16.).
Levy, D., 2006. An artificial cornea is in sight, thanks to biomimetic hydrogels. Stanford report. http://news.stanford.edu/news/2006/september13/cornea-091306.html (accessed 10.01.16.).
Li, W.-M., Chen, S.-Y., Liu, D.-M., 2013. In situ doxorubicin-CaP shell formation on amphiphilic gelatin-iron oxide core as a multifunctional drug delivery system with improved cytocompatibility, pH-responsive drug release and MR imaging. Acta Biomater. 9 (2), 5360–5368. http://www.ncbi.nlm.nih.gov/pubmed/23022876 (accessed 10.01.16.).
Liang, P., et al., 2013. Facile preparation of heparin/$CaCO_3$/CaP hybrid nano-carriers with controllable size for anticancer drug delivery. Colloids Surf. B: Biointerfaces 102, 783–788. http://www.sciencedirect.com/science/article/pii/S0927776512005048 (accessed 10.01.16.).
Lima, A.C., Sher, P., Mano, J.F., 2012. Production methodologies of polymeric and hydrogel particles for drug delivery applications. Expert Opin. Drug Deliv. 9 (2), 231–248. http://www.ncbi.nlm.nih.gov/pubmed/22250602 (accessed 10.01.16.).
Lima, A.C., et al., 2013. Biomimetic methodology to produce polymeric multilayered particles for biotechnological and biomedical applications. Small 9 (15), 2487–2492.
Loomba, L., Sekhon, B.S., 2015. Calcium phosphate nanoparticles and their biomedical potential. J. Nanomater. Mol. Nanotechnol. http://dx.doi.org/10.4172/2324-8777.1000154.
Lu, Y., et al., 2015. Assessing sequence plasticity of a virus-like nanoparticle by evolution toward a versatile scaffold for vaccines and drug delivery. Proc. Natl. Acad. Sci. U. S. A. 112 (40), 12360–12365. http://www.pnas.org/content/112/40/12360.abstract (accessed 22.02.16.).
Maestrelli, F., et al., 2011. Improvement of oxaprozin solubility and permeability by the combined use of cyclodextrin, chitosan, and bile components. Eur. J. Pharm. Biopharm. 78 (3), 385–393. http://www.ncbi.nlm.nih.gov/pubmed/21439375 (accessed 10.01.16).
Mandal, B., et al., 2013. Core-shell-type lipid-polymer hybrid nanoparticles as a drug delivery platform. Nanomed. Nanotechnol. Biol. Med. 9 (4), 474–491. http://dx.doi.org/10.1016/j.nano.2012.11.010.
Matsumoto, M., et al. (Eds.), 2012. Design for Innovative Value Towards a Sustainable Society. Springer, Dordrecht. http://www.springerlink.com/index/10.1007/978-94-007-3010-6 (accessed 15.12.15.).
Miladi, K., et al., 2014. Particles from preformed polymers as carriers for drug delivery. EXCLI J. 13, 28–57.
Mladenovska, K., et al., 2007. Colon-specific delivery of 5-aminosalicylic acid from chitosan-Ca-alginate microparticles. Int. J. Pharm. 342 (1–2), 124–136. http://www.ncbi.nlm.nih.gov/pubmed/17590293 (accessed 25.01.16.).
Mukaizawa, F., et al., 2009. Novel oral absorption system containing polyamines and bile salts enhances drug transport via both transcellular and paracellular pathways across Caco-2 cell monolayers. Int. J. Pharm. 367 (1–2), 103–108. http://www.ncbi.nlm.nih.gov/pubmed/18929635 (accessed 10.01.16.).
Naahidi, S., et al., 2013. Biocompatibility of engineered nanoparticles for drug delivery. J. Control. Release 166 (2), 182–194. http://dx.doi.org/10.1016/j.jconrel.2012.12.013.
Pandeeswar, M., Govindaraju, T., 2014. Bioinspired nanoarchitectonics of naphthalene diimide to access 2D sheets of tunable size, shape, and optoelectronic properties. J. Inorg. Organomet. Polym. Mater. 25 (2), 293–300. http://dx.doi.org/10.1007/s10904-014-0144-7.
Park, J.K., et al., 2008. Controlled release of donepezil intercalated in smectite clays. Int. J. Pharm. 359 (1–2), 198–204. http://www.ncbi.nlm.nih.gov/pubmed/18502063 (accessed 21.02.16.).

Park, K., 2014. The controlled drug delivery systems: past forward and future back. J. Control. Release 28 (190), 3–8.

Parodi, A., et al., 2013. Synthetic nanoparticles functionalized with biomimetic leukocyte membranes possess cell-like functions. Nat. Nanotechnol. 8 (1), 61–68. http://dx.doi.org/10.1038/nnano.2012.212.

Patel, P.V., et al., 2013. Self micro-emulsifying drug delivery system of tacrolimus: formulation, in vitro evaluation and stability studies. Int. J. Pharm. Invest. 3 (2), 95–104. http://www.pubmedcentral.nih.gov/articlerender.fcgi?artid=3757905&tool=pmcentrez&rendertype=abstract (accessed 18.02.15.).

Poon, Z., et al., 2011. Layer-by-layer nanoparticles with a pH-sheddable layer for in vivo targeting of tumor hypoxia. ACS Nano 5 (6), 4284–4292. http://dx.doi.org/10.1021/nn200876f.

Rahman, M.A., 2013. Role of excipients in successful development of self-emulsifying/microemulsifying drug delivery system (SEDDS/SMEDDS). Drug Dev. Ind. Pharm. 39, 1–19. http://www.ncbi.nlm.nih.gov/pubmed/22372916 (accessed 14.10.15.).

Ramachandran, R., Paul, W., Sharma, C.P., 2009. Synthesis and characterization of PEGylated calcium phosphate nanoparticles for oral insulin delivery. J. Biomed. Mater. Res. B Appl. Biomater. 88B (1), 41–48. http://www.ncbi.nlm.nih.gov/pubmed/18946870 (accessed 10.01.16.).

Ranzani, T., et al., 2015. A bioinspired soft manipulator for minimally invasive surgery. Bioinspir. Biomim. 10 (3), 035008. http://dx.doi.org/10.1088/1748-3190/10/3/035008.

Saha, S., Loo, S.C.J., 2015. Recent developments in multilayered polymeric particles—from fabrication techniques to therapeutic formulations. J. Mater. Chem. B 3 (17), 3406–3419. http://pubs.rsc.org/en/content/articlehtml/2015/tb/c5tb00086f (accessed 20.02.16.).

Sano, K., Minamisawa, T., Shiba, K., 2010. Autonomous silica encapsulation and sustained release of anticancer protein. Langmuir: ACS J. Surf. Colloids 26 (4), 2231–2234. http://www.ncbi.nlm.nih.gov/pubmed/20085330 (accessed 10.01.16.).

Seyda Bucak, B.Y., Sezer, A.D., 2012. Recent Advances in Novel Drug Carrier Systems. InTech, Rijeka. http://www.intechopen.com/books/recent-advances-in-novel-drug-carrier-systems/magnetic-nanoparticles-synthesis-surface-modifications-and-application-in-drug-delivery (accessed 10.12.15.).

Sharma, A., Kakkar, A., 2015. Designing dendrimer and miktoarm polymer based multi-tasking nanocarriers for efficient medical therapy. Molecules (Basel, Switzerland) 20 (9), 16987–17015. http://www.mdpi.com/1420-3049/20/9/16987/htm (accessed 06.12.15.).

Shi, J., et al., 2012. Biomimetic self-assembly of calcium phosphate templated by PNIPAAm nanogels for sustained smart drug delivery. Mater. Sci. Eng. C 32 (5), 1299–1306. http://dx.doi.org/10.1016/j.msec.2012.04.008.

Shimomura, M., 2010. The new trends in next generation biomimetics material technology: learning from biodiversity. Sci. Technol. Trends Q. Rev. 37, 53–75.

Shubhra, Q.T.H., et al., 2014. Poloxamers for surface modification of hydrophobic drug carriers and their effects on drug delivery. Polym. Rev. 54 (1), 112–138. http://dx.doi.org/10.1080/15583724.2013.862544.

Si, T., et al., 2012. Novel coaxial atomization processes for microfabrication of multilayered biodegradable microcapsules. In: Luo, Q., Gu, Y., Li, X.D. (Eds.), Photonics Asia. International Society for Optics and Photonics, Bellingham, WA, pp. 85531H. http://proceedings.spiedigitallibrary.org/proceeding.aspx?articleid=1485478 (accessed 20.02.16.).

Siebke, G., et al., 2014. A model for μ-biomimetic thermal infrared sensors based on the infrared receptors of *Melanophila acuminata*. Bioinspir. Biomim. 9 (3), 036012. http://www.ncbi.nlm.nih.gov/pubmed/24762777 (accessed 14.02.16.).

Steven, C.R., et al., 2014. Bioinspired silica as drug delivery systems and their biocompatibility. J. Mater. Chem. B 2 (31), 5028. http://pubs.rsc.org/en/content/articlehtml/2014/tb/c4tb00510d.

Stojančević, M., et al., 2014. Application of bile acids in drug formulation and delivery. Front. Life Sci. 7 (3–4), 112–122. http://dx.doi.org/10.1080/21553769.2013.879925.

Stroble, J.K., Stone, R.B., Watkins, S.E., 2009. An overview of biomimetic sensor technology. Sens. Rev. 29 (2), 112–119. https://www.researchgate.net/publication/239397331_An_overview_of_biomimetic_sensor_technology (accessed 16.02.16.).

Sun, Q., et al., 2004. Bioinspired synthesis of mesoporous silicas. Curr. Opin. Solid State Mater. Sci. 8 (2), 111–120. http://www.sciencedirect.com/science/article/pii/S1359028604000063.

Tan, W., et al., 2011. Molecular aptamers for drug delivery. Trends Biotechnol. 29 (12), 634–640. http://www.pubmedcentral.nih.gov/articlerender.fcgi?artid=3218254&tool=pmcentrez&rendertype=abstract (accessed 09.10.15.).

Tan, S., et al., 2015. Cell or cell membrane-based drug delivery systems. Theranostics 5 (8), 863–881. http://www.thno.org/v05p0863.htm.

Thakur, V.K., Thakur, M.K., 2015. Handbook of Polymers for Pharmaceutical Technologies, Bioactive and Compatible Synthetic/Hybrid Polymers. Wiley, New York. https://books.google.com/books?id=dTHKCgAAQBAJ&pgis=1 (accessed 10.01.16.).

Ur-Rehman, T., Tavelin, S., Gröbner, G., 2011. Chitosan in situ gelation for improved drug loading and retention in poloxamer 407 gels. Int. J. Pharm. 409 (1–2), 19–29. http://www.sciencedirect.com/science/article/pii/S0378517311001335 (accessed 04.03.16.).

Vauthier, C., Labarre, D., 2008. Modular biomimetic drug delivery systems. J. Drug Deliv. Sci. Technol. 18 (1), 59–68. http://www.sciencedirect.com/science/article/pii/S1773224708500086 (accessed 24.12.15.).

Wang, J., et al., 2013. Peptide decorated calcium phosphate/carboxymethyl chitosan hybrid nanoparticles with improved drug delivery efficiency. Int. J. Pharm. 446 (1–2), 205–210. http://www.ncbi.nlm.nih.gov/pubmed/23422273 (accessed 10.01.16.).

Wu, X., et al., 2007. Preparation and assessment of glutaraldehyde-crosslinked collagen-chitosan hydrogels for adipose tissue engineering. J. Biomed. Mater. Res. A 81 (1), 59–65. http://www.ncbi.nlm.nih.gov/pubmed/17109417 (accessed 02.12.13.).

Xiao, C.-D., Shen, X.-C., Tao, L., 2013. Modified emulsion solvent evaporation method for fabricating core-shell microspheres. Int. J. Pharm. 452 (1–2), 227–232. http://www.sciencedirect.com/science/article/pii/S0378517313004237 (accessed 20.02.16.).

Ye, W.-L., Zhao, Y.-P., Na, R., Li, F., Mei, Q.-B., Zhao, M.-G., Zhou, S.-Y., 2015. Actively targeted delivery of doxorubicin to bone metastases by a pH-sensitive conjugation. J. Pharm. Sci. 104, 2293–2303. http://dx.doi.org/10.1002/jps.24476.

Zhang, Y., Hong, H., Cai, W., 2011. Tumor-targeted drug delivery with aptamers. Curr. Med. Chem. 18 (27), 4185–4194. http://www.pubmedcentral.nih.gov/articlerender.fcgi?artid=3205327&tool=pmcentrez&rendertype=abstract (accessed 21.02.16.).

Zheng, J.P., et al., 2007. Study on ibuprofen/montmorillonite intercalation composites as drug release system. Appl. Clay Sci. 36 (4), 297–301. http://www.sciencedirect.com/science/article/pii/S0169131707000026 (accessed 21.02.16.).

Zhu, J., et al., 2014. Progress in aptamer-mediated drug delivery vehicles for cancer targeting and its implications in addressing chemotherapeutic challenges. Theranostics 4 (9), 931–944.

Zou, Y., et al., 2012. Development of an injectable two-phase drug delivery system for sequential release of antiresorptive and osteogenic drugs. J. Biomed. Mater. Res. B Appl. Biomater. 100 (1), 155–162. http://dx.doi.org/10.1002/jbm.b.31933.

Metamorphic biomaterials

3

V.F. Cardoso[*,†], C. Ribeiro*[*], S. Lanceros-Mendez*[*,‡,§]
[*]University of Minho, Braga, Portugal, [†]University of Minho, Guimarães, Portugal, [‡]BC Materials, Technology and Scientific Park of Bizkaia, Derio, Spain, [§]KERBASQUE, Basque Foundation for Science, Bilbao, Spain

Eppur si muove!

Galileo Galilei (1564–1642)

3.1 Introduction

Mother nature offers numerous inspirations for the design and development of new materials capable of responding to specific stimuli in a controllable, predictable, and reproducible way. In fact, many substances in living systems naturally vary their structures and behavior according to the conditions of the surrounding environment in order to maintain and regulate normal functions (Roy et al., 2010; Gil and Hudson, 2004). These variations include changes in shape, size, color, or stiffness and rely on complex feedback mechanisms. As a result, during the last decade, academic and industrial research has been motivated to develop new functional materials able to mimic the response capabilities of natural living systems and to develop applications for them (Zhai, 2013; Xia and Jiang, 2008).

Stimuli-responsive materials are defined as materials that can undergo change in a controlled fashion of one or more of their physicochemical properties, such as size, shape, solubility, permeability, electrical, mechanical, and optical, in response to single or multiple external stimuli, such as light, temperature, electrical and magnetic fields, pH, and biological signals (McCabe et al., 2009). Other denominations have been used for stimuli-responsive materials such as "environmental-sensitive," "smart," or "intelligent" materials. Such materials are playing an increasingly important role in a wide range of technological applications and devices in the biomedical, coating, and microelectronic fields (Thevenot et al., 2013), among others. The current literature describes a variety of inorganic materials characterized by stimuli-responsive behavior, including ceramics, alloys, and composites. However, most research relies on the design and development of polymer-based materials that can incorporate tailored and highly sensitive building blocks for all of the abovementioned stimuli (Gray and Bergbreiter, 1997). Different types of responsive polymers, such as bulk solids, thin-films/surfaces, solutions, gels, and nanoscale structures, have demonstrated great potential as controlled drug-delivery systems, therapeutic and diagnostic agents, artificial muscle actuators, (bio)sensors, active catheters, coatings capable of interacting with and to respond to their surrounding environment, among others (Zhai, 2013; Motornov et al., 2010; Liu and Urban, 2010; Roy and Gupta, 2003).

Bioinspired Materials for Medical Applications. http://dx.doi.org/10.1016/B978-0-08-100741-9.00003-6

Table 3.1 **Examples of stimuli-responsive polymer capabilities**

Function	Definition	References
Shape-changing	Shape changes in response to an external stimulus	Bogue (2014) and Bowman (2014)
Self-sensing	Detection and/or quantification in response to an external stimulus	Han et al. (2015) and Wee et al. (2005)
Self-actuating	Actuation in response to an external stimulus	Hwang and Lee (2006) and Datla et al. (2014)
Self-healing	Self-repair in response to damage	Wu et al. (2008) and Yang and Urban (2013)

Stimuli-responsive polymers can be divided into different categories according to their functions, as presented in Table 3.1.

Shape-changing polymers are the most mature of the technologies mentioned in Table 3.1 and may be characterized by variations in their shape when subjected to an external stimulus. It is important to note that the materials listed in the table and their related technologies are not mutually exclusive and therefore more than one function can be present in a specific material. For example, shape-changing polymers can often be combined with self-sensing or self-actuating materials. Shape-changing materials are the scope of the present review and will be discussed in more detailed. The common feature of those materials is that, independently of the external input, a morphological variation is obtained. Thus, they can be also identified as metamorphic materials.

3.2 Shape-changing polymers

Shape-changing materials include polymer-based materials that are capable of reversibly change their shape and/or dimensions in response to single or multiple external stimuli. They play a key role in a wide range of technological and biomedical fields, including diagnostic and therapeutic applications, tissue engineering, microelectronics, and even design and architecture (Rasmussen et al., 2012; Jeong and Gutowska, 2002). Some of them are able to change their dimensions maintaining their shape, while others change their shape without changing their dimensions. Others are still capable of changing both parameters simultaneously. Changes may take place in all dimensions to an equal or unequal extent depending on the distribution and arrangement of the responsive elements and the geometric shape. Stimuli could be classified as physical, chemical, or biological as described in Table 3.2.

Physical stimuli will affect the energy level and/or distribution within the materials and change the molecular interactions at a critical onset point (Gil and Hudson, 2004). Within the scope of this chapter, photoresponsive, thermoresponsive, electroresponsive, and magnetoresponsive polymers that respond to variation of light, temperature, electrical field, or magnetic field, respectively, will be discussed. Nevertheless, other

Table 3.2 Classes of stimuli-responsive polymers, regarding shape-changing polymers

	Shape-changing polymers	Principle of response	References
Physical	Photoresponsive	Light variation	Yu and Kobayashi (2010), Tomatsu et al. (2011), Wang and Zhang (2012), and Rwei et al. (2015)
	Thermoresponsive	Temperature variation	Pastuszka and MacKay (2016), Klouda (2015), Roy et al. (2013), and Ward and Georgiou (2011)
	Electroresponsive	Applied electric field	Pillay et al. (2014), Wei et al. (2014), Meng and Hu (2010), and Zhang and Choi (2014)
	Magnetoresponsive	Applied magnetic field	Xu and Gu (2014), Medeiros et al. (2011), and Filipcsei et al. (2007)
Chemical	pH-responsive	pH variation	Dai et al. (2008), Zhu and Chen (2015), Manchun et al. (2012), and Gao et al. (2010)
	Redox-responsive	Oxidation state variation	Huo et al. (2014), Gauthier (2014), and McCarley (2012)
Biological	Glucose-responsive	Variations of glucose levels	Wu et al. (2011), Peppas (2004), and Ma and Shi (2014)
	Enzyme-responsive	Catalytic action of enzymes	Zelzer et al. (2013), Hu et al. (2012), and de la Rica et al. (2012)

physical stimuli involving ultrasound and pressure have been also described (Zhao et al., 2013; Russina et al., 2015; Paris et al., 2015).

Recently, functional polymers that react to chemical and biological stimuli have been intensively investigated as these stimuli are inherently present in natural living systems. Chemical and biological responsive polymers can thus adapt their properties in response to interactions with specific entities commonly related with health or disease states, allowing in vivo applications in a more specific and localized way (Roy et al., 2010). Polymers that respond to relevant chemical stimuli, namely pH variations and redox gradients will also be discussed (Guragain et al., 2015; Cabane et al., 2012; Hoffman, 2013). Additionally, important biological stimuli including glucose levels and enzymes will also be presented. Other biochemical stimuli involving ionic strength, antigens, and inflammatory processes, among others, also have been reported (Qian et al., 2015; Berron et al., 2012; Miyata et al., 1999; Mahmoud et al., 2011).

3.2.1 Physical stimuli shape-responsive polymers

3.2.1.1 Photoresponsive polymers

Light is an environmental stimulus that allows noncontact control within a defined area or volume with high precision and accuracy by selecting appropriate wavelength, intensity, exposure time, and/or polarization, among other parameters (Seki, 2007).

Photoresponsive polymers are macromolecules combined with light-sensitive molecular units (chromophores) in their pendant groups or backbone. Therefore when irradiated by light, photoresponsive polymers show the ability to reversibly and repeatedly change their physical and/or chemical properties, such as geometrical structure, refractive index, dielectric constant, conformation, solubility, and surface wettability, among others (Guragain et al., 2015). In the case of shape-changing materials, photoresponsive polymers can generate light-driven deformations or shape-memory properties, exhibiting sophisticated arrangements including contraction/expansion, bending, creeping, and rotation (Wang et al., 2011). Typical chromophores are azobenzene, spiropyran, spirooxazine, stilbene, or nitrobenzyl groups, which have been incorporated into a variety of polymer systems, including poly(acrylic acid)—PAA, polyimide, polyamide, poly(ethyl acrylate), poly(ethylene oxide), poly(*N*-(2-hydroxypropyl)methacrylamide), poly(*N*-isopropylacrylamide)—PNIPAM, and poly(2-dimethylaminoethyl methacrylate)—PDMAEMA (Yu and Kobayashi, 2010; Tomatsu et al., 2011; Wang and Zhang, 2012). Despite the large variety of photoresponsive polymers that can be obtained combining specific chromophores with specific polymers, those containing azobenzene groups are the most widely studied. Azobenzene presents a reversible photoinduced trans-to-cis isomerization (Fig. 3.1) that is accompanied by a quick change in geometrical shape, electronic structure, and polarity (Bandara and Burdette, 2012; Seki, 2004).

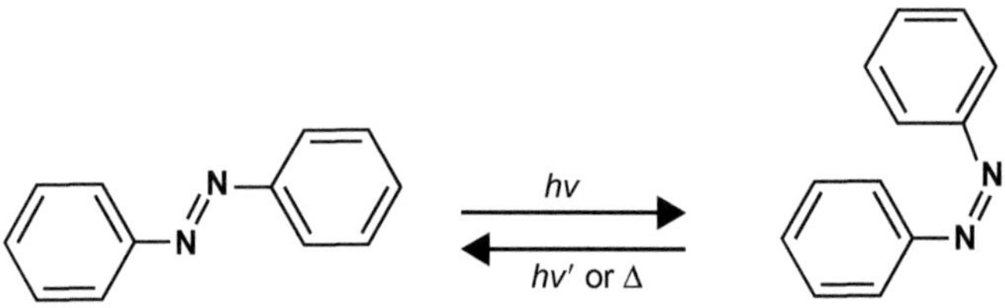

Fig. 3.1 Reversible photoinduced isomerization of azobenzene: (left) trans form and (right) cis form.

Photoresponsive polymers have been extensively studied for applications such as smart photomechanical transduction and actuation, bioactivity switching of proteins, reversible optical storage, tissue engineering, and drug-delivery systems (Guragain et al., 2015). In the specific case of biomedical applications, namely with in vivo applications, the light wavelength needs to be tuned to the so-called “biologically friendly windows,” the near infrared (IR) portion of the electromagnetic spectrum, which is less harmful and has a deeper penetration in living tissues than the ultraviolet/visible wavelengths. Therefore the IR radiation is minimally absorbed by cells/tissues and maximally by the photoresponsive polymers, which is essential, for example, in photoactivation of drug carriers within a living system (Cabane et al., 2012).

3.2.1.2 Thermoresponsive polymers

Thermoresponsive polymers have attracted great attention for biomedical applications, such as drug-delivery systems, tissue engineering, and smart switching systems for separation, permeation, actuation, and detachment control of biological entities (Gil and Hudson, 2004). In addition, they have also been used in catalysis, surface engineering, and information processing. Shape-memory polymers that respond to changes in the external conditions such as temperature also find broad applications in temperature sensing elements (Lin et al., 2010). Despite the fact that thermoresponsive polymers can be limited by issues related to heat transfer and consequently slow response, temperature has been widely used as a stimulus since its changes are applicable both in vitro and in vivo.

These materials are characterized by a critical temperature at which the hydrophobic and hydrophilic interactions between the polymer chains and the aqueous media abruptly change according to their composition, which induces the rupture of intra- and intermolecular hydrophobic and electrostatic interactions, resulting in collapse, shrinking, or expansion of the polymer chains (Cabane et al., 2012).

In this context, the polymer solution can feature a higher critical solution temperature—HCST (also called upper critical solution temperature—UCST) or a lower critical solution temperature—LCST. If the polymer solution has a phase separation below a specific temperature and shows a single phase above that temperature, the polymers generally present a HCST. Otherwise, the polymers exhibit a LCST at which a quick transition from a stable monophase to an instable biphase system occurs while increasing the temperature of the system. This phase separation takes place because of a reversible molecular coil-to-globule transition, minimizing considerably the free energy of the system. At this point, the solution becomes turbid due to the scattering of light caused by the phase separation between the collapsed polymer molecules and the expelled water during heating. Moreover, LCST depends on other parameters such as chain length, tacticity, incorporation of comonomers, or pressure (Gil and Hudson, 2004).

Intermolecular interactions (hydrogen bonding and hydrophobic forces) in water medium are also important properties of thermoresponsive polymers, which might create micelle aggregation, hydrogel shrinkage, or physical crosslinks.

Physically speaking, LCST represents the shared minima of the spinodal and coexistence curves in a binary system, namely polymer and solvent (Schattling et al., 2014). Typically, this phase transition phenomena are fully reversible and the polymer solution can recover the initial state.

From a technological point of view, LCST-based polymer systems are the most studied. They are commonly observed in highly polar media such as water and alcohols due to the hydrogen bonding in polymer-solvent interacting systems (Schattling et al., 2014). Examples of LCST-based polymers in aqueous solution are polyacrylamides, polyvinylethers, polyoxazolines, being the most studied PNIPAM because of its biocompatibility and its critical temperature that can be turned to the human body temperature by incorporating hydrophilic or hydrophobic comonomers into the polymer structure (Ward and Georgiou,

2011; Ridi et al., 2014). PNIPAM shrinks and becomes hydrophobic at temperatures above its LCST, and turns into swollen and hydrophilic state below its LCST (Tekin et al., 2011). Natural polymers have also shown thermoresponsive behaviors such as cellulose derivatives, chitosan, dextran, or even some proteins (Klouda and Mikos, 2008).

3.2.1.3 Electroactive polymers

Electroactive polymers are an increasingly important class of smart materials that can undergo structural deformations, such as swelling, shrinkage, and bending, in response to an electrical field. This kind of external stimulus has the advantage of allowing accurately controlled electrical to mechanical energy transformation through the precise selection of voltage, current, duration of the electrical pulses and interval between pulses (Murdan, 2003). Moreover, despite the sizable active structural deformation in response to an electrical stimulus, electroresponsive polymers show simple processability, down-scalability, low specific gravity and are, in most cases, inexpensive. These properties present a high potential in several biotechnological applications including biomechanics, artificial muscles, active catheters, (bio)sensors, actuators, and drug-delivery systems, among others (Roy et al., 2010; Gil and Hudson, 2004; Rajagopalan et al., 2010; Verbrugghe et al., 2015; Liu et al., 2011). In fact, electric signals have already been used in the form of iontophoresis and electroporation in the field of dermal and transdermal drug-delivery systems and safe limits of electrical field strengths for topical applications have already been determined (Murdan, 2003).

Electroresponsive polymers can be categorized into two main groups based on their primary activation mechanisms, namely electronic electroactive polymers—EEAPs and ionic electroactive polymers—IEAPs. EEAPs are driven by external electric fields and by Coulomb forces and include materials such as piezoelectric polymers, electrostrictive polymers, and dielectric elastomers (Martins et al., 2014; Cardoso et al., 2011). Although these polymers require typically high electrical field strengths in the order of 10–100 V μm^{-1} for electrostrictive polymers and dielectric elastomers, efforts to reduce driven electric fields are being carried out (Meng and Hu, 2010). Nevertheless, EEAPs feature attractive actuating performance due to their high efficiency, short response time, high durability, stability, and reliability. In turn, IEAPs are driven by the movement of ions or molecules and comprise polyelectrolyte gels, ionic polymer–metal composites, conducting polymers, and carbon nanotubes (although not polymeric). Such materials show the advantages of typically being activated by very low voltage of about 1–5 V. However, they can only typically be operated within a surrounding electrolyte medium (Meng and Hu, 2010; Verbrugghe et al., 2015).

Recently, new approaches are being explored using ionic liquids/electroactive polymer composites, allowing large deformations at low voltages to be obtained without the need of a surrounding electrolyte medium (Mejri et al., 2015; Leones et al., 2014; Akle et al., 2006). These systems display great potential for biomedical application as they overcome the stability issues of IEAPs and avoid the need for large applied field of EEAPs, leading also to much larger shape variations.

Among the most investigated electroresponsive polymers for biomedical applications are polyelectrolyte hydrogels based on both natural and synthetic polymers, with the ability to deform under an electric field due to anisotropic swelling or deswelling, as charged ions are directed towards the anode and cathode side of the gel (Murdan, 2003; Jackson and Stam, 2015). These water-swollen macromolecules feature many advantages. First of all, they present the unique ability to resemble natural biological tissues because of their hydrophilic nature, soft consistency, and three-dimensional (3D) polymeric network that allow large amounts of water. Moreover, they are stable in aqueous and biological fluids at physiological temperature, pH, and ionic strength, and many of them are biocompatible (Verbrugghe et al., 2015).

Furthermore, they cause minimal mechanical irritation to the surrounding tissue and reduced protein adsorption and cell adhesion are possible due to the rubbery nature of hydrogels and to the low interfacial tension between the gel surface and the aqueous surrounding fluids, respectively. Physically, they have the unique ability to absorb water, which allows them to swell/deswell to several thousand times their original volume, which in turn makes them extremely interesting for drug-delivery systems because of their ability to release specific volumes of drugs (Hoffman, 2013; Jackson and Stam, 2015). Finally, depending on the applications and sites of administration, hydrogels can acquire various shapes like rods, disks, films, and microparticles and their physical and chemical properties can vary with composition (Murdan, 2003; Verbrugghe et al., 2015). Typical natural polymers used to process electroresponsive polymers are chitosan, hyaluronic acid, and alginate, while PAA, poly(methacrylic acid)—PMAA and polyacrylonitrile have been used as synthetic polymers. Additionally, combinations of natural and synthetic components have been also used (Pillay et al., 2014; Liu et al., 2011).

However, a few neutral polymers have demonstrated high actuating deformation under electric filed in nonconducting media such as silicone and poly(dimethylsiloxane)—PDMS with titanium dioxide particles (Fig. 3.2) (Filipcsei et al., 2000). Moreover, piezoelectric polymers, such as the poly(vinylidene fluoride)—PVDF and its copolymers, feature interesting properties for sensors and actuators applications such as artificial

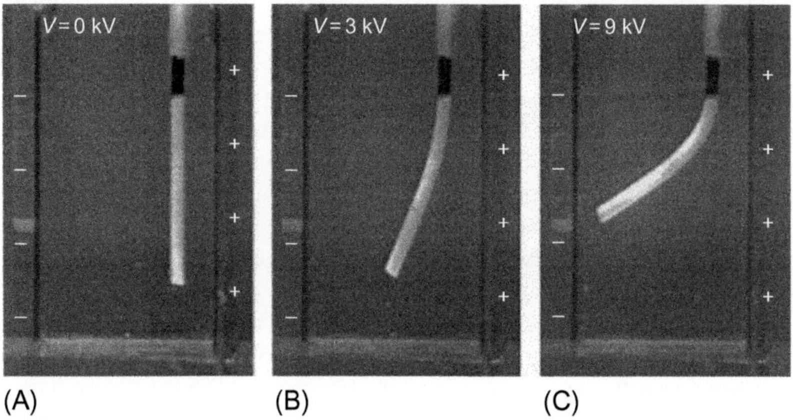

Fig. 3.2 Bending of a PDMS gel loaded with 10% of titanium dioxide particles as a function of uniform electric field strength: (A) 0 V; (B) 3 kV; (C) 9 kV.
Reprinted from Filipcsei, G., Fehér. J., Zrínyi, M., 2000. Electric field sensitive neutral polymer gels. J. Mol. Struct. 554 (1), 109–117, Copyright (2000) with permission from Elsevier.

muscles actuators and active catheters applications because of their excellent and controllable piezoelectric response together with their great combination of processability, mechanical and chemical resistance, thermal stability, and suitable mechanical properties (Ribeiro et al., 2015a; Ferreira et al., 2015; Nunes-Pereira et al., 2015).

3.2.1.4 Magnetoresponsive polymers

There is a growing interest in the use of magnetic fields as the selective stimuli for the development, fabrication, and application of smart materials. Magnetoresponsive polymers show a magnetic-active effect in response to a magnetic field.

This class of smart materials rely mostly on composites constituted by magnetic particles whose size (mainly nano-sized) allows them to become embedded into a polymer matrix to confer a magnetic response. A large range of compositions, shapes, dimensions, and surface properties of magnetic nanoparticles have been developed depending on the synthesis route and the intended application. Examples of magnetic nanoparticles include iron oxide Fe_3O_4 or γ-Fe_2O_3, "soft" metallic ion or "hard" magnetic compound, such as cobalt, nickel, iron nitride, iron platinum, and iron palladium. These magnetoresponsive polymers constitute interesting solutions for several biomedical applications not only because they can provide fast responses to external magnetic fields, but also because of the absence of electrical connections. Therefore, they can be spatially and temporally controlled externally providing a noninvasive approach by remote control (Ridi et al., 2014).

Rigid polymeric matrices filled with magnetic nanoparticles, often called magnetic plastics, were the first magnetic responsive materials and presented low flexibility and their size, shape, and elastic properties were practically unchanged in the presence of magnetic fields. Consequently, they have been successfully used in just a few applications, such as permanent magnets, magnetic cores, and connecting elements (Marchi et al., 2015).

Instead, highly flexible polymer matrices containing magnetic nanoparticles represent another possibility for magnetoresponsive polymer composites with enhanced functional properties (Liu et al., 2012). Besides their fast response, they can achieve large and homogeneous or nonhomogeneous deformations in response to external magnetic fields. Based on the polymer matrix employed, flexible magnetoresponsive polymers are subdivided into magnetoresponsive elastomers and magnetoresponsive polymer gels (also called ferrogels) (Meng and Hu, 2010). Poly(vinyl alcohol)—PVA, PNIPAM, acetoacetoxyethyl methacrylate, poly(ethylene glycol)—PEG have been used as polymer matrices in magnetoresponsive polymer gels, while silicones such as PDMS have been employed for magnetoresponsive elastomers (Thevenot et al., 2013; Czaun et al., 2008; Reinicke et al., 2010). Shape and size deformations of the elastomers-based polymer matrix take place instantaneously and reversibly when an external nonuniform magnetic field is applied and removed, respectively. This phenomenon occurs because the forces acting on the magnetic particles are transmitted directly to the polymer chains, coupling their shape.

In order to obtain a high magnetic response, elastomer composites should feature low elastic modulus, high initial susceptibility, and high saturation magnetization (Meng and Hu, 2010). In the case of magnetoresponsive polymer gels subject to a nonuniform magnetic field, wherein the average field gradient is perpendicular to the axis of the gel, the gel can undergo significant elongation, contraction, or curvature in less than a second in response to the applied field.

This new generation of soft responsive materials with elastic and magnetic properties has opened new opportunities in a vast range of biomedical applications (Roy et al., 2010). Apart from structural deformation, alternating magnetic fields allow regions in the proximity of the magnetoresponsive materials to be heated up. In fact, as the size of the magnetic nanoparticles is reduced below a critical diameter (normally 10 nm), they feature superparamagnetic properties, which allow the production of a hyperthermic effect at high frequency fields, which can consequently be used to thermally ablate pathological cells. Magnetoresponsive polymers have also been intensively investigated in applications such as controlled and targeted drug-delivery systems, artificial muscles, cancer therapy agents, microfluidics for the separation of specific biological entities, microelectronics, coating, among others (Marchi et al., 2015; Czaun et al., 2008).

Moreover, polymer-based magnetoelectric materials also appear as a promising research field due to the interplay of piezoelectric and magnetorestrictive effects of polymer and nanoparticles, respectively, which allow their use in a wide range of biomedical applications, such as those mentioned above, and also in magnetic storage media, and tunneling magnetoresistance (Martins and Lanceros-Méndez, 2013; Gonçalves et al., 2013).

Another class of magnetoresponsive materials comprises the molecular magnets, which feature a relatively weak magnetic response at extremely low temperatures and are still at an early stage of research (Marchi et al., 2015).

3.2.2 Chemical shape-responsive polymers

3.2.2.1 pH-responsive polymers

pH-responsive polymers are materials that contain ionizable groups in their backbone capable of donating or accepting protons upon an environmental change in pH. Ionic interactions are activated by pH change, which lead to the collapsing or extending of the polymer chains, induced by electrostatic repulsions of the generated charges (Gil and Hudson, 2004); pK_a defines the specific pH at which the degree of ionization is dramatically altered (Schattling et al., 2014); pH-responsive polymers are widely studied in the biomedical field since pH variations are presented in living tissues and also occur in some pathologies. The gastrointestinal tract is an interesting site to apply pH-responsive polymers since the stomach gastric juice exhibits a pH between 1 and 3 whereas the intestines feature a pH between 5 and 8 (Jeong and Gutowska, 2002). This variation has been used to design and develop new functional drug-delivery systems capable of contracting under stomach acid, thus protecting the drugs, and expanding at the intestinal pH in order to release the drugs locally, thus increasing the absorption efficiency. Moreover, chronic wounds show pH values between 5 and 7 and tumor tissues show lower pH than normal tissues. Thus, antitumor drugs encapsulated or conjugated onto carrier materials could be released in the acidic microenvironment of tumor tissues (Fig. 3.3) (Manchun et al., 2012; Cabane et al., 2012).

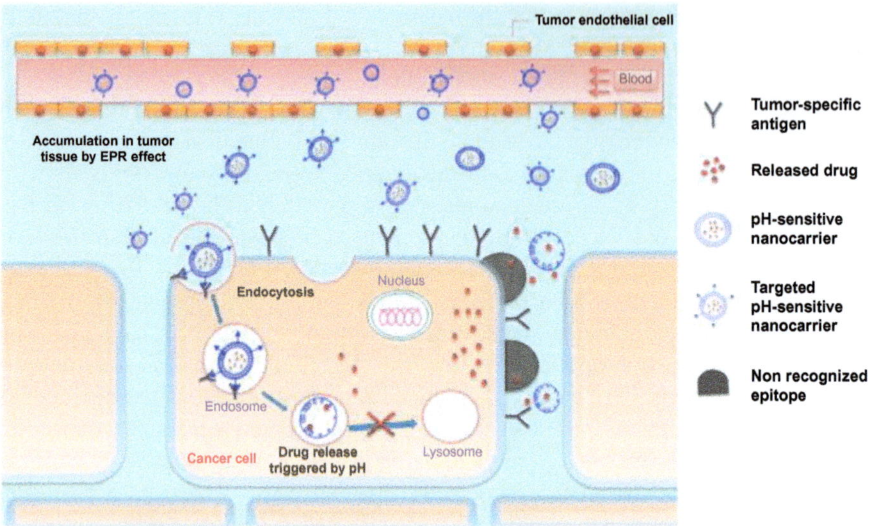

Fig. 3.3 Schematic illustration of pH-responsive nanocarriers targeting. pH-responsive nanocarriers accumulate in the tumor tissue via the enhanced permeability and retention effect through the leaky blood vessels. After pH-responsive nanocarriers accumulate in the tissue, the system is triggered to release the anticancer drug in response to extracellular pH stimuli, or is taken up by cancer cells after binding to target antigens on the surface of the cancer cells. In this latter case the drugs are released inside the cancer cells by intracellular pH stimuli. Reprinted from Manchun, S., Dass, C.R., Sriamornsak, P., 2012. Targeted therapy for cancer using pH-responsive nanocarrier systems. Life Sci. 90 (11–12), 381–387, Copyright (2012) with permission from Elsevier.

pH-responsive polymers can be divided into two types, polybases and polyacids. Polybases accept protons under acidic pH conditions. They are mostly constituted by amine, pyridine, or imidazone groups in their side chains. Examples of polybases are PDMAEMA, poly(2-diethylaminoethyl methacrylate), poly(2- or 4-vinylpyridine), poly(vinyl imidazole) and also biopolymers such as chitosan and synthetic polypeptides such as poly(histidine).

In contrast, polyacids release their protons under basic pH conditions (Schattling et al., 2014). Examples of polyacids are alginate, poly(glutamic acid), PAA, PMMA, poly(ethylacrylic acid), and poly(propylacrylic acid) and can contain groups, such as carboxyl or sulforamide, among others (Gil and Hudson, 2004; Cabane et al., 2012; Schattling et al., 2014). Polymers with the ability to degrade under acid or basic conditions can also be used as pH-responsive polymers for drug-delivery systems. Poly(ortho esters) and poly(β-amino esters)—PbAE are examples of pH-responsive biodegradable polymers, which suffer degradation under acidic conditions. Besides drug-delivery applications, pH-responsive polymers have also been used in gene delivery and gene therapy research (Jeong and Gutowska, 2002).

3.2.2.2 Redox-responsive polymers

A redox stimulus is an electrochemical signal addressing redox-sensitive groups, leading to a change in their oxidation state (Schattling et al., 2014). Redox-responsive polymers have been designed to respond to natural redox gradients in living tissues or to create smart carrier systems that release drugs at a given location and at a specific time, minimizing side effects in healthy cells/tissues (Gauthier, 2014).

The basic principle is to take advantage of the difference in redox potential between healthy and unhealthy cells/tissues. A specific class of redox-responsive polymers, which are used to develop redox-responsive bio-erodible or biodegradable systems, concerns those containing labile groups (Cabane et al., 2012). Polyanhydrides, PbAE, and poly(lactic-*co*-glycolic acid)—PLGA containing acid labile groups stimulate redox responsiveness. Poly(NiPAAm-*co*-Ru(bpy)$_3$) also have been used as representative redox-responsive polymer (Yoshida et al., 2000; Murase et al., 2009). The redox reaction of Ru(bpy)$_3$ alters the hydrophobic and hydrophilic properties of the polymer chains that results in their swelling and deswelling at the oxidized and reduced states, respectively (McCarley, 2012; Cabane et al., 2012). Other common redox-active derivates are ferrocene, disulfide, diselenide, boronic ester groups, and paramagnetic organic molecules, such as 2,2,6,6-tetramethylpiperidine-1-oxyl (Huo et al., 2014; Saleem et al., 2015; Brulisauer et al., 2014). Besides controlled and targeted release systems, redox-responsive polymers have been used in catalysis, energy, microfluidic, water purification, sensors and actuators applications (Huo et al., 2014; McCarley, 2012).

3.2.3 Biological shape-responsive polymers

3.2.3.1 Glucose-responsive polymers

Glucose-responsive polymers have received considerable attention in recent years because of their large biomedical market potential in both glucose sensing and insulin-delivery applications. Diabetes mellitus is a chronic disease characterized by an accumulation of glucose in the bloodstream due to insufficient production or inefficient usage of the hormone insulin (Ma and Shi, 2014). Patients suffering from diabetes mellitus require life-long and painful treatments that include regular monitoring of blood sugar concentration and periodic subcutaneously administration of insulin in order to prevent acute complications and even death. However, normal levels of blood glucose are difficult, if not impossible, to ensure with this treatment. Therefore new and alternative approaches are desirable, which can provide self-regulating insulin release in response to blood glucose levels, in a noninvasive manner.

In recent years, glucose-responsive polymers have been designed and developed in order to meet these specifications. They can rely on three different mechanisms, which include enzymatic oxidation of glucose by glucose oxidase—GOx, binding of glucose with lectins proteins and reversible covalent bond formation between glucose and boronic acids—BA (Wu et al., 2011; Wu and Zhou, 2013).

Glucose-responsive polymers based on GOx are one of the most reported biofeedback-controlled insulin-release system and rely on the conversion of glucose to gluconic acid and hydrogen peroxide by the enzymatic action of GOx in the presence of oxygen and water. Gluconic acid has the ability to trigger a response in pH-responsive polymers loaded or conjugated with GOx and insulin. The pH-response usually causes a change on their morphology, namely swelling or collapsing of the polymer chains, releasing insulin.

Many polymer matrices based on polyacids and polybases synthesized in the presence of GOx have been developed and tested for autonomous controlled release of insulin. Examples are PAA-modified cellulose, PMAA-graft-ethylene glycol, PAA-grafted PVDF, poly(methacrylic acid-*g*-ethylene glycol), and PDEAEM. Moreover, PEG grafts and chitosan have also been used as glucose-responsive polymers because of their nontoxic, nonimmunogenic, and biocompatible behaviors (Chu et al., 2004; Ravaine et al., 2008; Marek and Peppas, 2013). Polymers that respond to hydrogen peroxide variations instead of GOx have also been reported (Uchiyama et al., 2003).

Glycopolymers conjugated with specific lectins may be used as glucose-responsive polymers. Lectins are carbohydrate-binding proteins, macromolecules that are highly specific for sugar moieties. Therefore, glycoproteins tend to crosslink and/or aggregate in the presence of lectins, and reverse this process when critical levels of saccharide are exceeded. Concanavalin A—ConA has been one of the lectins mostly studied due to its sensitivity to glucose. ConA grafted to PEG, PLGA, carboxymethyl dextran, chitosan-modified poly(acrylonitrile-*co*-acrylic acid), and poly(ethylene glycol) dimethacrylate also have been reported (Hurkat et al., 2012; Sahota et al., 2015; Yin et al., 2010).

Although the two protein-based mechanisms referred to previously are highly specific to glucose, they can suffer denaturation under nonbiological conditions or when they are required to be used and stored for a long period of time, which can limit their applications in vivo (Cambre and Sumerlin, 2011). Therefore glucose-responsive polymers using synthetic components, such as BA that shows the ability to reversibly complex with sugars, can provide the necessary stability and durability for this type of application. Variations in pH or diol concentration (ie, glucose) can change the hydrophilicity of BA-based polymers by the conversion of neutral BA groups to anionic boronate esters. In fact, as the glucose levels increase, the ratio of the anionic form to the neutral form increases, as well as the hydrophilicity of the system (Guan and Zhang, 2013).

Most of the glucose-responsive polymers based on BA are hydrogels that swell or collapse in response to the hydropholicity increase in the presence of glucose. Examples are based on 3-acrylamidophenylboronic acids, *N*,*N*-3-dimethyl-1, 3-propanediamine, or *N*,*N*-dimethylacrylamide coupled with PVA by the BA groups present in the terpolymer (Roy et al., 2010). An alternative BA monomer 4-(1,6-dioxo-2,5-diaza-7-oxamyl)phenylboronic acid with a more physiological relevant pK_a of approximately 7.8 coupled to the thermoresponsive polymer PNIPAM that exhibit a phase transition temperature of approximately 40°C also have been considered as potential glucose-responsive polymer. The gel undergoes volume changes under physiological conditions in response to glucose concentration variations within the range of typical sugar levels (Cambre and Sumerlin, 2011).

3.2.3.2 Enzyme-responsive polymers

The design and development of enzyme-responsive polymers emerged recently as a promising new research area in stimuli-responsive materials and rely on polymers that suffer macroscopic property changes when triggered by the biocatalytic action of an enzyme (de la Rica et al., 2012).

Enzymes play an important role in many biological and metabolic pathways, including cell regulation in natural living systems (Hu et al., 2012). Moreover, reactions catalyzed by enzymes feature the incomparable advantages of unique selectivity and efficiency, they are operable under mild conditions and can be conducted in vitro, so that a nature-mimicking environment for the development of artificial systems completing cascade reactions can be performed (Roy et al., 2010; Hu et al., 2012). For example, polymer networks composed of alginate-loaded chitosan or dexamethasone-loaded chitosan microcapsules are sensitive to chitosanase. In addition, azoaromatic bonds are responsive to azoreductase (Cabane et al., 2012). Therefore, enzyme-responsive polymers allow a wide design flexibility and scope of applications.

Enzyme-responsive polymers are classically composed by enzyme-reactive moieties in the form of labile bonds along the main chain or side groups of the polymer or by functional groups that react under enzymatic conditions (Roy et al., 2010). Catalytic action of an enzyme can lead to morphological transitions, swelling/collapse of hydrogels, or surface modification of the polymer matrix. Therefore enzyme-responsive polymers are being intensively studied for controlled and triggered drug-delivery systems, biocatalysis, tissue engineering, and medical imaging, among other applications (Hu et al., 2012).

Enzyme-responsive polymers can be developed as enzyme-responsive polymeric assemblies, micro- and nanoparticles and hydrogels because of their similar properties to the extracellular matrix. Thus, a wide variety of hydrogels that suffer degradation in the presence of proteases for the release of encapsulated contents have been designed and tested for therapeutic purposes (Roy et al., 2010; de la Rica et al., 2012).

3.3 Representative applications

Once living systems have the ability to modify their conditions in order to respond to external stimulus, and in order to mimic this behavior, smart polymers arise as the class of materials more suitable for this approach. Among these smart polymers shape-changing or metamorphic materials have revealed interesting properties suitable for applications in the biomedical field.

As already mentioned, shape-changing polymers undergo shape variations or deformations in response to external stimuli, such as temperature, pH, light, electric or magnetic field or biological molecules, among others. These stimuli can be artificially controlled (ultrasound, light, magnetic or electric field, among others) or naturally promoted by an internal physiological environment (temperature or pH changes). From a biomedical point of view, the shape-changing materials sensitive to temperature or pH are among the most important systems. Body temperature represents a complex and nonlinear system subjected to internal and external variation (Kelly, 2006). It is essential that the internal temperature is maintained within specific limits for the normal functioning of the human body.

It is possible to find variations of pH along the gastrointestinal tract (Fallingborg, 1999; Evans et al., 1988) and also in some specific areas, such as in tumors (with lower pH and higher temperature than healthy cells) (Tannock and Rotin, 1989; Gerweck and Seetharaman, 1996), in muscle cells after muscle activity (Street et al., 2001; Stackhouse et al., 2001), or in the brain (Magnotta et al., 2012; Chesler and Chan, 1988). Furthermore, many cellular processes depend on pH, such as macromolecules synthesis, cell proliferation, metabolites transport, and enzymatic activity (Tannock and Rotin, 1989).

Besides temperature and pH stimulus, it is possible to detect mechanical stimuli occurring within the human body (Lim et al., 2006). The cells of the human body are constantly subjected to mechanical stimulations throughout life, such as fluid shear (Jen et al., 2000), hydrostatic and osmotic pressure (Ogawa, 2011), blood volume and pressure (Terracio et al., 1988). Furthermore, the effect of mechanical stimulus may be assessed with respect to extracellular matrix production (Chiquet et al., 2009), bone formation (Klein-Nulend et al., 2012), and gene expression (Chiquet et al., 2009).

In the next section, an overview of the main biomedical applications based on shape-changing materials in response to natural stimulus (temperature—thermoresponsive materials, pH—pH-responsive materials, and mechanical—mechano-electrical materials) will be presented.

3.3.1 Tissue engineering

Tissue engineering holds great promise for creating tissue models with the structural organization and functionality of native tissues being at the basis of regenerative medicine.

The use of shape-changing polymers has attracted increasing interest due to their advantages when compared to other polymers that act only as cell supports.

Thermoresponsive polymers in tissue engineering are mainly used as substrate for cell culture and as injectable gels for in situ scaffolding (Ward and Georgiou, 2011). In cell culture, the thermoresponsive ability of the polymers is mainly used to regulate the attachment and detachment of the cells from the surface (Gandhi et al., 2015), allowing the reutilization of the polymer surface for repeated cell culture (Nitschke et al., 2007; Tang et al., 2012) (Fig. 3.4). With this approach, micro- and nano-fabrication techniques have also been used to create thermoresponsive polymer-based platforms for tissue-engineering applications (Tekin et al., 2011). The substrates, also used in the field of cell sheet engineering, have been used to generate functional tissues, without any scaffolding material, minimizing the inflammation and immune rejection in vivo (da Silva et al., 2007). The first study under this scope was conducted in 1990 (Takezawa et al., 1990) and since then, cell sheet technology has been used to fabricate different types of tissues for various tissue-engineering applications, including nerve injury (Pesirikan et al., 2013), cardiac (Tekin et al., 2011; Shimizu et al., 2003;

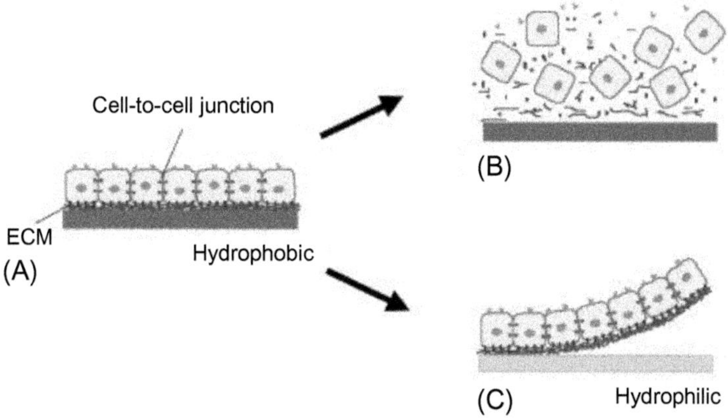

Fig. 3.4 Cell sheet release from temperature-responsive culture surfaces. (A) When cells are cultured confluently, the cells connect to each other via cell-to-cell junction proteins. (B) When harvested by protease treatments, cell-to-cell connections are disrupted and cells are released separately. (C) When PNIPAM-grafted surfaces are used, cell-to-cell connections are completely preserved and the cells are released as a contiguous cell sheet. Extracellular matrices retained underneath the cell sheets play a role as an adhesive agent.
Adapted from Shimizu, T., Yamato, M., Kikuchi, A., Okano, T., 2003. Cell sheet engineering for myocardial tissue reconstruction. Biomaterials 24 (13), 2309–2316, Copyright (2003), with permission from Elsevier.

Kawamura et al., 2012), hepatic (Tekin et al., 2011; Harimoto et al., 2002), bone (Pirraco et al., 2011; Long et al., 2014), corneal (Nishida et al., 2004; Teichmann et al., 2015; Yang et al., 2006), kidney (Kushida et al., 2001), and skin (Yamato et al., 2001).

Another application is based on thermoresponsive polymers mixed with the cells at room temperature and then injected into the body (~37°C). Due to the increase of the temperature and once the body temperature is above the polymer's LCST, the thermoresponsive polymer forms a physical gel in which the cells are encapsulated (Lu et al., 2007). Contrary to what happens in vitro, the in situ formation of the cell/scaffold allows the delivery of not only encapsulated cells, but also nutrients and growth factors to defects, through minimally invasive approaches (Gandhi et al., 2015).

The main form of thermoresponsive biomaterials for tissue engineering are hydrogels that are especially attractive as injectable biomaterials in cardiac tissue repair (Hasan et al., 2015; Cui et al., 2014), bone substitutes (Bongio et al., 2013), neuronal injury (Stabenfeldt et al., 2006), corneal tissue engineering (Hopkinson et al., 2008), adipose tissue engineering (Tan et al., 2009), muscle (Ding et al., 2013) and vascular (Jordan et al., 2005) tissue engineering.

PNIPAM shows a LCST very close to the body temperature, being therefore one of the most studied thermoresponsive polymers for biomedical applications. Various methods have been used to develop PNIPAM-coated substrates. Some of these surfaces were successfully used to generate cell sheets. However, some PNIPAM-coated surfaces are not suitable for the formation of tissue monolayers as they inhibit cell attachment at temperatures above LCST. Chitosan-based hydrogels have been also investigated as potential cell carriers for tissue-engineering applications (Klouda and Mikos, 2008). A list of the main thermoresponsive polymers published over the past 7 years was reviewed by Klouda (2015).

Many of the major cells and organ functions of the human body are controlled by electrical signals and as mechanical stimulus can be found in human body (Ribeiro et al., 2015b), mechano-electrical materials, namely piezoelectric materials, appear to be a promising choice for tissue-engineering applications. In these kinds of materials it is possible to apply electrical signals to the cells by mechano-electrical transduction (Fig. 3.5). Studies of the piezoelectric polymers used for tissue-engineering applications are mostly devoted to bone (Ribeiro et al., 2012, 2015c; Dubkova et al., 1999), neural (Delaviz et al., 2011; Evans et al., 2000) and muscle regeneration (Ribeiro et al., 2015a; Martins et al., 2013). Piezoelectric materials can be used in different topographies, such as films (Cardoso et al., 2012), fibers (Ribeiro et al., 2010; Correia et al., 2015), porous membranes (Nunes-Pereira et al., 2015; Cardoso et al., 2015), spheres (Correia et al., 2014), and 3D scaffolds (Correia et al., 2016).

Aiming to address the biomimetic conditions of the human body, such as the presence of piezoelectricity in bone, polymer-based piezoelectric materials have already proven their suitability in the bone-regeneration processes (Ribeiro et al., 2015b). This biomimetic approach is particularly relevant as bone is physiologically subjected to mechano-electrical solicitations related to walking, jumping, and running (Fukada and Yasuda, 1957). However, in some cases, the patient is immobilized due to bone fracture, and as a result the natural mechanical stimulus during walking does not occur naturally. In these cases, magnetoelectric composite materials provide an innovative tool, allowing the use of an external magnetic field to remotely control tissue stimulation (Ribeiro et al., 2016). Magnetoelectric composite materials have also been produced that are similar to the piezoelectric materials mentioned above (Martins and Lanceros-Méndez, 2013; Martins et al., 2015; Gonçalves et al., 2015a,b).

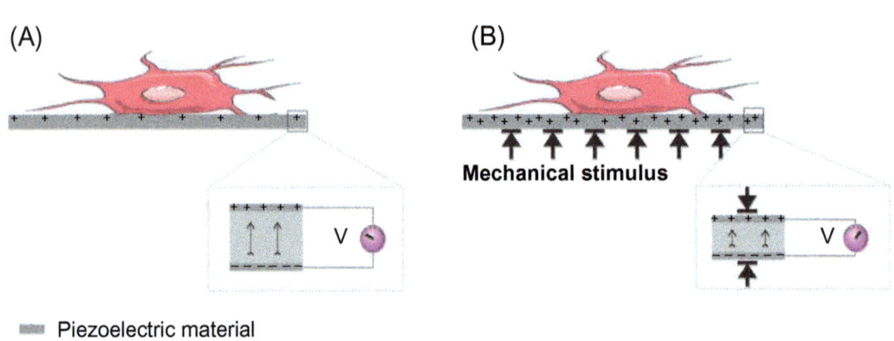

Fig. 3.5 Schematic representation of the piezoelectric effect (piezoelectric material representation at the bottom of the image) and corresponding cell culture on piezoelectric supports (A) without and (B) with mechanical stimulus, the later leading to an electrical potential variation in the materials which, in turn, influences cell response.
Adapted from Ribeiro, C., Sencadas, V., Correia, D.M., Lanceros-Méndez, S., 2015. Piezoelectric polymers as biomaterials for tissue engineering applications. Colloids Surf. B Biointerfaces 136, 46–55, Copyright (2015), with permission from Elsevier.

3.3.2 Drug-delivery systems

Drug delivery is the method developed for the administration of pharmaceutical compounds (drugs) to achieve a therapeutic effect in humans or animals. Key factors are to deliver the drug to the right area, at the right time, and at the right concentration (Gandhi et al., 2015). This can be achieved by introducing smart polymeric carriers that allow the drug delivery in response to a stimulus. The ideal drug-delivery system is the one in which the drug delivery is able to respond to small physiological variations and/or metabolic states (Almeida et al., 2012).

Thermoresponsive polymers and, in particular, LCST polymers, are the most studied and used in drug administration systems.

Different forms of carrier have been used such as, hydrogel, micro- and nano-spheres, micelles and fibers, among others.

With respect to hydrogels, the drug, therapeutic agents, or proteins are mixed with the polymer in its liquid state so they can be injected into the subcutaneous layer of the human body into the damaged area or tumor where they form a gel when the temperature increases (Almeida et al., 2012). These systems can be used to release chemotherapeutic agents into solid tumors (MacEwan et al., 2010), for the delivery of antimicrobial agents for the prevention/treatment of wound infection (Jones et al., 2008), for treating irregularly shaped tissue sites (eliminating the need for custom produced scaffold designs) (Bhattarai et al., 2010), to deliver angiogenesis-suppressing drugs to limit the nutrient/oxygen supply to the tumor cells (and in this way control the tumor growth) (Cho et al., 2011).

Thermosensitive monolithic hydrogels can be used to promote drug-delivery profiles identified as "ON–OFF." These systems can deliver the drug encapsulated in the presence of low temperatures (ON) and stop delivering when the temperature increases (OFF) (Soppimath et al., 2002) or vice versa (Shin et al., 1997) and have been used to deliver anticancer drugs (Kim et al., 2009).

Polymer spheres have been used especially to formulate protein drugs, such as elastin-based nano-spheres as carrier for the delivery of bone morphogenetic proteins (Bessa et al., 2010). Also, micelles are useful for encapsulating hydrophobic drugs and delivering them into an aqueous environment (Ward and Georgiou, 2011). The administration of synthetic hormones to decrease the adipose tissue deposits in skin has been achieved by the use of smart polymer nanofibers from a blend of PVA and PNIPAM (Azarbayjani et al., 2010).

The main advantage of the thermoresponsive polymer system is the avoidance of toxic organic solvents and the reduced systemic side effects, the capacity to deliver both hydrophilic and lipophilic drugs as well as sustained release properties (Priya James et al., 2014).

Ionic pH sensitive polymers are polyelectrolytes that contain in their structure acid (carboxylic or sulfonic) or basic (ammonium salts) groups, and their main feature is the ability to accept or release protons in response to pH changes (Almeida et al., 2012). In most cases, drugs need to be delivered in response to the pH value in the body, being desirable the administration of drugs in a controlled manner that precisely matches physiological needs at targeted location, predetermined release rate, and specific periods of time (Zhu and Chen, 2015). The pH changes within the human body. Thus, different organs, tissues, and cellular compartments present different pH values, which makes the pH a suitable stimulus for controlled drug delivery and these pH-based useful systems (Schmaljohann, 2006).

Different pH-responsive carrier forms have been used such as hydrogel, micro- and nano-spheres, micelles, and dendrimers.

This kind of system can be used, for example, for oral drug delivery where the polymer retains the drug in the presence of acid pH in the stomach and delivers it in the alkaline pH of the small intestine (Zhu and Chen, 2015), for example against *Helicobacter pylori* infection (Lin et al., 2009; Thamphiwatana et al., 2013).

The pH-responsive polymer systems offer an interesting opportunity for drug delivery in the optimization of cancer prevention and/or therapy, resulting in better tumor management. It is considered an ideal trigger for the delivery of anticancer drugs due to the fact that the pH at both primary and metastasized tumors is lower than the pH of normal tissue (Manchun et al., 2012). In this way, the design of pH-responsive carriers stable at physiological pH but deformed under acidic pH, significantly enhances the efficiency of therapies and minimizes the side effects. Recent studies have reported some promising pH-responsive carriers for tumor-selective delivery. For instance, pH-responsive micelles for the delivery of doxorubicin from tumor blood vessels into interstitia (Jin et al., 2014) or nano-spheres for the treatment of HeLa cancer cells (Guo et al., 2011) have been developed (Fig. 3.6).

Other applications of pH-responsive polymers for drug-delivery systems have also been explored such as the incorporation of fibroblast growth factors to improve angiogenesis in infracted myocardium (Garbern et al., 2011); the incorporation of ketoprofen for colon-targeted delivery (Kulkarni et al., 2012); intracellular delivery of ovalbumin to dendritic cells (a class of cells intimately involved with adaptive immunity) (Hu et al., 2007) and for controlling drug release in nocturnal asthma treatment (Tran et al., 2013).

Piezoelectric materials can be used for drug-delivery applications based on the same concept as discussed above for tissue-engineering applications. More precisely, these materials have been explored for the ibuprofen release (Salazar et al., 2015), for transdermal and subcutaneous drug delivery (Ochoa et al., 2012), to release antimicrobial agent during the healing period (Boschin et al., 2006; Tabary et al., 2007), or for wound dressing (He et al., 2015).

Magnetoelectric materials show ideal properties related to high drug loading, site-specificity, and precise on-demand controlled drug delivery (Kaushik et al., 2014). These materials have been used as carriers to release anti-HIV drug (Nair et al., 2013), for the delivery of antineoplastic drugs (in particular for ovarian cancer cells) (Guduru et al., 2013), or for the treatment of specific infectious and inflammatory diseases (Ikoba et al., 2015).

3.3.3 Gene therapy

Gene therapy is a technique for correcting defective genes that are responsible for specific genetic diseases. Specifically, the critical step is the appropriate delivery of the

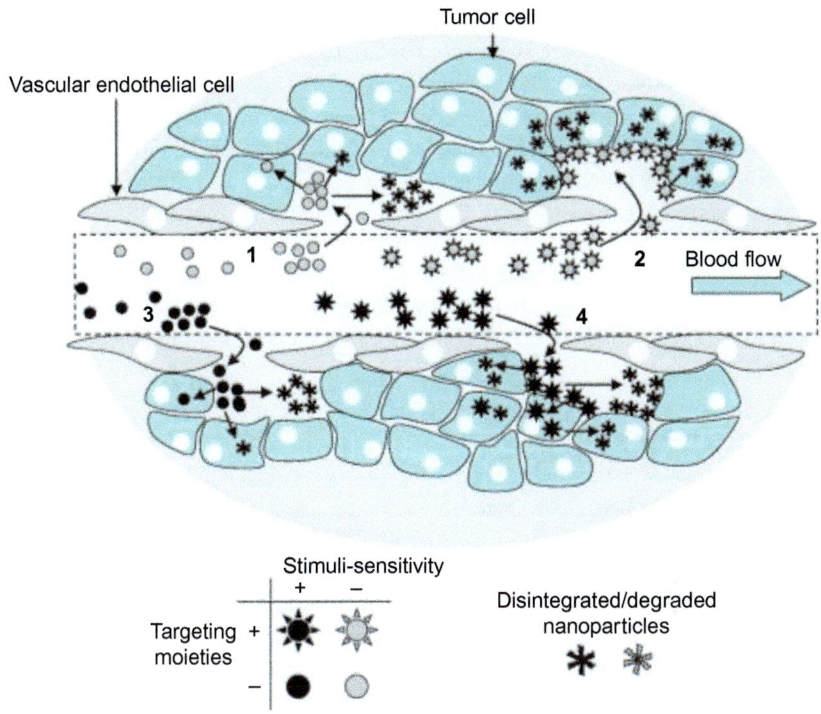

Fig. 3.6 Targeting strategies for cancer therapy. (1) Passive targeting can be achieved by enhanced permeation and retention (EPR) effect mediated by leaky vascular structures. Accumulation of macromolecular drugs or nanoparticles increases local drug concentration by degradation of drug carriers at the extracellular space or inside cells after endocytosis. (2) Active targeting mediated by targeting ligands specifically localizes drug carriers at desired cells or tissues. Due to the ligands, primary action mechanism is drug release inside cells after endocytosis. (3) Smart polymer systems loading therapeutic drugs also can be localized by EPR effect. Depending on disease, disintegration or degradation of the drug carrier to release drugs can occur. (4) Combination of targeting ligands and smart polymer systems provides a more effective release of encapsulated drugs. By environmental signals, drugs can be released at the extracellular space or inside target cells according to a predetermined program. Adapted from Kim, S., Kim, J.H., Jeon, O., Kwon, I.C., Park, K., 2009. Engineered polymers for advanced drug delivery. Eur. J. Pharm. Biopharm. 71 (3), 420–430, Copyright (2009), with permission from Elsevier.

therapeutic gene (deoxyribonucleic acid, DNA) into the cells that will repair, regulate, or replace the defective gene that causes the disease (Ward and Georgiou, 2011). With the introduction of thermoresponsive and pH-responsive polymers into polycationic carriers a very promising and more effective gene delivery can be obtained, including reduced immunogenicity and toxicity, increasing nuclear delivery, large DNA loading capacity and adjustable structures, among others (Hamidi et al., 2012).

Thermoresponsive and pH-responsive polymers have been mainly used to enhance the transfection efficiency by changing the temperature or pH, respectively, either during the complexation and/or during the incubation or transfection period (Ward and Georgiou, 2011; Takeda et al., 2004; Kwon et al., 2009; Haladjova et al., 2014; Iwai et al., 2013; Putnam et al., 2003; Singh et al., 2014).

Thermoresponsive system also have been employed as nonviral gene delivery vectors for retarding or regenerating the degenerative discs (Feng et al., 2015; Dang et al., 2006); as direct gene transfer of plasmid DNA (Twaites et al., 2005); to accelerate diabetic wound healing (Lee et al., 2003) and to cancer therapy (Cao et al., 2015; Su et al., 2015).

pH-responsive systems also have been applied for efficient cancer target gene therapy (Shi et al., 2014; Li et al., 2012; Sethuraman et al., 2006); for siRNA delivery (Meyer et al., 2008; Sato et al., 2012) and skin diseases (Donkuru et al., 2012).

3.4 Conclusions

Smart materials and in particular smart polymers represent a class of materials increasingly used for advanced applications. In particular, biomedical and biotechnological approaches specifically take advantage of metamorphic polymers to develop advanced tissue engineering, drug-delivery systems, and specific therapies. Some of these approaches are based on biomimetic approaches, some others rely on the specificity of the variations of temperature, pH, mechanical or electrical signals within the living body.

Robust proofs of concepts have been carried out, as well as specific therapeutic implementations. Despite those advances, which demonstrate the strong potential of smart polymer systems for advanced biomedical applications, there is a long and intense way to go in developing specific polymers and polymer composites with precise and tailored responses based on the deep knowledge of the biological functions they will support, take advantage from, repair, or heal. Shape and smart polymer-based materials, traditionally used for sensor and actuator applications, are "on the move" for a next generation of active therapies based on a better integration of biological functions and materials design.

Acknowledgments

The authors thank FEDER funds through the COMPETE 2020 Programme and National Funds through FCT – Portuguese Foundation for Science and Technology under Strategic Funding UID/FIS/04650/2013.This work is also funded by the FCT under grants SFRH/BPD/98109/2013 (VFC) and SFRH/BPD/90870/2012 (CR). The authors thank financial support from the Basque Government Industry Department under the ELKARTEK Program.

References

Akle, B.J., Bennett, M.D., Leo, D.J., 2006. High-strain ionomeric-ionic liquid electroactive actuators. Sens. Actuators A 126 (1), 173–181.

Almeida, H., Amaral, M.H., Lobão, P., 2012. Temperature and pH stimuli-responsive polymers and their applications in controlled and selfregulated drug delivery. J. Appl. Pharm. Sci. 2 (6), 01–10.

Azarbayjani, A.F., Venugopal, J.R., Ramakrishna, S., Lim, P.F.C., Chan, Y.W., Chan, S.Y., 2010. Smart polymeric nanofibers for topical delivery of levothyroxine. J. Pharm. Pharm. Sci. 13 (3), 400–410.

Bandara, H.M.D., Burdette, S.C., 2012. Photoisomerization in different classes of azobenzene. Chem. Soc. Rev. 41 (5), 1809–1825.

Berron, B.J., May, A.M., Zheng, Z., Balasubramaniam, V., Bowman, C.N., 2012. Antigen-responsive, microfluidic valves for single use diagnostics. Lab Chip 12 (4), 708–710.

Bessa, P.C., Machado, R., Nürnberger, S., Dopler, D., Banerjee, A., Cunha, A.M., et al., 2010. Thermoresponsive self-assembled elastin-based nanoparticles for delivery of BMPs. J. Control. Release 142 (3), 312–318.

Bhattarai, N., Gunn, J., Zhang, M., 2010. Chitosan-based hydrogels for controlled, localized drug delivery. Adv. Drug Deliv. Rev. 62 (1), 83–99.

Bogue, R., 2014. Smart materials: a review of capabilities and applications. Assem. Autom. 34 (1), 16–22.

Bongio, M., Nejadnik, M.R., Kasper, F.K., Mikos, A.G., Jansen, J.A., Leeuwenburgh, S.C.G., et al., 2013. Development of an in vitro confinement test to predict the clinical handling of polymer-based injectable bone substitutes. Polym. Test. 32 (8), 1379–1384.

Boschin, F., Blanchemain, N., Bria, M., Delcourt-Debruyne, E., Morcellet, M., Hildebrand, H.F., et al., 2006. Improved drug delivery properties of PVDF membranes functionalized with β-cyclodextrin—application to guided tissue regeneration in periodontology. J. Biomed. Mater. Res., Part A 79A (1), 78–85.

Bowman, C.N., 2014. Smart shape changing and shape morphing polymeric materials. Polymer 55 (23), 5847–5848 (Editorial).

Brulisauer, L., Gauthier, M.A., Leroux, J.C., 2014. Disulfide-containing parenteral delivery systems and their redox-biological fate. J. Control. Release 195, 147–154.

Cabane, E., Zhang, X.Y., Langowska, K., Palivan, C.G., Meier, W., 2012. Stimuli-responsive polymers and their applications in nanomedicine. Biointerphases 7 (1–4), 9 (Review).

Cambre, J.N., Sumerlin, B.S., 2011. Biomedical applications of boronic acid polymers. Polymer 52 (21), 4631–4643.

Cao, P., Sun, X., Liang, Y., Gao, X., Li, X., Li, W., et al., 2015. Gene delivery by a cationic and thermosensitive nanogel promoted established tumor growth inhibition. Nanomedicine 10 (10), 1585–1597. http://dx.doi.org/10.2217/nnm.15.20.

Cardoso, V.F., Minas, G., Costa, C.M., Tavares, C.J., Lanceros-Mendez, S., 2011. Micro and nano-films of poly(vinylidene fluoride) with controlled thickness, morphology and electroactive crystalline phase for sensor and actuator applications. Smart Mater. Struct. 20 (8), 087002.

Cardoso, V.F., Costa, C.M., Minas, G., Lanceros-Mendez, S., 2012. Improving the optical and electroactive response of poly(vinylidene fluoride-trifluoroethylene) spin-coated films for sensor and actuator applications. Smart Mater. Struct. 21 (8).

Cardoso, V.F., Lopes, A.C., Botelho, G., Lanceros-Méndez, S., 2015. Poly(vinylidene fluoride-trifluoroethylene) porous films: tailoring microstructure and physical properties by solvent casting strategies. Soft Mater. 13 (4), 243–253.

Chesler, M., Chan, C.Y., 1988. Stimulus-induced extracellular pH transients in the in vitro turtle cerebellum. Neuroscience 27 (3), 941–948.

Chiquet, M., Gelman, L., Lutz, R., Maier, S., 2009. From mechanotransduction to extracellular matrix gene expression in fibroblasts. Biochim. Biophys. Acta, Mol. Cell Res. 1793 (5), 911–920.

Cho, J.K., Hong, K.Y., Park, J.W., Yang, H.K., Song, S.C., 2011. Injectable delivery system of 2-methoxyestradiol for breast cancer therapy using biodegradable thermosensitive poly(organophosphazene) hydrogel. J. Drug Target. 19 (4), 270–280.

Chu, L.Y., Li, Y., Zhu, J.H., Wang, H.D., Liang, Y.J., 2004. Control of pore size and permeability of a glucose-responsive gating membrane for insulin delivery. J. Control. Release 97 (1), 43–53.

Correia, D.M., Gonçalves, R., Ribeiro, C., Sencadas, V., Botelho, G., Ribelles, J.L.G., et al., 2014. Electrosprayed poly(vinylidene fluoride) microparticles for tissue engineering applications. RSC Adv. 4 (62), 33013–33021.

Correia, D.M., Ribeiro, C., Sencadas, V., Botelho, G., Carabineiro, S.A.C., Ribelles, J.L.G., et al., 2015. Influence of oxygen plasma treatment parameters on poly(vinylidene fluoride) electrospun fiber mats wettability. Prog. Org. Coat. 85, 151–158.

Correia, D.M., Ribeiro, C., Sencadas, V., Vikingsson, L., Oliver Gasch, M., Gómez Ribelles, J.L., et al., 2016. Strategies for the development of three dimensional scaffolds from piezoelectric poly(vinylidene fluoride). Mater. Des. 92, 674–681.

Cui, H., Liu, Y., Cheng, Y., Zhang, Z., Zhang, P., Chen, X., et al., 2014. In vitro study of electroactive tetraaniline-containing thermosensitive hydrogels for cardiac tissue engineering. Biomacromolecules 15 (4), 1115–1123.

Czaun, M., Hevesi, L., Takafuji, M., Ihara, H., 2008. A novel approach to magneto-responsive polymeric gels assisted by iron nanoparticles as nano cross-linkers. Chem. Commun. 18, 2124–2126.

da Silva, R.M.P., Mano, J.F., Reis, R.L., 2007. Smart thermoresponsive coatings and surfaces for tissue engineering: switching cell-material boundaries. Trends Biotechnol. 25 (12), 577–583.

Dai, S., Ravi, P., Tam, K.C., 2008. pH-responsive polymers: synthesis, properties and applications. Soft Matter 4 (3), 435–449.

Dang, J.M., Sun, D.D.N., Shin-Ya, Y., Sieber, A.N., Kostuik, J.P., Leong, K.W., 2006. Temperature-responsive hydroxybutyl chitosan for the culture of mesenchymal stem cells and intervertebral disk cells. Biomaterials 27 (3), 406–418.

Datla, N.V., Konh, B., Koo, J.J.Y., Choi, D.J.W., Yu, Y., Dicker, A.P., et al., 2014. Polyacrylamide phantom for self-actuating needle-tissue interaction studies. Med. Eng. Phys. 36 (1), 140–145.

de la Rica, R., Aili, D., Stevens, M.M., 2012. Enzyme-responsive nanoparticles for drug release and diagnostics. Adv. Drug Deliv. Rev. 64 (11), 967–978.

Delaviz, H., Faghihi, A., Azizzadeh Delshad, A., Bahadori, Mh., Mohamadi, J., Roozbehi, A., 2011. Repair of peripheral nerve defects using a polyvinylidene fluoride channel containing nerve growth factor and collagen gel in adult rats. Cell J. (Yakhteh) 13 (3(Autumn)), 137–142.

Ding, K., Yang, Z., Zhang, Y.L., Xu, J.Z., 2013. Injectable thermosensitive chitosan/β-glycerophosphate/collagen hydrogel maintains the plasticity of skeletal muscle satellite cells and supports their in vivo viability. Cell Biol. Int. 37 (9), 977–987.

Donkuru, M., Wettig, S.D., Verrall, R.E., Badea, I., Foldvari, M., 2012. Designing pH-sensitive gemini nanoparticles for non-viral gene delivery into keratinocytes. J. Mater. Chem. 22 (13), 6232–6244.

Dubkova, V.I., Alekseenko, V.I., Chudakov, O.P., Glinnik, A.V., Maevskaya, O.I., 1999. Piezoelectric effect in composite material implants designed for bone tissue displacement. Inzh.-Fiz. Zh. 72 (5), 1008–1015.

Evans, D.F., Pye, G., Bramley, R., Clark, A.G., Dyson, T.J., Hardcastle, J.D., 1988. Measurement of gastrointestinal pH profiles in normal ambulant human-subjects. Gut 29 (8), 1035–1041.

Evans, G.R.D., Brandt, K., Niederbichler, A.D., Chauvin, P., Hermann, S., Bogle, M., et al., 2000. Clinical long-term in vivo evaluation of poly(L-lactic acid) porous conduits for peripheral nerve regeneration. J. Biomater. Sci. Polym. Ed. 11 (8), 869–878. http://dx.doi.org/10.1163/156856200744066.

Fallingborg, J., 1999. Intraluminal pH of the human gastrointestinal tract. Dan. Med. Bull. 46 (3), 183–196 (0907-8916 (Print)).

Feng, G., Chen, H., Li, J., Huang, Q., Gupte, M.J., Liu, H., et al., 2015. Gene therapy for nucleus pulposus regeneration by heme oxygenase-1 plasmid DNA carried by mixed polyplex micelles with thermo-responsive heterogeneous coronas. Biomaterials 52, 1–13.

Ferreira, C.G., Cardoso, V.F., Lopes, A.C., Botelho, G., Lanceros-Méndez, S., 2015. Tailoring microstructure and physical properties of poly(vinylidene fluoride–hexafluoropropylene) porous films. J. Mater. Sci. 50 (14), 5047–5058.

Filipcsei, G., Fehér, J., Zrínyi, M., 2000. Electric field sensitive neutral polymer gels. J. Mol. Struct. 554 (1), 109–117.

Filipcsei, G., Csetneki, I., Szilagyi, A., Zrinyi, M., 2007. Magnetic field-responsive smart polymer composites. Oligomers Polymer Composties Molecular Imprinting. Springer-Verlag, Berlin pp. 137–189.

Fukada, E., Yasuda, I., 1957. On the piezoelectric effect of bone. J. Phys. Soc. Jpn. 12 (10), 1158–1162.

Gandhi, A., Paul, A., Sen, S.O., Sen, K.K., 2015. Studies on thermoresponsive polymers: phase behaviour, drug delivery and biomedical applications. Asian J. Pharm. Sci. 10 (2), 99–107.

Gao, W.W., Chan, J.M., Farokhzad, O.C., 2010. pH-responsive nanoparticles for drug delivery. Mol. Pharm. 7 (6), 1913–1920.

Garbern, J.C., Minami, E., Stayton, P.S., Murry, C.E., 2011. Delivery of basic fibroblast growth factor with a pH-responsive, injectable hydrogel to improve angiogenesis in infarcted myocardium. Biomaterials 32 (9), 2407–2416.

Gauthier, M.A., 2014. Redox-responsive drug delivery. Antioxid. Redox Signal. 21 (5), 705–706 (Editorial).

Gerweck, L.E., Seetharaman, K., 1996. Cellular pH gradient in tumor versus normal tissue: potential exploitation for the treatment of cancer. Cancer Res. 56 (6), 1194–1198.

Gil, E.S., Hudson, S.M., 2004. Stimuli-responsive polymers and their bioconjugates. Prog. Polym. Sci. 29 (12), 1173–1222.

Gonçalves, R., Martins, P.M., Caparrós, C., Martins, P., Benelmekki, M., Botelho, G., et al., 2013. Nucleation of the electroactive β-phase, dielectric and magnetic response of poly(vinylidene fluoride) composites with Fe_2O_3 nanoparticles. J. Non-Cryst. Solids 361 (1), 93–99.

Gonçalves, R., Martins, P., Correia, D.M., Sencadas, V., Vilas, J.L., León, L.M., et al., 2015a. Development of magnetoelectric $CoFe_2O_4$/poly(vinylidene fluoride) microspheres. RSC Adv. 5 (45), 35852–35857.

Gonçalves, R., Martins, P., Moya, X., Ghidini, M., Sencadas, V., Botelho, G., et al., 2015b. Magnetoelectric $CoFe_2O_4$/polyvinylidene fluoride electrospun nanofibres. Nanoscale 7 (17), 8058–8061.

Gray, H.N., Bergbreiter, D.E., 1997. Applications of polymeric smart materials to environmental problems. Environ. Health Perspect. 105 (Suppl. 1), 55–63 (Research Support, Non-U.S. Gov't; Research Support, U.S. Gov't, Non-P.H.S.; Review).

Guan, Y., Zhang, Y.J., 2013. Boronic acid-containing hydrogels: synthesis and their applications. Chem. Soc. Rev. 42 (20), 8106–8121.

Guduru, R., Liang, P., Runowicz, C., Nair, M., Atluri, V., Khizroev, S., 2013. Magneto-electric nanoparticles to enable field-controlled high-specificity drug delivery to eradicate ovarian cancer cells. Sci. Rep. 3, 2953.

Guo, M., Que, C., Wang, C., Liu, X., Yan, H., Liu, K., 2011. Multifunctional superparamagnetic nanocarriers with folate-mediated and pH-responsive targeting properties for anticancer drug delivery. Biomaterials 32 (1), 185–194.

Guragain, S., Bastakoti, B.P., Malgras, V., Nakashima, K., Yamauchi, Y., 2015. Multi-stimuli-responsive polymeric materials. Chem. Eur. J. 21 (38), 13164–13174.

Haladjova, E., Toncheva-Moncheva, N., Apostolova, M.D., Trzebicka, B., Dworak, A., Petrov, P., et al., 2014. Polymeric nanoparticle engineering: from temperature-responsive polymer mesoglobules to gene delivery systems. Biomacromolecules 15 (12), 4377–4395. http://dx.doi.org/10.1021/bm501194g.

Hamidi, M., Shahbazi, M.A., Rostamizadeh, K., 2012. Copolymers: efficient carriers for intelligent nanoparticulate drug targeting and gene therapy. Macromol. Biosci. 12 (2), 144–164.

Han, B.G., Ding, S.Q., Yu, X., 2015. Intrinsic self-sensing concrete and structures: a review. Measurement 59, 110–128.

Harimoto, M., Yamato, M., Hirose, M., Takahashi, C., Isoi, Y., Kikuchi, A., et al., 2002. Novel approach for achieving double-layered cell sheets co-culture: overlaying endothelial cell sheets onto monolayer hepatocytes utilizing temperature-responsive culture dishes. J. Biomed. Mater. Res. 62 (3), 464–470.

Hasan, A., Khattab, A., Islam, M.A., Hweij, K.A., Zeitouny, J., Waters, R., et al., 2015. Injectable hydrogels for cardiac tissue repair after myocardial infarction. Adv. Sci. 2 (11), 1500122.

He, T., Wang, J., Huang, P., Zeng, B., Li, H., Cao, Q., et al., 2015. Electrospinning polyvinylidene fluoride fibrous membranes containing anti-bacterial drugs used as wound dressing. Colloids Surf. B: Biointerfaces 130, 278–286.

Hoffman, A.S., 2013. Stimuli-responsive polymers: biomedical applications and challenges for clinical translation. Adv. Drug Deliv. Rev. 65 (1), 10–16.

Hopkinson, A., Varghese, V.M., Kumary, T.V., Dua, H.S., 2008. A novel cytocompatible thermoresponsive co-polymer for corneal tissue engineering. Acta Ophthalmol. 86.

Hu, Y., Litwin, T., Nagaraja, A.R., Kwong, B., Katz, J., Watson, N., et al., 2007. Cytosolic delivery of membrane-impermeable molecules in dendritic cells using pH-responsive core–shell nanoparticles. Nano Lett. 7 (10), 3056–3064. http://dx.doi.org/10.1021/nl071542i.

Hu, J.M., Zhang, G.Q., Liu, S.Y., 2012. Enzyme-responsive polymeric assemblies, nanoparticles and hydrogels. Chem. Soc. Rev. 41 (18), 5933–5949.

Huo, M., Yuan, J., Tao, L., Wei, Y., 2014. Redox-responsive polymers for drug delivery: from molecular design to applications. Polym. Chem. 5 (5), 1519–1528. http://dx.doi.org/10.1039/C3PY01192E.

Hurkat, P., Jain, A., Shilpi, S., Gulbake, A., Jain, S.K., 2012. Concanavalin A conjugated biodegradable nanoparticles for oral insulin delivery. J. Nanopart. Res. 14, 1219.

Hwang, I.H., Lee, J.H., 2006. Self-actuating biosensor using a piezoelectric cantilever and its optimization. In: International Mems Conference 2006. Iop Publishing Ltd, Bristol, pp. 362–367.

Ikoba, U., Peng, H., Li, H., Miller, C., Yu, C., Wang, Q., 2015. Nanocarriers in therapy of infectious and inflammatory diseases. Nanoscale 7 (10), 4291–4305.

Iwai, R., Haruki, R., Nemoto, Y., Nakayama, Y., 2013. Enhanced transfection efficiency of poly(*N*,*N*-dimethylaminoethyl methacrylate)-based deposition transfection by combination with tris(hydroxymethyl)aminomethane. Bioconjug. Chem. 24 (2), 159–166. http://dx.doi.org/10.1021/bc300317e.

Jackson, N., Stam, F., 2015. Optimization of electrical stimulation parameters for electro-responsive hydrogels for biomedical applications. J. Appl. Polym. Sci. 132 (12), 41687.

Jen, C.J., Jhiang, S.-J., Chen, H.-I., 2000. Invited Review: effects of flow on vascular endothelial intracellular calcium signaling of rat aortas ex vivo. J. Appl. Physiol. 89 (4), 1657–1662.

Jeong, B., Gutowska, A., 2002. Lessons from nature: stimuli-responsive polymers and their biomedical applications. Trends Biotechnol. 20 (7), 305–311.

Jin, Z.H., Jin, M.J., Jiang, C.G., Yin, X.Z., Jin, S.Z., Quan, X.Q., et al., 2014. Evaluation of doxorubicin-loaded pH-sensitive polymeric micelle release from tumor blood vessels and anticancer efficacy using a dorsal skin-fold window chamber model. Acta Pharmacol. Sin. 35 (6), 839–845.

Jones, D.S., Lorimer, C.P., McCoy, C.P., Gorman, S.P., 2008. Characterization of the physicochemical, antimicrobial, and drug release properties of thermoresponsive hydrogel copolymers designed for medical device applications. J. Biomed. Mater. Res. B Appl. Biomater. 85B (2), 417–426.

Jordan, O., Doelker, E., Rüfenacht, D., 2005. Biomaterials used in injectable implants (liquid embolics) for percutaneous filling of vascular spaces. Cardiovasc. Intervent. Radiol. 28 (5), 561–569.

Kaushik, A., Jayant, R.D., Sagar, V., Nair, M., 2014. The potential of magneto-electric nanocarriers for drug delivery. Expert Opin. Drug Deliv. 11 (10), 1635–1646.

Kawamura, M., Miyagawa, S., Miki, K., Saito, A., Fukushima, S., Higuchi, T., et al., 2012. Feasibility, safety, and therapeutic efficacy of human induced pluripotent stem cell-derived cardiomyocyte sheets in a porcine ischemic cardiomyopathy model. Circulation 126 (11(Suppl. 1)), S29–S37.

Kelly, G., 2006. Body temperature variability (Part 1): a review of the history of body temperature and its variability due to site selection, biological rhythms, fitness, and aging. Altern. Med. Rev. 11 (4), 278–293.

Kim, S., Kim, J.H., Jeon, O., Kwon, I.C., Park, K., 2009. Engineered polymers for advanced drug delivery. Eur. J. Pharm. Biopharm. 71 (3), 420–430.

Klein-Nulend, J., Bacabac, R.G., Bakker, A.D., 2012. Mechanical loading and how it affects bone cells: the role of the osteocyte cytoskeleton in maintaining our skeleton. Eur. Cell Mater. 24, 278–291.

Klouda, L., 2015. Thermoresponsive hydrogels in biomedical applications a seven-year update. Eur. J. Pharm. Biopharm. 97, 338–349.

Klouda, L., Mikos, A.G., 2008. Thermoresponsive hydrogels in biomedical applications. Eur. J. Pharm. Biopharm. 68 (1), 34–45.

Kulkarni, R.V., Boppana, R., Krishna Mohan, G., Mutalik, S., Kalyane, N.V., 2012. pH-responsive interpenetrating network hydrogel beads of poly(acrylamide)-g-carrageenan and sodium alginate for intestinal targeted drug delivery: synthesis, in vitro and in vivo evaluation. J. Colloid Interface Sci. 367 (1), 509–517.

Kushida, A., Yamato, M., Kikuchi, A., Okano, T., 2001. Two-dimensional manipulation of differentiated Madin-Darby canine kidney (MDCK) cell sheets: the noninvasive harvest from temperature-responsive culture dishes and transfer to other surfaces. J. Biomed. Mater. Res. 54 (1), 37–46.

Kwon, J.S., Park, I.K., Cho, A.S., Shin, S.M., Hong, M.H., Jeong, S.Y., et al., 2009. Enhanced angiogenesis mediated by vascular endothelial growth factor plasmid-loaded thermo-responsive amphiphilic polymer in a rat myocardial infarction model. J. Control. Release 138 (2), 168–176.

Lee, P.-Y., Li, Z., Huang, L., 2003. Thermosensitive hydrogel as a Tgf-β1 gene delivery vehicle enhances diabetic wound healing. Pharm. Res. 20 (12), 1995–2000.

Leones, R., Costa, C.M., Machado, A.V., Esperança, J.M.S.S., Silva, M.M., Lanceros-Méndez, S., 2014. Effect of ionic liquid anion type in the performance of solid polymer electrolytes based on poly(vinylidene fluoride-trifluoroethylene). Electroanalysis 27 (2), 457–464.

Li, P., Liu, D., Miao, L., Liu, C., Sun, X., Liu, Y., et al., 2012. A pH-sensitive multifunctional gene carrier assembled via layer-by-layer technique for efficient gene delivery. Int. J. Nanomedicine 7, 925–939.

Lim, C.T., Zhou, E.H., Quek, S.T., 2006. Mechanical models for living cells—a review. J. Biomech. 39 (2), 195–216.

Lin, Y.-H., Chang, C.-H., Wu, Y.-S., Hsu, Y.-M., Chiou, S.-F., Chen, Y.-J., 2009. Development of pH-responsive chitosan/heparin nanoparticles for stomach-specific anti-*Helicobacter pylori* therapy. Biomaterials 30 (19), 3332–3342.

Lin, X.K., Chen, L., Zhao, Y.P., Dong, Z.Z., 2010. Synthesis and characterization of thermoresponsive shape-memory poly(stearyl acrylate-*co*-acrylamide) hydrogels. J. Mater. Sci. 45 (10), 2703–2707.

Liu, F., Urban, M.W., 2010. Recent advances and challenges in designing stimuli-responsive polymers. Prog. Polym. Sci. 35 (1–2), 3–23.

Liu, Y., Servant, A., Guy, O.J., Al-Jamal, K.T., Williams, P.R., Hawkins, K.M., et al., 2011. An electric-field responsive microsystem for controllable miniaturised drug delivery applications. In: Kaltsas, G., Tsamis, C. (Eds.), Eurosensors XXV. Elsevier Science Bv, Amsterdam.

Liu, Y.D., Hong, C.H., Choi, H.J., 2012. Polymeric colloidal magnetic composite microspheres and their magneto-responsive characteristics. Macromol. Res. 20 (12), 1211–1218.

Long, T., Zhu, Z., Awad, H.A., Schwarz, E.M., Hilton, M.J., Dong, Y., 2014. The effect of mesenchymal stem cell sheets on structural allograft healing of critical-sized femoral defects in mice. Biomaterials 35 (9), 2752–2759.

Lu, H.F., Targonsky, E.D., Wheeler, M.B., Cheng, Y.L., 2007. Thermally induced gelable polymer networks for living cell encapsulation. Biotechnol. Bioeng. 96 (1), 146–155.

Ma, R.J., Shi, L.Q., 2014. Phenylboronic acid-based glucose-responsive polymeric nanoparticles: synthesis and applications in drug delivery. Polym. Chem. 5 (5), 1503–1518.

MacEwan, S.R., Callahan, D.J., Chilkoti, A., 2010. Stimulus-responsive macromolecules and nanoparticles for cancer drug delivery. Nanomedicine 5 (5), 793–806. http://dx.doi.org/10.2217/nnm.10.50.

Magnotta, V.A., Heo, H.-Y., Dlouhy, B.J., Dahdaleh, N.S., Follmer, R.L., Thedens, D.R., et al., 2012. Detecting activity-evoked pH changes in human brain. Proc. Natl. Acad. Sci. U. S. A. 109 (21), 8270–8273.

Mahmoud, E.A., Sankaranarayanan, J., Morachis, J.M., Kim, G., Almutairi, A., 2011. Inflammation responsive logic gate nanoparticles for the delivery of proteins. Bioconjug. Chem. 22 (7), 1416–1421.

Manchun, S., Dass, C.R., Sriamornsak, P., 2012. Targeted therapy for cancer using pH-responsive nanocarrier systems. Life Sci. 90 (11–12), 381–387.

Marchi, S., Casu, A., Bertora, F., Athanassiou, A., Fragouli, D., 2015. Highly magneto-responsive elastomeric films created by a two-step fabrication process. ACS Appl. Mater. Interfaces 7 (34), 19112–19118.

Marek, S.R., Peppas, N.A., 2013. Insulin release dynamics from poly(diethylaminoethyl methacrylate) hydrogel systems. AIChE J. 59 (10), 3578–3585.

Martins, P., Lanceros-Méndez, S., 2013. Polymer-based magnetoelectric materials. Adv. Funct. Mater. 23 (27), 3371–3385.

Martins, P.M., Ribeiro, S., Ribeiro, C., Sencadas, V., Gomes, A.C., Gama, F.M., et al., 2013. Effect of poling state and morphology of piezoelectric poly(vinylidene fluoride) membranes for skeletal muscle tissue engineering. RSC Adv. 3 (39), 17938–17944.

Martins, P., Lopes, A.C., Lanceros-Mendez, S., 2014. Electroactive phases of poly(vinylidene fluoride): determination, processing and applications. Prog. Polym. Sci. 39 (4), 683–706.

Martins, P., Gonçalves, R., Lopes, A.C., Venkata Ramana, E., Mendiratta, S.K., Lanceros-Mendez, S., 2015. Novel hybrid multifunctional magnetoelectric porous composite films. J. Magn. Magn. Mater. 396, 237–241.
McCabe, J.F., Yan, Z.Q., Al Naimi, O.T., Mahmoud, G., Rolland, S.L., 2009. Smart materials in dentistry—future prospects. Dent. Mater. J. 28 (1), 37–43.
McCarley, R.L., 2012. Redox-Responsive Delivery Systems. In: Cooks, R.G., Yeung, E.S. (Eds.), Annual Review of Analytical Chemistry, vol. 5, pp. 391–411.
Medeiros, S.F., Santos, A.M., Fessi, H., Elaissari, A., 2011. Stimuli-responsive magnetic particles for biomedical applications. Int. J. Pharm. 403 (1–2), 139–161.
Mejri, R., Dias, J.C., Lopes, A.C., Hentati, S.B., Silva, M.M., Botelho, G., et al., 2015. Effect of ionic liquid anion and cation on the physico-chemical properties of poly(vinylidene fluoride)/ionic liquid blends. Eur. Polym. J. 71, 304–313.
Meng, H., Hu, J.L., 2010. A brief review of stimulus-active polymers responsive to thermal, light, magnetic, electric, and water/solvent stimuli. J. Intell. Mater. Syst. Struct. 21 (9), 859–885.
Meyer, M., Philipp, A., Oskuee, R., Schmidt, C., Wagner, E., 2008. Breathing life into polycations: functionalization with pH-responsive endosomolytic peptides and polyethylene glycol enables siRNA delivery. J. Am. Chem. Soc. 130 (11), 3272–3273. http://dx.doi.org/10.1021/ja710344v.
Miyata, T., Asami, N., Uragami, T., 1999. A reversibly antigen-responsive hydrogel. Nature 399 (6738), 766–769.
Motornov, M., Roiter, Y., Tokarev, I., Minko, S., 2010. Stimuli-responsive nanoparticles, nanogels and capsules for integrated multifunctional intelligent systems. Prog. Polym. Sci. 35 (1–2), 174–211.
Murase, Y., Maeda, S., Hashimoto, S., Yoshida, R., 2009. Design of a mass transport surface utilizing peristaltic motion of a self-oscillating gel. Langmuir 25 (1), 483–489.
Murdan, S., 2003. Electro-responsive drug delivery from hydrogels. J. Control. Release 92 (1–2), 1–17.
Nair, M., Guduru, R., Liang, P., Hong, J., Sagar, V., Khizroev, S., 2013. Externally controlled on-demand release of anti-HIV drug using magneto-electric nanoparticles as carriers. Nat. Commun. 4, 1707.
Nishida, K., Yamato, M., Hayashida, Y., Watanabe, K., Maeda, N., Watanabe, H., et al., 2004. Functional bioengineered corneal epithelial sheet grafts from corneal stem cells expanded ex vivo on a temperature-responsive cell culture surface. Transplantation 77 (3), 379–385.
Nitschke, M., Gramm, S., Götze, T., Valtink, M., Drichel, J., Voit, B., et al., 2007. Thermo-responsive poly(NiPAAm-*co*-DEGMA) substrates for gentle harvest of human corneal endothelial cell sheets. J. Biomed. Mater. Res. A 80A (4), 1003–1010.
Nunes-Pereira, J., Ribeiro, S., Ribeiro, C., Gombek, C.J., Gama, F.M., Gomes, A.C., et al., 2015. Poly(vinylidene fluoride) and copolymers as porous membranes for tissue engineering applications. Polym. Test. 44, 234–241.
Ochoa, M., Mousoulis, C., Ziaie, B., 2012. Polymeric microdevices for transdermal and subcutaneous drug delivery. Adv. Drug Deliv. Rev. 64 (14), 1603–1616.
Ogawa, R., 2011. Mechanobiology of scarring. Wound Repair Regen. 19, s2–s9.
Paris, J.L., Cabanas, M.V., Manzano, M., Vallet-Regi, M., 2015. Polymer-grafted mesoporous silica nanoparticles as ultrasound-responsive drug carriers. ACS Nano 9 (11), 11023–11033.
Pastuszka, M.K., MacKay, J.A., 2016. Engineering structure and function using thermoresponsive biopolymers. Wiley Interdiscip. Rev. Nanomed. Nanobiotechnol. 8 (1), 123–138.
Peppas, N.A., 2004. Is there a future in glucose-sensitive, responsive insulin delivery systems? J. Drug Deliv. Sci. Technol. 14 (4), 247–256.

Pesirikan, N., Chang, W., Zhang, X., Xu, J., Yu, X., 2013. Characterization of Schwann cells in self-assembled sheets from thermoresponsive substrates. Tissue Eng. Part A 19 (13–14), 1601–1609.

Pillay, V., Tsai, T.S., Choonara, Y.E., du Toit, L.C., Kumar, P., Modi, G., et al., 2014. A review of integrating electroactive polymers as responsive systems for specialized drug delivery applications. J. Biomed. Mater. Res., Part A 102 (6), 2039–2054.

Pirraco, R.P., Obokata, H., Iwata, T., Marques, A.P., Tsuneda, S., Yamato, M., et al., 2011. Development of osteogenic cell sheets for bone tissue engineering applications. Tissue Eng. Part A 17 (11–12), 1507–1515.

Priya James, H., John, R., Alex, A., Anoop, K.R., 2014. Smart polymers for the controlled delivery of drugs—a concise overview. Acta Pharm. Sin. B 4 (2), 120–127.

Putnam, D., Zelikin, A.N., Izumrudov, V.A., Langer, R., 2003. Polyhistidine–PEG:DNA nanocomposites for gene delivery. Biomaterials 24 (24), 4425–4433.

Qian, Y.C., Chen, P.C., Zhu, X.Y., Huang, X.J., 2015. Click synthesis of ionic strength-responsive polyphosphazene hydrogel for reversible binding of enzymes. RSC Adv. 5 (55), 44031–44040.

Rajagopalan, M., Jeon, J.H., Oh, I.K., 2010. Electric-stimuli-responsive bending actuator based on sulfonated polyetherimide. Sens. Actuators B 151 (1), 198–204.

Rasmussen, M.K., Pedersen, E.W., Petersen, M.G., Hornb, K., 2012. Shape-changing interfaces: a review of the design space and open research questions. In: Proceedings of the SIGCHI Conference on Human Factors in Computing Systems; Austin, Texas, USA. ACM, New York, NY, pp. 735–744.

Ravaine, V., Ancla, C., Catargi, B., 2008. Chemically controlled closed-loop insulin delivery. J. Control. Release 132 (1), 2–11.

Reinicke, S., Dohler, S., Tea, S., Krekhova, M., Messing, R., Schmidt, A.M., et al., 2010. Magneto-responsive hydrogels based on maghemite/triblock terpolymer hybrid micelles. Soft Matter 6 (12), 2760–2773.

Ribeiro, C., Sencadas, V., Ribelles, J.L.G., Lanceros-Méndez, S., 2010. Influence of processing conditions on polymorphism and nanofiber morphology of electroactive poly(vinylidene fluoride) electrospun membranes. Soft Mater. 8 (3), 274–287.

Ribeiro, C., Moreira, S., Correia, V., Sencadas, V., Rocha, J.G., Gama, F.M., et al., 2012. Enhanced proliferation of pre-osteoblastic cells by dynamic piezoelectric stimulation. RSC Adv. 2 (30), 11504–11509.

Ribeiro, C., Correia, D.M., Ribeiro, S., Sencadas, V., Botelho, G., Lanceros-Méndez, S., 2015a. Piezoelectric poly(vinylidene fluoride) microstructure and poling state in active tissue engineering. Eng. Life Sci. 15 (4), 351–356 (Review).

Ribeiro, C., Sencadas, V., Correia, D.M., Lanceros-Méndez, S., 2015b. Piezoelectric polymers as biomaterials for tissue engineering applications. Colloids Surf. B: Biointerfaces 136, 46–55. Review.

Ribeiro, C., Pärssinen, J., Sencadas, V., Correia, V., Miettinen, S., Hytönen, V.P., et al., 2015c. Dynamic piezoelectric stimulation enhances osteogenic differentiation of human adipose stem cells. J. Biomed. Mater. Res. A 103 (6), 2172–2175.

Ribeiro, C., Correia, V., Martins, P., Gama, F.M., Lanceros-Mendez, S., 2016. Proving the suitability of magnetoelectric stimuli for tissue engineering applications. Colloids Surf. B: Biointerfaces 140, 430–436.

Ridi, F., Bonini, M., Baglioni, P., 2014. Magneto-responsive nanocomposites: preparation and integration of magnetic nanoparticles into films, capsules, and gels. Adv. Colloid Interface Sci. 207, 3–13.

Roy, I., Gupta, M.N., 2003. Smart polymeric materials: emerging biochemical applications. Chem. Biol. 10 (12), 1161–1171 (Review).

Roy, D., Cambre, J.N., Sumerlin, B.S., 2010. Future perspectives and recent advances in stimuli-responsive materials. Prog. Polym. Sci. 35 (1–2), 278–301 (Review).
Roy, D., Brooks, W.L.A., Sumerlin, B.S., 2013. New directions in thermoresponsive polymers. Chem. Soc. Rev. 42 (17), 7214–7243 (Review).
Russina, O., Lo Celso, F., Triolo, A., 2015. Pressure-responsive mesoscopic structures in room temperature ionic liquids. Phys. Chem. Chem. Phys. 17 (44), 29496–29500.
Rwei, A.Y., Wang, W.P., Kohane, D.S., 2015. Photoresponsive nanoparticles for drug delivery. Nano Today 10 (4), 451–467 (Review).
Sahota, T., Tomlins, P., Taylor, M.J., 2015. Long-term stability of glucose responsive dextran methacrylate-concanavalin A methacrylamide gels as part of an implantable artificial pancreas. Int. J. Polym. Mater. Polym. Biomater. 64 (18), 946–954.
Salazar, H., Lima, A.C., Lopes, A.C., Botelho, G., Lanceros-Mendez, S., 2015. Poly(vinylidene fluoride-trifluoroethylene)/NAY zeolite hybrid membranes as a drug release platform applied to ibuprofen release. Colloids Surf. A Physicochem. Eng. Asp. 469, 93–99.
Saleem, M., Yu, H.J., Wang, L., Zain-ul-Abdin, Khalid, H., Akram, M., et al., 2015. Review on synthesis of ferrocene-based redox polymers and derivatives and their application in glucose sensing. Anal. Chim. Acta 876, 9–25 (Review).
Sato, Y., Hatakeyama, H., Sakurai, Y., Hyodo, M., Akita, H., Harashima, H., 2012. A pH-sensitive cationic lipid facilitates the delivery of liposomal siRNA and gene silencing activity in vitro and in vivo. J. Control. Release 163 (3), 267–276.
Schattling, P., Jochum, F.D., Theato, P., 2014. Multi-stimuli responsive polymers—the all-in-one talents. Polym. Chem. 5 (1), 25–36 (Review).
Schmaljohann, D., 2006. Thermo- and pH-responsive polymers in drug delivery. Adv. Drug Deliv. Rev. 58 (15), 1655–1670.
Seki, T., 2004. Dynamic photoresponsive functions in organized layer systems comprised of azobenzene-containing polymers. Polym. J. 36 (6), 435–454 (Review).
Seki, T., 2007. Smart photoresponsive polymer systems organized in two dimensions. Bull. Chem. Soc. Jpn. 80 (11), 2084–2109 (Review).
Sethuraman, V.A., Na, K., Bae, Y.H., 2006. pH-responsive sulfonamide/PEI system for tumor specific gene delivery: an in vitro study. Biomacromolecules 7 (1), 64–70. http://dx.doi.org/10.1021/bm0503571.
Shi, B., Zhang, H., Bi, J., Dai, S., 2014. Endosomal pH responsive polymers for efficient cancer targeted gene therapy. Colloids Surf. B: Biointerfaces 119, 55–65.
Shimizu, T., Yamato, M., Kikuchi, A., Okano, T., 2003. Cell sheet engineering for myocardial tissue reconstruction. Biomaterials 24 (13), 2309–2316.
Shin, H.S., Kim, S.Y., Lee, Y.M., 1997. Indomethacin release behaviors from pH and thermo-responsive poly(vinyl alcohol) and poly(acrylic acid) IPN hydrogels for site-specific drug delivery. J. Appl. Polym. Sci. 65 (4), 685–693.
Singh, B., Choi, Y.J., Park, I.K., Akaike, T., Cho, C.S., 2014. Chemical modification of chitosan with pH-sensitive molecules and specific ligands for efficient DNA transfection and siRNA silencing. J. Nanosci. Nanotechnol. 14 (1), 564–576.
Soppimath, K.S., Aminabhavi, T.M., Dave, A.M., Kumbar, S.G., Rudzinski, W.E., 2002. Stimulus-responsive "smart" hydrogels as novel drug delivery systems. Drug Dev. Ind. Pharm. 28 (8), 957–974.
Stabenfeldt, S.E., García, A.J., LaPlaca, M.C., 2006. Thermoreversible laminin-functionalized hydrogel for neural tissue engineering. J. Biomed. Mater. Res. A 77A (4), 718–725.
Stackhouse, S.K., Reisman, D.S., Binder-Macleod, S.A., 2001. Challenging the role of pH in skeletal muscle fatigue. Phys. Ther. 81 (12), 1897–1903.

Street, D., Bangsbo, J., Juel, C., 2001. Interstitial pH in human skeletal muscle during and after dynamic graded exercise. J. Physiol. 537 (Pt 3), 993–998.

Su, S., Tian, Y., Li, Y., Ding, Y., Ji, T., Wu, M., et al., 2015. "Triple-punch" strategy for triple negative breast cancer therapy with minimized drug dosage and improved antitumor efficacy. ACS Nano 9 (2), 1367–1378. http://dx.doi.org/10.1021/nn505729m.

Tabary, N., Lepretre, S., Boschin, F., Blanchemain, N., Neut, C., Delcourt-Debruyne, E., et al., 2007. Functionalization of PVDF membranes with carbohydrate derivates for the controlled delivery of chlorhexidin. Biomol. Eng. 24 (5), 472–476.

Takeda, N., Nakamura, E., Yokoyama, M., Okano, T., 2004. Temperature-responsive polymeric carriers incorporating hydrophobic monomers for effective transfection in small doses. J. Control. Release 95 (2), 343–355.

Takezawa, T., Mori, Y., Yoshizato, K., 1990. Cell culture on a thermo-responsive polymer surface. Biotechnology 8 (9), 854–856.

Tan, H., Ramirez, C.M., Miljkovic, N., Li, H., Rubin, J.P., Marra, K.G., 2009. Thermosensitive injectable hyaluronic acid hydrogel for adipose tissue engineering. Biomaterials 30 (36), 6844–6853.

Tang, Z., Akiyama, Y., Okano, T., 2012. Temperature-responsive polymer modified surface for cell sheet engineering. Polymer 4 (3), 1478–1498.

Tannock, I.F., Rotin, D., 1989. Acid pH in tumors and its potential for therapeutic exploitation. Cancer Res. 49 (16), 4373–4384.

Teichmann, J., Nitschke, M., Pette, D., Valtink, M., Gramm, S., Härtel, F.V., et al., 2015. Thermo-responsive cell culture carriers based on poly(vinyl methyl ether)—the effect of biomolecular ligands to balance cell adhesion and stimulated detachment. Sci. Technol. Adv. Mater. 16 (4), 045003.

Tekin, H., Sanchez, J.G., Tsinman, T., Langer, R., Khademhosseini, A., 2011. Thermoresponsive platforms for tissue engineering and regenerative medicine. AICHE J. 57 (12), 3249–3258.

Terracio, L., Miller, B., Borg, T.K., 1988. Effects of cyclic mechanical stimulation of the cellular components of the heart: in vitro. In Vitro Cell. Dev. Biol. 24 (1), 53–58.

Thamphiwatana, S., Fu, V., Zhu, J., Lu, D., Gao, W., Zhang, L., 2013. Nanoparticle-stabilized liposomes for pH-responsive gastric drug delivery. Langmuir: ACS J. Surf. Colloids 29 (39), 12228–12233.

Thevenot, J., Oliveira, H., Sandre, O., Lecommandoux, S., 2013. Magnetic responsive polymer composite materials. Chem. Soc. Rev. 42 (17), 7099–7116. http://dx.doi.org/10.1039/C3CS60058K.

Tomatsu, I., Peng, K., Kros, A., 2011. Photoresponsive hydrogels for biomedical applications. Adv. Drug Deliv. Rev. 63 (14–15), 1257–1266 (Review).

Tran, P.-L., Tran, T.-D., Vo, V., Lee, B.-J., 2013. pH-sensitive polymeric systems for controlling drug release in nocturnal asthma treatment. In: Toi, V.V., Toan, N.B., Dang Khoa, T.Q., Lien Phuong, T.H. (Eds.), 4th International Conference on Biomedical Engineering in Vietnam. Springer, Berlin/Heidelberg, pp. 304–308.

Twaites, B.R., de las Heras Alarcón, C., Lavigne, M., Saulnier, A., Pennadam, S.S., Cunliffe, D., et al., 2005. Thermoresponsive polymers as gene delivery vectors: cell viability, DNA transport and transfection studies. J. Control. Release 108 (2–3), 472–483.

Uchiyama, T., Kiritoshi, Y., Watanabe, J., Ishihara, K., 2003. Degradation of phospholipid polymer hydrogel by hydrogen peroxide aiming at insulin release device. Biomaterials 24 (28), 5183–5190.

Verbrugghe, P., Verhoeven, J., Coudyzer, W., Verbeken, E., Dubruel, P., Mendes, E., et al., 2015. An electro-responsive hydrogel for intravascular applications: an in vitro and in vivo evaluation. J. Mater. Sci. Mater. Med. 26 (11), 264.

Wang, G.J., Zhang, J., 2012. Photoresponsive molecular switches for biotechnology. J. Photochem. Photobiol. C: Photochem. Rev. 13 (4), 299–309.
Wang, W., Wang, X.Z., Cheng, F.T., Yu, Y.L., Zhu, Y.T., 2011. Light-driven soft actuators based on photoresponsive polymer materials. Prog. Chem. 23 (6), 1165–1173.
Ward, M.A., Georgiou, T.K., 2011. Thermoresponsive polymers for biomedical applications. Polymer 3 (3), 1215–1242 (Review).
Wee, K.W., Kang, G.Y., Park, J., Kang, J.Y., Yoon, D.S., Park, J.H., et al., 2005. Novel electrical detection of label-free disease marker proteins using piezoresistive self-sensing micro-cantilevers. Biosens. Bioelectron. 20 (10), 1932–1938 (Proceedings paper).
Wei, J.J., Ren, L.X., Tang, C.B., Su, Z.H., 2014. Electric-stimulus-responsive multilayer films based on a cobaltocenium-containing polymer. Polym. Chem. 5 (22), 6480–6488.
Wu, W.T., Zhou, S.Q., 2013. Responsive materials for self-regulated insulin delivery. Macromol. Biosci. 13 (11), 1464–1477 (Review).
Wu, D.Y., Meure, S., Solomon, D., 2008. Self-healing polymeric materials: a review of recent developments. Prog. Polym. Sci. 33 (5), 479–522 (Review).
Wu, Q., Wang, L., Yu, H.J., Wang, J.J., Chen, Z.F., 2011. Organization of glucose-responsive systems and their properties. Chem. Rev. 111 (12), 7855–7875.
Xia, F., Jiang, L., 2008. Bio-inspired, smart, multiscale interfacial materials. Adv. Mater. 20 (15), 2842–2858 (Review).
Xu, H.Y., Gu, N., 2014. Magnetic responsive scaffolds and magnetic fields in bone repair and regeneration. Front. Mater. Sci. 8 (1), 20–31 (Review).
Yamato, M., Utsumi, M., Kushida, A., Konno, C., Kikuchi, A., Okano, T., 2001. Thermo-responsive culture dishes allow the intact harvest of multilayered keratinocyte sheets without dispase by reducing temperature. Tissue Eng. 7 (4), 473–480.
Yang, Y., Urban, M.W., 2013. Self-healing polymeric materials. Chem. Soc. Rev. 42 (17), 7446–7467 (Review).
Yang, J., Yamato, M., Nishida, K., Hayashida, Y., Shimizu, T., Kikuchi, A., et al., 2006. Corneal epithelial stem cell delivery using cell sheet engineering: not lost in transplantation. J. Drug Target. 14 (7), 471–482. http://dx.doi.org/10.1080/10611860600847997.
Yin, R., Han, J., Zhang, J., Nie, J., 2010. Glucose-responsive composite microparticles based on chitosan, concanavalin A and dextran for insulin delivery. Colloids Surf. B: Biointerfaces 76 (2), 483–488.
Yoshida, R., Tanaka, M., Onodera, S., Yamaguchi, T., Kokufuta, E., 2000. In-phase synchronization of chemical and mechanical oscillations in self-oscillating gels. J. Phys. Chem. A 104 (32), 7549–7555.
Yu, H.F., Kobayashi, T., 2010. Photoresponsive block copolymers containing azobenzenes and other chromophores. Molecules 15 (1), 570–603 (Review).
Zelzer, M., Todd, S.J., Hirst, A.R., McDonald, T.O., Ulijn, R.V., 2013. Enzyme responsive materials: design strategies and future developments. Biomater. Sci. 1 (1), 11–39 (Review).
Zhai, L., 2013. Stimuli-responsive polymer films. Chem. Soc. Rev. 42 (17), 7148–7160 (Review).
Zhang, W.L., Choi, H.J., 2014. Stimuli-responsive polymers and colloids under electric and magnetic fields. Polymer 6 (11), 2803–2818 (Review).
Zhao, Y.Z., Du, L.N., Lu, C.T., Jin, Y.G., Ge, S.P., 2013. Potential and problems in ultrasound-responsive drug delivery systems. Int. J. Nanomedicine 8, 1621–1633 (Review).
Zhu, Y.J., Chen, F., 2015. pH-responsive drug-delivery systems. Chem. Asian J. 10 (2), 284–305.

Molecular signalling mechanisms of host–materials interactions

4

J.F. da Silva Domingues, T.G. Van Kooten*†

*Institute of Pharmacology and Structural Biology, CNRS UMR 5089, Toulouse Cedex, France, †University of Groningen, Groningen, The Netherlands

4.1 Introduction

The host response to biomaterials applied or in contact with the human body has been studied for decades, together with the study of diverse materials for medical applications. The term biocompatibility is strongly associated with the use of biomaterials and, although its meaning is often reduced to biosafety, in essence it encompasses a broad range of characteristics, many of which deal with the host response.

In order to properly discuss molecular signalling mechanisms of host–material interactions, it is necessary to define the terms biomaterials and biocompatibility. Considering the influence of David Williams in reaching a consensus about these issues, we adopt the views that he expressed in two keynote papers (Williams, 2008, 2009).

Biomaterials no longer constitute a class of tangible materials but rather a substance or system that both has mass and occupies space, and that directs the course of medical treatment. This concept relates to the classical implantable medical devices, but also extends to the fields of drug- and gene-delivery systems, nanomedicine, tissue engineering, nanotechnology, artificial organ systems, neuronal interfaces and three-dimensional (3D) printing applications, including biological elements such as living cells. Therefore an entire range from the nanometre level to macroscopically sized implants has to be covered.

This has consequences for how biocompatibility should be conceptualized. Williams (2008) proposed the following definition:

> *Biocompatibility refers to the ability of a biomaterial to perform its desired function with respect to a medical therapy, without eliciting any undesirable local or systemic effects in the recipient or beneficiary of that therapy, but generating the most appropriate beneficial cellular or tissue response in that specific situation, and optimizing the clinically relevant performance of that therapy.*

This definition has evolved over two decades of reviewing the literature and discussing with many peers in the field. It encompasses the new developments in a rapidly extending field of research, but also creates endless opportunities to perform further research as it has not been stated what the most appropriate beneficial response is. It is evident though that biocompatibility no longer refers to a material alone, but rather to the system comprising both the material and the host (Williams, 2014).

Bioinspired Materials for Medical Applications. http://dx.doi.org/10.1016/B978-0-08-100741-9.00004-8

Our understanding of host–material interactions is improving over time. The often recited foreign-body response associated with the use of biomaterials is slowly transforming into a tissue healing response that can be beneficial towards tissue engineering and regenerative medicine applications.

As pointed out by Brown et al. (2012), biomaterials have become more cell-friendly and are designed to be degradable; they often have highly engineered bulk and/or surface structures and involve the use of bioactive molecules. With this evolution, our immune system is targeted in ways different from the classical inert biomaterial implants.

Besides the innate immune system that has always been considered the main factor responsible for the biomaterial-associated host responses, the acquired immune system may also start to reveal an important role in these responses. Interestingly, these developments coincide with the emergence of new concepts in macrophage behaviour, where it is recognized that these cells that orchestrate the tissue response can adapt to different phenotypes ranging from the proinflammatory M1 (classically activated) to the prohealing M2 (alternatively activated), most likely in a continuous spectrum of activities (Scislowska-Czarnecka et al., 2012; Mosser and Edwards, 2008).

Biomaterials will always induce a complex biological reaction when implanted into living tissue. Even if not rejected in the strict immunological sense, the strong inflammation and fibrotic reactions observed at the implant site of different patients suggests that biomaterials affect the homeostasis of the host immune system (Franz et al., 2011). These host immune responses are mediated by a large number of molecular signals, including cytokines, antibodies and reactive radical species, and the involvement of different cell types, including macrophages, neutrophils, natural killer cells, T cells, B cells and dendritic cells (DCs) (Gardner et al., 2013). Therefore, when developing materials for biological use, it is essential to understand the molecular and cellular aspects controlling the complexity of the innate and adaptive immune system. In this chapter, we will discuss host–material interactions and the scientific developments as they stand in 2016, as well as their implications for the design of new biomaterial systems.

4.2 The foreign-body response

The foreign-body response has been the hallmark of the inflammatory response to the implantation and presence of biomaterials in the body. It is an integral part of the wound-healing response, which is classically described as the response of vascularized tissue to injury. Anderson (2001) published the now classical cascade of events associated with the implantation of biomaterials. First, the implantation of any biomaterial inflicts damage to the surrounding tissue which contributes to the initiation of an inflammatory response (innate immunity). As soon as the biomaterial is implanted, it is covered with a layer of proteins that regulate the activation and guide the interplay of the coagulation cascade, complement system, platelets and immune cells (Anderson et al., 1996, 2008).

Cell adhesion and subsequent coverage of the biomaterial surface can occur through integrin activity, as integrins are the major class of adhesion receptors of leukocytes (Anderson et al., 2008; Franz et al., 2011). Besides recognition of biomaterials by adhesion receptors, the activation of immune cells can also be mediated by danger signals, which include heat shock proteins, high mobility group box 1, ATP (adenosine triphosphate) and uric acid (Franz et al., 2011). These danger signals are released by dying cells to alert the host of associated tissue damage, therewith inducing inflammation.

Proteolytic enzymes may also leak from other injured cells and additionally trigger extracellular danger signals when adsorbing to biomaterials. Soluble or biomaterial-associated danger signals are recognized by innate immune cells through pattern recognition receptors (PRR), for example, scavenger receptors, toll-like receptors (TLR) and C-type lectins (Franz et al., 2011). The initial deposition of blood components on the biomaterial surface also works as a provisional matrix for the cell–material interface, which supplies structural, biochemical and cellular components to the processes of wound healing and the foreign-body reaction.

The first immune cells to recognize the foreign body and to be activated are the tissue resident leukocytes (mast cells, macrophages and lymphocytes). These local leukocytes are mainly involved in the local tissue function, homeostasis and immune surveillance, and in the presence of a foreign body they may release cytokines and chemokines that drive the recruitment of neutrophils (polymorphonuclear leukocytes) and inflammatory monocytes from the blood stream (Franz et al., 2011).

Neutrophils are the first recruited cells to reach the implantation site and are characteristic of the acute inflammatory response. They start releasing proteases, reactive oxygen species (ROS) and other enzymes with the intention of degrading the foreign body (Anderson et al., 1996; Franz et al., 2011; Gardner et al., 2013). Neutrophils are also a significant source of immunoregulatory signals, such as the chemokine interleukin-8 (IL-8) that is released to attract more neutrophils to the inflammation site, or monocyte chemotactic protein 1 (MCP-1) and macrophage inflammatory protein 1β (MIP-1β) which work as chemoattractants and activation factors for monocytes, macrophages, immature DCs and lymphocytes (Anderson et al., 1996).

Successful healing will depend on a complex balance between the signals released by neutrophils. For instance, the increased release of MCP-1 and MIP-1β suppresses the further infiltration of neutrophils in favour of a macrophage infiltration (Anderson et al., 2008). Neutrophils remain at the implantation site for a limited amount of time, with a peak at around 24 hours. Within 2 days after biomaterial implantation, neutrophils undergo apoptosis due to the decrease of activation signals and are eliminated by macrophages that had started to infiltrate the tissue. Macrophages may persist in the tissue as long as necessary, which can range from days to weeks to even months, depending on the inertness of the implant material.

DCs, macrophages and B cells are the three major cell types considered as professional antigen presentation cells (APCs). Professional APCs use PRRs to identify pathogen-associated molecular patterns and start a signalling cascade that leads to the upregulation of stimulatory molecules (such as CD80, CD86 and CD40), secretion of cytokines (such as TNF-α, TGF-β, IL-12 and IL-1) and increased surface expression of major histocompatibility complex-I and -II (MHC-I and MHC-II, respectively) (Khan and Reddy, 2014). Commonly, an acute inflammatory response to tissue damage resolves quickly in less than 2 weeks and the host tissue returns to normal homeostasis. However, if the foreign body or biomaterial remains present it will continue to trigger an ongoing inflammatory response, the blood- or lymph node-derived lymphocytes can be engaged and a chronic inflammation takes place.

A chronic inflammation in the presence of a biomaterial can be characterized by the presence of foreign-body giant cells, which result from the fusion of macrophages into giant cells with the intention of engulfing bigger bodies, a process that often is considered to be an act of frustration. These foreign-body giant cells may degrade biomaterials by the phagocytosis of larger particles, yet when the giant cells do not succeed in the engulfment of the foreign body they may enter a state of frustrated phagocytosis, which results in an enhanced degradative capacity (eg, localized secretion of protons, enzymes and ROS) accompanied by a reduction of the phagocytic activity of the giant cells (Gardner et al., 2013).

The true elimination of the foreign body generally is not achieved but the formation and maturation of a fibrous encapsulation can be considered as a successful elimination. This capsule actually resembles fibrosis. It consists of a small fraction of parallel arranged, elongated fibroblasts and a large fraction of similarly arranged collagen type I fibres (Franz et al., 2011; Scislowska-Czarnecka et al., 2012). By using degradable materials, the presence of a fibrous capsule may be avoided, but degradation mechanisms, kinetics and nature of the degradation products will influence the remainder of the inflammatory process. Nowadays, we are still implanting degradable materials that have been in use for more than 30 years. Despite intensive research on new degradable materials, which are tuned to optimal cell and tissue responses, new materials enter the market in a very slow pace (Furth et al., 2007). Still it is especially in this segment that development towards smart, functional biomaterials progresses at the highest speed.

When inspecting the definition of biocompatibility, provided by Williams (2008), it is noticeable that the presence of a fibrous capsule does not present the most appropriate beneficial cell or tissue response. For some applications this is exceptionally clear as the fibrous capsule intervenes with transport of signalling molecules or nutrients (eg, biosensors, pacemaker electrodes and cochlear implant electrodes). Moreover, it has been shown to be a risk factor when the fibroblasts in the capsule transform into myofibroblasts and start contracting the capsule, as observed for example in women having silicone breast implants (Steiert et al., 2013).

Therefore the presence of a significant fibrous capsule is generally seen as an unwanted outcome of the inflammatory process and it hinders the tissue regeneration or healing. Hence, biomaterial systems development is often aimed at minimizing the capsule formation or at generating ‘bio-tolerable’ implants that can permanently reside in the body and only elicit a low degree of inflammation (Ratner, 2011).

It is possible to incorporate drug release strategies that modulate the immune response as an integral part of the biomaterial or device, with the emphasis on antiinflammatory drugs (reviewed by Morais et al., 2010), but at the horizon it appears that novel opportunities arise to minimize inflammation without the use of drugs, as shown in this chapter. Of course others and more specific unwanted effects of inflammation have also been reported, such as the restenosis after stent implantation or the calcification of heart valve replacements, and complement activation and coagulation-related events on blood-contacting biomaterials (Onuki et al., 2008; Nilsson et al., 2007). However, these are very specific cases and will not be discussed in this chapter.

4.2.1 The role of adsorbed proteins in signalling

Proteins are abundantly present in the human body. Blood, for example, consists of a cellular fraction and a plasma fraction in more or less equal proportions, where the plasma contains many different proteins including the coagulation cascade members, the complement system proteins, adhesive proteins (such as vitronectin and fibronectin) and albumin. Plasma-derived serum is routinely being used in in vitro cell cultures in percentages ranging from 5% to 20%. It has been recognized for a long period of time that proteins colonize material surfaces directly with first contact. Actually, the proteins are the first colonizers of any material implanted in the body. Leo Vroman performed a series of experiments using a very simple lens-on-a-slide model (Vroman and Adams, 1986), in which he discovered that proteins compete for the limited amount of surface area and that proteins displace each other over time. Steele et al. (1995) elucidated the role of both fibronectin and vitronectin in cell adhesion to tissue culture polystyrene (TCPs) as opposed to polystyrene. The usual excellent cell adhesion on TCPs can be explained by a favourable 3D folding pattern of the fibronectin with an excellent availability of the RGD (arginyl-glycyl-aspartic) cell binding site with which the integrin $\alpha5\beta1$ can interact (Li et al., 2003). In the presence of all the serum proteins, the adsorption of fibronectin is minimal (Siani et al., 2015), but a favourable folding pattern positively influences cell adhesion. These studies demonstrate that, although the proteins cover the material surface, the surface characteristics determines the composition of the protein layer and also the individual folding patterns.

The effect of the adsorbed protein layer on cells is determined by the availability of cell binding sites for the diverse integrins that most cell types possess. The contacts established between the cells and the protein layer are often referred to as focal contacts, which actually is an assembly of a number of intracellular proteins closely associated with each other and activating each other through phosphorylation. The maturity and size of the focal contact depends on the integrin-ligand binding and on the aggregation of integrins in patches.

Maturation is associated with the formation of F-actin (actin filaments) stress fibres in the cell. Only an adequate maturation allows the potential cell proliferation and differentiation. When analysing the detailed molecular events in focal adhesion formation as a function of material surface properties, it becomes clear that the make-up of a focal adhesion can be highly variable, both in the ratios of the associated proteins present (such as vinculin and talin), as in the degree of phosphorylation in the different tyrosines within relevant proteins (Keselowsky and García, 2005). It is still not clear how we can translate these observations to explain the cell behaviour differences, yet it is evident that mature focal adhesions are of pivotal importance for downstream cell behaviour. Jeon et al. (2015) supported this evidence with a study of nanocrater-patterned surfaces that directed cells to areas where the adhesions could be formed.

The foreign-body response is strongly biased by the macrophage behaviour. The starting point, however, is still the layer of adsorbed proteins, in which fibrinogen is an important inducer of leukocyte recruitment. Keselowsky et al. (2007) reported on the importance of fibronectin in an in vivo study using plasma fibronectin (pFN) conditional knock-out mice. They have shown that fibronectin is also involved in the host response during the chronic inflammation phase and that depletion of pFN led to a twofold thicker fibrous capsule with a high presence of foreign-body giant cells.

4.2.1.1 Protein corona

The use of nanoparticles (NPs) plays an important role in nanomedical applications. These particles are biomaterials applied in the human body for both diagnostic and therapeutic purposes. As they are usually applied in the bloodstream, NPs are prone to collect an adsorbed protein layer in their surface, which is referred to as the protein corona (Nel et al., 2009). Although adsorbed protein layers are typically thin, they still measure several nanometres, which imply that the NPs size significantly increases with the presence of the protein corona. The use of nanosized structures drastically changes the way proteins adsorb and subsequently fold, not only with NPs but also with nanostructured material surfaces. Nel et al. (2009) argue that the folding of the proteins changes due to intimate interactions with the nanostructures that can be based on multiple mechanisms including hydrophobic, van der Waals, hydrodynamic, electrostatic, solvent, steric and polymer–bridging interactions. This can even result in the exposure of cryptic sites in the adsorbed proteins that normally are not seen by the immune surveillance cells, and that may initiate a specific immune response and unforeseen protein behaviour. The composition of the protein corona is influenced by material properties, as convincingly shown by Sakulkhu et al. (2014) in a study exposing superparamagnetic iron oxide nanoparticles (SPIONs), coated with different polymers, to foetal bovine serum and characterizing the adsorbed proteins. It is not a bold thought to presume that protein adsorption events on nanostructured materials induce cell behaviour that is often valued as beneficial for the host (reviewed by Bettinger et al., 2009).

4.2.2 Macrophages perform an orchestrating role

Anderson et al. (2008) pointed out that macrophages can be found in the inflammatory tissue surrounding an implant during a prolonged period of time, which highlights the key role of this cell type in orchestrating the tissue response to a biomaterial. Another way to look at this statement is that if we can control the macrophage activity spectrum we will be able to control the tissue response. The notion that a continuous range of macrophage phenotypes may exist supports this statement. In the past 10 years macrophages have been discussed in terms of their classically activated (M1) and antiinflammatory (M2) phenotypes.

M1 and M2 are known to be directly related to proinflammatory and homeostatic/wound healing respectively and are present both in innate and adaptive immune responses (Franz et al., 2011; Scislowska-Czarnecka et al., 2012; Galdiero and Mantovani, 2015). M2 is known to be clearly discerned from the well-characterized M1 cell type, yet it probably represents an even broader group of macrophages with activity spectra completely different from the M1 phenotype.

Actually, it has been proposed a redefinition of the M1/M2 paradigm or the establishment of a more comprehensive classification of macrophages based on the observations that macrophages adopt a certain phenotype derived from all interactions with tissues during their life span (Martinez and Gordon, 2014). M1 macrophages are well defined and known to be crucial for the host defence by secreting inflammatory cytokines, ROS and nitrogen radicals with the intention of eliminating pathogens. It is known that macrophages, both of primary origin and cell lines, can be differentiated into an M1 phenotype by stimulating with IFN-γ (interferon gamma), TNF-α (tumour necrosis factor alpha), the presence of natural killer cells and lipopolysaccharides (LPS).

Typical cytokines produced by M1 macrophages are TNF-α, IL-6, IL-1β, IL-12 (Scislowska-Czarnecka et al., 2012). On the other hand, M2 macrophages can be divided into macrophages with wound healing or regulatory functions. Wound-healing macrophages are typically present in response to IL-4, IL-13 and T helper 2 cells, and are known to be responsible for antiinflammatory activities and for promoting healing by influencing extracellular matrix production and fibroblasts activation.

Macrophages are fully equipped to produce virtually all types of collagens and the associated matrixmetalloproteinases (MMP) (Schnoor et al., 2008). Regulatory macrophages are responsible for limiting the inflammation and inhibiting immune responses and are triggered by signals such as apoptotic cells, prostaglandins, IL-10, glucocorticoids (Scislowska-Czarnecka et al., 2012; Mosser and Edwards, 2008). The expression of IL-10, CD206 and scavenger receptors are also associated with the M2 phenotype. Therefore M1 macrophages are usually involved in the early phase of the immune response, while M2 macrophages are mainly involved in the resolution phase. These effects were observed by Jones et al. (2007) in a study with in vitro cultures of human monocytes on polymers with different surface properties. They reported that the initial expression of IL-1β, IL-6, IL-8 and MIP-1β was gradually replaced by IL-10, over a time period of 10 days. On the other hand, human acute monocytic leukemia cell line (THP1)-derived M2 macrophages have been shown to shift towards the M1 phenotype upon the uptake of SPIONs (Laskar et al., 2013). This fuels the notion that macrophages may change their phenotype according to signal changes and the inflammation stage, yet it is still debatable whether in vivo the same phenotypic changes may occur or if there is the arrival of differently activated macrophages at different stages of the immune response. This debate is also supported by the studies of Van Putten et al. (2013), who reported an in vivo collagen-induced foreign-body reaction in rats where a large number of macrophages could not be categorized in either M1 or M2.

On the other hand, macrophages participate in several complex diseases such as cancer, atherosclerosis, insulin resistance in obesity and periodontal disease as reviewed by Brown et al. (2012). It appears that the M1 and M2 macrophage activity patterns are balanced in these diseases and that a phenotype switch is often needed to resolve the inflammatory response and create a functional recovery of tissue.

Macrophages do not seem to be trapped in a single differentiation status, that is, polarization. Macrophages keep an active communication with fibroblasts, which may be responsible for the macrophage phenotype switch during the development of the foreign response. Macrophages in turn can also influence the phenotype of fibroblasts. The release of MMP, transforming growth factor beta (TGF-β), platelet-derived growth factor, IL-1β and many other cytokines and growth factors represent the means for this macrophage–fibroblast communication.

This communication can be mimicked in vitro using coculture models where both cell types communicate either directly (juxtacrine), indirectly (paracrine) or by a conditioned media (one-way signalling). For instance, Ploeger et al. (2013) reported that human dermal fibroblasts are triggered to secrete the inflammatory cytokines IL-6, chemokine (C–C motif) ligand 2 (CCL2), CCL7, MMP1 and MMP3 when exposed to paracrine factors from M1 macrophages. When stimulated with the factors from M2 macrophages these cells started to proliferate and secrete collagen. Thus, the M1 and M2 phenotypes give rise to similar activity patterns in the dermal fibroblasts. Interestingly, the fibroblast phenotypes could be reversed by subsequent exposure to the paracrine factors secreted by the macrophages of the opposing phenotype. Macrophages can also be influenced by a proangiogenic environment in which they become M2 polarized, although this polarization can be reversed by the classical stimulation with LPS and IFN-γ (Ploeger et al., 2012). In fact, even conditioned media from the respective phenotype drive the cells into a similar phenotype. Ploeger et al. (2012) demonstrated that the soluble factors overruled the influence of the two dimensional (2D) extracellular matrix composition.

On the other hand, in in vitro studies, Holt et al. (2010) have reported on a panel of primary-derived and secondary-derived cells and observed that the foreign-body response in vivo was best simulated using primary cell cocultures. Furthermore, out of a broad selection of cytokines, the authors chose IL-6, TNF, MCP-1, CCL5, MIP-1α and MIP-1β as the most relevant signalling molecules to be further investigated due to their high concentrations (secreted above 40 pg/mL). These and other cytokines were also found by Zeng and Chen (2010) in a study with macrophage–fibroblast cocultures in hydrogels. The main aim of the study was to evaluate if cells derived from diabetic animals behaved differently from cells obtained from healthy animals. Interestingly, the authors reported that both fibroblasts and macrophages can produce these cytokines, but in cocultures a significant increase in the total amount of the molecules was observed when compared with monocultures. In this study, no reference was made to macrophage polarization.

4.2.3 Role of the adaptive immune system

The innate immune system has for a long time been recognized as the main system responsible for the host response to a biomaterial implantation, yet recently there is a growing interest in the role of the adaptive immune system in this response. Biomaterials have gradually evolved towards combinatorial materials, including biomolecular components, and therefore the interest in studying the complexity of the immune response has also increased.

The adaptive immune response is mainly defined by the response of T and B cells to specific antigens presented by professional APCs. APCs, such as DCs, work as a bridge between the innate and the adaptive immunity (Kou and Babensee, 2011). APCs have two major roles in the response to a foreign body, first the uptake, process and display of peptide epitopes from encountered antigens, second they are able to signal and direct T and B cells to respond in an appropriate manner. T and B cells become morphologically distinguishable only after activation by an antigen.

T cells develop in the thymus and can be mostly found in three stages, as naïve, effector and memory cells. A T cell becomes active and differentiated when three signals are in place. First, the T-cell receptor (TCR) from naïve T cells recognizes and attaches to a specific peptide, which is determined by the affinity of the unique TCRs for the peptide–MHC complex (Ploeger et al., 2013). The second signal is the co-stimulation, where the professional APCs provide a coactivation signal that is detected by molecules displayed in the surface of T cells (CD40L and CD28). For instance, Acharya et al. (2008) have shown in vitro the importance of APCs for the activation of T cells. In an in vitro coculture model of murine bone marrow-derived DCs with CD4+ T cells purified from a mice spleen, they have shown that DCs mediated the T-cell proliferation and CD4+ T-cell response. Finally, T cells can detect a third signal, the soluble cytokines, which guide the T cells to differentiate into different subsets, depending of the cytokines present in the microenvironment.

T cells can display, besides TCR, one of two co-receptors depending on the microenvironment cytokine profile, CD4 or CD8. CD8+ T cells, also termed cytotoxic T lymphocytes, are receptors that exclusively interact with the MHC class I molecules and are capable of secreting molecules that can trigger cell apoptosis. In contrast, CD4+ T cells are receptors that exclusively interact with the MHC-II molecules and are often termed helper T cells due to their ability to signal and influence other cells.

B cells develop high-affinity antibody repertoires analogous to T cells and TCRs, which form the humoral memory compartment. Similar to T cells, B cells recognize potential circulating antigens by surface receptors. After recognizing an antigen, the B cell internalizes and processes it for MHC-II presentation. T cells that recognize the presented peptide then signal back to the B cell (via CD40L and cytokines) to inform if the peptide has encoded a relevant antibody or not (Crotty, 2015).

Therefore B- and T-cell activation and proliferation are controlled in part by several transmembrane receptors and, as such, these proteins could be potential therapeutic targets. However, little is known about the identification and characterization of transmembrane receptors that regulate the adaptive immune response to biomaterials. One of the few studies about transmembrane receptors in a biomaterial context was done by Shankar et al. (2010). Cytotoxic T lymphocyte associated antigen receptor-4 (CTLA-4) is a protein receptor on the surface of T cells that acts as an 'off' switch when bound to CD80 or CD86 on the surface of antigen-presenting cells. In this study, Shankar et al. (2010) investigated the effect of self-assembled monolayers (SAM) surfaces on the maturation of DCs and, interestingly, they observed that a surface with –CH3 SAM induced not only a lower DC maturation, but also an increased expression of CTLA-4 on T cells. CTLA-4 comes out in this study as a potential mediator for inhibiting the T-cell responses to biomaterials.

4.2.4 Bacteria complicate the inflammatory response

In normal conditions, the acute and chronic inflammation in response to a biocompatible material can last weeks, months or even years, whereas normal wound healing without the presence of materials usually takes 2 weeks. The persistence of inflammation for more than 3 weeks may also be an indication of biomaterial-associated infection (BAI) (Anderson et al., 2008). Bacteria have a strong tendency to attach to surfaces and the critical first step in the development of bacterial infections involves the bacterial adhesion to host cells, extracellular matrix glycoproteins and biomaterial surfaces. Our immune system has evolved to efficiently tackle invading microorganisms as long as they are not associated with materials. Similarly, bacteria have developed mechanisms to evade our immune system. In this chapter, we do not aim to discuss all details of biomaterial–bacteria–host interactions, but we will expose briefly some stimulating observations of how the presence of a biomaterial can change the interactions between host cells and microorganisms.

Pathogen-associated molecular patterns are recognized by PRR of the host cells, which may induce inflammasome activity. Similar recognition exists for damage-associated molecular patterns by macrophages. Malik et al. (2011) demonstrated that the presence of particulate matter, such as wear debris, induces inflammasome formation in DCs and macrophages and that this also applies to nonparticulate, implanted biomaterials. Inflammasome activity seems to be associated with the presence of the foreign-body response. Molecular adhesion of bacteria–bacteria, bacteria–biomaterial surface and bacterial–phagocyte involves noncovalent intermolecular interactions governed by Lifshitz-van der Waals binding or electrostatic interactions between charged functional groups. Although individual secondary bonds and electrostatic interactions are relatively weak in physiological conditions, compared to primary chemical bonds, their combined effects can result in very strong binding between bacteria adhering on a biomaterial. In in vitro conditions, Da Silva Domingues et al. (2013) have shown that the long-range attraction between macrophages and bacteria were mainly dictated by van der Waals forces while short-range acid–base interactions dictated the overall phagocyte–microorganism macroscopic adhesion.

The thermodynamic conditions are therefore a driving force in the recognition of BAI by the host immune system. Additionally, the physicochemical nature of the biomaterial surface is decisive for the nature of the immune response to a biomaterial in combination with bacteria. As discussed before, in the presence of a foreign body the host may react with an exacerbated inflammation response, which in the presence of bacteria may work in favour of the phagocytosed bacteria. For instance, Boelens et al. (2000a) have shown that mice implanted with polyvinylpyrrolidone-grafted silicon elastomer and infected with *Staphylococcus epidermidis* developed an exacerbated proinflammatory response, with high production of the proinflammatory cytokine IL-1β and persistent *S. epidermidis* infection. Interestingly, the same authors have proven that by using an IL-1 receptor type I-deficient (IL-$1R^{-/-}$), the infection was reduced (Boelens et al., 2000b).

These studies reveal that the modulation of the immune system by inhibition of this molecular signal may be beneficial for the outcome of BAI situations. TLR, such as TLR2 and TLR9, are known to bind ligands that are present in *Staphylococcus aureus* biofilms, yet these recognition pathways do not seem to be utilized by host cells in in vivo catheter-associated biofilms (Thurlow et al., 2011). The macrophages revealed a limited phagocytic action and adopted an M2 phenotype, which points out for the modulation of the host immune system by the *S. aureus* presence. *S. aureus* were able to tune the classical inflammatory response and make macrophages less bactericidal by interfering with M1 polarization, as reviewed by Hanke and Kielian (2012). *S. epidermidis* biofilms associated with medical devices can also escape immune surveillance, as it was shown in a study of Schommer et al. (2011). They have shown that in the presence of J774A.1 murine macrophages, the evasion of *S. epidermidis* was related to the biofilm mode-of-growth and the associated presence of intercellular adhesins, polysaccharide intercellular adhesin, accumulation-associated protein and extracellular matrix binding protein. In this study, macrophages also turned away from the M1 phenotype.

The design of smart biomaterials that can promote tissue integration and at the same time inhibit microbial colonization has received increasing attention. As in the case of offering distinct adhesion sites for establishing focal adhesions, a similar approach can be taken for reducing bacterial adhesion. Optimal balances have to be sought by playing with the design parameters (Wang et al., 2014).

4.3 Molecular signalling mechanisms

Information on the release of cytokines in paracrine signalling during the inflammatory process can be found in numerous published studies (Glaros et al., 2009; Holt et al., 2010; Barron and Wynn, 2011; Duffield et al., 2013; Ploeger et al., 2013; Zhou et al., 2015). Several different cytokines and growth factors can be involved and integrated in complex maps of signalling pathways. In the end it may prove valuable to have all the dots connected, for example by performing in silico experiments and predict outcomes of implant designs. Nevertheless, in this chapter, we approach the issue of molecular signalling mechanisms from the point of view of what is known from in vivo and in vitro studies and what challenges our current understanding.

The central theme of discussion is the immune response, which with the use of more refined biomaterials tend to involve both the innate and adaptive immune system as elaborately reviewed by Franz et al. (2011). In the quest for reducing the fibrous capsule size, Majd et al. (2015) developed micropatterns of adhesive proteins on silicone implants and tested these patterns both in vitro using macrophages and fibroblasts and in vivo in a subcutaneous rat implantation model. They observed that unmodified silicone led to a thick alpha smooth muscle actin (αSMA) positive capsule containing profibrotic myofibroblasts and multiple giant cells after 30 days of implantation. Providing the silicone with a continuous collagen type I coating drastically reduced the numbers of giant cells, but only slightly reduced the capsule thickness with the presence of some αSMA. The real reduction occurred in the implants modified with a 4×2 μm micropattern of collagen indicating that tissue integration was markedly enhanced. This was corroborated by the low collagen density in the thin capsule found around the micropatterned silicone implant. In vitro experiments were conducted to shed some light on these observations, especially with respect to the fibroblast behaviour. It has been shown before that micropatterns created with adhesive proteins, such as collagen or fibronectin, influence the differentiation of fibroblasts to myofibroblasts (Kendall and Feghali-Bostwick, 2014).

These cells have been implemented in fibrosis processes including organ fibrosis through TGF-β, WNT and YAP/TAZ (Yes-associated protein/transcriptional coactivator with PDZ binding motif) signalling (Piersma et al., 2015). Their role in the fibrotic response including the adverse contraction of capsules around implants has been reviewed by Rolfe et al. (2011). From the adhesion perspective, Goffin et al. (2006) reported that the focal adhesion size in cells dictates formation of stress fibres containing αSMA and that this depends on the tension created in the stress fibres. These stress fibres have to be attached to relatively large focal adhesions, typically 8–30 μm long in this particular experiment. In this work, a relationship to substratum stiffness was also described, a topic we discuss as well in this chapter.

Majd et al. (2015) also measured the presence of αSMA fibres in fibroblasts cultured on different sizes of micropatterns containing fibronectin and confirmed that the larger patch sizes, starting with 2×10 μm, resulted in significant αSMA-containing stress fibre formation. Even in the presence of TGF-β1 the 2×4 μm micropattern barely elicited a αSMA positive response. So, assuming that this is the result of the macrophage–fibroblast interaction during 30 days in a subcutaneous location, the question arises: "why these differences in the foreign body response occur?"

The authors propose that the underlying mechanism involves the extent of cell adhesion, with no cell adhesion on bare silicone; excessive cell adhesion on the collagen-coated silicone and balanced cell adhesion on the micropattern, the later suppressing collagen production and αSMA expression. Although this is still quite a descriptive explanation it provides us with two important deliberations. First, it actually reminds us that inertness by itself does not exclude a tissue response and that it is therefore recommendable to choose the proactive approach to controlling the tissue response. It is interesting to note that bare silicone in the past was classified as an inert biomaterial. Second, it also suggests that it can be useful to test implant materials in vitro using the proper cell types and studying the proper cell responses.

Another challenging implant material is the porous templated scaffold in which the interconnected pores are all equal, but adjustable between 10 and 160 μm (reviewed by Bryers et al., 2012). Excellent healing in multiple in vivo environments was observed with pore sizes in the range of 30–40 μm regardless of the material of choice. Porous scaffold materials have been used to allow tissue ingrowth and tissue healing, especially in combination with the use of degradable scaffolds. The exquisitely clear maximum coincides with a high macrophage infiltration and therefore it has been proposed that these macrophages differentiate towards the healing phenotype (Madden et al., 2010). The results indicate that the material surface design and also bulk design can influence the macrophage phenotype and therewith the host response. However, the mechanisms of phenotype differentiation remain to be elucidated.

When looking into the nanometre dimensions, observational studies also reveal optimal cell behaviour in narrow ranges of nanofeatures. Dalby et al. (2007) demonstrated that human mesenchymal stem cells differentiated into osteoblasts producing a mature bone matrix on 120 nm diameter pits, but only when the pits were slightly randomized. Full randomization, as well as homogeneous square arrangements were much less convincing in the expression of osteopontin, osteocalcin and matrix mineralization. Many osteo-specific genes were upregulated on the slightly randomized nanopattern. In general, nanostructures enhance cell behaviour in a positive way, for example by drastically reducing the fibrotic capsule thickness in implant materials when compared with the solid counterpart (Cao et al., 2010).

Stiffness of materials has become an issue of high importance. It has been recognized that cell cultures performed on the gold standard TCP actually represent a highly artefactual situation. First of all, these cultures are 2D leading to flattened cell morphologies. Secondly, the substratum is a very stiff material, much stiffer than most of the tissues in our body. Furthermore, Cha et al. (2012) have highlighted developments in the design of biomaterials to control stem cell behaviour, which help in defining the stem cell niche responsible for either self-renewal or differentiation into the different lineages. They argue that in order to mimic the complexity of native stem cell niches, the physical and biomolecular elements need to be present when developing biomaterials.

Stiffness is therefore highly important to successfully direct the stem cell fate. Cells seem to have a mechanical memory for stiffness dosing as very nicely demonstrated by Yang et al. (2014). Human mesenchymal stem cells remembered their residence on previous substratum when transferred to a material possessing a different stiffness, an accomplishment mediated by YAP, TAZ and preosteogenic transcription factor RUNX2. Depending on the culture times, the effects were reversible, which indicates that cells can adapt, although not after long culture times.

These observations give rise to different possible questions. For instance, how reliable are studies examining cell–material interactions if the cells are precultured on, for example, TCPs? Do the cells inherit characteristics from the previous substratum, including stiffness-mediated effects? It may be necessary to culture and passage the cells on the materials of interest for a prolonged period of time before drawing conclusions about the cell–material interactions. Further evidence of the stiffness importance arise from the observation that stem cells use the mechanical information of the surrounding environment to steer their differentiation, as shown by Engler et al. (2006) for neurogenic, myogenic and osteogenic differentiation out of mesenchymal stem cells.

Smart designs of 3D materials are emerging more and more, for example, to study physical and molecular influences. Chwalek et al. (2014) showed that soft star-shaped poly(ethylene glycol)–heparin hydrogels (containing MMP-degradable sites, covalently bound integrin ligands and reversibly conjugated proangiogenic growth factors) convincingly induced capillary networks in several model systems, both with primary differentiated cells and with mesenchymal stem cells. It would be interesting to study how the foreign-body response is modulated by this kind of systems specifically with respect to macrophage behaviour. Would the macrophages be bypassed or would they interfere with the host response?

In summary, an immune response is generally tailored by specific cues such as exposure dose, molecular recognition patterns, physiological location, cellular trafficking and cell phenotypes.

4.4 Conclusion and future developments

As above mentioned, the immune system is able to recognize and respond to foreign bodies by the identification of structural molecular patterns on the surface of the material. Nowadays, biomaterial development focuses on harnessing these immunological cues to design biomaterials that modulate innate and adaptive immunity in a controlled manner. At the moment, the majority of biomaterial research that aims at the modulation of the immune system is based on the professional APCs. An important strategy is the use of both smart biomaterials and bioactive signalling molecules.

Smart biomaterials will likely be resorbable polymers tailored at the molecular level and able to respond to changes in the microenvironment and interactions with tissue cells. A great challenge for the future development of biomaterials is the controlled differentiation of target cells in the presence of biomaterials. Typically, differentiation is controlled by soluble growth factors and cytokines.

As discussed in this chapter, new strategies of biomaterial design reveal high potential for directing cell behaviour and should lead to important advances in biomaterial research. Implantation is also a critical factor from the clinical point of view of the biomaterial development.

New smart materials may be designed with biodegradable, shape-memory and stimuli-sensitive polymers and should be combined with minimal invasive surgery application of the materials. An important hurdle to overcome is the efficacy of biomaterial systems in the aged patient when replacing or supporting diseased tissues. The presence of a pathological condition may drastically change the outcome of the foreign-body response although this has barely been implemented in the in vitro and animal implantation studies reported in literature. There still is a lot to discover about how the immune system will deal with all the new biomaterial systems and strategies currently in the process of development. A multidisciplinary collaboration of clinical, biomedical and biological experts will be required to assess the merits of these developments.

Acknowledgment

J.F. da Silva Domingues, recipient of an ERS-EU RESPIRE2 Marie Sklodowska-Curie Postdoctoral Research Fellowship - Number MCF 7783-2014, with funding from the People Programme of the European Union's Seventh Framework Programme (FP7/2007-2013) under REA grant agreement 600368.

References

Acharya, A., Dolgova, N., Clare-Salzler, M., Keselowsky, B., 2008. Adhesive substrate-modulation of adaptive immune responses. Biomaterials 29 (36), 4736–4750.

Anderson, J., 2001. Biological responses to biomaterials. Annu. Rev. Mater. Res. 31, 81–110.

Anderson, J.M., Gristina, A.G., Hanson, S.R., Harker, L.A., Johnson, R.J., Merrit, K., Naylor, P.T., Schoen, F.J., 1996. Host reactions to biomaterials and their evaluation. In: Ratner, B., Hoffman, A., Schoen, F., Lemons, J. (Eds.), Biomaterials Science: An Introduction to Materials in Medicine. Elsevier Academic Press, London, pp. 165–214.

Anderson, J., Rodriguez, A., Chang, D., 2008. Foreign body reaction to biomaterials. Semin. Immunol. 20, 86–100.

Barron, L., Wynn, T., 2011. Fibrosis is regulated by Th2 and Th17 responses and by dynamic interactions between fibroblasts and macrophages. Am. J. Physiol. Gastrointest. Liver Physiol. 300, G723–G728.

Bettinger, C., Langer, R., Borenstein, J., 2009. Engineering substrate topography at the micro- and nanoscale to control cell function. Angew. Chem. Int. Ed. 48, 5406–5415.

Boelens, J., Dankert, J., Murk, J., Weening, J., Van der Poll, T., Dingemans, K., Koole, L., Laman, J., Zaat, S., 2000a. Biomaterial-associated persistence of *Staphylococcus epidermidis* in pericatheter macrophages. J. Infect. Dis. 181 (4), 1337–1349.

Boelens, J., Van Der Poll, T., Zaat, S., Murk, J., Weening, J., Dankert, J., 2000b. Interleukin-1 receptor type I gene-deficient mice are less susceptible to *Staphylococcus epidermidis* biomaterial-associated infection than are wild-type mice. Infect. Immun. 68, 6924–6931.

Brown, B., Ratner, B., Goodman, S., Amar, S., Badylak, S., 2012. Macrophage polarization: an opportunity for improved outcomes in biomaterials and regenerative medicine. Biomaterials 33 (15), 3792–3802.

Bryers, J., Giachelli, C., Ratner, B., 2012. Engineering biomaterials to integrate and heal: the biocompatibility paradigm shifts. Biotechnol. Bioeng. 109 (8), 1898–1911.

Cao, H., McHugh, K., Chew, S., Anderson, J., 2010. The topographical effect of electrospun nanofibrous scaffolds on the in vivo and in vitro foreign body reaction. J. Biomed. Mater. Res. A 93 (3), 1151–1159.

Cha, C., Liechty, W., Khademhosseini, A., Peppas, N., 2012. Designing biomaterials to direct stem cell fate. ACS Nano 6 (11), 9353–9358.

Chwalek, K., Tsurkan, M., Freudenberg, U., Werner, C., 2014. Glycosaminoglycan-based hydrogels to modulate heterocellular communication in in vitro angiogenesis models. Sci. Rep. 4, 4414.

Crotty, S., 2015. A brief history of T cell help to B cells. Nat. Rev. Immunol. 15, 185–189.

Da Silva Domingues, J., Van der Mei, H., Busscher, H., Van Kooten, T., 2013. Phagocytosis of bacteria adhering to a biomaterial surface in a surface thermodynamic perspective. PLoS One 8 (7), e70046.

Dalby, M., Gadegaard, N., Tare, R., Andar, A., Riehle, M., Herzyk, P., Wilkinson, C., Oreffo, R., 2007. The control of human mesenchymal cell differentiation using nanoscale symmetry and disorder. Nat. Mater. 6, 997–1003.

Duffield, J., Lupher, M., Thannickal, V., Wynn, T., 2013. Host responses in tissue repair and fibrosis. Annu. Rev. Pathol. Mech. Dis. 8, 241–276.

Engler, A., Sen, S., Sweeney, H., Discher, D., 2006. Matrix elasticity directs stem cell lineage specification. Cell 126 (4), 677–689.

Franz, S., Rammelt, S., Scharnweber, D., Simon, J., 2011. Immune responses to implants—a review of the implications for the design of immunomodulatory biomaterials. Biomaterials 32 (28), 6692–6709.

Furth, M., Atala, A., Van Dyke, M., 2007. Smart biomaterials design for tissue engineering and regenerative medicine. Biomaterials 28 (34), 5068–5073.

Galdiero, M., Mantovani, A., 2015. Macrophage plasticity and polarization: relevance to biomaterials. In: Badylak, S.F. (Ed.), Host Response to Biomaterials. The Impact of Host Response on Biomaterial Selection. Academic Press, Oxford, ISBN: 978-0-12-800196-7, pp. 117–130 (Chapter 6).

Gardner, A., Lee, S., Woods, E., Acharya, A., 2013. Biomaterials-based modulation of the immune system. BioMed. Res. Int. 2013, 732182.

Glaros, T., Larsen, M., Li, L., 2009. Macrophages and fibroblasts during inflammation, tissue damage and organ injury. Front. Biosci. 14, 3988–3993.

Goffin, J., Pittet, P., Csucs, G., Lussi, J., Meister, J., Hinz, B., 2006. Focal adhesion size controls tension-dependent recruitment of alpha-smooth muscle actin to stress fibers. J. Cell Biol. 172 (2), 259–268.

Hanke, M., Kielian, T., 2012. Deciphering mechanisms of staphylococcal biofilm evasion of host immunity. Front. Cell. Infect. Microbiol. 2, 62.

Holt, D., Chamberlain, L., Grainger, D., 2010. Cell–cell signaling in co-cultures of macrophages and fibroblasts. Biomaterials 31 (36), 9382–9394.

Jeon, H., Koo, S., Reese, W., Loskill, P., Grigoropoulos, C., Healy, K., 2015. Directing cell migration and organization via nanocrater-patterned cell–repellent interfaces. Nat. Mater. 14 (9), 918–923.

Jones, J., Chang, D., Meyerson, H., Colton, E., Kwon, I., Matsuda, T., Anderson, J., 2007. Proteomic analysis and quantification of cytokines and chemokines from biomaterial surface-adherent macrophages and foreign body giant cells. J. Biomed. Mater. Res. A 83A, 585–596.

Kendall, R., Feghali-Bostwick, C., 2014. Fibroblasts in fibrosis: novel roles and mediators. Front. Pharmacol. 5, 123.

Keselowsky, B., García, A., 2005. Quantitative methods for analysis of integrin binding and focal adhesion formation on biomaterial surfaces. Biomaterials 26 (4), 413–418.

Keselowsky, B., Bridges, A., Burns, K., Tate, C., Babensee, J., LaPlaca, M., García, A., 2007. Role of plasma fibronectin in the foreign body response to biomaterials. Biomaterials 28 (25), 3626–3631.

Khan, T., Reddy, S., 2014. Immunological principles regulating immunomodulation with biomaterials. Acta Biomater. 10, 1720–1727.

Kou, P., Babensee, J., 2011. Macrophage and dendritic cell phenotypic diversity in the context of biomaterials. J. Biomed. Mater. Res. A 96 (1), 239–260.

Laskar, A., Eilertsen, J., Li, W., Yuan, X., 2013. SPION primes THP1 derived M2 macrophages towards M1-like macrophages. Biochem. Biophys. Res. Commun. 441 (4), 737–742.

Li, F., Redick, S., Erickson, H., Moy, V., 2003. Force measurements of the $\alpha5\beta1$ integrin–fibronectin interaction. Biophys. J. 84, 1252–1262.

Madden, L., Mortisen, D., Sussman, E., Dupras, S., Fugate, J., Cuy, J., Hauch, K., Laflamme, M., Murry, C., Ratner, B., 2010. Proangiogenic scaffolds as functional templates for cardiac tissue engineering. Proc. Natl. Acad. Sci. U. S. A. 107 (34), 15211–15216.

Majd, H., Scherer, S., Boo, S., Ramondetti, S., Cambridge, E., Raffoul, W., Friedrich, M., Pittet, B., Pioletti, D., Hinz, B., Pietramaggiori, G., 2015. Novel micropatterns mechanically control fibrotic reactions at the surface of silicone implants. Biomaterials 54, 136–147.

Malik, A., Hoque, R., Ouyang, X., Ghani, A., Hong, E., Khan, K., Moore, L., Ng, G., Munro, F., Flavell, R., Shi, Y., Kyriakides, T., Mehal, W., 2011. Inflammasome components Asc and caspase-1 mediate biomaterial-induced inflammation and foreign body response. Proc. Natl. Acad. Sci. U. S. A. 108 (50), 20095–20100.

Martinez, F., Gordon, S., 2014. The M1 and M2 paradigm of macrophage activation: time for reassessment. F1000Prime Rep. 6, 13.

Morais, J., Papadimitrakopoulos, F., Burgess, D., 2010. Biomaterials/tissue interactions: possible solutions to overcome foreign body response. AAPS J. 12 (2), 188–196.

Mosser, D., Edwards, J., 2008. Exploring the full spectrum of macrophage activation. Nat. Rev. Immunol. 8, 958–969.

Nel, A., Mädler, L., Velegol, D., Xia, T., Hoek, E., Somasundaran, P., Klaessig, F., Castranova, V., Thompson, M., 2009. Understanding biophysicochemical interactions at the nano-bio interface. Nat. Mater. 8, 543–557.

Nilsson, B., Ekdahl, K., Mollnes, T., Lambris, J., 2007. The role of complement in biomaterial-induced inflammation. Mol. Immunol. 44 (1–3), 82–94.

Onuki, Y., Bhardwaj, U., Papadimitrakopoulos, F., Burgess, D., 2008. A review of the biocompatibility of implantable devices: current challenges to overcome foreign body response. J. Diabetes Sci. Technol. 2 (6), 1003–1015.

Piersma, B., Bank, R., Boersema, M., 2015. Signaling in fibrosis: TGF-β, WNT, and YAP/TAZ converge. Front. Med. (Lausanne) 2, 59.

Ploeger, D., Van Putten, S., Koerts, J., Van Luyn, M., Harmsen, M., 2012. Human macrophages primed with angiogenic factors show dynamic plasticity, irrespective of extracellular matrix components. Immunobiology 217 (3), 299–306.

Ploeger, D., Hosper, N., Schipper, M., Koerts, J., De Rond, S., Bank, R., 2013. Cell plasticity in wound healing: paracrine factors of M1/M2 polarized macrophages influence the phenotypical state of dermal fibroblasts. Cell Commun. Signal. 11, 29.

Ratner, B., 2011. The biocompatibility manifesto: biocompatibility for the twenty-first century. J. Cardiovasc. Transl. Res. 4 (5), 523–527.

Rolfe, B., Mooney, J., Zhang, B., Jahnke, S., Le, S.-J., Chau, Y.-Q., Huang, Q., Wang, H., Campbell, G., Campbell, J., 2011. The fibrotic response to implanted biomaterials: implications for tissue engineering, regenerative medicine and tissue engineering—cells and biomaterials. In: Eberli, D. (Ed.), Regenerative Medicine and Tissue Engineering—Cells and Biomaterials. InTech, Croatia, ISBN: 978-953-307-663-8, pp. 551–568 (Chapter 26).

Sakulkhu, U., Mahmoudi, M., Maurizi, L., Salaklang, J., Hofmann, H., 2014. Protein corona composition of superparamagnetic iron oxide nanoparticles with various physico-chemical properties and coatings. Sci. Rep. 4, 5020.

Schnoor, M., Cullen, P., Lorkowski, J., Stolle, K., Robenek, H., Troyer, D., Rauterberg, J., Lorkowski, S., 2008. Production of type VI collagen by human macrophages: a new dimension in macrophage functional heterogeneity. J. Immunol. 180 (8), 5707–5719.

Schommer, N., Christner, M., Hentschke, M., Ruckdeschel, K., Aepfelbacher, M., Rohde, H., 2011. *Staphylococcus epidermidis* uses distinct mechanisms of biofilm formation to interfere with phagocytosis and activation of mouse macrophage-like cells 774A.1. Infect. Immun. 79 (6), 2267–2276.

Scislowska-Czarnecka, A., Pamula, E., Tlalka, A., Kolaczkowska, E., 2012. Effects of aliphatic polyesters on activation of the immune system: studies on macrophages. J. Biomater. Sci. Polym. Ed. 23 (6), 715–738.

Shankar, S., Petrie, T., García, A., Babensee, J., 2010. Dendritic cell responses to self-assembled monolayers of defined chemistries. J. Biomed. Mater. Res. A 92 (4), 1487–1499.

Siani, A., Khaw, R., Manley, O., Tirella, A., Cellesi, F., Donno, R., Tirelli, N., 2015. Fibronectin localization and fibrillization are affected by the presence of serum in culture media. Sci. Rep. 5, 9278.

Steele, J., Dalton, B., Johnson, G., Underwood, P., 1995. Adsorption of fibronectin and vitronectin onto Primaria and tissue culture polystyrene and relationship to the mechanism of initial attachment of human vein endothelial cells and BHK-21 fibroblasts. Biomaterials 16 (14), 1057–1067.

Steiert, A., Boyce, M., Sorg, H., 2013. Capsular contracture by silicone breast implants: possible causes, biocompatibility, and prophylactic strategies. Med. Devices (Auckl.) 6, 211–218.

Thurlow, L., Hanke, M., Fritz, T., Angle, A., Aldrich, A., Williams, S., Engebretsen, I., Bayles, K., Horswill, A., Kielian, T., 2011. *Staphylococcus aureus* biofilms prevent macrophage phagocytosis and attenuate inflammation in vivo. J. Immunol. 186 (11), 6585–6596.

Van Putten, S., Ploeger, D., Popa, E., Bank, R., 2013. Macrophage phenotypes in the collagen-induced foreign body reaction in rats. Acta Biomater. 9 (5), 6502–6510.

Vroman, L., Adams, A., 1986. Adsorption of proteins out of plasma and solutions in narrow spaces. J. Colloid Interface Sci. 111 (2), 391–402.

Wang, Y., Da Silva Domingues, J., Subbiahdoss, G., Van der Mei, H., Busscher, H., Libera, M., 2014. Conditions of lateral surface confinement that promote tissue-cell integration and inhibit biofilm growth. Biomaterials 35 (21), 5446–5452.

Williams, D., 2008. On the mechanisms of biocompatibility. Biomaterials 29 (20), 2941–2953.

Williams, D., 2009. On the nature of biomaterials. Biomaterials 30 (30), 5897–5909.

Williams, D., 2014. There is no such thing as a biocompatible material. Biomaterials 35 (38), 10009–10014.

Yang, C., Tibbitt, M., Basta, L., Anseth, K., 2014. Mechanical memory and dosing influence stem cell fate. Nat. Mater. 13, 645–652.

Zeng, Q., Chen, W., 2010. The functional behavior of a macrophage/fibroblast co-culture model derived from normal and diabetic mice with a marine gelatin-oxidized alginate hydrogel. Biomaterials 31, 5772–5781.

Zhou, G., Loppnow, H., Groth, T., 2015. A macrophage/fibroblast co-culture system using a cell migration chamber to study inflammatory effects of biomaterials. Acta Biomater. 26, 54–63.

Multifunctional biomaterials and their bioinspired systems for bioactive molecules delivery

5

J.J.T.M. Swartjes[*,a]
[*]University of Groningen, Groningen, The Netherlands
[a]Current address: Ecole Polytechnique Fédérale de Lausanne (EPFL), Institut des Matériaux and Institut des Sciences et Ingénierie Chimiques, Laboratoire des Polymères Bâtiment MXD Station 12 CH-1015 Lausanne, Switzerland

5.1 Introduction

Even though the need for an implant or biomedical device sometimes starts at a young age due to disease or trauma, as life progresses, wear and tear increase the chances of failure of one or more bodily parts and its related functions. At that moment, biomaterials become indispensable for a continued quality of life throughout the individual's existence. As the life expectancy increases in modern first-world countries, the number of people requiring an implant or biomedical device to maintain their health increases accordingly (Mantripragada et al., 2013). Along with the modernization and progression of the healthcare systems in developing countries, this will result in a tremendous increase in the demand for biomaterials to adequately serve patients around the world (Basu, 2014).

In order for a biomaterial to properly fulfill or restore the bodily functions it is intended to, it must comply with a large number of requirements. These requirements are often complicated and change as per implant or device, making it impossible to generalize them. A bone implant, for example, needs to be able to bear a considerable amount of weight, while a tissue engineering scaffold often only needs to support cells, mostly for just limited periods of time (Wu et al., 2014). Additionally, some biomaterials are only used to transport or deliver other materials or (bio)molecules into specific places inside the body (Alvarez-Lorenzo and Concheiro, 2013).

While the requirements differ for each application, this does not limit biomaterials to only those that exhibit a single functionality. In fact, multifunctionality is a prerequisite in most applications. In the case of the previous example of the bone implant, it not only needs to be able to support the load of the bone it replaces, it also needs to integrate with the native tissue without causing problems. Therefore, bone cells need to grow into the material to secure the implant within the existing bone (Agarwal and García, 2015). Whereas this specific example involves a combination of structural and biological functions, multifunctionality also relates to multiple biological functions, which can encompass biocompatibility, improved recovery or infection prevention.

Bioinspired Materials for Medical Applications. http://dx.doi.org/10.1016/B978-0-08-100741-9.00005-X

Within this chapter, the focus on material functionality will be divided into two aspects; influencing tissue cells and influencing microorganisms. The need for specific functionality of a biomaterial towards human cells is dictated by the need for biocompatibility, but extended to improved integration, recovery and desired cell responses (de Souza Costa et al., 2014; Stadlinger et al., 2012). Whereas biomaterials often need to be attractive for tissue cells, or at least not harmful, it is highly important that this attractiveness does not translate to microorganisms, as this increases the chances of bacterial contamination (Bellis, 2011).

Whenever an implant or biomedical device is placed inside the human body, implantation is accompanied with significant risks (Campoccia et al., 2013; Goodman et al., 2013; Zimmerli and Sendi, 2011). One of these is the risk of developing a biomaterial associated infection (BAI) due to bacterial contamination during implantation, or postoperatively (Busscher et al., 2012). The infection rate of biomaterials strongly depends on the site of implantation, and even within specific implants, infection rates differ amongst hospitals, countries and continents (Lee et al., 2012; Merritt et al., 1979; Yue et al., 2015). Nevertheless, even the lowest estimated infection rate poses a significant risk to patients and with the rapidly increasing number of biomaterial implants and devices, the absolute number of infections will rise as a result. Whereas in many cases an infection can be resolved by replacing the implant, this procedure is at the very least costly, inconvenient and dangerous (Bjerkan et al., 2012; Hinds et al., 2012). In other cases, replacement of the implant is much harder and the chances of a recurrent infection increase considerably.

Infection starts with bacterial contamination and adhesion of bacteria to the implant or device surface (Hall-Stoodley and Stoodley, 2009). Bacteria prefer to live surface bound and as such they colonize objects placed inside the human body (Donlan, 2002; Høiby et al., 2011). Once bacteria have managed to invade the host and connect to the biomaterial, they start to grow biofilms. These biofilms are communities of organized bacteria communicating through signaling molecules and designed to significantly increase the chances of bacterial survival (Hall-Stoodley et al., 2004; Høiby et al., 2010).

By forming a dense network of cells and extracellular polymeric substances (EPS), biofilms limit the influx of antibiotics, while shielding themselves for the hosts immune system, resulting in severe resistance to eradication (Flemming and Wingender, 2010; Flemming et al., 2007; Hall-Stoodley and Stoodley, 2009). The dangers of infection and the subsequent difficulty of removing biofilms have led to the preventive administration of antibiotics during high-risk procedures (Schmidmaier et al., 2006). However, as the amount of bacteria resistant to antibiotics is rising and the discovery of new antibiotics is declining, BAI remains a serious issue and is expected to increase in significance (Bush et al., 2011; Laxminarayan et al., 2013; WHO, 2014).

As such, there is an ongoing search for preventive measures against bacterial contamination and biofilm formation. In this search, bioinspired approaches are becoming more and more popular, as nature has often solved problems that have proven to be far too complex for mankind to solve (Chen et al., 2012). There are many examples of naturally occurring surfaces that are nonfouling and even more peptides that show antibacterial activity (Waghu et al., 2014; Wong et al., 2011). Even though these systems are not always directly translatable to clinical applications, great inspiration can be taken from them.

This chapter will discuss multifunctional biomaterials inspired by biological systems directed at influencing tissue cells and microorganisms, separately, or a combination of both, by delivery of bioactive molecules. Delivery is here considered in the broad sense of the word, as materials can contain biomolecules that are released when appropriate, but also merely present the biomolecules at the target site. As the field of biomaterials and their related functions has expanded beyond comprehension, a selection of relevant and recent studies will be discussed to underline the importance of multifunctional materials.

5.2 Biomaterials influencing cellular response

Biomaterials and biomedical devices cannot be successful without eliciting the proper cell response for their respective application. The overall consensus is that materials should not induce cell damage or death, regardless of the place in the body or the tissue it contacts. However, severe differences in the desired cell response exist beyond this initial founding requirement. Implants requiring tissue integration need to be adhesive to cells, while catheters for transport of blood or other bodily fluids should not stimulate cells to adhere in order to prevent obstruction of the passing liquid. Additionally, besides adhesiveness, a whole arsenal of other cell responses can be induced by the right biological cues, ranging from differentiation to a specific cell type to the expression of genes and production of signaling molecules (Bellis, 2011; Kim and Peyton, 2012; Kwee and Mooney, 2015; Schaap-Oziemlak et al., 2014).

There is also a key material property involved in the provoked cell's response after implantation or cell seeding to a material; in an abundance of cell types, the cell response depends on the mechanical properties of the material they grow on (Schaap-Oziemlak et al., 2014). As the body has numerous cell types, constituting different tissues and performing different functions, each cell has its own particular preference for material characteristics (Branco da Cunha et al., 2014). Cells grow best and differentiate to the appropriate cell type when they are grown on materials resembling the native tissue they constitute. Cells making up hard structures in the body, such as bone, need to be grown on hard materials, while cells assembling into soft structures grow best on soft materials. Additionally, cells experiencing specific mechanical cues from the body need these cues provided to them in vitro as well; when trying to differentiate stem cells towards cardiac muscle cells, they need to receive similar electrical stimulation found in vivo, in order to stimulate differentiation (Nunes et al., 2013).

As mentioned before, tissue integration is one of the major challenges posed to bone implants. Despite the biocompatibility of titanium, which is the most common metal used for bone implants (long-term), integration remains a problem (Geetha et al., 2009; Junker et al., 2009). To improve tissue integration Zhou et al. used an approach based on bio-molecular self-assembly (Zhou et al., 2015). By constructing a chimeric peptide consisting of a peptide implant binding domain and a bone-inducing protein, rapid and complete surface coverage of cells on titanium implants was realized, including highly elevated levels of bone marker genes. This dual functional approach improved the cell response and differentiation of stem cells towards bone cells, without the need for complicated chemical attachment methods to secure the protein to the implant surface. Another method to induce differentiation of osteoblasts into bone cells involves the influence of strontium ions. In a recent study, a 3D structure of strontium and micro-arc oxidized titanium was covered with a polydopamine film (Liu et al., 2014). While the dopamine enhanced cell adhesion, the release of strontium ions from the underlying structure promoted the early stage of osteoblast differentiation as determined by the levels of alkaline phosphatase (ALP). Polydopamine also has been used previously to directly immobilize ALP on the surface of titanium. However, results showed that even though ALP expression and activity has been generally accepted as a marker for early osteogenic phenotype differentiation and even suggested to predict in vivo bone-forming capacity (Prins et al., 2014), direct immobilization of ALP has no such effect on osteogenic differentiation (Nijhuis et al., 2014). Dopamine is a popular bio-adhesive due to its nonspecificity and ability to attach to almost any surface or material.

Most applications make use of the polymerization of dopamine under alkaline conditions and ambient air, which induces oxidation and subsequent polymerization. In an attempt to provide more control over the oxidation process, Wang et al. explored the possibility of electro-polymerization of dopamine to modify cardiovascular stents (Wang et al., 2014). Using this alternative polymerization technique, they achieved a higher grafting density when compared to the classical approach and were able to covalently bind vascular endothelial growth factor (VEGF) to their complex 3D structures. In vitro studies demonstrated that their coating significantly promoted adhesion, proliferation, migration, nitric oxide secretion, and maintenance of normal phenotype of endothelial cells and even reduced neo-intimal formation in vivo.

Whereas dopamine is a general bio-adhesive, arginine-glycine-aspartate (RGD) is a commonly used peptide sequence specifically known to promote cellular adhesion. Salvagni et al. combined a RGD motif with an elastin-like penta-peptide to create a recombinant protein-based polymer that offers tissue cells a specific binding-site while optimizing the mechanical properties behavior of the coated surface (Salvagni et al., 2014). This construct was repeated six times, after which immobilization on titanium was achieved by variation of the elastin-like building block with an isoleucine substituted by a lysine, possessing a primary amine for covalent immobilization. As a result, ALP activity was significantly higher on modified titanium compared to control surfaces.

While titanium is the preferred material for healing or bridging bone defects, hydrogels are often studied as scaffolds for structures that require less mechanical rigidity. As such, polyethylene glycol (PEG)–peptide hydrogels have recently been used to create bio-mimetic scaffolds for regeneration of heart-valves (Zhang et al., 2015). In this study, PEG hydrogels were combined with tethered cell-adhesive RGD peptides, incorporating collagenase-degradable peptide PQ (GGGPQG; IWGQGK). The cell adhesive peptide was added to adhere cells to the otherwise nonadhesive PEG, while the peptide QP was added to increase the degradability of the polymer structure. Collagen is another common base for the preparation of hydrogels, as it is naturally occurring and therefore physico-chemically mimics the extracellular matrix (ECM) of cells, providing outstanding biocompatibility (Seliktar, 2012). The biomimetic nature of collagen hydrogels when used as a scaffold for mesenchymal stem cells (MSC) can induce expression of transcription factors related to preservation of pluripotency and selfrenewal, and the secretion of angiogenic cytokines (Rustad et al., 2012). The preservation of pluripotency is important to prevent restriction of stem cells to a specific phenotype in an early stage, while angiogenic cytokines are necessary to promote angiogenesis in tissue engineered scaffolds to induce vascularization. Additionally, besides taking advantage of the properties of collagen as an ECM mimic itself, hydrogels can be loaded with a great variety of biomolecules to induce the desired response in a range of target sites within the body (Choi et al., 2014; Mullen et al., 2015).

The overview of biomaterials and their elicited responses given here depicts the complexity of designing biomaterials. There is no simple way of adding components to influence cell response, as each application brings restrictions towards the required material properties. For most applications there are a steady number of commonly used materials that have been proven to form a solid base, which can be elegantly modified to improve performance, as long as the basic properties are not altered severely. However, there is no doubt that new base materials will be discovered offering additional platforms for a variety of modifications.

5.3 Biomaterials influencing microorganisms

As biomaterials are implanted in the body or used within a device designed to aid a specific bodily function, one of the greatest risks for the patient is for the biomaterial to become contaminated with bacteria (Ribeiro et al., 2012). Bacteria prefer to live on surfaces, creating biofilms that offer shelter and protection, rather than existing as single entities freely floating around (Donlan, 2002; Hall-Stoodley et al., 2004). Despite the percentage of infections gradually declining for decades and currently estimated by some to be as low as 2% for some specific applications, the absolute number of patients suffering from infection-related problems is enormous, and rising dramatically due to the increasing number of people requiring a biomedical implant or device (Widmer, 2001). The current impact, as well as the prospective increase in the number of BAI is the main reason for decades of research aimed at finding strategies to prevent and fight infection. Due to the current decrease in antibiotic efficiency caused by antibiotic-resistant strains and subsiding discovery of new antibiotic formulations, the number of studies aiming to solve the BAI problem without the use of antibiotics is increasing rapidly (Cooper and Shlaes, 2011; Høiby et al., 2010; WHO, 2014).

Looking at the huge number of successes in the reduction and prevention of bacterial adhesion and biofilm formation in vitro (Banerjee et al., 2011; Campoccia et al., 2013; Carvalho et al., 2013; Epstein et al., 2012; Swartjes et al., 2013, 2014a,b; Wong et al., 2011) and comparing them to the few concepts that have successfully been applied in clinical situations, the complexity of the problems associated with bacterial adhesion and biofilm formation becomes evident. This is partially attributable to the complexity of medical devices and implants, which all create interfaces between materials and biology.

Another part of the complexity stems from the incomplete understanding of bacterial adhesion mechanisms (Beaussart et al., 2013; Li et al., 2014; Sullan et al., 2015; Swartjes and Veeregowda, 2016). Previously, chemically altered surfaces containing large hydrophilic polymer chains, so-called polymer brushes, were regarded as a promising approach to solve the bacterial adhesion problem (Ayres, 2010; Bhairamadgi et al., 2014; Terada et al., 2006). However, clinical application so far has been restricted to relatively simple systems, such as contact lenses, endotracheal tubes and urinary catheters (Busscher et al., 2012).

The reason for calling these applications simple is the temporary nature of the devices, which are designed to be used for a short period of time; the contact with the receiver tissue is limited and they are not designed to be completely integrated, in contrast to other more complex implants. Additionally, in the case of endotracheal tubes and urinary catheters, the coated area is located in the lumen of the devices, offering an environment protected from direct contact with any hard materials that could displace the coating.

Breakdown of functional requirements for the use of these medical device examples again highlights the application specificity that is desired for implant and medical device coatings or modifications. It is highly unlikely that a single future solution will be found to solve all the microbial infection-related problems in the medical field dealing with devices and implants. This is strengthened by the fact that the primary bacterial species responsible for causing infection greatly differ depending on the site of the body receiving an implant or device. The microbiome of the oral cavity, for example, represents a completely different range of species when compared to the gut (Guarner and Malagelada, 2003; Wessel et al., 2014). However, this only supports the ongoing trend of seeking inspiration in the diversity provided by nature and using these bio-inspired approaches to fight bacteria.

Taking inspiration from nature in an effort to prevent the complications caused by bacteria, or microorganisms in general, can be carried out in many ways, for example, by using the mechanical strategies found in nature and applying them to prevent bacteria-related problems, or by using chemical natural resources such as biomolecules, peptides and proteins (Holmberg et al., 2013; Muszanska et al., 2011; Swartjes et al., 2013, 2014a). A strategy that might be considered to fall between these two strategies is the use of dopamine, or the related catechols (Lee et al., 2006, 2007).

The dopamine molecule is found to be largely responsible for the strong adhesiveness of marine mussels and over the years its use as a bio-adhesive has increased dramatically. The versatility of dopamine makes its use widespread, including among groups performing surface modifications designed to prevent bacterial adhesion (Huang et al., 2014a; Lee et al., 2007; Lepoittevin et al., 2015; Shi et al., 2016). The most common method of applying dopamine is through the formation of a polydopamine (PDA) layer by exposure of a surface to a dopamine solution under alkaline conditions and subsequently functionalizing the PDA modified surface with additional molecules. This method was applied by Lepoittevin et al. using stainless steel and poly(ethyleneterephthalate) surfaces, combined with end-functionalization of pentadecafluorooctanoyl chloride, thereby creating hydrophobic antifouling surfaces and decreasing the adhesion of *Pseudomonas aeruginosa* by up to 98% (Lepoittevin et al., 2015). Several approaches combine the application of PDA layers to material surfaces with the subsequent attachment of zwitterionic molecules (Huang et al., 2014a;

Li et al., 2008; Sundaram et al., 2014). Even though many of these approaches rely on the incorporation of sulfobetaine, a quaternary ammonium compound that is also highly hydrophilic, as the zwitterionic component (Huang et al., 2014a; Li et al., 2008; Sundaram et al., 2014), other molecules such as peptide sequences can be used as well (Cui et al., 2014). Whereas these studies used the aforementioned order of applying a PDA layer with subsequent functionalization, Huang et al. did not use dopamine as a linker molecule, but functionalized the dopamine molecules itself using sulfobetaine (Huang et al., 2014a). Interestingly, the study reports that binding was not performed under the usually applied alkaline environment, but instead required a low pH leading to hydrogen bonding with oxidized titanium surfaces, which were only converted to covalent bonds by subsequent rising of the pH.

Whereas dopamine as a bio-adhesive itself is not active against bacteria, but is used to intermediate between antiadhesives or antimicrobials and surfaces, there are many biomolecules that themselves exhibit profound effects against pathogens (Blackledge et al., 2013; Gomes et al., 2013; Harding and Reynolds, 2014; Salwiczek et al., 2014; Schlusselhuber et al., 2015; Swartjes et al., 2014a). Currently, the three main biomolecules studied for their potential use as antibacterial agents in relation to biomaterials are enzymes, quorum sensing inhibitors (QSI) and peptides (Kratochvil et al., 2015; Swartjes et al., 2014a).

Peptides exhibiting activity against bacteria are commonly referred to as antimicrobial peptides, or AMPs. This class is also by far the biggest and perhaps therefore the most promising of the biomolecules being considered for use in and on biomaterials (Fox, 2013). The list of peptides that are able to kill or inhibit the growth of bacteria is long and continues to expand (Waghu et al., 2014).

There are two main reasons for the continued discovery of new AMPs; first, new AMPs keep being discovered from different sources, of which the animal kingdom is an extremely important one. A large number of animal species, including insects, produce peptides that have antimicrobial properties (Andreu and Rivas, 1998; Brogden et al., 2003; Zasloff, 2002).

The second source of AMP discovery is by modification of already known peptides, with or without antimicrobial activity, and synthesis of completely new peptides, although these latter are most often still based on existing AMPs (Moghaddam et al., 2015; Sader et al., 2004; Scholl et al., 2012). The use of dopamine to intermediate between surfaces and antimicrobials and to secure their attachment has been mentioned above and is also used in combination with AMPs. The reactivity of dopamine has been combined with the AMP CWR11 (peptide sequence CWFWKWWRRRRR-NH2), for example, to coat polydimethylsiloxane (PDMS) in order to decrease bacterial adhesion and biofilm formation on catheter materials (Lim et al., 2015). This method displayed significant reduction in adhesion, as well as biofilm formation of *Escherichia coli*, *Staphylococcus aureus* and *P. aeruginosa*, but the uncontrolled nature of the polydopamine film and the subsequent conjugation of CWR11 lack any insight into the details of the antimicrobial activity.

Exact information about the coupling mechanism can be of importance, as shown by the covalent binding of Leucocin A to gold substrates (Etayash et al., 2014).

Switching between binding Leucocin A to gold by the N-, or the C-terminus changed the amount of bacteria that adhered to the surface, suggesting that each coupling direction allowed for different interactions between the immobilized peptide and added bacteria. Even though the differences found were small, controlled coupling gives the advantage of specific orientation, which is of importance with respect to AMP activity (Costa et al., 2011). Going into further depth regarding the important aspect of peptide presentation via surface immobilized strategies, a variety of reactive surfaces can be used to ensure different immobilization orientations of AMPs (Rapsch et al., 2014).

Preactivated surfaces of epoxy, aldehyde, NHS and PDITC have been used to immobilize peptides and identify their antimicrobial activities, revealing significant differences in antimicrobial activity between immobilization strategies using these different coupling mechanisms. Additionally, coupling of AMPs can also be combined with the use of polymer brushes, resulting in surfaces which are not only antifouling, but also express antimicrobial activity (Gao et al., 2011; Jiang and Xu, 2013; Yu et al., 2015).

Delivery of AMPs by release from implant materials avoids having to choose between coupling mechanisms and, depending on the application, can therefore be the preferred method of choice. The use of multilayers to capture AMPs and slowly release them into the surrounding area is advantageous because the release profile can be adjusted by adding layers or modifying layer thickness. Polysaccharide films releasing bound AMPs by enzymatic degradation of the layers inhibit bacterial growth more as the number of layers increased (Cado et al., 2013). In this case, more layers allowed for a higher content of AMPs, sustaining the release for a longer period of time. Another method of controlling the release of AMPs is to include a phospholipid layer, which offers a sustained and more controlled release of HHC-36 from calcium phosphate covered TiO_2 layers (Kazemzadeh-Narbat et al., 2013; Ma et al., 2012).

AMPs are considered by some to be the best candidates to replace antibiotics, as there is no known resistance build up after exposure to AMPs (di Luca et al., 2014; Hussain et al., 2006). However, there is another interesting class of biomolecules studied for their effect against bacterial adhesion and biofilm formation that has shown promising results. Being the smallest group of the aforementioned biomolecules, QSIs comprise a highly interesting class, especially considering their relatively recent discovery (Kalia, 2013). As a consequence, the majority of QSI studies focus on questions regarding the mechanisms and effects, resulting in far less studies concerning the application of QSI for biomedical applications. Nevertheless, it has been shown that covalent surface immobilization of dihydropirrolones (DHPs) via click chemistry can significantly reduce surface coverage of *P. aeruginosa* and *S. aureus* by inhibiting QS. Release of QSI by carboxymethylcellulose-coated surfaces and nano-porous superhydrophobic surfaces were effective in preventing bacterial adhesion as well, showing that for QSIs there are also different methods of delivery to be considered when designing materials for specific applications (Broderick et al., 2014; Kratochvil et al., 2015).

5.4 Bio-inspired materials influencing cellular response and microorganisms

As science advances, possibilities increase, and reinvention combined with adaptation leads to the development of complex materials performing multiple functions simultaneously. Hip implants have been used to replace worn out hips since approximately the 1950s and have been continuously improved to reach the defined shaped they have had for the last few decades (Gomez and Morcuende, 2005). Currently, most of the improvements that are studied no longer deal with the shape of the implant, but instead with promoting tissue integration and, perhaps even more importantly, how to prevent microbial infection. Titanium and stainless steel are the most used base materials for orthopedic implants, due to their material properties and relative good biocompatibility. However, despite the biocompatibility, there are ongoing efforts to find ways to increase bone integration to achieve an extended lifespan (Schmidt et al., 2001). At the same time, another major threat to orthopedic implants stems from bacterial contamination, especially within the last decade, as the number of bacteria expressing antibiotic resistance has increased dramatically. Solving both of these issues means that implants have to be designed to be multifunctional, improving tissue integration while discouraging bacterial adhesion (Fig. 5.1).

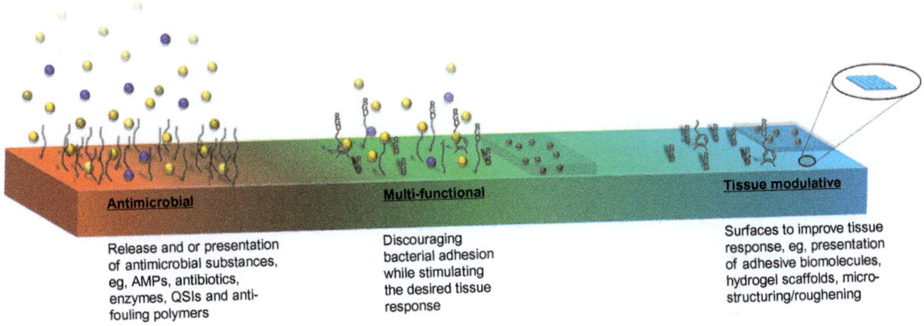

Fig. 5.1 Schematic representation of possible modifications for antimicrobial surfaces *(left)*, tissue modulative surfaces *(right)* and multifunctional surfaces *(middle)*. Antimicrobial surfaces can be achieved by the release and or by the surface display of antimicrobial substances, such as AMPS, antibiotics, enzymes, QSIs and antifouling polymers. A specific tissue response can be induced by the presentation of adhesive biomolecules, hydrogels scaffolds or micro-roughening, for example. Combining both of these approaches leads to multifunctional surfaces which discourage bacterial adhesion, or kill bacteria, while stimulating tissue cells to adhere, differentiate or express specific genes.

Antiadhesive coatings can be fabricated in many ways and at first sight might seem like an attractive solution to prevent bacterial contamination of an implant (Li et al., 2008; Swartjes et al., 2014a; Wang et al., 2011). However, generally speaking, besides preventing bacterial adhesion, antiadhesive coatings also discourage the adhesion of tissue cells and therefore hamper tissue integration. As a result, the type of implants requiring tissue integration is not suitable for application of purely antiadhesive coatings. To circumvent these issues with tissue integration, biologically inspired peptide sequences can be used to promote adhesion of tissue cells (Chua et al., 2008). These sequences, for example the RGD sequence, are not recognized by bacteria and therefore selectively attract tissue cells to inhabit the implant surface. RGD has been coupled to the end of the polymer chains in polymer brushes to complement the antifouling character, which keeps bacteria off the surface, with cell adhesive properties (Muszanska et al., 2014). The additional incorporation of AMPs to the polymer chains can enhance the functionality of these brushes even more, by including antimicrobial properties (Muszanska et al., 2014). These brushes consisted of Pluronic F-127 modified with the appropriate peptide sequences and were adsorbed onto silicone rubber by hydrophobic interactions. To achieve similar brush formation on glass surfaces, surface-initiated atom radical polymerization (ATRP) can be used to form a brush to which the RGD can be coupled subsequently (He et al., 2014).

Similarly, silk functionalization of antiadhesive poly(methacrylic acid) brushes on titanium increased cell adhesion, but maintained its antiadhesive properties towards bacteria (Zhang et al., 2008). In some cases, the base material already represents a tissue adhesive surface and creating patches of nonadhesive PEG "islands" at the right separation distance excludes bacterial adhesion without negative effects on tissue cell adhesion (Wang et al., 2011).

Other approaches include modification of the implant surface by different roughening methods. Treatment of 316L stainless steel by shot peening can induce hierarchical roughness, surface grain refinement and alter the mechanical properties, leading to a positive cell response while reducing the adherence towards Gram-positive bacteria (Bagherifard et al., 2015). Additionally, creating porous surfaces resembling native bone tissue can stimulate osteogenic differentiation and bone formation (Huang et al., 2014b; Huo et al., 2013).

The addition of multilevel nanostructured TiO_2 to carbon reinforced polyetherketone resulted in a nanoporous titanium layer stimulating fibroblast adhesion and displaying antibacterial properties (Wang et al., 2016). The porous bone-like surface of these materials consequently also makes them suitable for loading of antibacterial agents, creating a multifunctional implant with enhanced integration properties and decreased risk of bacterial contamination (Huang et al., 2014b).

Copper loading of porous bioactive-glass scaffold also leads to stimulation of cell responses, including osteogenic responses and angiogenesis (Wu et al., 2013). Besides the modulation of cell responses, copper loading also inhibited bacterial viability. Porous structures are not just suited for loading with antimicrobial agents, they can also be loaded with biomolecules stimulating differentiation of cells into the desired cell types (Chen et al., 2015).

Biomolecules themselves offer a tremendous spectrum of functionality that can be added to materials in an effort to induce the desired cell responses. A combination of ALP and chitosan immobilization to titanium, mediated by polydopamine, resulted in reductions in bacterial adhesion and stimulation of cellular ALP activity and calcium deposition of osteoblasts, human mesenchymal stem cells and human adipose-derived stem cells. Collagen is known to facilitate the adhesion of tissue cells and increase cell compatibility (Seliktar, 2012). Bronk et al. isolated a streptococcal collagen-mimetic protein and coated it on titanium to increase the cell compatibility, while it also discouraged bacterial colonization, offering a promising biomimetic strategy to improve implant success (Bronk et al., 2014). Other biomimetic strategies involve layer-by-layer assembly of heparin-like nanogels, loaded with Ag-nanoparticles to obtain materials that have high blood compatibility, decreased protein adsorption and prolonged clotting times, whilst also being antibacterial (Xia et al., 2014).

5.5 Conclusions

Nature remains a great source of inspiration for the development of biomaterials and strategies to combat biomedical problems. Whether it concerns structural features determining surface characteristics, or biomolecules directly extracted or derived from natural products, possible solutions are hidden in a considerable number of organisms. As biomaterials evolve, they often reach near perfection in certain aspects, only to expose weaknesses and challenges in others. The hip implant is such an example, having obtained its definite shape decades ago, but still the center of numerous studies, now focusing on surface properties trying to increase cellular interactions and diminish the risk of bacterial infection. Even though modern science has learned to focus on many aspects simultaneously, guiding towards more multidisciplinary research, there is no doubt that the materials currently being developed will offer the same challenges in the future, once the current goals have been achieved. As a result, multifunctional materials are being developed and older materials are being modified to add functionalities and try to perfect their functions.

One of the major challenges within the field of biomaterials, however, may be more complicated than the research itself. Some of the currently used biomaterials have an established history of use and have gained the confidence of many surgeons. When biomaterials are relatively successful, meaning success rates are high, proving the benefits of modifications can be a difficult challenge. From a statistical point of view, small improvements require large sample sizes to prove a decrease of the complications currently arising. Moreover, new or improved biomaterials will have even less chance of establishing themselves as a successful alternative if their use requires surgeons to adapt current procedures in order to use these new biomaterials. Since the established procedures are sometimes performed on a daily basis, a new procedure might require years of experience before it is performed with the same accuracy, confidence and success rate. Any implant modification which requires an adjustment of the implant procedure can therefore induce failure not related to the modification itself.

Even though it is important that scientists do not limit their possibilities in an early stage, as it will reduce creativity, these factors are a major determinant for successful translation of new strategies to clinical applications. Complicating the already difficult process of biomaterial design, it means that, where possible, multifunctionality and bio-inspired design should improve current implants and devices one step at a time, as this might increase the chances of successfully building towards perfected biomaterials.

References

Agarwal, R., García, A.J., 2015. Biomaterial strategies for engineering implants for enhanced osseointegration and bone repair. Adv. Drug Deliv. Rev. 94, 53–62. http://dx.doi.org/10.1016/j.addr.2015.03.013.

Alvarez-Lorenzo, C., Concheiro, A., 2013. Bioinspired drug delivery systems. Curr. Opin. Biotechnol. 24, 1167–1173. http://dx.doi.org/10.1016/j.copbio.2013.02.013.

Andreu, D., Rivas, L., 1998. Animal antimicrobial peptides: an overview. Biopolymers 47, 415–433. http://dx.doi.org/10.1002/(SICI)1097-0282(1998)47:6<415::AID-BIP2>3.0.CO;2-D.

Ayres, N., 2010. Polymer brushes: applications in biomaterials and nanotechnology. Polym. Chem. 1, 769–777. http://dx.doi.org/10.1039/B9PY00246D.

Bagherifard, S., Hickey, D.J., de Luca, A.C., Malheiro, V.N., Markaki, A.E., Guagliano, M., et al., 2015. The influence of nanostructured features on bacterial adhesion and bone cell functions on severely shot peened 316L stainless steel. Biomaterials 73, 185–197. http://dx.doi.org/10.1016/j.biomaterials.2015.09.019.

Banerjee, I., Pangule, R.C., Kane, R.S., 2011. Antifouling coatings: recent developments in the design of surfaces that prevent fouling by proteins, bacteria, and marine organisms. Adv. Mater. 23, 690–718. http://dx.doi.org/10.1002/adma.201001215.

Basu, B., 2014. Orthopaedic biomaterials: current status and future perspective. Mater. Technol. 29, B2–B3. http://dx.doi.org/10.1179/1066785713Z.000000000196.

Beaussart, A., El-Kirat-Chatel, S., Herman, P., Alsteens, D., Mahillon, J., Hols, P., et al., 2013. Single-cell force spectroscopy of probiotic bacteria. Biophys. J. 104, 1886–1892. http://dx.doi.org/10.1016/j.bpj.2013.03.046.

Bellis, S.L., 2011. Advantages of RGD peptides for directing cell association with biomaterials. Biomaterials 32, 4205–4210. http://dx.doi.org/10.1016/j.biomaterials.2011.02.029.

Bhairamadgi, N.S., Pujari, S.P., Leermakers, F.A.M., Van Rijn, C.J.M., Zuilhof, H., 2014. Adhesion and friction properties of polymer brushes: fluoro versus non fluoro polymer brushes at varying thickness. Langmuir 30, 2068–2076.

Bjerkan, G., Witso, E., Nor, A., Viset, T., Loseth, K., Lydersen, S., et al., 2012. A comprehensive microbiological evaluation of fifty-four patients undergoing revision surgery due to prosthetic joint loosening. J. Med. Microbiol. 61, 572–581. http://dx.doi.org/10.1099/jmm.0.036087-0.

Blackledge, M.S., Worthington, R.J., Melander, C., 2013. Biologically inspired strategies for combating bacterial biofilms. Curr. Opin. Pharmacol. 13, 699–706. http://dx.doi.org/10.1016/j.coph.2013.07.004.

Branco da Cunha, C., Klumpers, D.D., Li, W.A., Koshy, S.T., Weaver, J.C., Chaudhuri, O., et al., 2014. Influence of the stiffness of three-dimensional alginate/collagen-I interpenetrating networks on fibroblast biology. Biomaterials 35, 8927–8936. http://dx.doi.org/10.1016/j.biomaterials.2014.06.047.

Broderick, A.H., Stacy, D.M., Tal-Gan, Y., Kratochvil, M.J., Blackwell, H.E., Lynn, D.M., 2014. Surface coatings that promote rapid release of peptide-based AgrC inhibitors for attenuation of quorum sensing in *Staphylococcus aureus*. Adv. Healthc. Mater. 3, 97–105. http://dx.doi.org/10.1002/adhm.201300119.

Brogden, K.A., Ackermann, M., McCray, P.B., Tack, B.F., 2003. Antimicrobial peptides in animals and their role in host defences. Int. J. Antimicrob. Agents 22, 465–478. http://dx.doi.org/10.1016/S0924-8579(03)00180-8.

Bronk, J.K., Russell, B.H., Rivera, J.J., Pasqualini, R., Arap, W., Höök, M., et al., 2014. A multifunctional streptococcal collagen-mimetic protein coating prevents bacterial adhesion and promotes osteoid formation on titanium. Acta Biomater. 10, 3354–3362. http://dx.doi.org/10.1016/j.actbio.2014.04.005.

Bush, K., Courvalin, P., Dantas, G., Davies, J., Eisenstein, B., Huovinen, P., et al., 2011. Tackling antibiotic resistance. Nat. Rev. Microbiol. 9, 894–896. http://dx.doi.org/10.1038/nrmicro2693.

Busscher, H.J., van der Mei, H.C., Subbiahdoss, G., Jutte, P.C., van den Dungen, J.A.M., Zaat, S.A.J., et al., 2012. Biomaterial-associated infection: locating the finish line in the race for the surface. Sci. Transl. Med. 4, 153rv10. http://dx.doi.org/10.1126/scitranslmed.3004528.

Cado, G., Aslam, R., Séon, L., Garnier, T., Fabre, R., Parat, A., et al., 2013. Self-defensive biomaterial coating against bacteria and yeasts: polysaccharide multilayer film with embedded antimicrobial peptide. Adv. Funct. Mater. 23, 4801–4809. http://dx.doi.org/10.1002/adfm.201300416.

Campoccia, D., Montanaro, L., Arciola, C.R., 2013. A review of the biomaterials technologies for infection-resistant surfaces. Biomaterials 34, 8533–8554. http://dx.doi.org/10.1016/j.biomaterials.2013.07.089.

Carvalho, I., Henriques, M., Carvalho, S., 2013. New strategies to fight bacterial adhesion. In: Méndez-Vilas, A. (Ed.), Microbial Pathogens and Strategies for Combating Them: Science, Technology and Education, vol. 1. Badajoz, Formatex, pp. 170–178.

Chen, P.Y., McKittrick, J., Meyers, M.A., 2012. Biological materials: functional adaptations and bioinspired designs. Prog. Mater. Sci. 57, 1492–1704. http://dx.doi.org/10.1016/j.pmatsci.2012.03.001.

Chen, L., Chen, C., Qiao, X., Yu, K., Xie, L., Cao, J., et al., 2015. Effect of porous titanium coated with IGF-1 and TGF-β1 loaded gelatin microsphere on function of MG63 cells. Trans. Nonferrous Met. Soc. China 25, 2974–2985. http://dx.doi.org/10.1016/S1003-6326(15)63924-3.

Choi, J., Jeong, Y., Gilad, A., Kim, T., Oh, M.H., Hyeon, T., et al., 2014. Engineered collagen hydrogels for the sustained release of biomolecules and imaging agents: promoting the growth of human gingival cells. Int. J. Nanomedicine 9, 5189–5201. http://dx.doi.org/10.2147/IJN.S71304.

Chua, P.-H., Neoh, K.-G., Kang, E.-T., Wang, W., 2008. Surface functionalization of titanium with hyaluronic acid/chitosan polyelectrolyte multilayers and RGD for promoting osteoblast functions and inhibiting bacterial adhesion. Biomaterials 29, 1412–1421. http://dx.doi.org/10.1016/j.biomaterials.2007.12.019.

Cooper, M.A., Shlaes, D., 2011. Fix the antibiotics pipeline. Nature 472, 32. http://dx.doi.org/10.1038/472032a.

Costa, F., Carvalho, I.F., Montelaro, R.C., Gomes, P., Martins, M.C.L., 2011. Covalent immobilization of antimicrobial peptides (AMPs) onto biomaterial surfaces. Acta Biomater. 7, 1431–1440. http://dx.doi.org/10.1016/j.actbio.2010.11.005.

Cui, J., Ju, Y., Liang, K., Ejima, H., Lörcher, S., Gause, K.T., et al., 2014. Nanoscale engineering of low-fouling surfaces through polydopamine immobilisation of zwitterionic peptides. Soft Matter 10, 2656–2663. http://dx.doi.org/10.1039/C3SM53056F.

de Souza Costa, C.A., Hebling, J., Scheffel, D.L.S., Soares, D.G.S., Basso, F.G., Ribeiro, A.P.D., 2014. Methods to evaluate and strategies to improve the biocompatibility of dental materials and operative techniques. Dent. Mater. 30, 769–784. http://dx.doi.org/10.1016/j.dental.2014.04.010.

di Luca, M., Maccari, G., Nifosi, R., 2014. Treatment of microbial biofilms in the post-antibiotic era: prophylactic and therapeutic use of antimicrobial peptides and their design by bioinformatics tools. Pathog. Dis. 70, 257–270. http://dx.doi.org/10.1111/2049-632X.12151.

Donlan, R.M., 2002. Biofilms: microbial life on surfaces. Emerg. Infect. Dis. 8, 881–890. http://dx.doi.org/10.3201/eid0809.020063.

Epstein, A.K., Wong, T.-S., Belisle, R.A., Boggs, E.M., Aizenberg, J., 2012. Liquid-infused structured surfaces with exceptional anti-biofouling performance. Proc. Natl. Acad. Sci. 109, 13182–13187. http://dx.doi.org/10.1073/pnas.1201973109.

Etayash, H., Norman, L., Thundat, T., Stiles, M., Kaur, K., 2014. Surface-conjugated antimicrobial peptide leucocin a displays high binding to pathogenic gram-positive bacteria. ACS Appl. Mater. Interfaces 6, 1131–1138. http://dx.doi.org/10.1021/am404729c.

Flemming, H., Wingender, J., 2010. The biofilm matrix. Nat. Rev. Microbiol. 8, 623–633. http://dx.doi.org/10.1038/nrmicro2415.

Flemming, H.C., Neu, T.R., Wozniak, D.J., 2007. The EPS matrix: the "House of biofilm cells". J. Bacteriol. 189, 7945–7947. http://dx.doi.org/10.1128/JB.00858-07.

Fox, J.L., 2013. Antimicrobial peptides stage a comeback. Nat. Biotechnol. 31, 379–382. http://dx.doi.org/10.1038/nbt.2572.

Gao, G., Lange, D., Hilpert, K., Kindrachuk, J., Zou, Y., Cheng, J.T.J., et al., 2011. The biocompatibility and biofilm resistance of implant coatings based on hydrophilic polymer brushes conjugated with antimicrobial peptides. Biomaterials 32, 3899–3909. http://dx.doi.org/10.1016/j.biomaterials.2011.02.013.

Geetha, M., Singh, A.K., Asokamani, R., Gogia, A.K., 2009. Ti based biomaterials, the ultimate choice for orthopaedic implants—a review. Prog. Mater. Sci. 54, 397–425. http://dx.doi.org/10.1016/j.pmatsci.2008.06.004.

Gomes, J., Grunau, A., Lawrence, A.K., Eberl, L., Gademann, K., 2013. Bioinspired surfaces against bacterial infections. Chimia 67, 275–278. http://dx.doi.org/10.2533/chimia.2013.275.

Gomez, P.F., Morcuende, J.A., 2005. A historical and economic perspective on Sir John Charnley, Chas F. Thackray Limited, and the early arthoplasty industry. Iowa Orthop. J. 25, 30–37.

Goodman, S.B., Yao, Z., Keeney, M., Yang, F., 2013. The future of biologic coatings for orthopaedic implants. Biomaterials 34, 3174–3183. http://dx.doi.org/10.1016/j.biomaterials.2013.01.074.

Guarner, F., Malagelada, J.-R., 2003. Gut flora in health and disease. Lancet 360, 512–519. http://dx.doi.org/10.1016/S0140-6736(03)12489-0.

Hall-Stoodley, L., Stoodley, P., 2009. Evolving concepts in biofilm infections. Cell. Microbiol. 11, 1034–1043. http://dx.doi.org/10.1111/j.1462-5822.2009.01323.x.

Hall-Stoodley, L., Costerton, J.W., Stoodley, P., 2004. Bacterial biofilms: from the natural environment to infectious diseases. Nat. Rev. Microbiol. 2, 95–108. http://dx.doi.org/10.1038/nrmicro821.

Harding, J.L., Reynolds, M.M., 2014. Combating medical device fouling. Trends Biotechnol. 32, 140–146. http://dx.doi.org/10.1016/j.tibtech.2013.12.004.

He, F., Luo, B., Yuan, S., Liang, B., Choong, C., Pehkonen, S.O., 2014. PVDF film tethered with RGD-click-poly(glycidyl methacrylate) brushes by combination of direct surface-initiated ATRP and click chemistry for improved cytocompatibility. RSC Adv. 4, 105–117. http://dx.doi.org/10.1039/c3ra44789h.

Hinds, P.R., Wilson, S.K., Sadeghi-Nejad, H., 2012. Dilemmas of inflatable penile prosthesis revision surgery: what practices achieve the best outcomes and the lowest infection rates? (CME). J. Sex. Med. 9, 2483–2491. http://dx.doi.org/10.1111/j.1743-6109.2012.02932.x. quiz 2492.

Høiby, N., Bjarnsholt, T., Givskov, M., Molin, S., Ciofu, O., 2010. Antibiotic resistance of bacterial biofilms. Int. J. Antimicrob. Agents 35, 322–332. http://dx.doi.org/10.1016/j.ijantimicag.2009.12.011.

Høiby, N., Ciofu, O., Johansen, H.K., Song, Z., Moser, C., Jensen, P.Ø., et al., 2011. The clinical impact of bacterial biofilms. Int. J. Oral Sci. 3, 55–65. http://dx.doi.org/10.4248/IJOS11026.

Holmberg, K.V., Abdolhosseini, M., Li, Y., Chen, X., Gorr, S.-U., Aparicio, C., 2013. Bioinspired stable antimicrobial peptide coatings for dental applications. Acta Biomater. 9, 8224–8231. http://dx.doi.org/10.1016/j.actbio.2013.06.017.

Huang, C.-J., Wang, L.-C., Shyue, J.-J., Chang, Y.-C., 2014a. Developing antifouling biointerfaces based on bioinspired zwitterionic dopamine through ph-modulated assembly. Langmuir 30, 12638–12646. http://dx.doi.org/10.1021/la503191b.

Huang, Y., Zha, G., Luo, Q., Zhang, J., Zhang, F., Li, X., et al., 2014b. The construction of hierarchical structure on Ti substrate with superior osteogenic activity and intrinsic antibacterial capability. Sci. Rep. 4, 6172. http://dx.doi.org/10.1038/srep06172.

Huo, K., Zhang, X., Wang, H., Zhao, L., Liu, X., Chu, P.K., 2013. Osteogenic activity and antibacterial effects on titanium surfaces modified with Zn-incorporated nanotube arrays. Biomaterials 34, 3467–3478. http://dx.doi.org/10.1016/j.biomaterials.2013.01.071.

Hussain, R., Joannou, C.L., Siligardi, G., 2006. Identification and characterization of novel lipophilic antimicrobial peptides derived from naturally occurring proteins. Int. J. Pept. Res. Ther. 12, 269–273. http://dx.doi.org/10.1007/s10989-006-9033-4.

Jiang, H., Xu, F.-J., 2013. Biomolecule-functionalized polymer brushes. Chem. Soc. Rev. 42, 3394–3426. http://dx.doi.org/10.1039/c2cs35453e.

Junker, R., Dimakis, A., Thoneick, M., Jansen, J.A., 2009. Effects of implant surface coatings and composition on bone integration: a systematic review. Clin. Oral Implants Res. 20, 185–206. http://dx.doi.org/10.1111/j.1600-0501.2009.01777.x.

Kalia, V.C., 2013. Quorum sensing inhibitors: an overview. Biotechnol. Adv. 31, 224–245. http://dx.doi.org/10.1016/j.biotechadv.2012.10.004.

Kazemzadeh-Narbat, M., Lai, B.F.L., Ding, C., Kizhakkedathu, J.N., Hancock, R.E.W., Wang, R., 2013. Multilayered coating on titanium for controlled release of antimicrobial peptides for the prevention of implant-associated infections. Biomaterials 34, 5969–5977. http://dx.doi.org/10.1016/j.biomaterials.2013.04.036.

Kim, H.-D., Peyton, S.R., 2012. Bio-inspired materials for parsing matrix physicochemical control of cell migration: a review. Integr. Biol. 4, 37. http://dx.doi.org/10.1039/c1ib00069a.

Kratochvil, M.J., Tal-Gan, Y., Yang, T., Blackwell, H.E., Lynn, D.M., 2015. Nanoporous superhydrophobic coatings that promote the extended release of water-labile quorum sensing inhibitors and enable long-term modulation of quorum sensing in *Staphylococcus aureus*. ACS Biomater. Sci. Eng. 1, 1039–1049. http://dx.doi.org/10.1021/acsbiomaterials.5b00313.150922080044007.

Kwee, B.J., Mooney, D.J., 2015. Manipulating the intersection of angiogenesis and inflammation. Ann. Biomed. Eng. 43, 628–640. http://dx.doi.org/10.1007/s10439-014-1145-y.

Laxminarayan, R., Duse, A., Wattal, C., Zaidi, A.K.M., Wertheim, H.F.L., Sumpradit, N., et al., 2013. Antibiotic resistance-the need for global solutions. Lancet Infect. Dis. 13, 1057–1098. http://dx.doi.org/10.1016/S1473-3099(13)70318-9.

Lee, H., Scherer, N.F., Messersmith, P.B., 2006. Single-molecule mechanics of mussel adhesion. Proc. Natl. Acad. Sci. U. S. A. 103, 12999–13003. http://dx.doi.org/10.1073/pnas.0605552103.

Lee, H., Dellatore, S.M., Miller, W.M., Messersmith, P.B., 2007. Mussel-inspired surface chemistry for multifunctional coatings. Science 318, 426–430. http://dx.doi.org/10.1126/science.1147241.

Lee, G.M., Kleinman, K., Soumerai, S.B., Tse, A., Cole, D., Fridkin, S.K., et al., 2012. Effect of nonpayment for preventable infections in U.S. Hospitals. N. Engl. J. Med. 367, 1428–1437. http://dx.doi.org/10.1056/NEJMsa1202419.

Lepoittevin, B., Bedel, S., Dragoé, D., Bruzaud, J., Barthés-Labrousse, M.-G., Mazerat, S., et al., 2015. Antibacterial surfaces obtained through dopamine and fluorination functionalizations. Prog. Org. Coat. 82, 17–25. http://dx.doi.org/10.1016/j.porgcoat.2015.01.007.

Li, G., Xue, H., Cheng, G., Chen, S., Zhang, F., Jiang, S., 2008. Ultralow fouling zwitterionic polymers grafted from surfaces covered with an initiator via an adhesive mussel mimetic linkage. J. Phys. Chem. B 112, 15269–15274. http://dx.doi.org/10.1021/jp8058728.

Li, J., Busscher, H.J., Swartjes, J.J.T.M., Chen, Y., Harapanahalli, A.K., Norde, W., et al., 2014. Residence-time dependent cell wall deformation of different *Staphylococcus aureus* strains on gold measured using surface-enhanced-fluorescence. Soft Matter 10, 7638–7646. http://dx.doi.org/10.1039/C4SM00584H.

Lim, K., Chua, R.R.Y., Ho, B., Tambyah, P.A., Hadinoto, K., Leong, S.S.J., 2015. Development of a catheter functionalized by a polydopamine peptide coating with antimicrobial and antibiofilm properties. Acta Biomater. 15, 127–138. http://dx.doi.org/10.1016/j.actbio.2014.12.015.

Liu, Y.-T., Kung, K.-C., Yang, C.-Y., Lee, T.-M., Lui, T.-S., 2014. Engineering three-dimensional structures using bio-inspired dopamine and strontium on titanium for biomedical application. J. Mater. Chem. B 2, 7927–7935. http://dx.doi.org/10.1039/C4TB00822G.

Ma, M., Kazemzadeh-Narbat, M., Hui, Y., Lu, S., Ding, C., Chen, D.D.Y., et al., 2012. Local delivery of antimicrobial peptides using self-organized TiO_2 nanotube arrays for peri-implant infections. J. Biomed. Mater. Res. A 100, 278–285. http://dx.doi.org/10.1002/jbm.a.33251.

Mantripragada, V.P., Lecka-Czernik, B., Ebraheim, N.A., Jayasuriya, A.C., 2013. An overview of recent advances in designing orthopedic and craniofacial implants. J. Biomed. Mater. Res. A 101, 3349–3364. http://dx.doi.org/10.1002/jbm.a.34605.

Merritt, K., Shafer, J.W., Brown, S.A., 1979. Implant site infection rates with porous and dense materials. J. Biomed. Mater. Res. 13, 101–108. http://dx.doi.org/10.1002/jbm.820130111.

Moghaddam, M.M., Aghamollaei, H., Kooshki, H., Barjini, K.A., Mirnejad, R., Choopani, A., 2015. The development of antimicrobial peptides as an approach to prevention of antibiotic resistance. Rev. Med. Microbiol. 26, 98–110. http://dx.doi.org/10.1097/MRM.0000000000000032.

Mullen, L.M., Best, S.M., Ghose, S., Wardale, J., Rushton, N., Cameron, R.E., 2015. Bioactive IGF-1 release from collagen–GAG scaffold to enhance cartilage repair in vitro. J. Mater. Sci. Mater. Med. 26, 2. http://dx.doi.org/10.1007/s10856-014-5325-y.

Muszanska, A.K., Busscher, H.J., Herrmann, A., van der Mei, H.C., Norde, W., 2011. Pluronic-lysozyme conjugates as anti-adhesive and antibacterial bifunctional polymers for surface coating. Biomaterials 32, 6333–6341. http://dx.doi.org/10.1016/j.biomaterials.2011.05.016.

Muszanska, A.K., Rochford, E.T.J., Gruszka, A., Bastian, A.A., Busscher, H.J., Norde, W., et al., 2014. Antiadhesive polymer brush coating functionalized with antimicrobial and RGD peptides to reduce biofilm formation and enhance tissue integration. Biomacromolecules 15, 2019–2026. http://dx.doi.org/10.1021/bm500168s.

Nijhuis, A.W.G., Van Den Beucken, J.J.J.P., Jansen, J.A., Leeuwenburgh, S.C.G., 2014. In vitro response to alkaline phosphatase coatings immobilized onto titanium implants using electrospray deposition or polydopamine-assisted deposition. J. Biomed. Mater. Res. A 102, 1102–1109. http://dx.doi.org/10.1002/jbm.a.34776.

Nunes, S.S., Miklas, J.W., Radisic, M., 2013. Maturation of stem cell-derived human heart tissue by mimicking fetal heart rate. Future Cardiol. 9, 751–754. http://dx.doi.org/10.2217/fca.13.71.

Prins, H.-J., Braat, A.K., Gawlitta, D., Dhert, W.J.A., Egan, D.A., Tijssen-Slump, E., et al., 2014. In vitro induction of alkaline phosphatase levels predicts in vivo bone forming capacity of human bone marrow stromal cells. Stem Cell Res. 12, 428–440. http://dx.doi.org/10.1016/j.scr.2013.12.001.

Rapsch, K., Bier, F.F., Tadros, M., von Nickisch-Rosenegk, M., 2014. Identification of antimicrobial peptides and immobilization strategy suitable for a covalent surface coating with biocompatible properties. Bioconjug. Chem. 25, 308–319. http://dx.doi.org/10.1021/bc4004469.

Ribeiro, M., Monteiro, F.J., Ferraz, M.P., 2012. Infection of orthopedic implants with emphasis on bacterial adhesion process and techniques used in studying bacterial-material interactions. Biomatter 2, 176–194. http://dx.doi.org/10.4161/biom.22905.

Rustad, K.C., Wong, V.W., Sorkin, M., Glotzbach, J.P., Major, M.R., Rajadas, J., et al., 2012. Enhancement of mesenchymal stem cell angiogenic capacity and stemness by a biomimetic hydrogel scaffold. Biomaterials 33, 80–90. http://dx.doi.org/10.1016/j.biomaterials.2011.09.041.

Sader, H.S., Fedler, K.A., Rennie, R.P., Stevens, S., Jones, R.N., 2004. Omiganan pentahydrochloride (MBI 226), a topical 12-amino-acid cationic peptide: spectrum of antimicrobial activity and measurements of bactericidal activity. Antimicrob. Agents Chemother. 48, 3112–3118. http://dx.doi.org/10.1128/AAC.48.8.3112-3118.2004.

Salvagni, E., Berguig, G., Engel, E., Rodriguez-Cabello, J.C., Coullerez, G., Textor, M., et al., 2014. A bioactive elastin-like recombinamer reduces unspecific protein adsorption and enhances cell response on titanium surfaces. Colloids Surf. B Biointerfaces 114, 225–233. http://dx.doi.org/10.1016/j.colsurfb.2013.10.008.

Salwiczek, M., Qu, Y., Gardiner, J., Strugnell, R.A., Lithgow, T., McLean, K.M., et al., 2014. Emerging rules for effective antimicrobial coatings. Trends Biotechnol. 32, 82–90. http://dx.doi.org/10.1016/j.tibtech.2013.09.008.

Schaap-Oziemlak, A.M., Kühn, P.T., van Kooten, T.G., van Rijn, P., 2014. Biomaterial–stem cell interactions and their impact on stem cell response. RSC Adv. 4, 53307–53320. http://dx.doi.org/10.1039/C4RA07915A.

Schlusselhuber, M., Humblot, V., Casale, S., Méthivier, C., Verdon, J., Leippe, M., et al., 2015. Potent antimicrobial peptides against *Legionella pneumophila* and its environmental host, *Acanthamoeba castellanii*. Appl. Microbiol. Biotechnol. 99, 4879–4891. http://dx.doi.org/10.1007/s00253-015-6381-z.

Schmidmaier, G., Lucke, M., Wildemann, B., Haas, N.P., Raschke, M., 2006. Prophylaxis and treatment of implant-related infections by antibiotic-coated implants: a review. Injury 37, S105–S112. http://dx.doi.org/10.1016/j.injury.2006.04.016.

Schmidt, C., Ignatius, A.A., Claes, L.E., 2001. Proliferation and differentiation parameters of human osteoblasts on titanium and steel surfaces. J. Biomed. Mater. Res. 54, 209–215.

Scholl, D., Gebhart, D., Williams, S.R., Bates, A., Mandrell, R., 2012. Genome sequence of *E. coli* O104:H4 leads to rapid development of a targeted antimicrobial agent against this emerging pathogen. PLoS One 7, 1–5. http://dx.doi.org/10.1371/journal.pone.0033637.

Seliktar, D., 2012. Designing cell-compatible hydrogels. Science 336, 13–17. http://dx.doi.org/10.1126/science.1214804.

Shi, H., Xue, L., Gao, A., Fu, Y., Zhou, Q., Zhu, L., 2016. Fouling-resistant and adhesion-resistant surface modification of dual layer PVDF hollow fiber membrane by dopamine and quaternary polyethyleneimine. J. Membr. Sci. 498, 39–47. http://dx.doi.org/10.1016/j.memsci.2015.09.065.

Stadlinger, B., Pourmand, P., Locher, M.C., Schulz, M.C., 2012. Systematic review of animal models for the study of implant integration, assessing the influence of material, surface and design. J. Clin. Periodontol. 39, 28–36. http://dx.doi.org/10.1111/j.1600-051X.2011.01835.x.

Sullan, R.M.A., Li, J.K., Crowley, P.J., Brady, L.J., Dufrêne, Y.F., 2015. Binding forces of *Streptococcus mutans* P1 adhesin. ACS Nano 9, 1448–1460. http://dx.doi.org/10.1021/nn5058886.

Sundaram, H.S., Han, X., Nowinski, A.K., Ella-Menye, J.R., Wimbish, C., Marek, P., et al., 2014. One-Step dip coating of zwitterionic sulfobetaine polymers on hydrophobic and hydrophilic surfaces. ACS Appl. Mater. Interfaces 6, 6664–6671. http://dx.doi.org/10.1021/am500362k.

Swartjes, J.J.T.M., Veeregowda, D.H., 2016. Implications for anisotropic behavior of nanoscale forces in bacterial attachment. Biophys. Rep. 1, 120–126. http://dx.doi.org/10.1007/s41048-016-0019-2.

Swartjes, J.J.T.M., Das, T., Sharifi, S., Subbiahdoss, G., Sharma, P.K., Krom, B.P., et al., 2013. A functional DNase i coating to prevent adhesion of bacteria and the formation of biofilm. Adv. Funct. Mater. 23, 2843–2849. http://dx.doi.org/10.1002/adfm.201202927.

Swartjes, J.J.T.M., Sharma, P.K., van Kooten, T., van der Mei, H.C., Mahmoudi, M., Busscher, H.J., et al., 2014a. Current developments in antimicrobial surface coatings for biomedical applications. Curr. Med. Chem. 21, 1. http://dx.doi.org/10.2174/09298673216661409161 21355.

Swartjes, J.J.T.M., Veeregowda, D.H., Van Der Mei, H.C., Busscher, H.J., Sharma, P.K., 2014b. Normally oriented adhesion versus friction forces in bacterial adhesion to polymer-brush functionalized surfaces under fluid flow. Adv. Funct. Mater. 24, 4435–4441. http://dx.doi.org/10.1002/adfm.201400217.

Terada, A., Yuasa, A., Kushimoto, T., Tsuneda, S., Katakai, A., Tamada, M., 2006. Bacterial adhesion to and viability on positively charged polymer surfaces. Microbiology 152, 3575–3583. http://dx.doi.org/10.1099/mic.0.28881-0.

Waghu, F.H., Gopi, L., Barai, R.S., Ramteke, P., Nizami, B., Idicula-Thomas, S., 2014. CAMP: collection of sequences and structures of antimicrobial peptides. Nucleic Acids Res. 42, 1154–1158. http://dx.doi.org/10.1093/nar/gkt1157.

Wang, Y., Subbiahdoss, G., Swartjes, J.J.T.M., van der Mei, H.C., Busscher, H.J., Libera, M., 2011. Length-scale mediated differential adhesion of mammalian cells and microbes. Adv. Funct. Mater. 21, 3916–3923. http://dx.doi.org/10.1002/adfm.201100659.

Wang, J., Li, B., Li, Z., Ren, K., Jin, L., Zhang, S., et al., 2014. Electropolymerization of dopamine for surface modification of complex-shaped cardiovascular stents. Biomaterials 35, 7679–7689. http://dx.doi.org/10.1016/j.biomaterials.2014.05.047.

Wang, X., Lu, T., Wen, J., Xu, L., Zeng, D., Wu, Q., et al., 2016. Selective responses of human gingival fibroblasts and bacteria on carbon fiber reinforced polyetheretherketone with multilevel nanostructured TiO2. Biomaterials 83, 207–218. http://dx.doi.org/10.1016/j.biomaterials.2016.01.001.

Wessel, S.W., Chen, Y., Maitra, A., van den Heuvel, E.R., Slomp, A.M., Busscher, H.J., et al., 2014. Adhesion forces and composition of planktonic and adhering oral microbiomes. J. Dent. Res. 93, 84–88. http://dx.doi.org/10.1177/0022034513511822.

WHO. 2014. Antimicrobial resistance: global report on surveillance. p. 232. doi:1.4.2014.

Widmer, A.F., 2001. New developments in diagnosis and treatment of infection in orthopedic implants. Clin. Infect. Dis. 33 (Suppl 2), S94–S106. http://dx.doi.org/10.1086/321863.

Wong, T.-S., Kang, S.H., Tang, S.K.Y., Smythe, E.J., Hatton, B.D., Grinthal, A., et al., 2011. Bioinspired self-repairing slippery surfaces with pressure-stable omniphobicity. Nature 477, 443–447. http://dx.doi.org/10.1038/nature10447.

Wu, C., Zhou, Y., Xu, M., Han, P., Chen, L., Chang, J., et al., 2013. Copper-containing mesoporous bioactive glass scaffolds with multifunctional properties of angiogenesis capacity, osteostimulation and antibacterial activity. Biomaterials 34, 422–433. http://dx.doi.org/10.1016/j.biomaterials.2012.09.066.

Wu, S., Liu, X., Yeung, K.W.K., Liu, C., Yang, X., 2014. Biomimetic porous scaffolds for bone tissue engineering. Mat. Sci. Eng. R Rep. 80, 1–36. http://dx.doi.org/10.1016/j.mser.2014.04.001.

Xia, Y., Cheng, C., Wang, R., Qin, H., Zhang, Y., Ma, L., et al., 2014. Surface-engineered nanogel assemblies with integrated blood compatibility, cell proliferation and antibacterial property: towards multifunctional biomedical membranes. Polym. Chem. 5, 5906–5919. http://dx.doi.org/10.1039/C4PY00870G.

Yu, K., Lo, J.C.Y., Mei, Y., Haney, E.F., Siren, E., Kalathottukaren, M.T., et al., 2015. Toward infection-resistant surfaces: achieving high antimicrobial peptide potency by modulating the functionality of polymer brush and peptide. ACS Appl. Mater. Interfaces 7, 28591–28605. http://dx.doi.org/10.1021/acsami.5b10074.

Yue, C., Zhao, B., Ren, Y., Kuijer, R., Van Der Mei, H.C., Busscher, H.J., et al., 2015. The implant infection paradox: why do some succeed when others fail? Opinion and discussion paper. Eur. Cells Mater. 29, 303–313.

Zasloff, M., 2002. Antimicrobial peptides of multicellular organisms. Nature 415, 389–395. http://dx.doi.org/10.1038/415389a.

Zhang, F., Zhang, Z., Zhu, X., Kang, E.-T., Neoh, K.-G., 2008. Silk-functionalized titanium surfaces for enhancing osteoblast functions and reducing bacterial adhesion. Biomaterials 29, 4751–4759. http://dx.doi.org/10.1016/j.biomaterials.2008.08.043.

Zhang, X., Xu, B., Puperi, D.S., Yonezawa, A.L., Wu, Y., Tseng, H., et al., 2015. Integrating valve-inspired design features into poly(ethylene glycol) hydrogel scaffolds for heart valve tissue engineering. Acta Biomater. 14, 11–21. http://dx.doi.org/10.1016/j.actbio.2014.11.042.

Zhou, Y., Snead, M.L., Tamerler, C., 2015. Bio-inspired hard-to-soft interface for implant integration to bone. Nanomedicine 11, 431–434. http://dx.doi.org/10.1016/j.nano.2014.10.003.

Zimmerli, W., Sendi, P., 2011. Pathogenesis of implant-associated infection: the role of the host. Semin. Immunopathol. 33, 295–306. http://dx.doi.org/10.1007/s00281-011-0275-7.

Perspectives of bioinspired materials in regenerative medicine

6

G.P. Chaves Filho, S.M.G. Moreira
Universidade Federal do Rio Grande do Norte, Natal, Brazil

6.1 Introduction

Problems related to organs or tissue donor availability have in recent decades driven active research in regenerative medicine and tissue regeneration due to their potential to restore the functionality of a damaged organ or tissue (Ninan et al., 2015; Pashuck and Stevens, 2012). To achieve this ambitious goal, scientists, engineers, and physicians are working together to recreate the cellular microenvironment found in healthy tissues (Stoppel et al., 2015).

Several strategies have been proposed and tested, including the application of biochemical and biophysical cues, as well as the use of stem cells (Lv et al., 2015). However, no matter what strategy is adopted, it tends to involve the use of a biomaterial, which should be in the right form to guarantee successful tissue regeneration. Biomaterials are used to produce scaffolds that are primarily used as tissues substitutes, but scaffolds can further act as delivery vehicles for therapeutic molecules (eg, growth factors, proteins, and other molecules), providing a sustained and tunable drug-release profile, without the need for multiple and high-dosage treatments. They can also be used as a cell delivery system, where they can provide physical support for cells and ensure their retention and distribution at the site of transplantation (Tam et al., 2014; Pashuck and Stevens, 2012).

Essentially, in order to produce an excellent scaffold, the biomaterial besides being biocompatible, must support cell growth and/or cell differentiation, thus allowing the retention of metabolic functions, in a similar manner as in the cellular original microenvironment. Furthermore, it should promote integration with the host tissue and allow vascularization (Martino et al., 2015). Hence, it is of vital importance to engineer and optimize the microenvironment around cells through the careful selection of biomaterials, biomolecules, and cells.

The natural extracellular matrix (ECM), with its multitude of evolved cell-instructive and cell-responsive properties, not only provides inspiration and guidelines for biomaterials design, but it is also used to produce natural scaffolds (Brown and Badylak, 2014; Ahn et al., 2015). Thus, biological materials used for scaffold production include: (1) those comprising an intact ECM, obtained through decellularization; (2) those comprising its individual components; and (3) hybrid materials incorporating synthetic and biologic components (Brown and Badylak, 2014; Keane et al., 2015). In addition, during in vivo degradation of ECM-based scaffolds, several embedded cytokines and chemokines are released, generating bioactive cryptic peptides, which promote the modulation of innate immune response and recruitment of endogenous

Bioinspired Materials for Medical Applications. http://dx.doi.org/10.1016/B978-0-08-100741-9.00006-1

stem/progenitor cells to the site of the scaffold, thus functioning as scaffold-mediated inductive processes (Turner and Badylak, 2015). ECM-based scaffolds have shown some interesting and useful biological activities for regenerative proposes, such as angiogenesis promotion, antimicrobial (Brennan et al., 2006; Badylak et al., 2009), and immunomodulatory activity (Daly et al., 2012a). Moreover, these scaffolds can be combined with cells or bioactive molecules to further improve biological response. Currently, there are more than 60 commercially available biologic scaffold products, derived from a wide variety of tissues (both allogeneic and xenogeneic) and companies that continue to commercialize new materials (Valerio et al., 2015).

Along with biological materials, synthetic materials are also being investigated for the production of scaffolds. Remarkably, polymeric materials, which can be prepared with affordable nanoarchitectures, are widely used due to their resemblance with ECM fibrous structure (Ulery et al., 2011). There are two major polymeric products used in the preparation of scaffolds: (1) natural polymers, including polysaccharides (eg, bacterial cellulose, dextrin, chitosan, chitin, and alginate) (Shao et al., 2015; Sun and Tan, 2013; Goncalves et al., 2015; Moreira et al., 2010), and proteins (eg, collagen, fibrin, silk, and elastin) (Chattopadhyay and Raines, 2014; Losi et al., 2013; Gil et al., 2013; Calamak et al., 2014; Girotti et al., 2015); and (2) synthetic polymers, such as polyglycolic acid (PGA), polylactic acid (PLA), poly(orthoesters), polyethylene glycol (PEG), poly-lactic-*co*-glycolic acid (PLGA), polyurethane, poly-e-caprolactone (PCL), among others (Ulery et al., 2011). Several of these polymers are approved by the Food and Drug Administration (FDA) for clinical use (Stoppel et al., 2015).

Another group of materials used for the preparation of scaffolds include biominerals, ceramics, and metals (Naleway et al., 2015).

To take advantage and overcome the limitations presented by each distinct group of materials (natural vs synthetic), a wide variety of composite materials and interpenetrating networks have been combined to achieve the desired results (Stoppel et al., 2015). Composites of natural materials, such as silk and collagen or chitosan and alginate, as well as blends of natural and synthetic systems, such as alginate-polyacrylamide-PCL interpenetrating networks, were developed. In addition, mixtures of polymeric and nonpolymeric materials such as collagen and hydroxyapatite (HA) or carbon nanotubes (CNTs) (Sun et al., 2015; Lee et al., 2015) and hybrid variants of these materials have emerged through synthetic designs and genetic engineering of peptide-based biopolymers (Girotti et al., 2015). Table 6.1 lists some of the materials used in regenerative medicine and their main gains and drawbacks.

A range of biomimetic materials fabricated as hydrogels, membranes, meshes, nanoparticles, and other structures have now been developed as tissue models, scaffolds, or templates for regenerative medicine (Mirazul Islam et al., 2015; Demirel et al., 2015; Naleway et al., 2015).

Among the various tissue engineering solutions, three-dimensional (3D) scaffolds that may be delivered noninvasively as injectable, space-filling liquids, and solidify at body conditions, are intensely investigated (Drury and Mooney, 2003; Godwin et al., 2014).

Next, main advances in bioinspired materials used in skin, bone, nerve, and cardiac tissues regeneration will be presented.

Table 6.1 Classification of biomaterial currently used in regenerative medicine and their principal features

Biomaterial classification	Material	Examples of scaffolds preparations	Principal features	References
Natural	Polymers	Polysaccharides—as bacterial cellulose, dextrin, chitosan, chitin, alginate—and proteins—as collagen, fibrin, silk, elastin	Provides innate biological guidance to cells, which favors cell attachment and promotes chemotactic responses	Stoppel et al. (2015), Barsotti et al. (2011), and Ulery et al. (2011)
Synthetic	Ceramics	Hydroxyapatite, tricalcium phosphate, bioactive glass, and calcium silicate	Resorbed materials, presenting conductive, and inductive properties	Bachar et al. (2013), Tampieri et al. (2014), and Vimalnath et al. (2015)
	Metals	Titanium, zirconium, and magnesium	Tensile strength, fatigue strength, and fracture toughness	Chaya et al. (2015), Patel et al. (2014), and Sun et al. (2013)
	Polymers	Polyglycolic acid, polylactic acid, poly(orthoesters), polyethylene glycol, poly-lactic-*co*-glycolic acid, polyurethane, and poly-e-caprolactone	Tunable properties (physical, chemical, and biological) to match the requirements of specific applications	Ulery et al. (2011), Maitz (2015), and Rashidi et al. (2014)
Hybrid and composite	Composites of natural materials; blends of natural and synthetic systems; mixture of polymeric and nonpolymeric materials	Silk and collagen or chitosan and alginate, alginate-polyacrylamide, collagen and hydroxyapatite or carbon nanotubes, among others	Mechanical and biological properties enhanced to overcome materials limitations	Ninan et al. (2015), Tampieri et al. (2014), Patel et al. (2014), and Jiang et al. (2013)

6.2 Skin Regeneration

As the largest organ of the body, the skin provides critical barrier and protective functions. It is composed mainly of three layers (epidermis, dermis, and hypodermis) and skin appendages, including hair follicles and sebaceous glands (Borena et al., 2015; Takeo et al., 2015; Lee et al., 2014). Generally, a defect in the skin's structure or function is referred to as a wound (Ninan et al., 2015) and wound healing is a complex well-developed and multiphase process that works through a sequential series of events including hemostasis, inflammation, proliferation, and remodeling (Gil et al., 2013; Norouzi et al., 2015; Ninan et al., 2015). Therefore, activation of local and systemic cells, growth factors, cytokines, and ECM components is involved, aiming at skin closure preferably by restoring tissue integrity through regeneration (Turner and Badylak, 2015; Calamak et al., 2014; Borena et al., 2015).

Burns, frostbite, trauma, malignancy, infection, and congenital defects can present with various degrees of skin damage and the patient's condition could be an extra concern (eg, cases of diabetic patient with nonhealing wounds), evidencing the level of knowledge of the healing processes that is needed (Rowan et al., 2015; Yanez et al., 2015). Nevertheless, depending on the extent of the skin damage, a wound dressing may be adequate to absorb wound exudates, prevent contamination, and apply sufficient pressure to encourage homeostasis (Turner and Badylak, 2015).

In the case of deeper injuries or large damaged areas, a skin substitute may be required. In these cases, autologous transplantation has been the golden-standard procedure, in spite of presenting several drawbacks (Bonvallet et al., 2015; Jayarama Reddy et al., 2013). Therefore, engineered skin substitutes represent a promising alternative capable of facilitating acute and chronic wounds healing, as well as burns treatment (Varkey et al., 2015; Norouzi et al., 2015; Ferreira et al., 2014).

Recognition of the ECM's importance in wound healing has led to the development of products that aim to stimulate or replace ECM functions. Therefore an ideal scaffold should provide an effective temporary barrier that not only mimics the native skin environment but also promotes healing and minimizes scarring (Norouzi et al., 2015). In this context, the ultimate aim must be to focus on the development of biologically responsive scaffolds combined with cells and multiple biomolecules resembling structural and biochemical cues of the natural ECM, in order to accomplish fully functional regeneration of skin tissue, avoiding grafting, scaffold replacement over time, or permanent pharmacotherapy (Ninan et al., 2015; Turner and Badylak, 2015; Norouzi et al., 2015).

There are many skin substitute technologies that are either available clinically or undergoing some stage of preclinical tests. Quite often, to develop those products that are clinically used today, scientists obtain inspiration from many interesting aspects of skin anatomy, immunology, and physiology (Rowan et al., 2015; Varkey et al., 2015; Yellowlees, 1990).

Natural ECM-derived scaffolds are promising materials, with specific immunomodulatory properties, capable of promoting regeneration (Valerio et al., 2015; Turner and Badylak, 2015). Some examples already commercialized include acellular dermis

(Collamend); urinary bladder matrix (UBM, commercialized as Matristem) (Valerio et al., 2015); and small intestinal submucosa (SIS, commercialized as OASIA wound matrix) (Zheng et al., 2005). ECM-derived products could also present different forms, for instance UBM is available as powder (MatriStem MicroMatrix, ACell, Inc., MD, USA) and sheet form (MatriStem Burn and Wound Matrices, ACell, Inc.) (Valerio et al., 2015).

Collagen-based materials are most often used for scaffold production for skin regeneration. There are several collagen-based products with different architecture (eg, sponge, fiber, powder, composite dressing, and hydrolyzed collagen) approved and commercialized (Chattopadhyay and Raines, 2014).

Despite their regenerative properties, ECM-derived materials often present low mechanical strength and fast degradation rates (Bonvallet et al., 2015). Therefore, several combinations have been described, using natural products (eg, Dynamatrix, BioDesign Grafts) or mixtures of natural and synthetic materials (eg, Integra) to obtain scaffolds with cell-instructive cues and, at the same time, suitable mechanical properties (Halim et al., 2010). The incorporation of biologics other than ECM, such as growth or angiogenic factors, and use of scaffold with preseeded cells, also represents a major area of interest (You and Han, 2014). Examples include cellularized graft-like products, such as Dermagraft (Hart et al., 2012), Apligraf (Curran and Plosker, 2002), and TransCyte (Amani et al., 2006). These products are generally composed of a polymer scaffold patch preseeded with human fibroblasts (Skardal et al., 2012).

Losi et al. described a biosynthetic scaffold composed of a fibrin layer for growth factors delivery, and a polyether-urethane–polydimethylsiloxane (PEtU–PDMS) layer to offer structural support and mechanical strength improvement of fibrin gel. PEtU–PDMS/fibrin scaffolds were loaded with bioactive vascular endothelial growth factor (VEGF) and basic fibroblastic growth factor (bFGF) and then released in a controlled and sustained manner, resulting in local angiogenesis stimulation and acceleration of wound healing in murine full-thickness skin wound (Losi et al., 2013). Recently, using a genetically diabetic mouse, they demonstrated that this scaffold loaded with platelet lysate can promote wound healing in vivo through simultaneous delivery of multiple active substances, suggesting its potential for treatment of diabetic foot ulcers (Losi et al., 2015).

As mentioned, 3D-biopolymeric scaffolds have extensive applications in tissue engineering because of their nanoscaled structural design, similar to native ECM, giving high surface to volume ratio, promoting cell adhesion, and interconnected pores, thereby facilitating nutrient transport and waste removal, among other advantages. A number of fabrication techniques (eg, electrospinning, selfassembly, phase separation, drawing, and template synthesis) have been employed to produce nanofibers using synthetic and natural compounds or mixtures of both (Norouzi et al., 2015; Bonvallet et al., 2015). Further, scaffolds based on different biomaterials represent a successful approach to regenerate cutaneous tissue since they provide structural support to cell functions, including adhesion, proliferation, and differentiation, and subsequent development of new tissue without scar formation (Losi et al., 2013, 2015; Ferreira et al., 2014; Shi et al., 2015).

Electrospinning is considered to be a straightforward and multifunctional technique to produce ultrafine fibers with diameters in the range of nano to micrometers (Zhao et al., 2015a; Bonvallet et al., 2015). In addition, cells can be seeded and biomolecules incorporated within 3D scaffolds in a precise order to produce a functional multilayer material (Pereira et al., 2013; Lin et al., 2015; Mahjour et al., 2015; Yanez et al., 2015).

Although fibroin-based materials are most explored as suture closure, they are described for the preparation of 3D-blended scaffolds (Nayak and Kundu, 2014; Bhardwaj et al., 2015; Nayak et al., 2013). Sheikh and collaborators using a cold-plate electrospinning approach produced 3D silk fibroin nanofiber scaffolds with high porosity, controlled thickness, and easy contouring for facial shape, allowing cell attachment and infiltration, showing that this is a promising methodology for producing 3D nanofibrous scaffolds (Sheikh et al., 2015).

Hydrogels, including those combined with nano and microarchitecture materials, are also applied in skin regeneration approaches (Griffin et al., 2015; Cam et al., 2015; Nayak and Kundu, 2014; Molinos et al., 2012). In particular, sericin-hydrogels were used to grow fibroblasts and keratinocytes and their potential as skin equivalents was demonstrated (Nayak et al., 2013). Several in vivo studies have looked at the production of biomaterials using sericin, a protein derived from the silkworm cocoon, with the capacity to stimulate collagen production in wounds, which led to activation of reepithelialization (Siritienthong et al., 2012; Siritientong et al., 2014; Aramwit et al., 2013), and antiinflammatory activity (Aramwit et al., 2010; Vyas and Vasconez, 2014). Sericin can be combined with other materials (eg, polyvinyl alcohol (PVA), poly(γ-glutamic acid) (γ-PGA)) and it seems promising from in vivo wound healing experiments (Shi et al., 2015), even when compared with the clinically available wound dressing known as "Bactigras" (Siritientong et al., 2014).

Griffin et al. described the production of an injectable hydrogel that exempts material degradation prior to tissue ingrowth. This scaffold combines injectability and microporosity, providing a stably linked interconnected network of micropores that allow cell migration and in vivo bulk integration with surrounding tissue (Fig. 6.1). Furthermore, these properties could change clinical wound treatment by acting as a moldable skin substitute and as a synthetic alternative to grafting. In addition, its injectable nature allows its application to any wound size and shape (Griffin et al., 2015).

Multilayered materials are being developed for application in the healing of compromised wounds. This system is based on sequential release of complementary bioactive components to enhance the activation of dermal tissue regeneration. Recently, a layer-by-layer approach was used to produce a 3D cell/fiber composed by nanofibers of blended PCL, type I collagen, and human skin cells (fibroblasts and keratinocytes). The assembled cell/nanofiber constructs, without or with keratinocyte layers, were cultured to form dermal substitutes or bilayer skin substitutes that were evaluated in nude mice (Mahjour et al., 2015).

A trilayered chitosan-based scaffold was successfully constructed to replicate striation of a full-thickness skin more accurately than a single- or bilayered scaffold, which needed weeks of coculturing of fibroblasts and keratinocytes to achieve similar patterns. Additionally, this composite was able to quickly absorb water and stayed

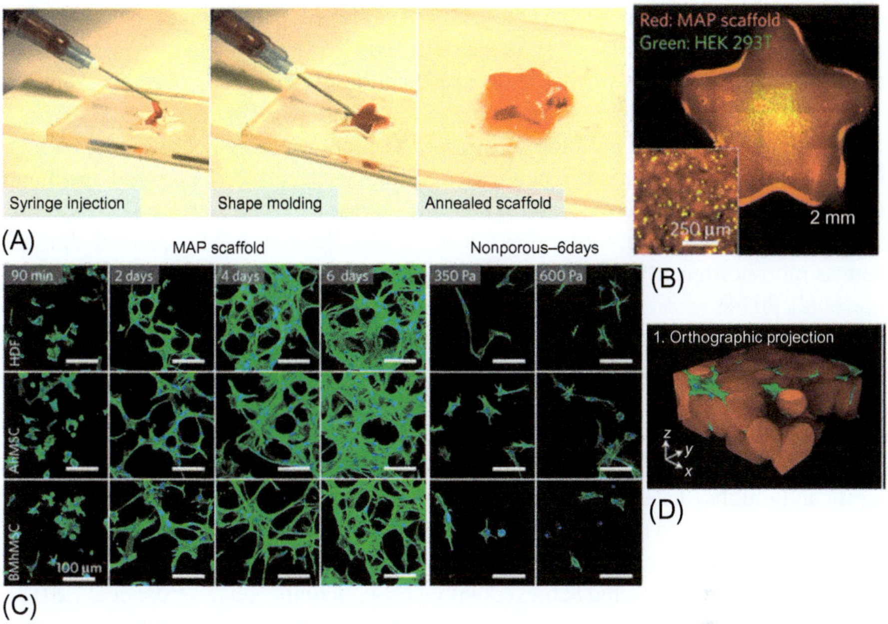

Fig. 6.1 Microporous annealed particle (MAP) scaffolds for wound healing application. (A) MAP scaffolds *(red)* are moldable to macroscale shapes, and can be injected to form complex shapes that are maintained after annealing. (B) This process can be performed in the presence of live cells *(green)*. (C) Fluorescent images demonstrating the formation of 3D cellular networks during 6 days of culture in MAP scaffolds *(red)* in vitro as well as nonporous gels (after 6 days), showing MAP scaffolds facilitate 3D cellular network formation and proliferation in vitro. Schematic illustrating how to read images of 3D cell growth and network formation presented in (D). *HDF*, human dermal fibroblasts; *AhMSC*, adipose-derived human mesenchymal stem cells; *BMhMSC*, bone marrow-derived human mesenchymal stem cells. Adapted with permission from Macmillan Publishers Ltd: (Nature materials) (Griffin et al., 2015) copyright (2015).

intact throughout the course of the 14-day cell culture tests. Fibroblasts seeded on both sides of scaffolds were able to proliferate and stayed separated by the thin film (Lin et al., 2015).

Recent advances in 3D-bioprinting techniques offer significant advantages in comparison with conventional skin tissue engineering, including capacity of dispensing live cells, soluble factors, and phase-changing hydrogels in a desired pattern while maintaining very high cell viability, allowing shape- and form-retention, flexibility, reproducibility, and high culture throughput (Gao and Cui, 2015; Koch et al., 2010, 2012; Murphy and Atala, 2014).

A laser-assisted bioprinting technique was used to create a fully cellularized skin substitute. Fibroblasts and keratinocytes were positioned on top of a stabilizing matrix and in vivo tests showed printed keratinocytes formed a multilayered epidermis with starting differentiation and stratum corneum. Keratinocytes proliferation was mainly detected in the suprabasal layers and printed fibroblasts partly stayed on top of the underlying matrix, where they produced collagen, while part of them migrated into the matrix. In vivo results further showed formation of some blood vessels from the wound bed and wound edges in the direction of printed cells (Michael et al., 2013).

Lee et al. demonstrated 3D-bioprinting potential for tissue engineering using human skin as a prototypical example. They used keratinocytes and fibroblasts as constituent cells to represent the epidermis and dermis, and collagen to represent the skin's dermal matrix. After optimization of the conditions, results showed that 3D-printed skin tissue was morphologically and biologically representative of in vivo human skin tissue (Lee et al., 2014).

Regeneration of functional skin in situ is another advantage of using 3D-bioprinting techniques. Thereby, bioprinting technology (inkjet approach) was used to treat full-thickness skin wounds in nu/nu mice. Mesenchymal stem cells (MSC) from amniotic fluid (AFS) and bone mesenchymal stem cells (BMSCs) were suspended in fibrin-collagen gel and "printed" over the wound site. Gel-containing cells presented significantly higher level of wound closure and reepithelialization compared to those treated with gel only. In addition, cell-treated wounds showed higher angiogenic induction, presenting microvessel density and capillary diameters greater than skin treated with gel, the best results being achieved with AFS-containing gel (Skardal et al., 2012).

In skin regeneration it is clear that 3D-bioprinting techniques, which allow the production of stratified materials containing different polymer combinations, biological factors and cells, present a huge potential in future strategies because the obtained materials can better mimic skin tissue, allowing vascularization, cell colonization, and differentiation. Several methodologies can be applied to produce this kind of material and, as stated earlier, several polymers have interesting properties for these applications. Bacterial cellulose (BC), which is produced by several bacteria strains (eg, *Acetobacter xylinum*), with high purity, using nonexpensive methodologies and with a desired shape (Czaja et al., 2006, 2007; Lin and Dufresne, 2014), is a nanofibrous material with a hydrophilic nature and large surface, capable of holding a large amount of water; this set of properties makes it an hydrogel with appealing mechanical features. Furthermore, BC is hemocompatible and does not present genotoxicity, meaning that BC does not induce gene mutations, changes in chromosome structure, or other DNA changes (Moreira et al., 2009; Andrade et al., 2010, 2011) and it can be obtained with different characteristics and be combined with other materials and/or biological factors, giving the possibility to produce scaffolds according to the required applications (Li et al., 2015b; Goncalves et al., 2015).

6.3 Bone regeneration

Bone is a complex hierarchical structure composed of cells, an organic matrix and inorganic salts. The organic matrix primarily consists of collagenous proteins (90%) and noncollagenous proteins, including osteocalcin, osteonectin, osteopontin, fibronectin, bone sialoprotein II, bone morphogenetic proteins (BMPs), and growth factors (Reznikov et al., 2014; Liedert et al., 2005). The inorganic material is mainly constituted by carbonate HA in the form of thin plate-shaped crystals (Reznikov et al., 2014). This tissue structure is continuously remodeled through the concerted actions of bone cells, osteoblasts and osteoclasts, responsible for bone formation and bone resorption, respectively (Florencio-Silva et al., 2015).

On the macroscale structure, two distinct bone types can be identified, namely, cancellous and cortical bone. Cortical bone is the dense bone tissue, with low porosity, that forms the shell surrounding bones, whereas the interior part of bone, enclosed by the cortical shell, is filled with cancellous bone that is metabolically more active, remodeled more often and composed of trabecular struts that form the porous structure filled with marrow (Rho et al., 1998).

Diseases, trauma, injury, and aging may severely affect bone integrity and its repair is extremely sensitive to mechanical conditions at the site of the repair process (Liedert et al., 2005). Thus, repair of bone defects remains a significant clinical challenge, which justifies the substantial investment in bone regenerative biomaterials research (Stevens et al., 2008).

Several biomaterials, including bioceramics, biopolymers, and metals, have been used to produce implantable scaffold for bone tissue engineering and regenerative medicine, as summarized on Fig. 6.2 (Amini et al., 2012; Li et al., 2014). Bioceramics, such as HA and bioglasses, have been well investigated due to their effectiveness.

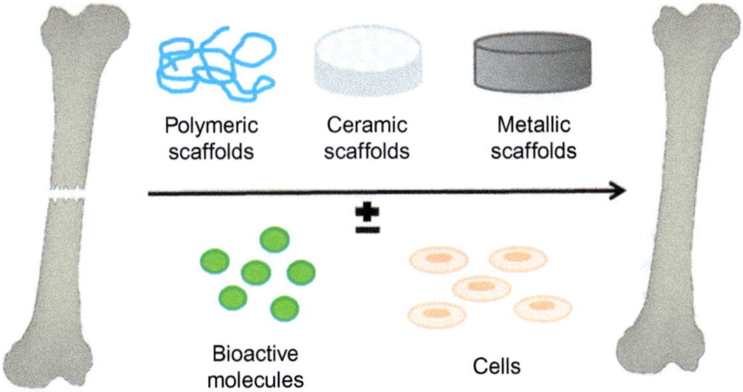

Fig. 6.2 Scaffold-based regeneration of skeletal tissues to meet clinical challenges.
Adapted from Li, J.J., Kaplan, D.L., Zreiqat, H., 2014. Scaffold-based regeneration of skeletal tissues to meet clinical challenges. J. Mater. Chem. B. 2, 7272–7306, with permission of The Royal Society of Chemistry.

HA, the main bone mineral component, can be regarded as an appropriate matrix for bone regeneration. HA-scaffolds improve osteogenic differentiation of MSC and other preosteoblastics lineages by their osteoconductivity properties (Jung et al., 2014; Krishnamurithy et al., 2015). However, it was shown that MSC seeding in HA-scaffolds could not improve bone regeneration compared to noncell-seeded HA-scaffolds (Rathbone et al., 2014).

The first clinical investigation using 90-Y HA produced in a medium flux research reactor showed effectiveness in terms of pain control, functional improvement, and prevention of disease progression in a single patient suffering from rheumatoid arthritis in one of the knee joints, representing a potential step forward toward effective therapy of those patients (Vimalnath et al., 2015). Some other composite scaffolds based on HA were synthesized in association with other materials. In the last decade, nano- and microstructured synthetic HA-based biomaterials have been intensely investigated for bone replacement in combination with chitosan (Chen et al., 2015), polyamide 66 (PA66) (Xiong et al., 2014), iron (Fe^{+2}, Fe^{+3})-doped with collagen (Tampieri et al., 2014) and magnetic iron oxides and multiwalled carbon nanotubes (MWCNTs) (Pistone et al., 2014).

An organic–inorganic hybrid microsphere of chitosan/nano-HA was prepared by high-voltage static microcapsule forming device. Results showed the greater capacity of osteoblasts for adhesion and proliferation in an environment of composite microspheres (Chen et al., 2015). A scaffold of nanoHA-PA66 with a size of 500 μm and 75–85% of porosity was formed by injection molding techniques, which provided a 3D microstructure that could facilitate cell adhesion, differentiation, and proliferation and, later on, helped fiber vascular and nerve colonization with new bone formation at 12 weeks, similar to the surrounding host bone (Xiong et al., 2014). A hybrid bioinspired scaffold made of iron (Fe^{+2}, Fe^{+3})-doped HA nanocrystals and collagen (prepared by freeze-drying process) affected cell proliferation and increased the osteogenic markers expression, when a static magnetic field was applied (Tampieri et al., 2014). The synthesized HA nanocomposites combined with magnetic iron oxides and MWCNTs produced by wet chemical precipitation, under basic conditions, showed biocompatibility and capacity to promote osteogenesis and delivery of clodronate, an inhibitor of osteoclastogenesis (Pistone et al., 2014). Carbon-based materials, such as CNTs and carbon nanofibers (CNFs), exhibit excellent mechanical and electrical properties and their use for bone regeneration is an emerging field (Dubey et al., 2015). For instance, MWCNTs induced the production of numerous vascular channels in formed tissue and in areas of new ossification, at 4 weeks postimplantation (Barrientos-Duran et al., 2014).

Carbon-based materials were also associated with other materials like PLGA (Gupta et al., 2015) and nano-HA/superhydrophilic for application in bone regeneration (Lobo et al., 2013). In vivo, SWCNT/PLGA composites showed similar biocompatibility to PLGA and high mechanical strength, mimicking the microstructure of human trabecular bone (Gupta et al., 2015). Nano-HA/superhydrophilic vertically aligned MWCNT nanocomposites promoted early ECM calcification (24 hours), in vitro, and bone regeneration with lamellar bone formation, after 9 weeks in vivo (Lobo et al., 2013).

Carbon-based materials were also used as an efficient carrier for delivery of therapeutic proteins and drugs. Folic acid (FA) was conjugated to amidated MWCNs to produce functionalized-MWCNTs (f-MWCNTs). Then methotrexate (MTX) was loaded into the pristine and f-MWCNTs to investigate their targeting capacity. The biodistribution studies showed MTX concentration was significantly higher in arthritic joints from folate f-MWCNTs as compared to free drug or drug-loaded in naked MWCNTs (Kayat et al., 2016).

Titanium (Ti) coated with graphene oxide (GO) and loaded with BMP-2 efficiently promotes in vitro osteogenic differentiation of human BMSCs and further promotes new robust bone formation in calvarial defect mouse models in comparison with Ti, Ti/GO, or Ti/BMP-2 implants (La et al., 2013).

Bioglass material is a glass ceramic often used in bone regeneration that was first introduced by Hench in 1969. The most recurrent and important of these materials is the 45S5 Bioglass, which is composed by 45% SiO_2, 24.5% NaO, 24.5% CaO, and 6% P_2O_2 (Jones, 2015).

Research using bioglass for drug delivery and bone tissue repair has significantly grown (Wu and Chang, 2012). Bioglass coated with PLGA-containing vancomycin-loaded microgels promotes the formation of HA in simulated body fluid and provides a rapid drug delivery, favoring antibacterial activity at the wound site (Olalde et al., 2013). Chitosan-polyvinyl pyrrolidone/45S5 Bioglass (CS-PVP/BG) scaffolds, fabricated by foam replication and chemical cross-linking techniques, also present sustained vancomycin release capacity. This material showed resistance to enzymatic degradation and cytocompatibility with MC3T3-E1 osteoblastic cells (Yao et al., 2015). Additionally, a considerable antibacterial activity against some important Gram-positive agents responsible for orthopedic infections was achieved by material coating with selenium nanoparticles or PLGA/selenium particles (Stevanovic et al., 2015).

Bioglass has been included in other matrices to improve their mechanical properties and biocompatibility. The interaction of bioglass with poly(octanediol citrate) impregnated with gallium promoted stiffness and decreased weight loss. Furthermore, osteoblast cells were well attached and grew on these composites, and a collagen synthesis increase was observed, particularly when 10% of bioglass was used (Zeimaran et al., 2015). Biocomposite scaffolds of lithium (Li)-containing mesoporous bioglass and monomethoxy poly(ethylene glycol)-poly(D,L-lactide-*co*-glycolide)-poly(L-lysine) (mPEG-PLGA-*b*-PLL) copolymer significantly promoted new bone formation, displaying good osteogenesis capacity in vivo (Cai et al., 2015).

Several ions were also used to dope bioglasses and to enhance their biological properties, including strontium (Zhao et al., 2015b), boron (Haro Durand et al., 2015), manganese (Miola et al., 2014), zinc (Saino et al., 2011), fluoride, and nitrogen (Bachar et al., 2013). When bioglass-contained strontium was used, the produced scaffold exhibited apatite-forming ability and stimulated MC3T3-E1 cell proliferation and differentiation, showing a good osteogenic capability. Notably, new blood vessel formation was stimulated, which is an important feature in tissue regeneration (Zhao et al., 2015b). Boron is also used as dopant to enhance vascularization. A 45S5 bioglass material doped with 2% B_2O_3 stimulated vascularization and angiogenesis of chorioallantoic membrane (a vascular membrane found in eggs of some amniotes, such as birds, used as angiogenic model) of an embryonic quail, by significantly increasing $\alpha v\beta 3$-integrin expression (Haro Durand et al., 2015). Bachar and coworkers demonstrate the effects of nitrogen and fluoride addition to bioglass. Results showed that incorporation of nitrogen into a material promotes an increase of its density, glass transition temperature, hardness, and elastic modulus, whereas fluoride incorporation decreases thermal property values, which is undesirable for most applications, although mechanical property was maintained. An association of both fluoride and nitrogen was utilized to confer better mechanical properties to the material (Bachar et al., 2013).

A new class of bioactive glasses, the calcium-magnesium sulfophosphates might be explored as a tissue engineering material. So far, good cytocompatibility and biodegradability properties were described, but further characterization is needed (Bassett et al., 2014).

Taken together, the results indicate that bioglass multifunctional scaffolds, incorporating selected biopolymer coatings and ions present great potential for application in bone tissue regeneration.

Biocomposite scaffolds based on natural polymers (mainly alginate, chitosan, collagen, hyaluronic acid (HyA), and silk), some of them containing osteoconductive properties, are often used in bone regenerative approaches (Pina et al., 2015). Additionally, their bone regeneration ability can be optimized by the incorporation of growth factors (Jahan and Tabrizian, 2016). Collagen scaffolds, for example, supplemented with BMP-2 and chitosan showed in vitro and in vivo biocompatibility and may enhance, at a reduced cost, the safety and efficacy of therapeutic implants in terms of large bone repair (Eap et al., 2014). The addition of MSCs microtissues and BMP-7 (instead of BMP-2) to the same collagen scaffold accelerated bone regeneration in vivo and suggested the potential of the technology based on cell contact dependent on growth factors release. This technology is advantageous because it needs lower growth factors amounts in comparison with the current simplistic approaches used in clinics (Schiavi et al., 2015).

The drug-release capacity is also explored for natural polymers in combinations of two or more materials. For instance, 3D-scaffolds produced by combination of chitosan and HyA were developed for controlled and sustained release of immobilized BMP-2, increasing osteogenic markers in MC3T3-E1 cells (Nath et al., 2015). The coeletrospinning-electrospraying approach was used for fabrication of collagen nanofibers scaffold (10–100nm of diameter) and nano-HA agglomerates and their in vitro cytocompatibility using MC3T3-E1 osteoblasts was demonstrated (Ribeiro et al., 2014). Biomimetic spiral-cylindrical scaffold based on hybrid chitosan/cellulose/nano-HA membrane exhibited the highest cell viability and osteocalcin production when 60% of nano-HA was used. In vivo tests on white rabbits resulted in bone regeneration and osseointegration, evidencing that this material has potential for large bone defects treatment (Jiang et al., 2013).

Silk fibroin-based scaffolds, like fibroin/PCL nano/microfibrous composite, were fabricated by the hybrid electrospinning method and showed improved properties in comparison with PCL microfibrous scaffolds, providing a suitable environment for MSC proliferation, adhesion, and differentiation into osteoblasts, in vitro. Moreover, in a rabbit calvarial defect model this material promoted new bone formation (Kwak et al., 2015). Silk fibroin membranes are an alternative to the widely used collagen membranes, once similar volumes of bone regeneration were observed with the advantage of lower cost and zero risk of infection (Kim et al., 2014).

Metals are commonly used in bone regenerative medicine due to their strong mechanical properties and biocompatibility. The most used are titanium (Ti)-, zirconium (Zr)-, and magnesium (Mg)-based materials.

Ti surface modified in oxygen-containing environments forms titania (TiO_2), which was used in a nanosized form for decorating Ti nanotubes. This material showed good cytocompatibility (Huo et al., 2014), antibacterial properties, and greater stem cell osteogenic capacity (Mozaffarian et al., 2015). The addition of BMP-2 into Ti implants stimulated healing and facilitated the formation of the characteristic bone tissue structures (Pavlova et al., 2014; Wen et al., 2016).

In the case of Zr, a material consisting of Zr dioxide disk was functionalized with photocured HyA hydrogels, containing two different amounts of BMP-2 and growth differentiation factor-5 (GDF-5). Similar antiinflammatory activity and similar behavior of drug-release, up to 28 days, was observed (Bae et al., 2013). In addition, Mg–calcium phosphorus compound was used to coat degradable Zr cylinders, resulting in a better implant toleration in comparison with uncoated implants. Moreover, large amounts of cells, rich fibrillar collagen, and calcium and phosphorus products were found on the surface of this material (Sun et al., 2013).

A new class of metals based on degradable Mg is promising for the reduction of long-term complications. These materials combine strength and degradability, offering many potential advantages over current scaffold technologies, which make them ideal for bone fixation. In vivo study, with white rabbits model, demonstrated that the Mg device degradation does not inhibit fracture healing and enhance bone formation around devices, suggesting a role for Mg in cell differentiation and bone growth (Chaya et al., 2015). In addition, Mg corrosive products (micron-size Mg particles) showed no adverse effect on either bone quality or quantity, suggesting this material may promote bone regeneration without inducing inflammation (Guo et al., 2016).

3D-bioprinting is a promising technology for bone regeneration, because it combines rapid prototyping to produce a scaffold with the desired shape and intrinsic structure and the introduction of several living cell types that can form bone tissue, once implanted (Fedorovich et al., 2011). 3D-technology combining mesoporous confinement range, surface chemical groups, and gradual degradation of poly(3-hydroxybutyrate-*co*-3-hydroxyhexanoate) was utilized to produce a composite drug-loaded cylindrical scaffold with slow release of isoniazid and rifampicin. Molecule release was effectively sustained for 12 weeks in local tissues in a rabbit model. In addition, good osteogenic potential was enhanced in a rabbit bone defect model (Elliott Donaghue and Shoichet, 2015).

PLGA-based thermoresponsive microparticulate material was produced at ambient conditions using a bioprinting technique. Materials showed yield stresses up to 1.22 MPa and Young's moduli up to 57.3 MPa, which are within the range displayed by human cancellous bone. Protein-releasing microspheres could be incorporated into bioprinted constructs with sustained release throughout 15 days and a high degree of protein activity measured up to day 9 (Sawkins et al., 2015).

6.4 Nerve regeneration

The nervous system is a complex collection of nerves and specialized cells called neurons that transmit signals between different parts of the body. Structurally, the nervous system has two components: the central nervous system (CNS), made up of the brain, spinal cord, and retina (Tam et al., 2014), and peripheral nervous system (PNS), which consists of sensory neurons, ganglia (clusters of neurons), and nerves that connect to one another and to the CNS. Due to differences in injury response, PNS has greater potential than CNS for regeneration. Thus, PNS has an intrinsic ability for repair and regeneration as compared with the very limited repair ability of CNS, mainly due to the establishment of an inhibitory environment around the lesion site and to the formation of a dense scar tissue (Shrestha et al., 2014; Assuncao-Silva et al., 2015).

Although an injured peripheral nerve can regenerate spontaneously, its regenerative capacity is limited in large defects and severe injury (Pateman et al., 2015; Faroni et al., 2015; Ahn et al., 2015), so autografts still remain the gold standard for nerve defect reconstruction. However, autograft availability and morbidity at the donor site may hamper the successful application of this technique (Gu et al., 2014; Manoli et al., 2014; Sabongi et al., 2015). Consequently, tissue engineered nerve grafts (TENGs) have emerged as a potential alternative to autologous nerve grafts (Sabongi et al., 2015). Generally, new TENGs approaches combine biomaterials (both natural and synthetic), bioactive molecules, physical cues, and cells to achieve neural repair (Faroni et al., 2015; Li et al., 2015c; Samal et al., 2015; Tam et al., 2014; Pateman et al., 2015; Sabongi et al., 2015).

A variety of stem cell types, such as BMSCs, adipose-derived stem cells (ADSCs), muscle-derived stem cells, stem cells from human exfoliated deciduous teeth (SHED), among others, have been applied not only due to their differentiation capability but also because their ability to secrete various trophic factors (Georgiou et al., 2013, 2015; Ding et al., 2010; Kolar and Kingham, 2014; Lavasani et al., 2014; Mohammadi et al., 2013; Sugimura-Wakayama et al., 2015).

6.4.1 Peripheral nerve regeneration

When peripheral nerve injury results in a substantial nerve gap where tension-free neurorrhaphy (suturing the two parts of a severed nerve) is impossible, interposition of some form of graft between nerve stumps is required to bridge the gap and support axonal regrowth (Gu et al., 2014). Although artificial nerve conduits, such as single hollow tubes, are commercially available for connecting transected peripheral nerves, they are not thought to be suitable as a physical guide for a long defect regeneration (Sabongi et al., 2015); therefore a number of TENGs alternatives have been assessed in a preclinical setting (Ahn et al., 2015; Eguchi et al., 2015; Pateman et al., 2015; Gu et al., 2014; Xie et al., 2015; Zhu et al., 2016).

Among natural TENGs options, decellularized allografts presented favorable results. Brooks et al. showed the safety of Avance Nerve Graft (AxoGen, Inc.) for nerve reconstruction (Brooks et al., 2012). Recently, AxoGen© claimed Avance Nerve Graft has no disadvantages related to immunogenicity due to its decellularized and cleansed ECM procedure (Cinteza et al., 2015). Thus, several examples of biological nerve guides have been successfully translated to the clinics (Geuna, 2015; Manoli et al., 2014; Tos et al., 2012; Brooks et al., 2012; Johnson et al., 2011; Kokkalis et al., 2011).

ECM-derived molecules (eg, collagen, laminin, fibrin, fibronectin, and hyaluronan) instead of decellularized allografts are also used. For instance, Neurotube, NeuroGen,

NeuroFlex, NeuroMax, NeuroWrap, and NeuroMend, all based in collagen Type I, are commercially available (Gu et al., 2014; Xie et al., 2015; Tan et al., 2012).

Tubulization techniques have been developed to bridge nerve gaps and numerous experimental and clinical trials investigated their potential (Pateman et al., 2015; Kim et al., 2012; Daly et al., 2012b; Gu et al., 2014; Isaacs et al., 2014). Initially, a nerve guidance conduit or nerve guidance channel (NGC) consisted of an empty cylindrical tube. Unlike the first materials, which were preferentially inert and nondegradable (eg, silicon) (Li et al., 2015a), the materials used today are biodegradable, with complex configurations, in which an NGC has either an internal microarchitecture or a multiple component composition within its lumen, in order to mimic the architecture of nerves for promoting neural cells adhesion, proliferation, migration, and function (Fig. 6.3) (Wood et al., 2013; Lee et al., 2012; Gu et al., 2014).

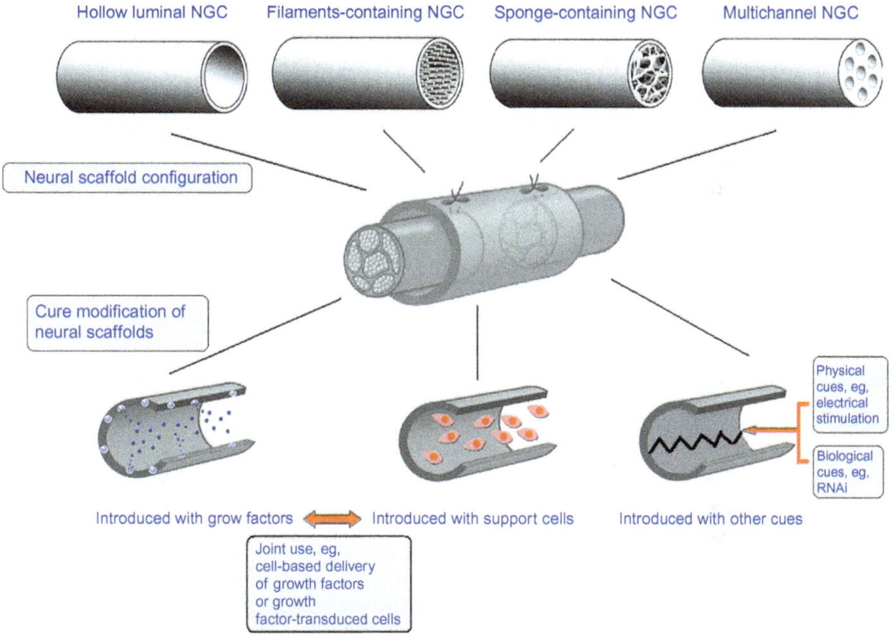

Fig. 6.3 A schematic diagram showing how an ideal tissue engineered nerve graft (TENG) is constructed by incorporating a diverse array of physical and biological cues to a neural scaffold with different configurations.
Reprinted from Gu, X., Ding, F., Williams, D.F., 2014. Neural tissue engineering options for peripheral nerve regeneration. Biomaterials 35, 6143–6156. Copyright (2014), with permission from Elsevier.

There are several different classes of biodegradable synthetic polymers used for peripheral nerve repair (eg, aliphatic polyesters, polyphosphoesters, polyurethanes, and piezoelectric polymers) and some of them are approved for clinical use, such as PGA (Neurotube) and PLC (Neurolac) (Li et al., 2015a; Tan et al., 2012).

In the last decade, biomaterial approaches have sought to replicate the native degradability of natural biomaterials, thereby stimulating the regeneration processes (Lutolf and Hubbell, 2005). In this context, GDNF (glial cell-derived neurotrophic factor)-containing PLGA-based microspheres were loaded into fibrin gels for treating a delayed injury in rat common fibular nerves. GDNF-containing microspheres improved the regeneration of common fibular nerves and reinnervation of extensor digitorum longus muscles, indicating that the number of motoneurons that regenerated their axons increased even after a delayed injury repair (Wood et al., 2013). Roam and colleagues produced an almost completely synthetic NGC based on PLGA-heparin-laminin microspheres, which allows soluble GDNF delivery with a controlled kinetics, cell-initiated degradability, and cell attachment. These modular plasmin-sensitive microspheres were formed inside silicone conduits using 3D-printed holders. Furthermore, in vivo results, using 13-mm rats sciatic nerve gap, confirmed NGCs degradability and biocompatibility and their ability to promote axonal regeneration (Roam et al., 2015).

The effects of conditioned media derived from SHED (SHED-CM) were also investigated on peripheral nerve regeneration. In vitro studies showed the neuritogenesis stimulation of dorsal root ganglia and increase of Schwann cells (SCs) viability by SHED-CM. Moreover, SHED-CM enhanced tube formation in an angiogenesis assay and silicon conduits containing SHED-CM increased the number of myelinated axons and axon-to-fiber ratio on a 10-mm rat sciatic nerve gap model, at 12 weeks after nerve transection surgery. This suggests that SHEDs may secrete various trophic factors, which enhance peripheral nerve regeneration through multiple mechanisms (Sugimura-Wakayama et al., 2015).

Cell delivery-approaches are also improved when cells are adhered or imbibed in a biomaterial/scaffold. Zhou et al. used an acellular nerve scaffold filled with BMSCs and SCs to enhance regeneration of a 10-mm sciatic nerve defect. Results consistently showed that BMSCs and SCs, when loaded together in an acellular nerve scaffold, enhanced functional recovery of the sciatic nerve; furthermore, their beneficial effect on sciatic injury regeneration was similar to the autograft, although never exceeding it. This study is nonetheless a step forward in the search for alternatives to nerve autografts (Zhou et al., 2015).

Among material properties, fiber orientation may have a role in nerve regeneration. In this context, Georgiou and colleagues described an electrospinning alternative for the production of an aligned cellular biomaterial. They produce sheets of engineered neural tissue (EngNT) through selfalignment of SCs within a collagen gel followed by stabilization using plastic compression (Georgiou et al., 2013). In vitro experiments demonstrated the EngNT ability to support robust neuronal regeneration only when living SCs were present. Additionally, authors used a critical-sized defect of 15-mm gap in rat sciatic nerve to compare EngNT regenerative ability with both Neurowrap (Integra) and a nerve graft. After 8 weeks postimplantation, considerably more tissue was present at the repair midpoint in EngNT as compared to empty conduits. Recently, the same group described a similar approach using ADSCs differentiated (dADSC) to a SCs-like phenotype, in vitro, instead of using primary SCs. The ability of EngNT-dADSC to support and guide neurite regeneration was demonstrated (Georgiou et al., 2015). Yet, EngNT did not support neuronal regeneration from proximal to distal stump, indicating that further optimizations are needed. Nonetheless, EngNT seems a promising material for neural regeneration.

Novel material options are being explored as matrix fillers in NGCs. Recently, a sericin/silicone-based NGC was fabricated and used as a long-term implant in vivo. Sericin conduit wrapped with a silicone conduit was used for the bridging repair of a 5-mm gap in a rat sciatic nerve transection model. These double conduits achieved functional recovery comparable to autologous nerve graft and, importantly, positive results were mainly attributed to sericin (Xie et al., 2015).

In the last decade we have experienced an increasing interest and an improved understanding of the application of nanotechnology to the nervous system. CNTs are increasingly being used in neurological applications, as components of implants, electrodes, or delivery vehicles, due to their unique chemical, mechanical, structural, and electrical properties (Nunes et al., 2012; Kafa et al., 2015). In this context, new combinations of synthetic materials, such as CNTs, phosphate glass microfibers (PGFs), PLA, PVA, polypyrrole (PPy), were used for the production of NGCs with electrical properties (Ribeiro et al., 2015; Ahn et al., 2015; Kim et al., 2012). Recently, Ahn and collaborators evaluated the functions of CNT-interfaced NGCs in the regeneration of a 10-mm gap of a transected rat sciatic nerve. They chemically tethered CNTs onto aligned PGFs surface and placed them into PLA tubes. 3D-scaffolds significantly improved (1) the number of regenerating axons crossing the scaffold, (2) the cross-sectional area of reinnervated muscles, and (3) the electrophysiological function, through the interfacing with CNTs (Ahn et al., 2015).

Other combinations using CNTs to prepare NGCs might prevent the secondary neurogenic muscular atrophy by improving the reestablishment of the neuromuscular junction (Ribeiro et al., 2015).

6.4.2 Central nerve injury repair and regeneration

CNS complexity has limited the development of successful therapeutic strategies. Further, it is well known that drugs/biologics diffusion across blood–brain barrier (BBB) is very limited using common delivery methods (oral and intravenous), pointing out the need of new therapeutic solutions (Tam et al., 2014; Li et al., 2015c). Moreover, as the multifactorial inhibitory environment of injured CNS suggests, combinatorial approaches using biomaterials as cell/biomolecules carriers would be more effective enhancing both cell survival and integration after cell transplantation and achieving local delivery to the brain, thereby circumventing the BBB and the systemic side effects (Assuncao-Silva et al., 2015; Elliott Donaghue et al., 2014, 2015; Liu et al., 2015a).

Among biomaterials used in CNS regeneration, hydrogels, often combined with nanoparticles and fibrous-based materials, are appealing 3D-scaffolds because of their physicochemical properties and high water content, which resembles the cell tissue microenvironment. Moreover, those materials can be combined with several bioactive molecules, which can be released in a controlled manner (Samal et al., 2015; Tam et al., 2014; Elliott Donaghue and Shoichet, 2015).

There are several examples of polymers used to produce hydrogels. Among them, ECM-derived proteins and synthetic polymers (eg, PLGA, PEG) are widely described (Liu et al., 2015a; Chen et al., 2015). Moreover, hydrogels can be prepared as injectable scaffolds, which allow in situ application (Zhu and Marchant, 2011; Chen et al., 2015; Visser et al., 2015; Liu et al., 2015a).

Chen et al. developed a hydrogel based on synthetic polymers—hydroxyl ethyl methacrylate [2-(methacryloyloxy)ethyl] trimethylammonium chloride (HEMA-MOETACL)—combined with bFGF and demonstrated its synergic effect on regeneration using rats submitted to a complete spinal cord transection. The bFGF/HEMA-MOETACL hydrogel sustained bFGF delivery to injured spinal cord and supported the ingrowth of regenerating tissue, promoting nerve tissue regeneration and functional recovery (Chen et al., 2015).

A drug delivery system (DDS) to encapsulate and release bioactive neurotrophin-3 (NT-3) into the injured spinal cord was developed. With a single injection of DDS—composed of biodegradable polymeric nanoparticles dispersed in a hyaluronan/methyl cellulose hydrogel—into the intrathecal space of the spinal cord with a thoracic clip compression, NT-3 diffused ventrally through the cord and was detectable in the spinal cord during 28 days. Delivery of NT-3 resulted in significant axon growth with no effect on the astroglial response and promoted functional improvements at 21 days (Elliott Donaghue et al., 2015).

Altogether, the results indicate that encapsulated growth factors or neurotrophin delivery is a promising approach for CNS repair.

As previously mentioned, CNTs present appealing properties for neurological applications (Nunes et al., 2012; Ahn et al., 2015; Chen et al., 2013b; Sun et al., 2015). Among them, nanotopographical and electrical conductivity may mediate neural modulation (Fabbro et al., 2013). Moreover, CNTs surface tunability and their ability to translocate plasma membranes make functionalized-CNTs (f-CNTs) promising intracellular delivery systems for CNS therapeutics or diagnostics (Bussy et al., 2015; Kafa et al., 2015). Thus, several reports show the f-CNTs potential benefits in stroke and spinal-cord-injured models (Lee et al., 2011; Al-Jamal et al., 2011; Mattson et al., 2000; Roman et al., 2011). In a very recent study, amino-functionalized MWNTs (f-MWNTs) were investigated concerning their ability to cross the BBB following intravenous injection. The f-MWNT exhibited significant brain uptake at 5 min after injection in mice. Furthermore, capillary depletion confirmed the presence of f-MWNT in brain capillaries and parenchyma fractions. Altogether, the results indicate that f-MWNT has potential to be used as nanocarrier for delivery of drugs and biologics into the brain, after systemic administration (Kafa et al., 2015).

Another material investigated for neuroregeneration is graphene, which along with CNT is a carbon allotrope with excellent physical properties and the ability to interface with neurons and neuronal circuits (John et al., 2015; Li et al., 2011). The large surface area and the possibility of conjugating different biomolecules onto its surface make graphene a suitable nanoscaffold for holding small-molecule drugs, genes, antibodies, proteins, DNAs, and small interfering RNAs (Chen et al., 2013b; John et al., 2015).

Li and collaborators reported the first utilization, in vitro, of 3D-graphene porous foam (3D-GF), as a novel scaffold for NSCs. The 3D-GF supported NSC growth, cells retention at an active proliferation state and enhanced NSC differentiation toward astrocytes and especially neurons. In addition, a good electrical coupling of 3D-GFs with differentiated NSCs for efficient electrical stimulation was observed, indicating the potential of this scaffold as a platform for NSC research, neural tissue engineering, and neural prostheses (Li et al., 2013).

Despite the promising results obtained with CNTs and graphene-based materials, concerns about their safety still need to be clarified (Bussy et al., 2015; Bardi et al., 2013).

CNS and PNS regenerations are complex processes that, despite many advancements and innovations, still have suboptimal outcomes especially related with functional recovery. One of the biggest limitations in translation to clinics of an innovative nerve repair and regeneration treatment remains its validation using an adequate nerve damage experimental model, which allows the prediction of a therapeutic agent and/or tissue engineering strategy effectiveness (Geuna, 2015).

6.5 Cardiac regeneration

Cardiovascular diseases (CVD) are a leading cause of death worldwide, as treatments for CVD are still limited in the category of detection and advanced therapies (Mozaffarian et al., 2015). In this context, cardiovascular regenerative medicine wisely involves and integrates the use of cells, biomaterials, scaffolds, and bioreactors toward establishing environments that mimic the natural environment to promote cardiac regeneration (Freytes et al., 2014).

Stem cell therapy offers the promise of organ repair and regeneration on demand. However, the vast majority of cells delivered into the heart by conventional means are lost within the first 24 hours (Cheng et al., 2012), highlighting the need for the development of injectable vehicles for cardiac repair purposes. HyA:Serum (HyA:Ser) hydrogels have been synthesized as a metabolic scaffold for the injection of encapsulated cells. This scaffold presented the ability to promote rapid cell adhesion, increase the cellular uptake, and induce rapid restoration of cellular bioenergetics, in vitro and in vivo. Besides, in vivo studies showed total scaffold degradability up to 14 days (Chan et al., 2015). HyA (FDA approved) degradation products promote angiogenesis, which is an important feature in transplanted cell engraftment and cardiac regeneration success (Portalska et al., 2014). Fibrin is another FDA approved material that is biocompatible and has the ability to serve as a vehicle capable of improving the survival of transplanted cells while reducing infarct expansion and promoting neovascularization in ischemic myocardium (Christman et al., 2004). Additionally, some fibrin degradation products have important properties, like healing enhancement or protective effect against myocardial reperfusion injury (Barsotti et al., 2011).

Gelatin is also used as a vehicle for cell therapy. Hyaluronan–gelatin hydrogel showed capacity to enhance cell retention and efficacy when administered after myocardial infarction. In addition, bEGF has been delivered with gelatin microspheres to induce angiogenesis and improve cardiac function (Smith et al., 2013). A strategy based on hyaluronan–gelatin, which embeds cardiovascular-derived cells, resulted in high engraftment and superior functional benefits to those of each component alone and it is a promising strategy that could be rapidly translated to clinical procedures as this material has entered human testing (Cheng et al., 2012).

Several approaches have used engineered scaffolds to mimic the architecture of the native myocardium tissue and precisely regulate cardiac cell functions. In this sense, electrospinning was used to fabricate elastomeric biodegradable poly(glycerol-sebacate) (PGS):gelatin scaffolds with a wide range of chemical composition, stiffness, and anisotropy. Furthermore, nanofibrous aligned scaffolds, consisting of 33 wt.% PGS, induced optimal synchronous contractions of cardiomyocytes (CMs), whilst significantly enhancing cellular alignment (Kharaziha et al., 2013). Recently, a nanofibrous PLA scaffold was also developed in an attempt to mimic natural ECM to support cardiac tissue formation from cardiovascular progenitor cells. Subcutaneous implantation of cell/scaffold constructs in a nude mouse model showed that scaffolds favorably supported the survival of grafted cells (Liu et al., 2015b).

A singular approach based on ECM, using decellularized tissues and injection of their digested products, offers the advantage of biomimetic promotion of native biochemical and structural matrix composition and the potential to develop autologous therapies. Importantly, decellularization of biological matrices induces the loss of major histocompatibility complex (MHC), thereby reducing the risks of immunological responses (Boccafoschi et al., 2015; Moroni and Mirabella, 2014; Singelyn and Christman, 2010). Thus, protocols to obtain decellularization matrices remain under study. A combination of detergents and DNase seems an optimal protocol to obtain decellularization scaffolds with better biodegradability and improved capacity to retain adipose tissue-derived progenitor cells (APCs) per unit of surface (Perea-Gil et al., 2015). Two types of SIS gels have been studied as materials for cardiac repair in a murine model, presenting distinct capacities for cardiac repair depending on bFGF presence, with the best result in its presence (Okada et al., 2010). Additionally, an emulsion of SIS increased neovascularization and preserved cardiac function (Zhao et al., 2010). VentriGel (Ventrix, San Diego, CA), an injectable hydrogel derived from ECM porcine myocardial, is progressing toward clinical trials after successful preclinical study in animal models. Findings demonstrated pathologic remodeling attenuation and improvement in contractile function. Moreover, hemocompatibility studies showed that this hydrogel (at relevant concentrations) does not affect clotting times or platelet activation (Seif-Naraghi et al., 2013).

Conductive and electroactive materials have the potential to enhance engineered cardiac tissue functions. SWNTs were incorporated into gelatin hydrogel scaffolds to construct 3D-engineer cardiac tissues (ECTs). SWNTs could provide favorable cellular microenvironment, in vitro, for cardiac contraction and expression of electrochemical-associated proteins. *In vivo* studies showed that ECTs were structurally integrated with the host myocardium (Zhou et al., 2014). In another study, the conductive polypyrrole–polycaprolactone (PPy–PCL) film was used as a platform for CMs culture, improving cell–cell communication mediated by formation of connexin-43 and enhancing higher velocities for calcium wave propagation (Spearman et al., 2015). Altogether, the results indicate that conductive materials provide a promising therapeutic perspective in cardiac tissue engineering/regeneration.

3D-printing is also a promising technique for the development of cardiac tissues, specifically the myocardium, heart valves, and coronary arteries, once it has inherent ability to build structures with arbitrary geometry and heterogeneous material properties (Mosadegh et al., 2015). A rational design of bioprinted trileaflet valve hydrogels based on methacrylate-gelatin and methacrylate-HyA showed good accuracy and properties to regulate encapsulated human aortic valvular interstitial cells (HAVE) with high cell viability and remodeling potential through cells by depositing their own ECM (Duan et al., 2014). A heart valve with two types of cells, aortic root sinus smooth muscle cells (SMCs) and aortic valve leaflet interstitial cells (VICs), encapsulated into root and leaflet regions was fabricated by 3D-printing. Cell viability was achieved over 7 days in culture, while tensile biomechanics of cell-laden hydrogels were maintained (Duan et al., 2013). Simultaneous printing of human microvascular endothelial cells (HMVECs) with fibrin scaffold induces cells to align themselves inside the channels and proliferate, establishing confluent linings to microvasculature formation (Cui and Boland, 2009).

One of the greatest challenges in regenerative medicine is CMs supplying tissue with sufficient oxygen and nutrients through vascularization. Growth factors are potent signaling molecules that act in a coordinated manner in physiological processes, such as tissue healing or angiogenesis, and are commonly used to stimulate endogenous blood vessel growth into damaged myocardium. Growth factor signaling, such as VEGF, EGF, and bFGF, can be successfully immobilized onto scaffold to improve angiogenesis, wound healing, and cell survival. Moreover, the combination of two or more growth factors could achieve a better effect (Miyagi et al., 2011; Wang et al., 2010). Thereby, coimmobilizing specific ratios of EGF and VEGF onto a chondroitin sulfate coating demonstrated a synergistic effect on cell survival when compared with each growth factor applied alone (Lequoy et al., 2016).

Nevertheless, it is clear that the approaches showed so far mitigated success and the delivery of angiogenic growth factors results in a highly disorganized and leaky vasculature formation. Thus, engineering methods have been combined in an attempt to design scaffolds with suitable properties to guide the tubulogenesis (Zhao et al., 2014). Cylinders of poly(ethylene glycol) diacrylate (PEGDA) hydrogel were fabricated, using a computational model, and were able to release VEGF and create vasculature with a predefined micropattern. Printed hydrogel bars had spacing large enough to locally increase VEGF concentration in the implanted tissue (Rich et al., 2014). A collagen–chitosan hydrogel was used for Tβ4 encapsulation, allowing its controlled release over 28 days. This approach was able to elicit localized and prolonged recruitment and differentiation of endothelial cells and smooth muscle cells into epicardial capillary outgrowths, in vitro, and augmented angiogenesis, in vivo, after subcutaneous injection (Chiu et al., 2012). The use of a DNA plasmid (pDNA) to produce growth factors in transfected cells provides a powerful alternative to purified protein delivery. Electrospun fibers with encapsulated pDNA-calcium phosphate nanoparticles encoding VEGF (pVEGF) and bFGF (pbFGF) demonstrated a better density profile of mature blood vessels than those containing individual plasmid and also induced lower cytotoxicity and less inflammation after implantation when compared with commonly used pDNA polyplexes with poly(ethyleneimine) (Chen et al., 2013a). The nanoparticle-based delivery systems of nucleotides, instead of purified protein, are also efficient in *in vivo* delivery models of modified mRNA (modeRNA). Formulated lipidoid nanoparticles (FLNP) were used to inject about 1–10 μg enhanced green fluorescent protein (eGFP) mRNA into a rat model and a dose-dependent of eGFPmRNA levels in the heart tissue was observed 20 hours after injection, unlike naked modRNA. Intracoronary administration of 10 μg FLNP/eGFPmodRNA also proved successful and these findings were recently confirmed in a pilot study using direct injection into pig myocardia, as well as percutaneous intracoronary delivery (Turnbull et al., 2016).

Although the general strategy for cardiac tissue engineering is focused on the combination of suitable cells for cardiac therapy with a 3D-scaffold, the creation of an appropriate cell environment is a central issue to improve effectiveness of cellular cardiomyoplasty (Zimmermann et al., 2006; Jawad et al., 2007). A scaffold-free cardiac tissue engineering technology was used to promote functional and vascularized cardiac tissue that could be successfully transplanted into the nude rat heart. Addition of fibroblasts and endothelial cells augmented cardiac spheroid formation and also promoted angiogenesis with contractile capabilities and formation of new blood vessels organized in a reticular pattern, with the advantage of reducing the incidence of an inflammatory response related to toxic events and the risk of infection introduced by classic soluble biodegradable scaffolds (Noguchi et al., 2016). Overall, the results obtained so far suggest that this is a promising technique in cardiac tissue engineering.

6.6 Final remarks

Nowadays, synthetic materials that mimic one or more of the natural structural design elements have been developed using different materials and several processing routes. Recent advances in the understanding of cell–matrix interactions and the role of ECM in regulation of cellular behavior have inspired researchers to design dynamic or responsive materials for regenerative medicine (Boekhoven and Stupp, 2014). However, compared to biologically derived acellular grafts and autografts, completely synthetic materials existing today are promising but still far from optimal, and it is now clear that no material or approach will solve all the challenges of regenerative medicine.

Among materials whose applications have been studied, those able to respond to a specific stimulus or condition (eg, light, pH, magnetic field, electricity, and among others) present a huge potential in regenerative medicine because upon stimulation they can change their bioactivity (de Jong et al., 2004; Minkenberg et al., 2011; Grzybowski et al., 2000). This is a critical aspect, since living tissues are complex dynamic systems composed by cells and macromolecules, thereby stimuli-responsive scaffolds that allow such multistep bioactivity display are a promising approach for the production of next-generation materials.

Materials such as natural and synthetic polymers, metals, ceramic, and glass have been used for a long time for the development of scaffolds and micro/nanoparticles, and many material combinations resulted in improved systems for particular applications. However, in the last decade, several new materials with interesting characteristics have been described. Among them carbon-based materials, such as MWCN and graphene, have emerged as promising materials for the development of new systems for regeneration of tissues that are related with electrical stimulus, such as nerve, muscle, cardiac, and bone due to their conductivity properties. Notwithstanding their promising results, several aspects of their biocompatibility and genotoxicity must be clarified. Another group of materials recently investigated in terms of biomedical applications are the supramolecular materials that offer the opportunity to create structures similar to those found in living systems, which combine order and dynamics through the reversibility of intermolecular bonds (Boekhoven and Stupp, 2014). The future development of bioinspired materials for use in medicine will clearly involve supramolecular approaches.

It is also clear that 3D systems are a better option when compared with monolayer systems because they more efficiently mimic living tissues and organs. Studies have shown that bioprinting of simple tissue structures is possible; however, constructing more complex and composite tissue structures (eg, solid organs) remains a challenge, mainly due to the lack of mechanical strength and integrity in the printed constructs, which is related with the innate properties of hydrogels (Seol et al., 2014). Nevertheless, 3D-bioprinting has already been used for the generation and transplantation of several tissues, including multilayered skin, bone, vascular grafts, tracheal splints, heart tissue, and cartilaginous structures (Murphy and Atala, 2014). In this sense, while printing fully functioning organs seems to be incredible at present, these technologies show enormous potential and great promise to become an essential tool in the future.

Finally, regarding biomaterial design, it is important to keep in mind that their performance in preclinical trials should also be related to the translation of results obtained from in vitro to in vivo applications. Thus, besides biocompatibility and regenerative properties, other characteristics should be considered if the material is to offer an appealing option for medical applications: preferentially, it must be widely available, cheap, durable, and stable, with a precise biodegradability profile, and it must exhibit no antigenicity. Therefore it has become clear that different approaches will induce different impacts on tissue reconstruction and a single strategy will hardly fulfill all regenerative medicine's needs. Thus it is likely that for each application a combination of different approaches may be required.

Acknowledgment

Gildácio Filho had financial support from the Institutional Program of Scientific Initiation Grants of CNPq–PIBIC/CNPq, Brazil.

References

Ahn, H.S., Hwang, J.Y., Kim, M.S., Lee, J.Y., Kim, J.W., Kim, H.S., Shin, U.S., Knowles, J.C., Kim, H.W., Hyun, J.K., 2015. Carbon-nanotube-interfaced glass fiber scaffold for regeneration of transected sciatic nerve. Acta Biomater. 13, 324–334.

Al-Jamal, K.T., Gherardini, L., Bardi, G., Nunes, A., Guo, C., Bussy, C., Herrero, M.A., Bianco, A., Prato, M., Kostarelos, K., Pizzorusso, T., 2011. Functional motor recovery from brain ischemic insult by carbon nanotube-mediated siRNA silencing. Proc. Natl. Acad. Sci. U. S. A. 108, 10952–10957.

Amani, H., Dougherty, W.R., Blome-Eberwein, S., 2006. Use of transcyte and dermabrasion to treat burns reduces length of stay in burns of all size and etiology. Burns 32, 828–832.

Amini, A.R., Laurencin, C.T., Nukavarapu, S.P., 2012. Bone tissue engineering: recent advances and challenges. Crit. Rev. Biomed. Eng. 40, 363–408.

Andrade, F.K., Costa, R., Domingues, L., Soares, R., Gama, M., 2010. Improving bacterial cellulose for blood vessel replacement: functionalization with a chimeric protein containing a cellulose-binding module and an adhesion peptide. Acta Biomater. 6, 4034–4041.

Andrade, F.K., Silva, J.P., Carvalho, M., Castanheira, E.M., Soares, R., Gama, M., 2011. Studies on the hemocompatibility of bacterial cellulose. J. Biomed. Mater. Res. A 98, 554–566.

Aramwit, P., Kanokpanont, S., Nakpheng, T., Srichana, T., 2010. The effect of sericin from various extraction methods on cell viability and collagen production. Int. J. Mol. Sci. 11, 2200–2211.

Aramwit, P., Siritienthong, T., Srichana, T., Ratanavaraporn, J., 2013. Accelerated healing of full-thickness wounds by genipin-crosslinked silk sericin/PVA scaffolds. Cells Tissues Organs 197, 224–238.

Assuncao-Silva, R.C., Gomes, E.D., Sousa, N., Silva, N.A., Salgado, A.J., 2015. Hydrogels and cell based therapies in spinal cord injury regeneration. Stem Cells Int. 2015, 948040.

Bachar, A., Mercier, C., Tricoteaux, A., Hampshire, S., Leriche, A., Follet, C., 2013. Effect of nitrogen and fluorine on mechanical properties and bioactivity in two series of bioactive glasses. J. Mech. Behav. Biomed. Mater. 23, 133–148.

Badylak, S.F., Freytes, D.O., Gilbert, T.W., 2009. Extracellular matrix as a biological scaffold material: structure and function. Acta Biomater. 5, 1–13.

Bae, M.S., Kim, J.E., Lee, J.B., Heo, D.N., Yang, D.H., Kim, J.H., Kwon, K.R., Bang, J.B., Bae, H., Kwon, I.K., 2013. ZrO(2) surface chemically coated with hyaluronic acid hydrogel loading GDF-5 for osteogenesis in dentistry. Carbohydr. Polym. 92, 167–175.

Bardi, G., Nunes, A., Gherardini, L., Bates, K., Al-Jamal, K.T., Gaillard, C., Prato, M., Bianco, A., Pizzorusso, T., Kostarelos, K., 2013. Functionalized carbon nanotubes in the brain: cellular internalization and neuroinflammatory responses. PLoS One 8. e80964.

Barrientos-Duran, A., Carpenter, E.M., Zur Nieden, N.I., Malinin, T.I., Rodriguez-Manzaneque, J.C., Zanello, L.P., 2014. Carboxyl-modified single-wall carbon nanotubes improve bone tissue formation in vitro and repair in an in vivo rat model. Int. J. Nanomedicine 9, 4277–4291.

Barsotti, M.C., Felice, F., Balbarini, A., di Stefano, R., 2011. Fibrin as a scaffold for cardiac tissue engineering. Biotechnol. Appl. Biochem. 58, 301–310.

Bassett, D.C., Meszaros, R., Orzol, D., Woy, M., Zhang, Y.L., Tiedemann, K., Wondraczek, L., Komarova, S., Barralet, J.E., 2014. A new class of bioactive glasses: calcium-magnesium sulfophosphates. J. Biomed. Mater. Res. A 102, 2842–2848.

Bhardwaj, N., Sow, W.T., Devi, D., Ng, K.W., Mandal, B.B., Cho, N.J., 2015. Silk fibroin-keratin based 3D scaffolds as a dermal substitute for skin tissue engineering. Integr. Biol. (Camb) 7, 53–63.

Boccafoschi, F., Botta, M., Fusaro, L., Copes, F., Ramella, M., Cannas, M., 2015. Decellularized biological matrices: an interesting approach for cardiovascular tissue repair and regeneration. J. Tissue Eng. Regen. Med. http://dx.doi.org/10.1002/term.2103.
Boekhoven, J., Stupp, S.I., 2014. 25th anniversary article: supramolecular materials for regenerative medicine. Adv. Mater. 26, 1642–1659.
Bonvallet, P.P., Schultz, M.J., Mitchell, E.H., Bain, J.L., Culpepper, B.K., Thomas, S.J., Bellis, S.L., 2015. Microporous dermal-mimetic electrospun scaffolds pre-seeded with fibroblasts promote tissue regeneration in full-thickness skin wounds. PLoS One 10. e0122359.
Borena, B.M., Martens, A., Broeckx, S.Y., Meyer, E., Chiers, K., Duchateau, L., Spaas, J.H., 2015. Regenerative skin wound healing in mammals: state-of-the-art on growth factor and stem cell based treatments. Cell. Physiol. Biochem. 36, 1–23.
Brennan, E.P., Reing, J., Chew, D., Myers-Irvin, J.M., Young, E.J., Badylak, S.F., 2006. Antibacterial activity within degradation products of biological scaffolds composed of extracellular matrix. Tissue Eng. 12, 2949–2955.
Brooks, D.N., Weber, R.V., Chao, J.D., Rinker, B.D., Zoldos, J., Robichaux, M.R., Ruggeri, S.B., Anderson, K.A., Bonatz, E.E., Wisotsky, S.M., Cho, M.S., Wilson, C., Cooper, E.O., Ingari, J.V., Safa, B., Parrett, B.M., Buncke, G.M., 2012. Processed nerve allografts for peripheral nerve reconstruction: a multicenter study of utilization and outcomes in sensory, mixed, and motor nerve reconstructions. Microsurgery 32, 1–14.
Brown, B.N., Badylak, S.F., 2014. Extracellular matrix as an inductive scaffold for functional tissue reconstruction. Transl. Res. 163, 268–285.
Bussy, C., Al-Jamal, K.T., Boczkowski, J., Lanone, S., Prato, M., Bianco, A., Kostarelos, K., 2015. Microglia determine brain region-specific neurotoxic responses to chemically functionalized carbon nanotubes. ACS Nano 9, 7815–7830.
Cai, Y., Guo, L., Shen, H., An, X., Jiang, H., Ji, F., Niu, Y., 2015. Degradability, bioactivity, and osteogenesis of biocomposite scaffolds of lithium-containing mesoporous bioglass and mPEG-PLGA-b-PLL copolymer. Int. J. Nanomedicine 10, 4125–4136.
Calamak, S., Erdogdu, C., Ozalp, M., Ulubayram, K., 2014. Silk fibroin based antibacterial bionanotextiles as wound dressing materials. Mater. Sci. Eng. C Mater. Biol. Appl. 43, 11–20.
Cam, C., Zhu, S., Truong, N.F., Scumpia, P.O., Segura, T., 2015. Systematic evaluation of natural scaffolds in cutaneous wound healing. J. Mater. Chem. B Mater. Biol. Med. 3, 7986–7992.
Chan, A.T., Karakas, M.F., Vakrou, S., Afzal, J., Rittenbach, A., Lin, X., Wahl, R.L., Pomper, M.G., Steenbergen, C.J., Tsui, B.M.W., Elisseeff, J.H., Abraham, M.R., 2015. Hyaluronic acid-serum hydrogels rapidly restore metabolism of encapsulated stem cells and promote engraftment. Biomaterials 73, 1–11.
Chattopadhyay, S., Raines, R.T., 2014. Review collagen-based biomaterials for wound healing. Biopolymers 101, 821–833.
Chaya, A., Yoshizawa, S., Verdelis, K., Myers, N., Costello, B.J., Chou, D.T., Pal, S., Maiti, S., Kumta, P.N., Sfeir, C., 2015. In vivo study of magnesium plate and screw degradation and bone fracture healing. Acta Biomater. 18, 262–269.
Chen, F., Wan, H., Xia, T., Guo, X., Wang, H., Liu, Y., Li, X., 2013a. Promoted regeneration of mature blood vessels by electrospun fibers with loaded multiple pDNA-calcium phosphate nanoparticles. Eur. J. Pharm. Biopharm. 85, 699–710.
Chen, Y., Star, A., Vidal, S., 2013b. Sweet carbon nanostructures: carbohydrate conjugates with carbon nanotubes and graphene and their applications. Chem. Soc. Rev. 42, 4532–4542.
Chen, B., He, J., Yang, H., Zhang, Q., Zhang, L., Zhang, X., Xie, E., Liu, C., Zhang, R., Wang, Y., Huang, L., Hao, D., 2015. Repair of spinal cord injury by implantation of bFGF-incorporated HEMA-MOETACL hydrogel in rats. Sci. Rep. 5, 9017.

Cheng, K., Blusztajn, A., Shen, D., Li, T.S., Sun, B., Galang, G., Zarembinski, T.I., Prestwich, G.D., Marbán, E., Smith, R.R., Marbán, L., 2012. Functional performance of human cardiosphere-derived cells delivered in an in situ polymerizable hyaluronan-gelatin hydrogel. Biomaterials 33, 5317–5324.

Chiu, L.L., Reis, L.A., Momen, A., Radisic, M., 2012. Controlled release of thymosin beta4 from injected collagen-chitosan hydrogels promotes angiogenesis and prevents tissue loss after myocardial infarction. Regen. Med. 7, 523–533.

Christman, K.L., Vardanian, A.J., Fang, Q., Sievers, R.E., Fok, H.H., Lee, R.J., 2004. Injectable fibrin scaffold improves cell transplant survival, reduces infarct expansion, and induces neovasculature formation in ischemic myocardium. J. Am. Coll. Cardiol. 44, 654–660.

Cinteza, D., Persinaru, I., Maciuceanu Zarnescu, B.M., Ionescu, D., Lascar, I., 2015. Peripheral nerve regeneration—an appraisal of the current treatment options. Maedica (Buchar) 10, 65–68.

Cui, X., Boland, T., 2009. Human microvasculature fabrication using thermal inkjet printing technology. Biomaterials 30, 6221–6227.

Curran, M.P., Plosker, G.L., 2002. Bilayered bioengineered skin substitute (Apligraf): a review of its use in the treatment of venous leg ulcers and diabetic foot ulcers. BioDrugs 16, 439–455.

Czaja, W., Krystynowicz, A., Bielecki, S., Brown Jr., R.M., 2006. Microbial cellulose—the natural power to heal wounds. Biomaterials 27, 145–151.

Czaja, W.K., Young, D.J., Kawecki, M., Brown Jr., R.M., 2007. The future prospects of microbial cellulose in biomedical applications. Biomacromolecules 8, 1–12.

Daly, K.A., Liu, S., Agrawal, V., Brown, B.N., Johnson, S.A., Medberry, C.J., Badylak, S.F., 2012a. Damage associated molecular patterns within xenogeneic biologic scaffolds and their effects on host remodeling. Biomaterials 33, 91–101.

Daly, W., Yao, L., Zeugolis, D., Windebank, A., Pandit, A., 2012b. A biomaterials approach to peripheral nerve regeneration: bridging the peripheral nerve gap and enhancing functional recovery. J. R. Soc. Interface 9, 202–221.

Demirel, M.C., Cetinkaya, M., Pena-Francesch, A., Jung, H., 2015. Recent advances in nanoscale bioinspired materials. Macromol. Biosci. 15, 300–311.

de Jong, J.J.D., Lucas, L.N., Kellogg, R.M., van Esch, J.H., Feringa, B.L., 2004. Reversible, light-driven, transcription of supramolecular into molecular chirality. Science 304, 278–281.

Ding, F., Wu, J., Yang, Y., Hu, W., Zhu, Q., Tang, X., Liu, J., Gu, X., 2010. Use of tissue-engineered nerve grafts consisting of a chitosan/poly(lactic-co-glycolic acid)-based scaffold included with bone marrow mesenchymal cells for bridging 50-mm dog sciatic nerve gaps. Tissue Eng. Part A 16, 3779–3790.

Drury, J.L., Mooney, D.J., 2003. Hydrogels for tissue engineering: scaffold design variables and applications. Biomaterials 24, 4337–4351.

Duan, B., Hockaday, L.A., Kang, K.H., Butcher, J.T., 2013. 3D bioprinting of heterogeneous aortic valve conduits with alginate/gelatin hydrogels. J. Biomed. Mater. Res. A 101, 1255–1264.

Duan, B., Kapetanovic, E., Hockaday, L.A., Butcher, J.T., 2014. Three-dimensional printed trileaflet valve conduits using biological hydrogels and human valve interstitial cells. Acta Biomater. 10, 1836–1846.

Dubey, N., Bentini, R., Islam, I., Cao, T., Castro Neto, A.H., Rosa, V., 2015. Graphene: a versatile carbon-based material for bone tissue engineering. Stem Cells Int. 2015, 804213.

Eap, S., Ferrand, A., Schiavi, J., Keller, L., Kokten, T., Fioretti, F., Mainard, D., Ladam, G., Benkirane-Jessel, N., 2014. Collagen implants equipped with 'fish scale'-like nanoreservoirs of growth factors for bone regeneration. Nanomedicine (Lond.) 9, 1253–1261.

Eguchi, Y., Ohtori, S., Sekino, M., Ueno, S., 2015. Effectiveness of magnetically aligned collagen for neural regeneration in vitro and in vivo. Bioelectromagnetics 36, 233–243.
Elliott Donaghue, I., Shoichet, M.S., 2015. Controlled release of bioactive PDGF-AA from a hydrogel/nanoparticle composite. Acta Biomater. 25, 35–42.
Elliott Donaghue, I., Tam, R., Sefton, M.V., Shoichet, M.S., 2014. Cell and biomolecule delivery for tissue repair and regeneration in the central nervous system. J. Control. Release 190, 219–227.
Elliott Donaghue, I., Tator, C.H., Shoichet, M.S., 2015. Sustained delivery of bioactive neurotrophin-3 to the injured spinal cord. Biomater. Sci. 3, 65–72.
Fabbro, A., Prato, M., Ballerini, L., 2013. Carbon nanotubes in neuroregeneration and repair. Adv. Drug Deliv. Rev. 65, 2034–2044.
Faroni, A., Mobasseri, S.A., Kingham, P.J., Reid, A.J., 2015. Peripheral nerve regeneration: experimental strategies and future perspectives. Adv. Drug Deliv. Rev. 82–83, 160–167.
Fedorovich, N.E., Alblas, J., Hennink, W.E., Oner, F.C., Dhert, W.J., 2011. Organ printing: the future of bone regeneration? Trends Biotechnol. 29, 601–606.
Ferreira, A.M., Mattu, C., Ranzato, E., Ciardelli, G., 2014. Bioinspired porous membranes containing polymer nanoparticles for wound healing. J. Biomed. Mater. Res. A 102, 4394–4405.
Florencio-Silva, R., Sasso, G.R., Sasso-Cerri, E., Simoes, M.J., Cerri, P.S., 2015. Biology of bone tissue: structure, function, and factors that influence bone cells. Biomed. Res. Int. 2015, 421746.
Freytes, D.O., Godier-Furnemont, A., Duan, Y., O'Neill, J.D., Vunjak-Novakovic, G., 2014. Biomaterial scaffolds for cardiac regeneration and repair derived from native heart matrix. In: Li, R.-K., Weisel, R.D. (Eds.), Cardiac Regeneration and Repair. Woodhead Publishing, Cambridge.
Gao, G., Cui, X., 2015. Three-dimensional bioprinting in tissue engineering and regenerative medicine. Biotechnol. Lett. 38, 203–211.
Georgiou, M., Bunting, S.C., Davies, H.A., Loughlin, A.J., Golding, J.P., Phillips, J.B., 2013. Engineered neural tissue for peripheral nerve repair. Biomaterials 34, 7335–7343.
Georgiou, M., Golding, J.P., Loughlin, A.J., Kingham, P.J., Phillips, J.B., 2015. Engineered neural tissue with aligned, differentiated adipose-derived stem cells promotes peripheral nerve regeneration across a critical sized defect in rat sciatic nerve. Biomaterials 37, 242–251.
Geuna, S., 2015. The sciatic nerve injury model in pre-clinical research. J. Neurosci. Methods 243, 39–46.
Gil, E.S., Panilaitis, B., Bellas, E., Kaplan, D.L., 2013. Functionalized silk biomaterials for wound healing. Adv. Healthc. Mater. 2, 206–217.
Girotti, A., Orbanic, D., Ibanez-Fonseca, A., Gonzalez-Obeso, C., Rodriguez-Cabello, J.C., 2015. Recombinant technology in the development of materials and systems for soft-tissue repair. Adv. Healthc. Mater. 4, 2423–2455.
Godwin, J., Kuraitis, D., Rosenthal, N., 2014. Extracellular matrix considerations for scar-free repair and regeneration: insights from regenerative diversity among vertebrates. Int. J. Biochem. Cell Biol. 56, 47–55.
Goncalves, S., Rodrigues, I.P., Padrao, J., Silva, J.P., Sencadas, V., Lanceros-Mendez, S., Girao, H., Gama, F.M., Dourado, F., Rodrigues, L.R., 2015. Acetylated bacterial cellulose coated with urinary bladder matrix as a substrate for retinal pigment epithelium. Colloids Surf. B Biointerfaces 139, 1–9.
Griffin, D.R., Weaver, W.M., Scumpia, P.O., di Carlo, D., Segura, T., 2015. Accelerated wound healing by injectable microporous gel scaffolds assembled from annealed building blocks. Nat. Mater. 14, 737–744.

Grzybowski, B.A., Stone, H.A., Whitesides, G.M., 2000. Dynamic self-assembly of magnetized, millimeter-sized objects rotating at a liquid-air interface. Nature 405, 1033–1036.

Gu, X., Ding, F., Williams, D.F., 2014. Neural tissue engineering options for peripheral nerve regeneration. Biomaterials 35, 6143–6156.

Guo, C., Li, J., She, C., Shao, X., Teng, B., Feng, J., Zhang, J.V., Ren, P.G., 2016. Bioeffects of micron-size magnesium particles on inflammatory cells and bone turnover in vivo and in vitro. J. Biomed. Mater. Res. B Appl. Biomater. 104, 923–931.

Gupta, A., Liberati, T.A., Verhulst, S.J., Main, B.J., Roberts, M.H., Potty, A.G., Pylawka, T.K., El-Amin III, S.F., 2015. Biocompatibility of single-walled carbon nanotube composites for bone regeneration. Bone Joint Res. 4, 70–77.

Halim, A.S., Khoo, T.L., Mohd Yussof, S.J., 2010. Biologic and synthetic skin substitutes: an overview. Indian J. Plast. Surg. 43, S23–S28.

Haro Durand, L.A., Vargas, G.E., Romero, N.M., Vera-Mesones, R., Porto-Lopez, J.M., Boccaccini, A.R., Zago, M.P., Baldi, A., Gorustovich, A., 2015. Angiogenic effects of ionic dissolution products released from a boron-doped 45S5 bioactive glass. J. Mater. Chem. B 3, 1142–1148.

Hart, C.E., Loewen-Rodriguez, A., Lessem, J., 2012. Dermagraft: use in the treatment of chronic wounds. Adv. Wound Care 1, 138–141.

Huo, K., Gao, B., Fu, J., Zhao, L., Chu, P.K., 2014. Fabrication, modification, and biomedical applications of anodized TiO2 nanotube arrays. RSC Adv. 4, 17300–17324.

Isaacs, J., Mallu, S., Yan, W., Little, B., 2014. Consequences of oversizing: nerve-to-nerve tube diameter mismatch. J. Bone Joint Surg. Am. 96, 1461–1467.

Jahan, K., Tabrizian, M., 2016. Composite biopolymers for bone regeneration enhancement in bony defects. Biomater. Sci. 4, 25–39.

Jawad, H., Ali, N.N., Lyon, A.R., Chen, Q.Z., Harding, S.E., Boccaccini, A.R., 2007. Myocardial tissue engineering: a review. J. Tissue Eng. Regener. Med. 1, 327–342.

Jayarama Reddy, V., Radhakrishnan, S., Ravichandran, R., Mukherjee, S., Balamurugan, R., Sundarrajan, S., Ramakrishna, S., 2013. Nanofibrous structured biomimetic strategies for skin tissue regeneration. Wound Repair Regen. 21, 1–16.

Jiang, H., Zuo, Y., Zou, Q., Wang, H., Du, J., Li, Y., Yang, X., 2013. Biomimetic spiral-cylindrical scaffold based on hybrid chitosan/cellulose/nano-hydroxyapatite membrane for bone regeneration. ACS Appl. Mater. Interfaces 5, 12036–12044.

John, A.A., Subramanian, A.P., Vellayappan, M.V., Balaji, A., Mohandas, H., Jaganathan, S.K., 2015. Carbon nanotubes and graphene as emerging candidates in neuroregeneration and neurodrug delivery. Int. J. Nanomedicine 10, 4267–4277.

Johnson, P.J., Newton, P., Hunter, D.A., Mackinnon, S.E., 2011. Nerve endoneurial microstructure facilitates uniform distribution of regenerative fibers: a post hoc comparison of midgraft nerve fiber densities. J. Reconstr. Microsurg. 27, 83–90.

Jones, J.R., 2015. Reprint of: review of bioactive glass: from Hench to hybrids. Acta Biomater. 23 (Suppl.), S53–S82.

Jung, O., Hanken, H., Smeets, R., Hartjen, P., Friedrich, R.E., Schwab, B., Grobe, A., Heiland, M., Al-Dam, A., Eichhorn, W., Sehner, S., Kolk, A., Woltje, M., Stein, J.M., 2014. Osteogenic differentiation of mesenchymal stem cells in fibrin-hydroxyapatite matrix in a 3-dimensional mesh scaffold. In Vivo 28, 477–482.

Kafa, H., Wang, J.T., Rubio, N., Venner, K., Anderson, G., Pach, E., Ballesteros, B., Preston, J.E., Abbott, N.J., Al-Jamal, K.T., 2015. The interaction of carbon nanotubes with an in vitro blood-brain barrier model and mouse brain in vivo. Biomaterials 53, 437–452.

Kayat, J., Mehra, N.K., Gajbhiye, V., Jain, N.K., 2016. Drug targeting to arthritic region via folic acid appended surface-engineered multi-walled carbon nanotubes. J. Drug. Target. 24, 318–327.

Keane, T.J., Dziki, J., Castelton, A., Faulk, D.M., Messerschmidt, V., Londono, R., Reing, J.E., Velankar, S.S., Badylak, S.F., 2015. Preparation and characterization of a biologic scaffold and hydrogel derived from colonic mucosa. J. Biomed. Mater. Res. B Appl. Biomater.

Kharaziha, M., Nikkhah, M., Shin, S.R., Annabi, N., Masoumi, N., Gaharwar, A.K., Camci-Unal, G., Khademhosseini, A., 2013. PGS: gelatin nanofibrous scaffolds with tunable mechanical and structural properties for engineering cardiac tissues. Biomaterials 34, 6355–6366.

Kim, Y.P., Lee, G.S., Kim, J.W., Kim, M.S., Ahn, H.S., Lim, J.Y., Kim, H.W., Son, Y.J., Knowles, J.C., Hyun, J.K., 2012. Phosphate glass fibres promote neurite outgrowth and early regeneration in a peripheral nerve injury model. J. Tissue Eng. Regener. Med. 9, 236–246.

Kim, J.Y., Yang, B.E., Ahn, J.H., Park, S.O., Shim, H.W., 2014. Comparable efficacy of silk fibroin with the collagen membranes for guided bone regeneration in rat calvarial defects. J. Adv. Prosthodont. 6, 539–546.

Koch, L., Kuhn, S., Sorg, H., Gruene, M., Schlie, S., Gaebel, R., Polchow, B., Reimers, K., Stoelting, S., Ma, N., Vogt, P.M., Steinhoff, G., Chichkov, B., 2010. Laser printing of skin cells and human stem cells. Tissue Eng. Part C Methods 16, 847–854.

Koch, L., Deiwick, A., Schlie, S., Michael, S., Gruene, M., Coger, V., Zychlinski, D., Schambach, A., Reimers, K., Vogt, P.M., Chichkov, B., 2012. Skin tissue generation by laser cell printing. Biotechnol. Bioeng. 109, 1855–1863.

Kokkalis, Z.T., Pu, C., Small, G.A., Weiser, R.W., Venouziou, A.I., Sotereanos, D.G., 2011. Assessment of processed porcine extracellular matrix as a protective barrier in a rabbit nerve wrap model. J. Reconstr. Microsurg. 27, 19–28.

Kolar, M.K., Kingham, P.J., 2014. Regenerative effects of adipose-tissue-derived stem cells for treatment of peripheral nerve injuries. Biochem. Soc. Trans. 42, 697–701.

Krishnamurithy, G., Murali, M.R., Hamdi, M., Abbas, A.A., Raghavendran, H.B., Kamarul, T., 2015. Proliferation and osteogenic differentiation of mesenchymal stromal cells in a novel porous hydroxyapatite scaffold. Regen. Med. 10, 579–590.

Kwak, M.H., Kim, J.E., Go, J., Koh, E.K., Song, S.H., Son, H.J., Kim, H.S., Yun, Y.H., Jung, Y.J., Hwang, D.Y., 2015. Bacterial cellulose membrane produced by Acetobacter sp. A10 for burn wound dressing applications. Carbohydr. Polym. 122, 387–398.

La, W.G., Park, S., Yoon, H.H., Jeong, G.J., Lee, T.J., Bhang, S.H., Han, J.Y., Char, K., Kim, B.S., 2013. Delivery of a therapeutic protein for bone regeneration from a substrate coated with graphene oxide. Small 9, 4051–4060.

Lavasani, M., Thompson, S.D., Pollett, J.B., Usas, A., Lu, A., Stolz, D.B., Clark, K.A., Sun, B., Peault, B., Huard, J., 2014. Human muscle-derived stem/progenitor cells promote functional murine peripheral nerve regeneration. J. Clin. Invest. 124, 1745–1756.

Lee, H.J., Park, J., Yoon, O.J., Kim, H.W., Lee Do, Y., Kim Do, H., Lee, W.B., Lee, N.E., Bonventre, J.V., Kim, S.S., 2011. Amine-modified single-walled carbon nanotubes protect neurons from injury in a rat stroke model. Nat. Nanotechnol. 6, 121–125.

Lee, J.Y., Giusti, G., Friedrich, P.F., Archibald, S.J., Kemnitzer, J.E., Patel, J., Desai, N., Bishop, A.T., Shin, A.Y., 2012. The effect of collagen nerve conduits filled with collagen-glycosaminoglycan matrix on peripheral motor nerve regeneration in a rat model. J. Bone Joint Surg. Am. 94, 2084–2091.

Lee, V., Singh, G., Trasatti, J.P., Bjornsson, C., Xu, X., Tran, T.N., Yoo, S.S., Dai, G., Karande, P., 2014. Design and fabrication of human skin by three-dimensional bioprinting. Tissue Eng. Part C Methods 20, 473–484.

Lee, J.W., Park, J.W., Khang, D., 2015. Analysis of osteoblast differentiation on polymer thin films embedded with carbon nanotubes. PLoS One 10, e0129856.

Lequoy, P., Murschel, F., Liberelle, B., Lerouge, S., de Crescenzo, G., 2016. Controlled co-immobilization of EGF and VEGF to optimize vascular cell survival. Acta Biomater. 29, 239–247.

Li, N., Zhang, X., Song, Q., Su, R., Zhang, Q., Kong, T., Liu, L., Jin, G., Tang, M., Cheng, G., 2011. The promotion of neurite sprouting and outgrowth of mouse hippocampal cells in culture by graphene substrates. Biomaterials 32, 9374–9382.

Li, N., Zhang, Q., Gao, S., Song, Q., Huang, R., Wang, L., Liu, L., Dai, J., Tang, M., Cheng, G., 2013. Three-dimensional graphene foam as a biocompatible and conductive scaffold for neural stem cells. Sci. Rep. 3, 1604.

Li, J.J., Kaplan, D.L., Zreiqat, H., 2014. Scaffold-based regeneration of skeletal tissues to meet clinical challenges. J. Mater. Chem. B 2, 7272–7306.

Li, R., Chen, L., Fu, J., Liu, Z., Wang, S., Pan, Y., 2015a. Promoting peripheral nerve regeneration with biodegradable poly (DL-lactic acid) films. Int. J. Clin. Exp. Pathol. 8, 8057–8065.

Li, Y., Wang, S., Huang, R., Huang, Z., Hu, B., Zheng, W., Yang, G., Jiang, X., 2015b. Evaluation of the effect of the structure of bacterial cellulose on full thickness skin wound repair on a microfluidic chip. Biomacromolecules 16, 780–789.

Li, Y.H., Feng, L., Zhang, G.X., Ma, C.G., 2015c. Intranasal delivery of stem cells as therapy for central nervous system disease. Exp. Mol. Pathol. 98, 145–151.

Liedert, A., Kaspar, D., Augat, P., Ignatius, A., Claes, L., 2005. Mechanobiology of bone tissue and bone cells. In: Kiseleva, I., Kamkin, A. (Eds.), Mechanosensitivity in Cells and Tissues. Academia, Academia Publishing House Ltd., Moscow.

Lin, N., Dufresne, A., 2014. Nanocellulose in biomedicine: current status and future prospect. Eur. Polym. J. 59, 302–325.

Lin, H.Y., Chen, S.H., Chang, S.H., Huang, S.T., 2015. Tri-layered chitosan scaffold as a potential skin substitute. J. Biomater. Sci. Polym. Ed. 26, 855–867.

Liu, C., Huang, Y., Pang, M., Yang, Y., Li, S., Liu, L., Shu, T., Zhou, W., Wang, X., Rong, L., Liu, B., 2015a. Tissue-engineered regeneration of completely transected spinal cord using induced neural stem cells and gelatin-electrospun poly (lactide-co-glycolide)/polyethylene glycol scaffolds. PLoS One 10, e0117709.

Liu, Q., Tian, S., Zhao, C., Chen, X., Lei, I., Wang, Z., Ma, P.X., 2015b. Porous nanofibrous poly(l-lactic acid) scaffolds supporting cardiovascular progenitor cells for cardiac tissue engineering. Acta Biomater. 26, 105–114.

Lobo, A.O., Siqueira, I.A., Das Neves, M.F., Marciano, F.R., Corat, E.J., Corat, M.A., 2013. In vitro and in vivo studies of a novel nanohydroxyapatite/superhydrophilic vertically aligned carbon nanotube nanocomposites. J. Mater. Sci. Mater. Med. 24, 1723–1732.

Losi, P., Briganti, E., Errico, C., Lisella, A., Sanguinetti, E., Chiellini, F., Soldani, G., 2013. Fibrin-based scaffold incorporating VEGF- and bFGF-loaded nanoparticles stimulates wound healing in diabetic mice. Acta Biomater. 9, 7814–7821.

Losi, P., Briganti, E., Sanguinetti, E., Burchielli, S., Al Kayal, T., Soldani, G., 2015. Healing effect of a fibrin-based scaffold loaded with platelet lysate in full-thickness skin wounds. J. Bioact. Compat. Polym. 30, 222–237.

Lutolf, M.P., Hubbell, J.A., 2005. Synthetic biomaterials as instructive extracellular microenvironments for morphogenesis in tissue engineering. Nat. Biotechnol. 23, 47–55.

Lv, H., Li, L., Zhang, Y., Chen, Z., Sun, M., Xu, T., Tian, L., Lu, M., Ren, M., Liu, Y., Li, Y., 2015. Union is strength: matrix elasticity and microenvironmental factors codetermine stem cell differentiation fate. Cell Tissue Res. 361, 657–668.

Mahjour, S.B., Fu, X., Yang, X., Fong, J., Sefat, F., Wang, H., 2015. Rapid creation of skin substitutes from human skin cells and biomimetic nanofibers for acute full-thickness wound repair. Burns. 41, 1764–1774.

Maitz, M.F., 2015. Applications of synthetic polymers in clinical medicine. Biosurf. Biotribol. 1, 161–176.
Manoli, T., Schulz, L., Stahl, S., Jaminet, P., Schaller, H.E., 2014. Evaluation of sensory recovery after reconstruction of digital nerves of the hand using muscle-in-vein conduits in comparison to nerve suture or nerve autografting. Microsurgery 34, 608–615.
Martino, M.M., Brkic, S., Bovo, E., Burger, M., Schaefer, D.J., Wolff, T., Gurke, L., Briquez, P.S., Larsson, H.M., Gianni-Barrera, R., Hubbell, J.A., Banfi, A., 2015. Extracellular matrix and growth factor engineering for controlled angiogenesis in regenerative medicine. Front. Bioeng. Biotechnol. 3, 45.
Mattson, M.P., Haddon, R.C., Rao, A.M., 2000. Molecular functionalization of carbon nanotubes and use as substrates for neuronal growth. J. Mol. Neurosci. 14, 175–182.
Michael, S., Sorg, H., Peck, C.T., Koch, L., Deiwick, A., Chichkov, B., Vogt, P.M., Reimers, K., 2013. Tissue engineered skin substitutes created by laser-assisted bioprinting form skin-like structures in the dorsal skin fold chamber in mice. PLoS One 8, e57741.
Minkenberg, C.B., Li, F., van Rijn, P., Florusse, L., Boekhoven, J., Stuart, M.C.A., Koper, G.J.M., Eelkema, R., van Esch, J.H., 2011. Responsive vesicles from dynamic covalent surfactants. Angew. Chem. Int. Ed. 50, 3421–3424.
Miola, M., Brovarone, C.V., Maina, G., Rossi, F., Bergandi, L., Ghigo, D., Saracino, S., Maggiora, M., Canuto, R.A., Muzio, G., Verne, E., 2014. In vitro study of manganese-doped bioactive glasses for bone regeneration. Mater. Sci. Eng. C Mater. Biol. Appl. 38, 107–118.
Mirazul Islam, M., Cepla, V., He, C., Edin, J., Rakickas, T., Kobuch, K., Ruzele, Z., Jackson, W.B., Rafat, M., Lohmann, C.P., Valiokas, R., Griffith, M., 2015. Functional fabrication of recombinant human collagen-phosphorylcholine hydrogels for regenerative medicine applications. Acta Biomater. 12, 70–80.
Miyagi, Y., Chiu, L.L., Cimini, M., Weisel, R.D., Radisic, M., Li, R.K., 2011. Biodegradable collagen patch with covalently immobilized VEGF for myocardial repair. Biomaterials 32, 1280–1290.
Mohammadi, R., Azizi, S., Amini, K., 2013. Effects of undifferentiated cultured omental adipose-derived stem cells on peripheral nerve regeneration. J. Surg. Res. 180, e91–e97.
Molinos, M., Carvalho, V., Silva, D.M., Gama, F.M., 2012. Development of a hybrid dextrin hydrogel encapsulating dextrin nanogel as protein delivery system. Biomacromolecules 13, 517–527.
Moreira, S., Silva, N.B., Almeida-Lima, J., Rocha, H.A., Medeiros, S.R., Alves Jr., C., Gama, F.M., 2009. BC nanofibres: in vitro study of genotoxicity and cell proliferation. Toxicol. Lett. 189, 235–241.
Moreira, S., Gil Da Costa, R.M., Guardão, L., Gärtner, F., Vilanova, M., Gama, M., 2010. In vivo biocompatibility and biodegradability of dextrin-based hydrogels. J. Bioact. Compat. Polym. 25, 141–153.
Moroni, F., Mirabella, T., 2014. Decellularized matrices for cardiovascular tissue engineering. Am. J. Stem Cells 3, 1–20.
Mosadegh, B., Xiong, G., Dunham, S., Min, J.K., 2015. Current progress in 3D printing for cardiovascular tissue engineering. Biomed. Mater. 10, 034002.
Mozaffarian, D., Benjamin, E.J., Go, A.S., Arnett, D.K., Blaha, M.J., Cushman, M., de Ferranti, S., Despres, J.P., Fullerton, H.J., Howard, V.J., Huffman, M.D., Judd, S.E., Kissela, B.M., Lackland, D.T., Lichtman, J.H., Lisabeth, L.D., Liu, S., Mackey, R.H., Matchar, D.B., Mcguire, D.K., Mohler 3rd, E.R., Moy, C.S., Muntner, P., Mussolino, M.E., Nasir, K., Neumar, R.W., Nichol, G., Palaniappan, L., Pandey, D.K., Reeves, M.J., Rodriguez, C.J., Sorlie, P.D., Stein, J., Towfighi, A., Turan, T.N., Virani, S.S., Willey, J.Z., Woo, D., Yeh,

R.W., Turner, M.B., 2015. Heart disease and stroke statistics—2015 update: a report from the American Heart Association. Circulation 131, e29–e322.

Murphy, S.V., Atala, A., 2014. 3D bioprinting of tissues and organs. Nat. Biotechnol. 32, 773–785.

Naleway, S.E., Porter, M.M., Mckittrick, J., Meyers, M.A., 2015. Structural design elements in biological materials: application to bioinspiration. Adv. Mater. 27, 5455–5476.

Nath, S.D., Abueva, C., Kim, B., Lee, B.T., 2015. Chitosan-hyaluronic acid polyelectrolyte complex scaffold crosslinked with genipin for immobilization and controlled release of BMP-2. Carbohydr. Polym. 115, 160–169.

Nayak, S., Kundu, S.C., 2014. Sericin-carboxymethyl cellulose porous matrices as cellular wound dressing material. J. Biomed. Mater. Res. A 102, 1928–1940.

Nayak, S., Dey, S., Kundu, S.C., 2013. Skin equivalent tissue-engineered construct: co-cultured fibroblasts/ keratinocytes on 3D matrices of sericin hope cocoons. PLoS One 8, e74779.

Ninan, N., Muthiah, M., Park, I.-K., Wong, T.W., Thomas, S., Grohens, Y., 2015. Natural polymer/inorganic material based hybrid scaffolds for skin wound healing. Polym. Rev. 55, 453–490.

Noguchi, R., Nakayama, K., Itoh, M., Kamohara, K., Furukawa, K., Oyama, J.I., Node, K., Morita, S., 2016. Development of a three-dimensional pre-vascularized scaffold-free contractile cardiac patch for treating heart disease. J. Heart Lung. Transplant. 35, 137–145.

Norouzi, M., Boroujeni, S.M., Omidvarkordshouli, N., Soleimani, M., 2015. Advances in skin regeneration: application of electrospun scaffolds. Adv. Healthc. Mater. 4, 1114–1133.

Nunes, A., Bussy, C., Gherardini, L., Meneghetti, M., Herrero, M.A., Bianco, A., Prato, M., Pizzorusso, T., Al-Jamal, K.T., Kostarelos, K., 2012. In vivo degradation of functionalized carbon nanotubes after stereotactic administration in the brain cortex. Nanomedicine (Lond.) 7, 1485–1494.

Okada, M., Payne, T.R., Oshima, H., Momoi, N., Tobita, K., Huard, J., 2010. Differential efficacy of gels derived from small intestinal submucosa as an injectable biomaterial for myocardial infarct repair. Biomaterials 31, 7678–7683.

Olalde, B., Garmendia, N., Saez-Martinez, V., Argarate, N., Nooeaid, P., Morin, F., Boccaccini, A.R., 2013. Multifunctional bioactive glass scaffolds coated with layers of poly(D, L-lactide-co-glycolide) and poly(n-isopropylacrylamide-co-acrylic acid) microgels loaded with vancomycin. Mater. Sci. Eng. C Mater. Biol. Appl. 33, 3760–3767.

Pashuck, E.T., Stevens, M.M., 2012. Designing regenerative biomaterial therapies for the clinic. Sci. Transl. Med. 4, 160sr4.

Patel, K.D., Kim, T.H., Lee, E.J., Han, C.M., Lee, J.Y., Singh, R.K., Kim, H.W., 2014. Nanostructured biointerfacing of metals with carbon nanotube/chitosan hybrids by electrodeposition for cell stimulation and therapeutics delivery. ACS Appl. Mater. Inter. 6, 20214–20224.

Pateman, C.J., Harding, A.J., Glen, A., Taylor, C.S., Christmas, C.R., Robinson, P.P., Rimmer, S., Boissonade, F.M., Claeyssens, F., Haycock, J.W., 2015. Nerve guides manufactured from photocurable polymers to aid peripheral nerve repair. Biomaterials 49, 77–89.

Pavlova, T.V., Pavlova, L.A., Nesterov, A.V., Kolesnikov, D.A., Shchyogolev, A.I., 2014. Comparative characterization of the skull bones after implantation of titanium biocomposites containing BMP-2 in their coating structure. Bull. Exp. Biol. Med. 158, 274–277.

Perea-Gil, I., Uriarte, J.J., Prat-Vidal, C., Gálvez-Montón, C., Roura, S., Llucià-Valldeperas, A., Soler-Botija, C., Farré, R., Navajas, D., Bayes-Genis, A., 2015. In vitro comparative study of two decellularization protocols in search of an optimal myocardial scaffold for recellularization. Am. J. Transl. Res. 7, 558–573.

Pereira, R.F., Barrias, C.C., Granja, P.L., Bartolo, P.J., 2013. Advanced biofabrication strategies for skin regeneration and repair. Nanomedicine (Lond.) 8, 603–621.
Pina, S., Oliveira, J.M., Reis, R.L., 2015. Natural-based nanocomposites for bone tissue engineering and regenerative medicine: a review. Adv. Mater. 27, 1143–1169.
Pistone, A., Iannazzo, D., Panseri, S., Montesi, M., Tampieri, A., Galvagno, S., 2014. Hydroxyapatite-magnetite-MWCNT nanocomposite as a biocompatible multifunctional drug delivery system for bone tissue engineering. Nanotechnology 25, 425701.
Portalska, K.J., Teixeira, L.M., Leijten, J.C., Jin, R., Van Blitterswijk, C., de Boer, J., Karperien, M., 2014. Boosting angiogenesis and functional vascularization in injectable dextran-hyaluronic acid hydrogels by endothelial-like mesenchymal stromal cells. Tissue Eng. Part A 20, 819–829.
Rashidi, H., Yang, J., Shakesheff, K.M., 2014. Surface engineering of synthetic polymer materials for tissue engineering and regenerative medicine applications. Biomater. Sci. 2, 1318–1331.
Rathbone, C.R., Guda, T., Singleton, B.M., Oh, D.S., Appleford, M.R., Ong, J.L., Wenke, J.C., 2014. Effect of cell-seeded hydroxyapatite scaffolds on rabbit radius bone regeneration. J. Biomed. Mater. Res. A 102, 1458–1466.
Reznikov, N., Shahar, R., Weiner, S., 2014. Bone hierarchical structure in three dimensions. Acta Biomater. 10, 3815–3826.
Rho, J.Y., Kuhn-Spearing, L., Zioupos, P., 1998. Mechanical properties and the hierarchical structure of bone. Med. Eng. Phys. 20, 92–102.
Ribeiro, N., Sousa, S.R., Van Blitterswijk, C.A., Moroni, L., Monteiro, F.J., 2014. A biocomposite of collagen nanofibers and nanohydroxyapatite for bone regeneration. Biofabrication 6, 035015.
Ribeiro, J., Pereira, T., Caseiro, A.R., Armada-Da-Silva, P., Pires, I., Prada, J., Amorim, I., Amado, S., Franca, M., Goncalves, C., Lopes, M.A., Santos, J.D., Silva, D.M., Geuna, S., Luis, A.L., Mauricio, A.C., 2015. Evaluation of biodegradable electric conductive tube-guides and mesenchymal stem cells. World J. Stem Cells 7, 956–975.
Rich, M.H., Lee, M.K., Baek, K., Jeong, J.H., Kim, D.H., Millet, L.J., Bashir, R., Kong, H., 2014. Material-mediated proangiogenic factor release pattern modulates quality of regenerated blood vessels. J. Control. Release 196, 363–369.
Roam, J.L., Yan, Y., Nguyen, P.K., Kinstlinger, I.S., Leuchter, M.K., Hunter, D.A., Wood, M.D., Elbert, D.L., 2015. A modular, plasmin-sensitive, clickable poly(ethylene glycol)-heparin-laminin microsphere system for establishing growth factor gradients in nerve guidance conduits. Biomaterials 72, 112–124.
Roman, J.A., Niedzielko, T.L., Haddon, R.C., Parpura, V., Floyd, C.L., 2011. Single-walled carbon nanotubes chemically functionalized with polyethylene glycol promote tissue repair in a rat model of spinal cord injury. J. Neurotrauma 28, 2349–2362.
Rowan, M.P., Cancio, L.C., Elster, E.A., Burmeister, D.M., Rose, L.F., Natesan, S., Chan, R.K., Christy, R.J., Chung, K.K., 2015. Burn wound healing and treatment: review and advancements. Crit. Care 19, 243.
Sabongi, R.G., Fernandes, M., Dos Santos, J.B., 2015. Peripheral nerve regeneration with conduits: use of vein tubes. Neural Regen. Res. 10, 529–533.
Saino, E., Grandi, S., Quartarone, E., Maliardi, V., Galli, D., Bloise, N., Fassina, L., de Angelis, M.G., Mustarelli, P., Imbriani, M., Visai, L., 2011. In vitro calcified matrix deposition by human osteoblasts onto a zinc-containing bioactive glass. Eur. Cell. Mater. 21, 59–72. discussion 72.
Samal, J., Hoban, D.B., Naughton, C., Concannon, R., Dowd, E., Pandit, A., 2015. Fibrin-based microsphere reservoirs for delivery of neurotrophic factors to the brain. Nanomedicine (Lond.) 10, 765–783.

Sawkins, M.J., Mistry, P., Brown, B.N., Shakesheff, K.M., Bonassar, L.J., Yang, J., 2015. Cell and protein compatible 3D bioprinting of mechanically strong constructs for bone repair. Biofabrication 7, 035004.

Schiavi, J., Keller, L., Morand, D.N., de Isla, N., Huck, O., Lutz, J.C., Mainard, D., Schwinte, P., Benkirane-Jessel, N., 2015. Active implant combining human stem cell microtissues and growth factors for bone-regenerative nanomedicine. Nanomedicine (Lond.) 10, 753–763.

Seif-Naraghi, S.B., Singelyn, J.M., Salvatore, M.A., Osborn, K.G., Wang, J.J., Sampat, U., Kwan, O.L., Strachan, G.M., Wong, J., Schup-Magoffin, P.J., Braden, R.L., Bartels, K., Dequach, J.A., Preul, M., Kinsey, A.M., Demaria, A.N., Dib, N., Christman, K.L., 2013. Safety and efficacy of an injectable extracellular matrix hydrogel for treating myocardial infarction. Sci. Transl. Med. 5, 173ra25.

Seol, Y.J., Kang, H.W., Lee, S.J., Atala, A., Yoo, J.J., 2014. Bioprinting technology and its applications. Eur. J. Cardiothorac. Surg. 46, 342–348.

Shao, W., Liu, H., Liu, X., Sun, H., Wang, S., Zhang, R., 2015. pH-responsive release behavior and anti-bacterial activity of bacterial cellulose-silver nanocomposites. Int. J. Biol. Macromol. 76, 209–217.

Sheikh, F.A., Ju, H.W., Lee, J.M., Moon, B.M., Park, H.J., Lee, O.J., Kim, J.H., Kim, D.K., Park, C.H., 2015. 3D electrospun silk fibroin nanofibers for fabrication of artificial skin. Nanomedicine 11, 681–691.

Shi, L., Yang, N., Zhang, H., Chen, L., Tao, L., Wei, Y., Liu, H., Luo, Y., 2015. A novel poly-(gamma-glutamic acid)/silk-sericin hydrogel for wound dressing: synthesis, characterization and biological evaluation. Mater. Sci. Eng. C Mater. Biol. Appl. 48, 533–540.

Shrestha, B., Coykendall, K., Li, Y., Moon, A., Priyadarshani, P., Yao, L., 2014. Repair of injured spinal cord using biomaterial scaffolds and stem cells. Stem Cell Res. Ther. 5, 91.

Singelyn, J.M., Christman, K.L., 2010. Injectable materials for the treatment of myocardial infarction and heart failure: the promise of decellularized matrices. J. Cardiovasc. Transl. Res. 3, 478–486.

Siritienthong, T., Ratanavaraporn, J., Aramwit, P., 2012. Development of ethyl alcohol-precipitated silk sericin/polyvinyl alcohol scaffolds for accelerated healing of full-thickness wounds. Int. J. Pharm. 439, 175–186.

Siritientong, T., Angspatt, A., Ratanavaraporn, J., Aramwit, P., 2014. Clinical potential of a silk sericin-releasing bioactive wound dressing for the treatment of split-thickness skin graft donor sites. Pharm. Res. 31, 104–116.

Skardal, A., Mack, D., Kapetanovic, E., Atala, A., Jackson, J.D., Yoo, J., Soker, S., 2012. Bioprinted amniotic fluid-derived stem cells accelerate healing of large skin wounds. Stem. Cells Transl. Med. 1, 792–802.

Smith, R.R., Marbán, E., Marbán, L., 2013. Enhancing retention and efficacy of cardiosphere-derived cells administered after myocardial infarction using a hyaluronan-gelatin hydrogel. Biomatter 3, e24490.

Spearman, B.S., Hodge, A.J., Porter, J.L., Hardy, J.G., Davis, Z.D., Xu, T., Zhang, X., Schmidt, C.E., Hamilton, M.C., Lipke, E.A., 2015. Conductive interpenetrating networks of polypyrrole and polycaprolactone encourage electrophysiological development of cardiac cells. Acta Biomater. 109–120.

Stevanovic, M., Filipovic, N., Djurdjevic, J., Lukic, M., Milenkovic, M., Boccaccini, A., 2015. 45S5Bioglass(R)-based scaffolds coated with selenium nanoparticles or with poly(lactide-co-glycolide)/selenium particles: processing, evaluation and antibacterial activity. Colloids Surf. B Biointerfaces 132, 208–215.

Stevens, B., Yang, Y., Mohandas, A., Stucker, B., Nguyen, K.T., 2008. A review of materials, fabrication methods, and strategies used to enhance bone regeneration in engineered bone tissues. J. Biomed. Mater. Res. B Appl. Biomater. 85, 573–582.

Stoppel, W.L., Ghezzi, C.E., Mcnamara, S.L., Black 3rd, L.D., Kaplan, D.L., 2015. Clinical applications of naturally derived biopolymer-based scaffolds for regenerative medicine. Ann. Biomed. Eng. 43, 657–680.

Sugimura-Wakayama, Y., Katagiri, W., Osugi, M., Kawai, T., Ogata, K., Sakaguchi, K., Hibi, H., 2015. Peripheral nerve regeneration by secretomes of stem cells from human exfoliated deciduous teeth. Stem Cells Dev. 24, 2687–2699.

Sun, J., Tan, H., 2013. Alginate-based biomaterials for regenerative medicine applications. Materials 6, 1285.

Sun, J., Wang, J., Jiang, H., Chen, M., Bi, Y., Liu, D., 2013. In vivo comparative property study of the bioactivity of coated Mg-3Zn-0.8Zr alloy. Mater. Sci. Eng. C Mater. Biol. Appl. 33, 3263–3272.

Sun, H., Lu, S., Jiang, X.X., Li, X., Li, H., Lin, Q., Mou, Y., Zhao, Y., Han, Y., Zhou, J., Wang, C., 2015. Carbon nanotubes enhance intercalated disc assembly in cardiac myocytes via the beta1-integrin-mediated signaling pathway. Biomaterials 55, 84–95.

Takeo, M., Lee, W., Ito, M., 2015. Wound healing and skin regeneration. Cold Spring Harb. Perspect. Med. 5, a023267.

Tam, R.Y., Fuehrmann, T., Mitrousis, N., Shoichet, M.S., 2014. Regenerative therapies for central nervous system diseases: a biomaterials approach. Neuropsychopharmacology 39, 169–188.

Tampieri, A., Iafisco, M., Sandri, M., Panseri, S., Cunha, C., Sprio, S., Savini, E., Uhlarz, M., Herrmannsdorfer, T., 2014. Magnetic bioinspired hybrid nanostructured collagen-hydroxyapatite scaffolds supporting cell proliferation and tuning regenerative process. ACS Appl. Mater. Interfaces 6, 15697–15707.

Tan, A., Rajadas, J., Seifalian, A.M., 2012. Biochemical engineering nerve conduits using peptide amphiphiles. J. Control. Release 163, 342–352.

Tos, P., Battiston, B., Ciclamini, D., Geuna, S., Artiaco, S., 2012. Primary repair of crush nerve injuries by means of biological tubulization with muscle-vein-combined grafts. Microsurgery 32, 358–363.

Turnbull, I.C., Eltoukhy, A.A., Fish, K.M., Nonnenmacher, M., Ishikawa, K., Chen, J., Hajjar, R.J., Anderson, D.G., Costa, K.D., 2016. Myocardial delivery of lipidoid nanoparticle carrying modRNA induces rapid and transient expression. Mol. Ther. 24, 66–75.

Turner, N.J., Badylak, S.F., 2015. The use of biologic scaffolds in the treatment of chronic nonhealing wounds. Adv. Wound Care 4, 490–500.

Ulery, B.D., Nair, L.S., Laurencin, C.T., 2011. Biomedical applications of biodegradable polymers. J. Polym. Sci. B Polym. Phys. 49, 832–864.

Valerio, I.L., Campbell, P., Sabino, J., Dearth, C.L., Fleming, M., 2015. The use of urinary bladder matrix in the treatment of trauma and combat casualty wound care. Regen. Med. 10, 611–622.

Varkey, M., Ding, J., Tredget, E.E., 2015. Advances in skin substitutes-potential of tissue engineered skin for facilitating anti-fibrotic healing. J. Funct. Biomater. 6, 547–563.

Vimalnath, K.V., Chakraborty, S., Rajeswari, A., Sarma, H.D., Nuwad, J., Pandey, U., Kamaleshwaran, K., Shinto, A., Dash, A., 2015. Radiochemistry, pre-clinical studies and first clinical investigation of 90Y-labeled hydroxyapatite (HA) particles prepared utilizing 90Y produced by (n, gamma) route. Nucl. Med. Biol. 42, 455–464.

Visser, J., Melchels, F.P., Jeon, J.E., Van Bussel, E.M., Kimpton, L.S., Byrne, H.M., Dhert, W.J., Dalton, P.D., Hutmacher, D.W., Malda, J., 2015. Reinforcement of hydrogels using three-dimensionally printed microfibres. Nat. Commun. 6, 6933.

Vyas, K., Vasconez, H., 2014. Wound healing: biologics, skin substitutes, biomembranes and scaffolds. Healthcare 2, 356.

Wang, H., Zhang, X., Li, Y., Ma, Y., Zhang, Y., Liu, Z., Zhou, J., Lin, Q., Wang, Y., Duan, C., Wang, C., 2010. Improved myocardial performance in infarcted rat heart by co-injection of basic fibroblast growth factor with temperature-responsive chitosan hydrogel. J. Heart Lung Transplant. 29, 881–887.

Wen, B., Kuhn, L., Charles, L., Pendrys, D., Shafer, D., Freilich, M., 2016. Comparison of bone morphogenetic protein-2 delivery systems to induce supracrestal bone guided by titanium implants in the rabbit mandible. Clin. Oral. Implants. Res. 27, 676–685.

Wood, M.D., Gordon, T., Kim, H., Szynkaruk, M., Phua, P., Lafontaine, C., Kemp, S.W., Shoichet, M.S., Borschel, G.H., 2013. Fibrin gels containing GDNF microspheres increase axonal regeneration after delayed peripheral nerve repair. Regen. Med. 8, 27–37.

Wu, C., Chang, J., 2012. Mesoporous bioactive glasses: structure characteristics, drug/growth factor delivery and bone regeneration application. Interface Focus 2, 292–306.

Xie, H., Yang, W., Chen, J., Zhang, J., Lu, X., Zhao, X., Huang, K., Li, H., Chang, P., Wang, Z., Wang, L., 2015. A silk sericin/silicone nerve guidance conduit promotes regeneration of a transected sciatic nerve. Adv. Healthc. Mater. 4, 2195–2205.

Xiong, Y., Ren, C., Zhang, B., Yang, H., Lang, Y., Min, L., Zhang, W., Pei, F., Yan, Y., Li, H., Mo, A., Tu, C., Duan, H., 2014. Analyzing the behavior of a porous nano-hydroxyapatite/polyamide 66 (n-HA/PA66) composite for healing of bone defects. Int. J. Nanomedicine 9, 485–494.

Yanez, M., Rincon, J., Dones, A., de Maria, C., Gonzales, R., Boland, T., 2015. In vivo assessment of printed microvasculature in a bilayer skin graft to treat full-thickness wounds. Tissue Eng. Part A 21, 224–233.

Yao, Q., Li, W., Yu, S., Ma, L., Jin, D., Boccaccini, A.R., Liu, Y., 2015. Multifunctional chitosan/polyvinyl pyrrolidone/45S5 Bioglass(R) scaffolds for MC3T3-E1 cell stimulation and drug release. Mater. Sci. Eng. C Mater. Biol. Appl. 56, 473–480.

Yellowlees, W.W., 1990. A comment on "Fish and meat in men's diet" by G. Williams. Nutr. Health 6, 211–212.

You, H.J., Han, S.K., 2014. Cell therapy for wound healing. J. Korean Med. Sci. 29, 311–319.

Zeimaran, E., Pourshahrestani, S., Pingguan-Murphy, B., Kadri, N., Rothan, H., Yusof, R., Towler, M., Djordjevic, I., 2015. Fabrication and characterization of poly(octanediol citrate)/gallium-containing bioglass microcomposite scaffolds. J. Mater. Sci. 50, 2189–2201.

Zhao, Z.Q., Puskas, J.D., Xu, D., Wang, N.P., Mosunjac, M., Guyton, R.A., Vinten-Johansen, J., Matheny, R., 2010. Improvement in cardiac function with small intestine extracellular matrix is associated with recruitment of C-kit cells, myofibroblasts, and macrophages after myocardial infarction. J. Am. Coll. Cardiol. 55, 1250–1261.

Zhao, Y., Feric, N.T., Thavandiran, N., Nunes, S.S., Radisic, M., 2014. The role of tissue engineering and biomaterials in cardiac regenerative medicine. Can. J. Cardiol. 30, 1307–1322.

Zhao, H., Ren, X., Zhang, Y., Huang, L., 2015a. Influence of self-assembly regenerated silk fibroin nanofibers on the properties of electrospun materials. Biomed. Mater. Eng. 26 (Suppl. 1), S89–S94.

Zhao, S., Zhang, J., Zhu, M., Zhang, Y., Liu, Z., Tao, C., Zhu, Y., Zhang, C., 2015b. Three-dimensional printed strontium-containing mesoporous bioactive glass scaffolds for repairing rat critical-sized calvarial defects. Acta Biomater. 12, 270–280.

Zheng, M.H., Chen, J., Kirilak, Y., Willers, C., Xu, J., Wood, D., 2005. Porcine small intestine submucosa (SIS) is not an acellular collagenous matrix and contains porcine DNA: possible implications in human implantation. J. Biomed. Mater. Res. B Appl. Biomater. 73, 61–67.

Zhou, J., Chen, J., Sun, H., Qiu, X., Mou, Y., Liu, Z., Zhao, Y., Li, X., Han, Y., Duan, C., Tang, R., Wang, C., Zhong, W., Liu, J., Luo, Y., Xing, M., Wang, C., 2014. Engineering the heart: evaluation of conductive nanomaterials for improving implant integration and cardiac function. Sci. Rep. 4, 3733.

Zhou, L.N., Zhang, J.W., Liu, X.L., Zhou, L.H., 2015. Co-graft of bone marrow stromal cells and schwann cells into acellular nerve scaffold for sciatic nerve regeneration in rats. J. Oral Maxillofac. Surg. 73, 1651–1660.

Zhu, J., Marchant, R.E., 2011. Design properties of hydrogel tissue-engineering scaffolds. Expert Rev. Med. Devices 8, 607–626.

Zhu, L., Liu, T., Cai, J., Ma, J., Chen, A.M., 2015. Repair and regeneration of lumbosacral nerve defects in rats with chitosan conduits containing bone marrow mesenchymal stem cells. Injury. 46, 2156–2163.

Zimmermann, W.H., Melnychenko, I., Wasmeier, G., Didie, M., Naito, H., Nixdorff, U., Hess, A., Budinsky, L., Brune, K., Michaelis, B., Dhein, S., Schwoerer, A., Ehmke, H., Eschenhagen, T., 2006. Engineered heart tissue grafts improve systolic and diastolic function in infarcted rat hearts. Nat. Med. 12, 452–458.

Advanced techniques for characterizing bioinspired materials

7

*R. Machado**, V. Sencadas*†

*University of Minho, Braga, Portugal, †University of Wollongong, Wollongong, NSW, Australia

7.1 Introduction

Materials science can be defined as the study of the relationship between materials processing, their structure, and their properties, and the interplay of these parameters (Fig. 7.1). Materials characterization is a powerful tool for understanding how the different parameters involved in the early stages of design and processing, influence their structure and performance.

The next sections provide a brief discussion of the most useful characterization techniques used to understand material basic properties; from its mechanical performance and fatigue-cycle studies to its chemical, morphological structure, and thermal properties.

At the end of the chapter, we provide some suggestions of further readings for a better comprehension of the materials' properties, as well as to assist in the design of novel processing methodologies and characterization techniques that can be used to explain and correlate materials features with their potential applications.

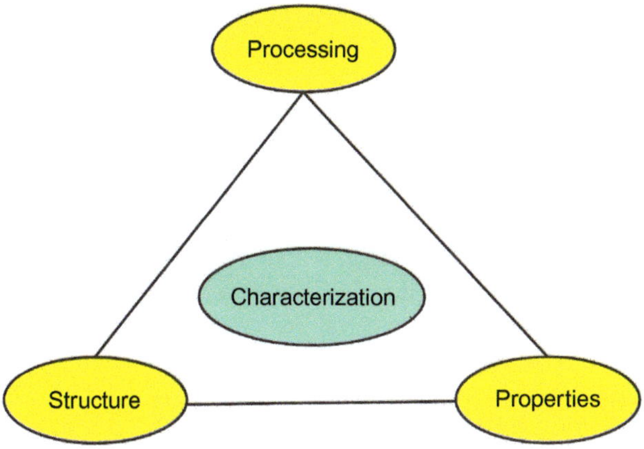

Fig. 7.1 Relationship between the materials properties and the characterization.

Bioinspired Materials for Medical Applications. http://dx.doi.org/10.1016/B978-0-08-100741-9.00007-3

7.2 Mechanical properties

The mechanical properties are some of the most important physical properties that need to be assessed in order to understand a material performance, not only at a laboratorial level but, more importantly, to explain and predict behavior in daily applications.

In order to discuss the quantitatively mechanical performance, it is necessary to derive mathematical expressions that relate the stress (σ) and strain (ε). When a material with uniform cross-section is stretched under a unidirectional stress, the overall sample volume will remain constant. Nevertheless, some changes do occur. As can be observed from Fig. 7.2, when the material is stretched under a tensile stress, the length of the material increases, while the dimensions in directions *Y* and *Z* decrease. The change in sample length in the stress (σ) direction is called deformation (ε) and is given by:

$$\varepsilon = \frac{\Delta L}{L_0} = \frac{L - L_0}{L_0} \tag{7.1}$$

where $\Delta L = L - L_0$, being L the length after deformation, and L_0 the initial length of the sample.

Considering that an ideal elastic solid obeys Hooke's law:

$$\sigma = E\varepsilon \tag{7.2}$$

where E is known as the material *Young's modulus* or *elasticity modulus*, the material stress can be obtained by:

$$\sigma = \frac{F}{A} \tag{7.3}$$

where F is the force applied to the material and A is the cross-sectional area of the sample, given by $A = t \times w$, being t the thickness and the w the width of the sample.

When a material is stretched, one of the dimensions increases and the other two will decrease. The ratio between the changes in the linear strain produced in the perpendicular direction (ε_{perp}), due to the tensile stress producing the tensile strain (ε), is called the Poisson's ration (υ), and is defined by:

$$\upsilon = -\frac{\varepsilon_{perp}}{\varepsilon} \tag{7.4}$$

The minus signal is introduced in order to make υ positive for most of the materials, for which ε_{perp} has the opposite sign to that of the tensile strain (Bower, 2002).

According to the Hooke's law (Eq. 7.2), the application of a stress leads to an instantaneous response strain on the material and once the stress is removed the strain instantaneously reverts to zero. Nevertheless, polymeric materials may often deviate from this ideal behavior, mainly because their mechanical response presents a/an (Bower, 2002; Sperling, 2006):

i. *time-dependence* response
ii. *nonrecovery* of strain on removal of the stress, ie, *yield*

iii. *nonlinearity* of response (ε is not proportional to σ), which does not imply no recovery
iv. *large strain* without fracture
v. *anisotropy* of response.

Fig. 7.2 depicts the representative stress–strain (σ vs ε) plot for a polymeric material with the five main regions that can generally be identified during the mechanical measurement (Bower, 2002; Sperling, 2006):

1. When a constant stress is applied to a polymeric material, deformation starts to occur. The polymer chains that originally are randomly organized start to move in the direction of the applied stress, until they reach a maximum stress—the yielding point. While for small loads the material behavior is linear viscoelastic, with increasing load the behavior becomes progressively nonlinear.
2. At the yielding point, the deformation becomes irreversible since the stress induces a plastic flow. The polymer chains start to disentangle and align in the direction of the applied mechanical stress with a necking region starting to appear in the center of the sample.
3. An increase in the strain leads to a decrease of the stress due to polymer chain disentanglement and alignment in the direction of the applied strain. At this point, a visible necking region is visible in the center of the sample.
4. After the necking formation, the stress reaches a plateau, and in this region, the necking starts to grow towards the edges of the sample due to the continuous alignment of the polymer chains in the direction of the stress—this stage is called the cold draw process, leading to highly aligned polymer chains.
5. Due to the high alignment of the polymer chains, and in order to maintain the experimental strain rate constant, there is an increase of the stress until the mechanical failure of the polymer; this stage is also known as strain-hardening.

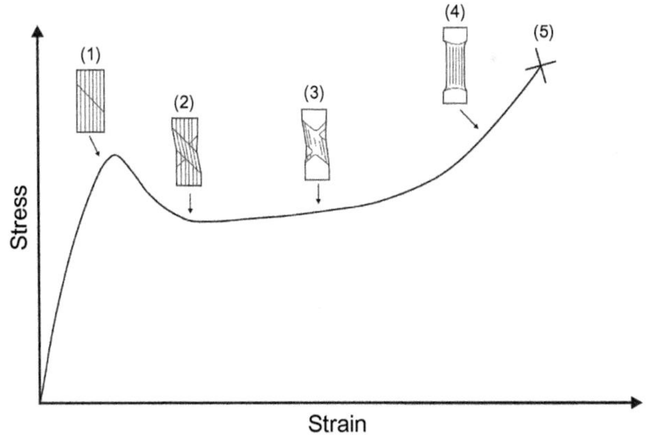

Fig. 7.2 Representative stress–strain plot for a polymeric material. The numbers in parentheses represent the different stages that occur during mechanical experiment in polymeric samples.

The mechanical properties of some natural and synthetic polymers are presented in Table 7.1.

Table 7.1 Mechanical properties of some natural and synthetic polymer materials

Material	E (MPa)[a]	UTS (MPa)[b]	ε_{break} (%)[c]	Reference
Gelatin films	20 ± 12	3 ± 1.5	25 ± 12	Bigi et al. (2001)
Silk-elastin-like protein (film)	3197 ± 326	70.5 ± 7.9	42.4 ± 22.3	Machado et al. (2015)
Silk-elastin-like protein (random fibers)	142 ± 48	14 ± 2	22 ± 6	Machado et al. (2013)
α-Elastin (random fibers)	0.33 ± 0.01	*	*	Araujo et al. (2014)
Polyhydroxybutyrate	3500	40	6	Goodfellow (2015)
Poly(lactic acid)	1610 ± 80	61.5 ± 3.80	5.2 ± 0.5	Zhang and Sun (2004)

[a] E, elasticity modulus.
[b] UTS, ultimate tensile strength.
[c] ε_{break}, strain-to-failure.
* Not available.

Fig. 7.3 presents the general mechanical behavior of different polymer materials. A polymer single-crystal fiber presents a very high tensile strength and a low strain at break, whereas an elastomer presents a very low tensile strength and high strain at break.

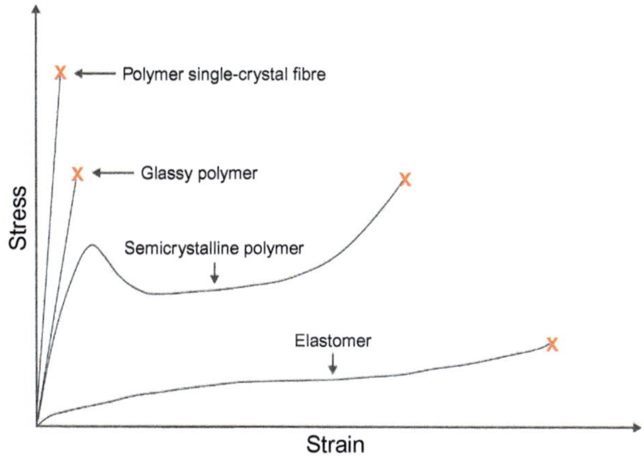

Fig. 7.3 Schematic stress–strain curves of different polymers, drawn approximately to scale (Bower, 2002).

7.3 Mechanical fatigue

Fatigue is one of the most important issues to address in materials science. Nevertheless, in the characterization of soft materials, it is a topic often underestimated and not completely explored. As the use of soft materials is growing fast, there is an emerging interest in understanding, modeling, and predicting the fatigue behavior and life cycle of a material. Fatigue failure can be interpreted as the failure of a certain structure under the action of repeated fluctuating stresses or strains. These induce progressive, localized, and permanent microstructural changes caused by cyclic plastic deformations that may culminate in the formation of cracks and subsequent final fracture (Erber et al., 1993). Mathematical models were first developed to establish the relationship between fatigue or damage accumulation, property degradation, loading variables, and applied cycles (Bower, 2002). These techniques proved to be fairly reliable and simple to use in many circumstances, making them attractive to the design engineer for life cycle predictions of developed structures.

While the application of one small plastic strain does not cause remarkable changes in the microstructure of a material, multiple repetitions of the plastic strain can lead to cumulative damage, which eventually results in fatigue failure (Anand and Parks, 2004). Therefore fatigue experiments are performed by submitting the material specimens to a cyclic varying load or displacement (Fig. 7.4). The material can be submitted to different shapes of time variation for the applied stress or strain, such as sine, triangular, or other more complex wave geometries, depending on the application characteristics.

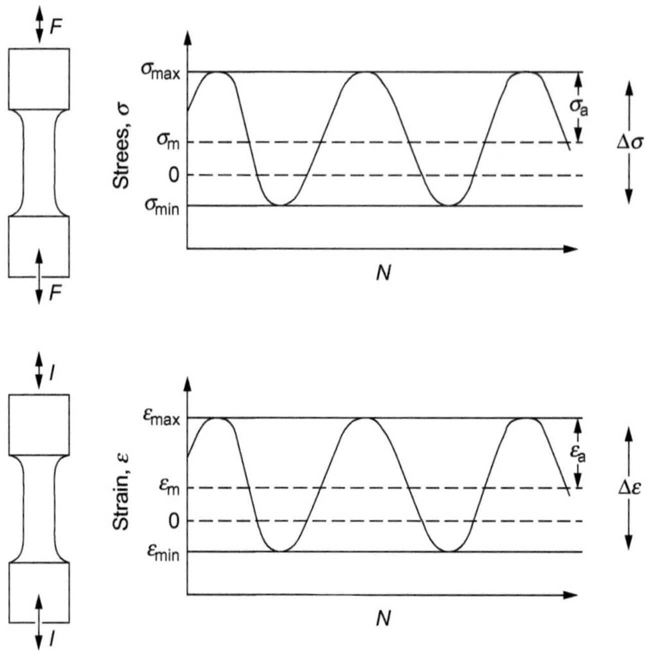

Fig. 7.4 Fatigue testing (Ashby and Jones, 2012).

In polymeric materials, the linear relationship between the stress and strain (elasticity) is only valid for very small deformations. Nevertheless, inelasticity is always present even though it may be detectable only by fine measurements (Frunz and Diaconescu, 2006). As a consequence of inelasticity, when a cyclic stress is applied, the plastic contribution for the mechanical response increases giving origin to a hysteresis closed loop during the cyclic mechanical loading (Fig. 7.5). This loop evolves with the number of stress cycles, its shape changing with increasing number of fatigue cycles (*N*), until finally fail (when $N = N_f$—the number of cycles to failure) (Ashby and Jones, 2012). As the area within the loop equals the amount of energy dissipated

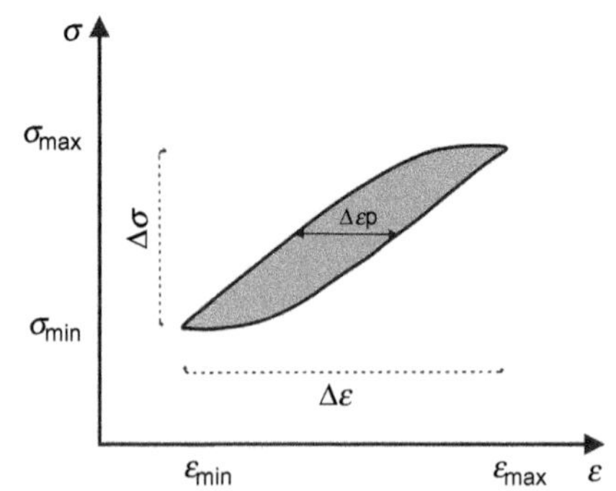

Fig. 7.5 Schematic of a mechanical hysteresis loop.

in the material and since sustained hysteresis relates to the rate of damage accumulation, the study of the hysteresis loop offers useful information on a material state (Frunz and Diaconescu, 2006; Erber et al., 1993).

7.3.1 Coffin–Manson model—plastic strain range—life model

The Coffin–Manson mathematical relationship has been used to model crack growth in metals due to repeated temperature cycling. This model establishes a relation between the width of hysteresis loops and the number of loading cycles required to produce failure; linking the hysteresis energy dissipation, the accumulation of material damage, and the average number of loading cycles leading to failure (Erber et al., 1993).

In order to determine the plastic strain range ($\Delta\varepsilon_p$), graphically represented by the width of the hysteresis loop (Fig. 7.5), the elastic strain range ($\Delta\varepsilon_e$) is subtracted from the total strain range ($\Delta\varepsilon_t$) (Kanchanomai and Mutoh, 2004). The relationship between the plastic strain range and the number of cycles to produce failure follows the following equation:

$$\left(N_\mathrm{f}\right)^{\alpha} \times \Delta\varepsilon_\mathrm{t} = \theta \tag{7.5}$$

where N_f is the fatigue life, α is the fatigue ductility exponent, and θ is the fatigue ductility coefficient (Kanchanomai and Mutoh, 2004). The result of the low-cycle fatigue according to the Coffin–Manson model is near a straight line for most common materials.

A modified equation was proposed at a later date, in order to model and predict the fatigue life for different experimental frequencies:

$$\left(N_\mathrm{f} \times \upsilon^{k-1}\right)^{\alpha} \times \Delta\varepsilon_\mathrm{t} = \theta \tag{7.6}$$

where υ and k are the frequency and frequency exponent, respectively, evaluated from the fatigue life-frequency relationship (Kanchanomai and Mutoh, 2004). According to the Coffin–Manson modified model, the relationship between the plastic strain range and frequency can be fit to a single curve. Nevertheless, the effect of the temperature in the material fatigue life is not predicted by this model, which implies the measurement of the fatigue parameter should be performed at desired temperatures.

7.3.2 Smith–Watson–Topper model

According to the Smith–Watson–Topper (SWT) model, the fatigue life cycle for any situation of mean stress depends on the product between the maximum stress and the total deformation (Ashby and Jones, 2012):

$$\frac{\Delta\varepsilon_\mathrm{t}}{2} = \varepsilon_\mathrm{a} = \frac{\Delta\varepsilon_\mathrm{e}}{2} + \frac{\Delta\varepsilon_\mathrm{p}}{2} = \frac{\sigma_\mathrm{f}'}{E}\left(2N_\mathrm{f}\right)^{b} + \varepsilon_\mathrm{f}'\left(2N_\mathrm{f}\right)^{c} \tag{7.7}$$

where $\frac{\Delta\varepsilon}{2}$ is the strain amplitude, ε_f' is the fatigue ductility coefficient, c is the fatigue ductility exponent and E is the material Young modulus. In this model, the material fatigue is based on the strain-life approach, where the cyclic response of the material is within the elastic-plastic stress–strain range, and can only be used to predict the fatigue life at zero mean stress (Ince and Glinka, 2011).

7.3.3 Morrow energy model—plastic strain energy density-life model

The plastic strain energy density can be physically interpreted as the energy of distortion associated with the change in shape of a volume element and is related to failure, particularly under conditions of ductile behavior, as it often occurs in many of the polymeric materials submitted to cyclic mechanical solicitation (Kanchanomai and Mutoh, 2004). According to the mathematical model proposed by Morrow (American Society for Testing and Materials, 1965), the strain energy density can be evaluated numerically as the inner area of the saturated hysteresis loop for the uniaxial fatigue experiments (Fig. 7.6), and is expressed mathematically as:

$$N_f^n \times W_p = C \tag{7.8}$$

where W_p is the plastic density energy, N_f is the fatigue life, and m and C are the fatigue exponent and coefficient, respectively. Morrow's model was modified in order to predict the effect of experimental frequency in the material fatigue life cycle, according to:

$$\left(N_f \times \upsilon^{k-1}\right)^m \times W_p = C \tag{7.9}$$

where υ and k are the frequency and frequency exponent, respectively, also proposed by the Coffin–Manson model for fatigue life-frequency relationship (Kanchanomai and Mutoh, 2004).

The above theories where developed to explain and predict mainly metallic materials fatigue life cycle, but they also proved to be suitable for predicting polymers fatigue behavior.

Scaffolds and membranes used for tissue and biomedical engineering are often under cyclic loading during in vitro or in vivo experiments. For example, poly-ε-caprolactone (PCL) macroporous scaffolds were produced by dissolving the polymer in a suitable solvent in the presence of poly(methyl methacrylate) spheres as a sacrificial porogen (Panadero et al., 2013). The scaffolds were cut into disks of 6 mm diameter and a thickness of approximately 2 mm, and submitted to a cyclic mechanical compression loading at a fixed strain of 15%, in order to mimic the cartilage deformation during walking. Panadero et al. (2013) found that the number of mechanical load-unload cycles can increase up to five times in water-immersed samples with all pores filled with water, when compared with those in dry conditions. This increased performance was attributed to the more uniform stress distribution that occurs when the sample is filled with water, and also to the incompressibility of water that supports a significant part of the mechanical cyclic loading. In their work, fibrin and water were also used to fill the pores leading to similar results. Fig. 7.6 represents the trabeculae PCL sample morphology with fibrin filling the pore structure; the mechanical loading-unloading cycles also applied to the samples. Based on experimental data, and using the fitting parameters obtained from Morrow's model, the mechanical life cycle performance was calculated and compared to the experimental results. In this model, a perfect correlation occurs when the data points lie on the solid diagonal line, and when the experimental data deviate no more than 10% from the theoretical line (American Society for Testing and Materials, 1965; Kanchanomai and Mutoh, 2004; Panadero et al., 2013). The findings suggest that the Morrow's theoretical model can be used to explain the polymer fatigue life behavior for the PCL trabecular scaffold under different conditions (Fig. 7.6).

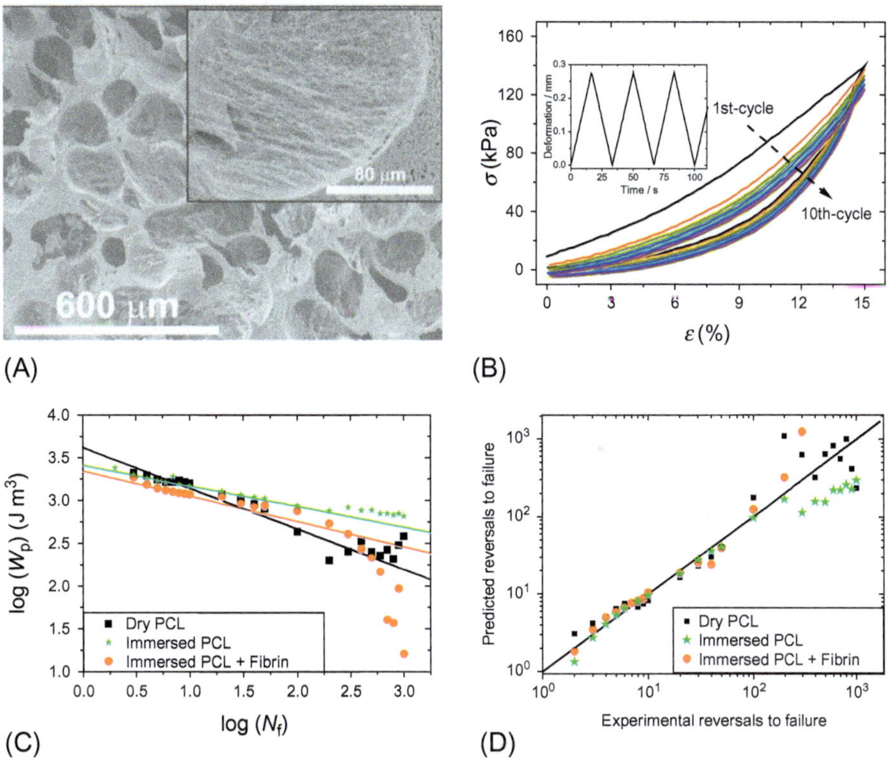

Fig. 7.6 (A) PCL sample microstructure with fibrin filling the pore structure. (B) Sample characteristic hysteresis loops with inset showing the cyclic mechanical loading applied. (C) Relationship between the overall equivalent behavior similar to plastic strain energy density and number of load-recovery cycles of PCL samples. (D) Comparison of predicted with experimentally fatigue behavior calculated according to the Morrow's model. Adapted from Panadero, J.A., Vikingsson, L., Gomez Ribelles, J.L., Sencadas, V., Lanceros-Mendez, S., 2013. Fatigue prediction in fibrin poly-ε-caprolactone macroporous scaffolds, J. Mech. Behav. Biomed. Mater. 28, 55–61.

In another experiment, the PCL porous matrix was filled with poly(vinyl alcohol) (PVA) and showed that the presence of the cross-linked PVA inside of the PCL macropores leads to an increase of the Young's modulus (Panadero et al., 2015b). However, the mechanical fatigue behavior predicted by the Morrow's model revealed that the PCL–PVA scaffolds had a poor performance when compared to the PCL samples filled with fibrin and water, likely due to complex changes in the porous structure and local interactions among the different phases, eg, PCL, PVA, and water.

Based on the previous results obtained for the different trabecular PCL scaffolds, the authors studied the effect of the mechanical fatigue cycle using murine bone marrow cell (KUM5 cells) culture. They applied a fixed strain of 15% at a frequency of 1 Hz during 30 and 90 min of stillness and real-time polymerase chain reaction (PCR) was performed to identify the cell expression of characteristic markers of several components of the extra cellular matrix (ECM) (Panadero et al., 2015a). The fatigue cycle measurements performed in the bioreactor showed that the mechanical behavior of the PCL constructs with ECM produced by the cells is different from the one reported above (Panadero et al., 2015a), but the overall fatigue cycle can be described by the Morrow's model, which is an important finding that could help in future scaffold design.

7.4 Fourier transform infrared spectroscopy (FTIR)

Infrared radiation is an electromagnetic radiation with wavelengths (υ) between 0.7 and 500 μm, corresponding to radiations with wavenumbers ($\nu = 1/\lambda$) between 1.4×10^4 and $20\,\text{cm}^{-1}$, which specifies the number of waves per centimeter.

When a molecule is submitted to infrared radiation, the absorption of such radiation leads to vibrational and/or rotational movements. Infrared absorption occurs when the *ac* electric field frequency associated to the incident radiation matches the changes of frequency in the vibration or rotation movements of the molecule that is absorbing the electromagnetic radiation (Stuart, 2004). When this matching occurs, the electromagnetic radiation is absorbed, promoting a change in the molecule vibration amplitude, which also affects the dipolar moment during absorption—also called the *transition dipole* or *transition moment* (Bower and Maddams, 1989). The absorbed energy is subsequently lost by the molecule, either in the form of reradiation or, more usually, by being transferred to other molecules of the material in the form of heat energy (Bower, 2002).

Essentially, an infrared spectrometer consists of the following elements (Bower and Maddams, 1989):

- **i.** A source of radiation with a continuous spectrum over a wide range of infrared wavelengths
- **ii.** A means of dispersing the radiation into its constituent wavelengths
- **iii.** A sample holder, allowing the radiation to pass through the sample or to be reflected
- **iv.** An infrared detector capable of measuring over the range of wavelengths of interest
- **v.** An acquisition and recording system.

The most common system used to study polymers is the *Fourier-transform* spectrometer, where all wavelengths pass through the sample to the detector simultaneously. The total transmitted intensity is measured as a function of the displacement of one of the mirrors in a double-beam interferometer, usually of the Michelson type. The separation of the wavelengths is subsequently done mathematically, by employing a Fourier transform on the intensity versus displacement data (Bower and Maddams, 1989).

7.4.1 Normal modes of vibration

A basic model to describe the interaction of the infrared radiation with matter is that of looking to a molecule as a system of masses joined by bonds behaving like springs (Fig. 7.7). Taking the example of the diatomic molecules, these exhibit three degrees of translational freedom and two degrees of rotational freedom. The atoms in the molecules can also move relative to one another, meaning that the bond lengths can vary, or one atom can move out of its present plane. Briefly, this is the definition of the bending and vibrational movements, which are referred to collectively as vibrations (Campbell et al., 2000; Bower and Maddams, 1989; Bower, 2002).

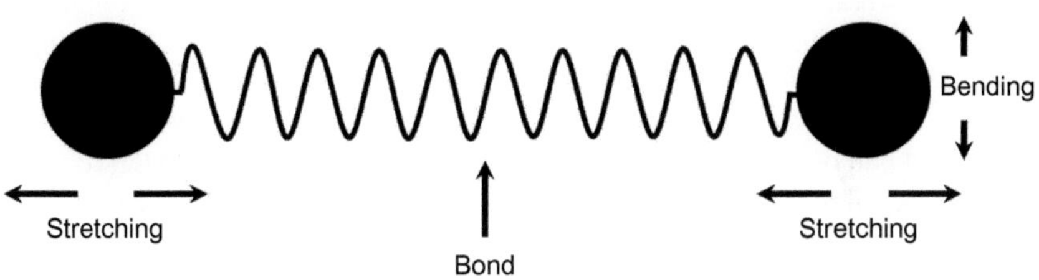

Fig. 7.7 Schematic representation of vibration modes in a diatomic molecule.

For a molecule consisting of N atoms, the number of vibrational degrees of freedom is $3N-6$, leading to the same number of normal modes of vibration. For linear molecules, where low rotational modes are equivalent, the number of vibrational degrees of freedom is represented by $3N-5$ (Campbell et al., 2000; Stuart, 2004). The degrees of freedom for polyatomic molecules, eg, polymers, are summarized in Table 7.2.

Whereas a diatomic molecule has only one mode of vibration, which corresponds to the stretching motion, a nonlinear B-A-B type triatomic molecule has three modes, two of which correspond to stretching motions, with the remaining corresponding to a bending motion. A linear type triatomic molecule has four vibration modes, two of which have the same frequency, and are said to be *degenerate* (Stuart, 2004).

Table 7.2 Degrees of freedom for polyatomic molecules

Type of degrees of freedom	Linear	Nonlinear
Translational	3	3
Rotational	2	3
Vibrational	$3N-5$	$3N-6$
Total	$3N$	$3N$

From Stuart, B.H., 2004. Introduction. Infrared Spectroscopy: Fundamentals and Applications. John Wiley and Sons, Chichester.

For a simple diatomic molecule, the vibration can be modeled as two masses, m_1 and m_2, joined by a spring, with deformation obeying to the Hooke's law (Eq. 7.2). The vibration frequency is then expressed by:

$$\nu = \frac{1}{2\pi}\left(\frac{k}{\mu}\right)^{1/2} \tag{7.10}$$

where, k is the spring constant and μ is the reduced mass, given by:

$$\mu = \frac{m_1 m_2}{m_1 + m_2} \tag{7.11}$$

From Eqs. (7.10), (7.11), one can observe that a molecule can only absorb radiation when the infrared radiation reaching the sample is of the same frequency as one of the fundamental modes of vibration of the molecule. In other words, a small part of the molecule has vibrational motion, while the rest is left unaffected.

Molecular vibrations can involve either changes in bond length—stretching, or bond angle—bending. Some bonds can stretch in-phase (symmetric stretching) or out-of-phase (asymmetric stretching) while the other vibrations contributing to the infrared are generically referred to as bending vibrations. Fig. 7.8 presents the molecular vibrations that can occur in an infrared measurement of a polymeric material.

Asymmetric vibrations produce a displacement of the dipoles leading to a change in the dipole moment of the molecule, making these ones "infrared active." On the other hand, symmetrical vibrations are weaker because they don't produce a change

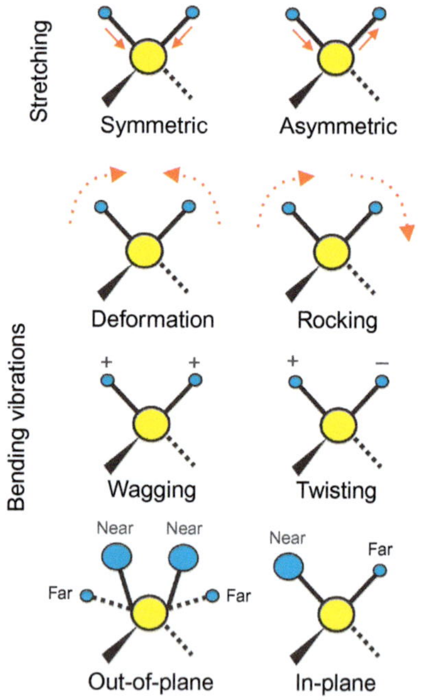

Fig. 7.8 Representation of the most common infrared vibrations observed in a polymeric molecule.

in the dipole moment, and, consequently, usually are inactive in infrared (Campbell et al., 2000; Stuart, 2004).

A polymeric molecule can contain tens of thousands of atoms and, consequently, the number of normal modes of vibration may be significantly higher. The infrared spectrum of a polymer may thus be expected to be tremendously complicated. However, polymeric materials are made from a large number of chemically identical units and many of the vibrations are equivalent, reducing the number of distinguishable vibrational states, which simplifies the problem of assignments (Fig. 7.9) (Stuart, 2004; Bower and Maddams, 1989).

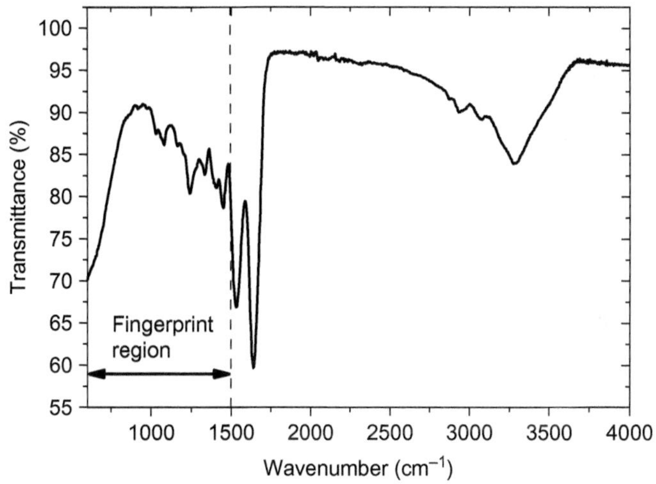

Fig. 7.9 Infrared spectrum of a fish gelatine sample.

The region between 1550 and 500 cm^{-1} usually contains a very complicated series of absorptions, frequently overlapping each other, mainly due to all kinds of bending vibrations (Fig. 7.8). This area of the spectra is called the *fingerprint* region (Fig. 7.9) and is characteristic of each polymeric material, and could therefore be used to identify the chemical compound.

Infrared spectroscopy is a very useful and powerful characterization technique providing information about the chemical and physical structure of a polymer, because any two regions of the material that differ in the way the repeating units are arranged, may exhibit detectable differences in the IR spectra (Bower and Maddams, 1989; Bower, 2002). In Table 7.3 the most common vibrational modes found for polymers are summarized.

7.4.2 Quantitative analysis

When the infrared radiation passes through an absorbing medium (Fig. 7.10), it may be expressed in terms of the Lambert–Beer law:

$$A = \log\left(\frac{I}{I_0}\right) = kct \tag{7.12}$$

Table 7.3 Characteristic vibration modes for common groups found in polymers

Type of vibration	Characteristic frequency (cm^{-1})
O–H {stretching}	3650–3000
N–H {stretching}	3500–3300
C–H {stretching}	3200–2800
S–H {stretching}	2600–2550
C≡N {stretching}	2255–2220
C≡C {stretching}	2250–2100
C=O {stretching}	1820–1680
C=C {stretching}	1900–1500
C=N {stretching}	1680–1610
N=N {stretching}—aliphatic	1580–15,500
N=N {stretching}—aromatic	1440–410
C–NO_2 {stretching}	1590–1530 {asymmetric}
	1380–1340 {symmetric}
C–SO_2–C {stretching}	1350–1310 {asymmetric}
	1160–1120 {symmetric}
C=S {stretching}	1250–1000
CH_2 {bending}	1470–1400
CH_3 {bending}	1380
C–C {stretching}—aromatic	1600, 1580, 1500, 1450, 1000
C–C {stretching}—alicyclic	1300–600
C–O–C {stretching}	1150–1060 {asymmetric}
	970–800 {symmetric}
Si–O–Si {stretching}	1100–1000 {asymmetric}
	550–540 {symmetric}
O–O {stretching}	900–845
S–S {stretching}	550–430
C–Cl {stretching}	800–550
C–Br {stretching}	700–550
C–I {stretching}	660–480

Adapted from Schrader, B., 2008. Infrared and Raman Spectroscopy: Methods and Applications, Wiley, New York; Campbell, D., Pethrick, R.A., White, J.R., 2000. Polymer Characterization: Physical Techniques, second ed. Taylor & Francis, Abingdon.

where A is the absorbance; I_0 is the incident light; I is the intensity at a thickness; t in the absorbing medium; c is the concentration of absorbing species; and k is a constant for the material termed the absorptivity or extinction coefficient (Campbell et al., 2000).

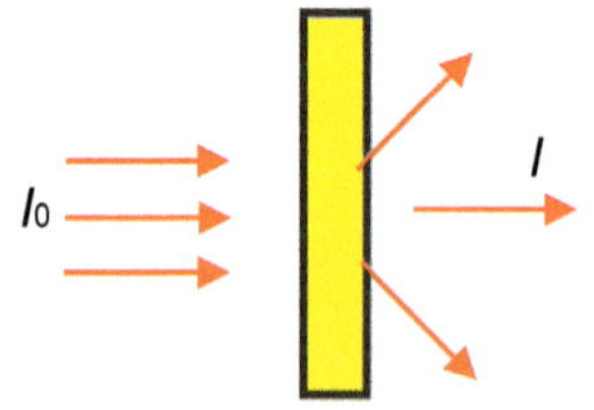

Fig. 7.10 Illustration of Lambert–Beer law.

Values of absorbance range from zero, when there is no absorption ($I = I_0$) to infinity when all incident light is completely absorbed ($I = 0$) (Campbell et al., 2000).

The IR absorption spectrum of a polymer sample is usually plotted as a percentage of the transmittance (I/I_0) or absorbance against a wavelength or wavenumber of infrared radiation. If the sample is very thick, the transmittance will approach zero and the absorbance will tend to infinity for all wavelengths. In order to avoid this issue, it is necessary to work with samples with thickness in the range of 30–300 μm (Bower, 2002).

Modern spectrometers are computer controlled, allowing not only to measure the IR spectra of the sample, but also to perform complex mathematical calculations with the data. As an example, they permit comparing the unknown polymer substance spectra with standard data of different polymers and other chemical substances present in the software database, ultimately leading to an identification of the polymer and its composition.

7.4.3 Polymer molecular orientation

One of the most important features of infrared spectroscopy is the simplicity of the measurement, which is usually a nondestructive characterization technique that also allows quantifying different material characteristics. The most important of those is the determination of polymer chain orientation, which will deeply influence the material performance.

As mentioned earlier, an infrared absorption band is associated with a particular vibration mode of the polymer bonds. For each one of these modes there is a particular direction within the polymer chain, which is the direction of the absorption dipole μ, also called *infrared-transition dipole* or *transition moment axis* (Bower and Maddams, 1989; Bower, 2002).

The IR radiation is absorbed by a particular functional group of the polymer chain only if the radiation frequency matches the frequency of vibration of the molecule, and a component of the electric vector E of the incident radiation I must be parallel to the transition-dipole axis. If a polymer chain is oriented, so should the dipole axes; in other words, sample absorption will depend on the polarization of the incident radiation.

In order to determine the polymer chain orientation, infrared measurements of transmittance or absorbance must be performed with polarized IR radiation, parallel or perpendicular to the mechanical draw direction, for a particular absorption band of the spectrum. Fig. 7.11 shows the FTIR spectra obtained for two orthogonal polarization directions, parallel and perpendicular to the draw direction of a poly(vinylidene fluoride) (PVDF) polymer sample. It is possible to observe that the overall spectra are similar with neither modes being totally suppressed nor new modes seeming to appear. Nevertheless, the amount of IR radiation absorbed by some particular modes are clearly different for IR spectra obtained with radiation polarized in the perpendicular or parallel to the polymer draw direction (Fig. 7.11).

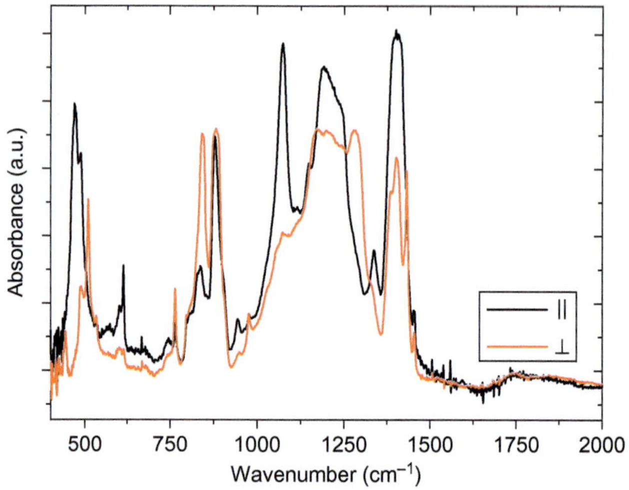

Fig. 7.11 Detail of the FTIR spectra obtained for a PVDF uniaxial stretched sample. FTIR was collected with the IR radiation polarized in the polymer draw (||) and perpendicular direction (⊥).

Assuming that reflectance and/or scattering do not contribute significantly to the differences in the attenuation and is only due to absorbance, the Lambert–Beer law (Eq. 7.12) can be modified in order to obtain the absorbance for the two IR polarized directions:

$$A_{\parallel} = k_{\parallel}ct$$
$$A_{\perp} = k_{\perp}ct \qquad (7.13)$$

where, $A_{\parallel}$ and $A_{\perp}$ are the absorbance of the polarized light in the parallel and perpendicular to the polymer stretching direction, respectively; $k_{\parallel}$ and $k_{\perp}$ are proportional to the average fractions of the incident energy per unit of area absorbed by a single absorber, for radiation polarized parallel or perpendicular to the polymer draw direction, respectively.

The absorption of the IR radiation is associated to changes in the oscillating dipole μ associated to the vibration mode. Considering that $A_{\parallel} \propto \langle \mu_{\parallel}^2 \rangle$ and $A_{\perp} \propto \langle \mu_{\perp}^2 \rangle$, where $\mu_{\parallel}$ and $\mu_{\perp}$ are the components of the oscillating dipole in the parallel and perpendicular to the draw direction in the plane of the sample (Fig. 7.12).

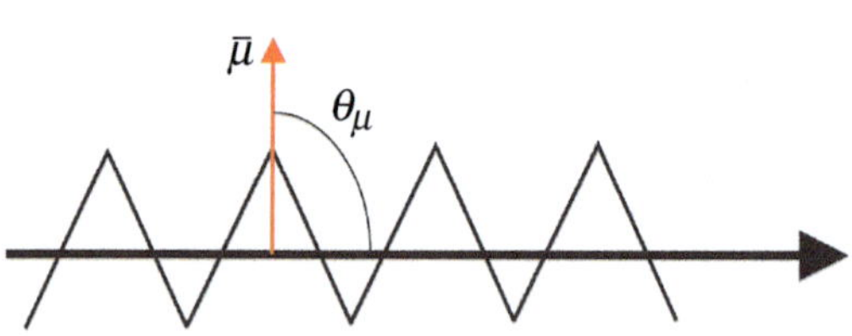

Fig. 7.12 Definition of the angle between the transition dipole μ with respect to the long axis of the polymer molecule (Gedde, 2001, p. 207).

Thus:

$$A_{\parallel} = C\left\langle \cos^2\theta_\mu \right\rangle \tag{7.14}$$

and assuming uniaxial symmetry:

$$A_{\perp} = C\left\langle \sin^2\theta_\mu \cos^2\theta_\mu \right\rangle = \frac{1}{2}C\left\langle \sin^2\theta_\mu \right\rangle \tag{7.15}$$

where:

$$C = A_{\parallel} + 2A_{\perp} = 3A_{iso} \tag{7.16}$$

where A_{iso} is the absorbance of an isotropic sample with same thickness and the simplification of Eq. (7.15) is due to the random orientation of the oscillating dipole μ (Bower, 2002). Replacing C in Eq. (7.14):

$$\left\langle \cos^2\theta_\mu \right\rangle = \frac{A_{\parallel}}{A_{\parallel} + 2A_{\perp}} \tag{7.17}$$

The ratio between the $A_{\parallel}$ and $A_{\perp}$ is called dichroic ratio, D:

$$D = \frac{A_{\parallel}}{A_{\perp}} \tag{7.18}$$

Replacing D in Eq. (7.17), one obtains:

$$\left\langle \cos^2\theta_\mu \right\rangle = \frac{D}{D+2} \tag{7.19}$$

Thus, the polymer chains main orientation can be defined by the Herman's orientation function, f, given by:

$$f = \frac{(D-1)(D_0+2)}{(D+1)(D_0-2)} \tag{7.20}$$

where D_0 is the dichroic ratio for a sample with perfect uniaxial orientation and is dependent of the angle between the oscillating dipole μ of the considered vibrational band and the local chain axis segment of the polymer:

$$D_0 = 2\cot^2\theta_\mu \tag{7.21}$$

Absorption bands associated with a perpendicular transition dipole moment have $D_0 = 0$, and the Herman's orientation factor is given by:

$$f = 2\frac{(1-D)}{(D+2)} \tag{7.22}$$

One of the main attractions of the IR technique is that the dichroism of the absorption bands assigned to different groups, and orientation of the different groups of the monomer can be determined (Gedde, 2001). Herman's mathematical model predicts that related to the direction of interest, well-aligned polymer chains had a value of 1, and perpendicular aligned chains had a value of −0.5, while for random aligned polymer chains $f = 0$, as illustrated in Fig. 7.13.

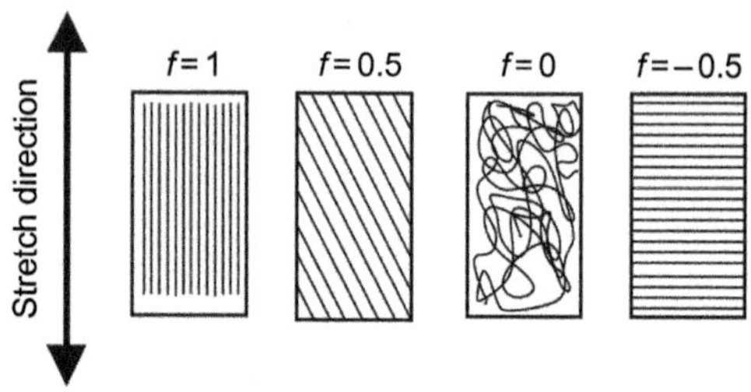

Fig. 7.13 Schematic representation of the Herman's orientation factor, related to polymer chain stretching direction.

The orientation of the uniaxial drawn PVDF was measured by Sencadas et al. (2009). In their work, the vibrational modes at 765 and 510 cm^{-1} were chosen, because they are related to the crystalline α and β-phases of the polymer and both are very well defined CF_2 bond vibrations relative to the direction of the polymer chain, and the reorientation of the chains could be monitored independently, for each crystalline phase. In their work, they reported that there was a change of the Herman's orientation factor from 0, for a perfect random polymer chains obtained from cooling the polymer from the melt, to −0.47 for the sample stretched five times its original length. By determining the position of the CF_2 dipole, the alignment of polymer chains in relation to the mechanical draw direction was indirectly measured. Their results were validated by measuring the polymer chain orientation by X-ray diffraction techniques (Branciforti et al., 2007), and the values reported are consistent with the ones obtained by FTIR measurements.

7.5 Thermal characterization techniques

7.5.1 Differential scanning calorimetry

Differential scanning calorimetry (DSC) is a direct analytical experimental technique that measures the heat flux $\partial q / \partial t$ to or from a sample specimen as well as enthalpy changes as a function of temperature or time. This method is not a passive experimental technique because there is a change of material structure, eg, crystallinity, morphology, etc., during the measurement. In DSC, the samples can also be submitted to annealing, aging, curing, or even to erase the previous material thermal history (Kämpf, 1986).

The present discussion will focus on the physical principles of the measurement and how to interpret the recorded data under nonisothermal conditions. This technique is also useful to study the polymer crystallization kinetics; however, this topic is beyond the scope of this discussion. Fully detailed description and physical principles involved in polymer crystallization kinetics can be found in Bower (2002) and Sperling (2006).

The apparatus basically consists of two furnaces with controlled atmosphere and independent temperature controller, heating elements, and individual thermocouples (Fig. 7.14). The sample and the reference sample (usually air) are placed inside small independent crucibles made from a high thermal conductive material, generally aluminum, but other materials can also be found such as gold, platinum, graphite, or even copper.

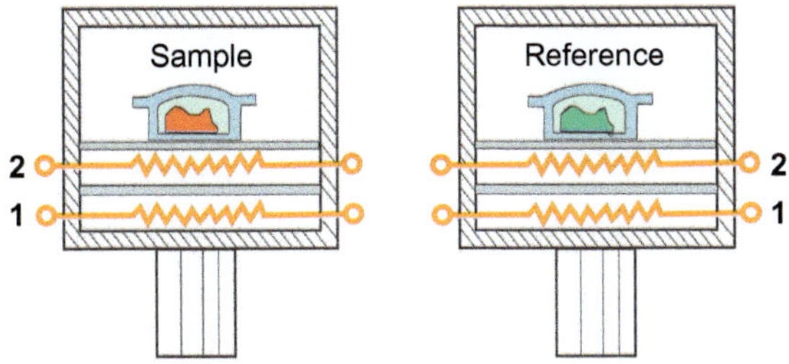

Fig. 7.14 A schematic drawing of a differential scanning calorimeter. The number 1 represents the heating/cooling system and the number 2 exemplifies the thermocouples (Lobo and Bonilla, 2003).

The user-defined thermal program is applied to the sample and reference in the same conditions, especially the same heating and/or cooling rate, and the temperature of each pan is recorded independently. As an example, consider if the sample was ice, and a constant heating rate is applied for the reference and the sample. When the ice starts to melt, and during the entire melting process, the sample temperature remains constant while the reference temperature continues to increase. When the ice melting process finishes the temperature of the sample starts to increase. By subtracting the temperature profile recorded for the sample and for the reference material, it is possible to calculate the amount of energy supplied to the sample during melting (Fig. 7.15).

Despite being a destructive characterization technique, DSC is fast and easy to operate, and only a small amount of sample (in the milligram scale) and a good physical contact between the sample and the base of the crucible is needed to reduce operation errors (Fig. 7.16). The main sources of operation mistakes/errors during a DSC measurement are related to a bad calibration of the thermocouples, sample contamination from the surroundings, the presence of moisture and/or residual solvents and inaccurate sample mass.

7.5.2 Thermogram analysis

If a polymer sample is submitted to a heat cycle at a constant heating rate and pressure, then the specific heat (C) of the polymer can be defined as:

$$C = \frac{Q}{m\Delta T} \tag{7.23}$$

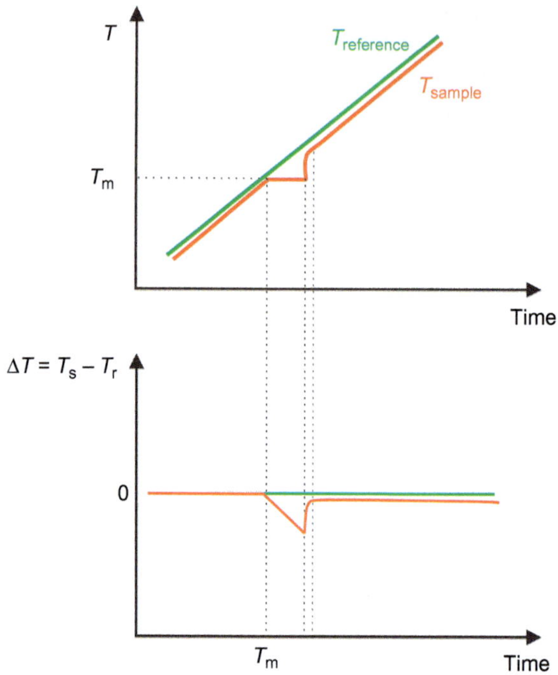

Fig. 7.15 Diagram of the temperature profile applied to the reference and to the sample during a DSC measurement. T_r, temperature of the reference sample; T_s, temperature of sample (NETZSCH, 2015).

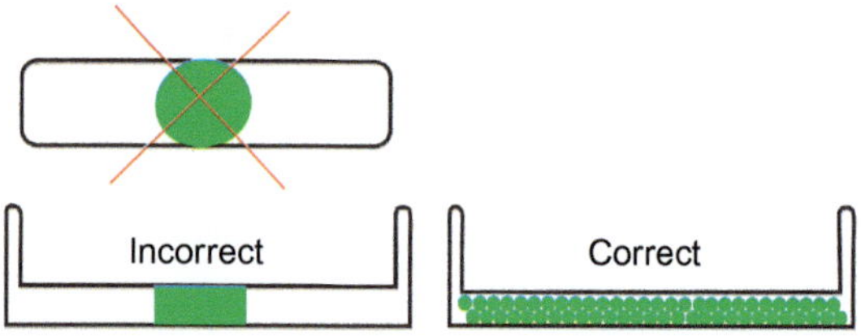

Fig. 7.16 Sample preparation for a DSC experiment (NETZSCH, 2015).

where Q is the amount of heat added (heat flow), m is the mass of the sample, and ΔT is the change in temperature. The heat of the melting (H_m) is defined as the amount of heat per unit of mass needed to change a substance from the solid state to a liquid state at its melting point. As the melting process is an endothermic reaction, it is represented by a positive peak in the DSC curve, considering the y-axis range setting of the heating flow (Fig. 7.17). The heat of melting can be calculated from the DSC plot by determination of the area under the melting transition, according to Eq. (7.24):

$$H_m = \frac{Q}{m} \tag{7.24}$$

From the analysis of the DSC plot (Fig. 7.17), one can acquire information from the different thermal events occurring in the polymer during the heating or cooling stages in the DSC measurement.

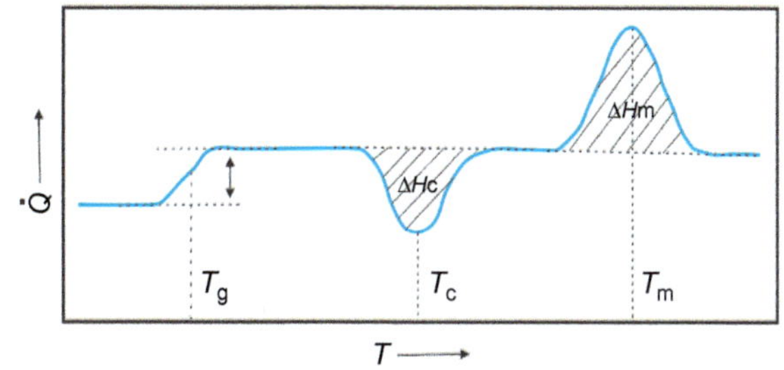

Fig. 7.17 Illustration of a DSC thermogram during the heating scan for a polymer sample. T_g, glass transition; T_c, cold-crystallization temperature; T_m, melting temperature.

In Fig. 7.17, the process that occurs at lower temperatures is called the glass transition (T_g). Below this temperature the polymer chains are in a "frozen" state and only local cooperative movements are allowed. When the temperature reaches the polymer glass transition, the movement of the polymer chains is promoted, softening the material, and is graphically represented by a slope/shift in the baseline (represented by T_g in Fig. 7.17). The calculation of the glass transition temperature can be done in different ways. The most common is the half C_p or half-height of the shifted baseline as illustrated in Fig. 7.17 (Lobo and Bonilla, 2003).

After glass transition, increasing the temperature may lead to a cold-crystallization process (T_c), which is a thermal event observed for some polymers. This occurs due to the high mobility of the polymer chains that organize in a more packed structure, releasing energy of the system. It is an exothermic process and therefore is represented by a negative peak in the thermogram with the area of the cold-crystallization peak being proportional to the energy required to pack the polymer in a more organized state—ΔH_c (Fig. 7.17).

Finally, as the temperature increases even further, the polymer crystalline regions reach the melting transition with the area of the melting peak being proportional to the amount of energy required to melt the crystalline regions of the polymer, also known as the melting enthalpy—ΔH_m, which can be used to calculate the percent of crystallinity present in the material.

The degree of crystallinity (X_c) for a given polymer is determined by applying the following equation:

$$X_c = \frac{\Delta H_m - \Delta H_c}{\Delta H_m^0} \times 100 \tag{7.25}$$

where ΔH_m^0 is a reference value and represents the heat of melting for a 100% crystalline polymer sample. It has been established for most common engineering polymers and some of these are in Table 7.4.

Depending on the sample thermal history, a cold-crystallization exothermic peak may or may not be observed during the DSC, and if it does not appear the value of $\Delta H_c = 0$.

Table 7.4 Heating for the melting of a 100% crystalline polymer sample

Polymer	Acronym	ΔH_m^0 (J/g)
Polypropylene	PP	207.1
Polyethylene	PE	293.6
Poly(ethylene terephthalate)	PET	140.1
Polyamide-6	PA6	230.1
Polyamide 12	PA12	209.3
Poly(lactic acid)	PLA	93.0
Poly(hydroxybutyrate)	PHB	146.0

Adapted from Mark, J.E., 2007. Physical Properties of Polymers Handbook. Springer, New York.

7.5.3 Thermogravimetric analysis

By definition, thermogravimetric analysis (TGA) is the measurement of the weight of a polymer sample as a function of temperature, time and/or atmosphere at a controlled temperature program. Usually, the evolution of the mass is measured in a high sensitive balance, under a well-defined atmosphere (inert or reactive gas) and plotted against temperature. TGA is used not only for polymeric materials, but also to characterize materials used in various environmental, food, pharmaceutical, and petrochemical applications. An example of a TGA plot is presented in Fig. 7.18.

The thermogram in Fig. 7.18 reveals several information parameters related to polymer degradation. In the case of poly(lactic acid) (PLA), the mass remains constant until pyrolysis starts to occur. The initial degradation temperature ($T_{initial}$) is defined as the temperature at which the material degradation begins, and is represented in the thermogram as the point at which there is a sudden decrease in mass from the initial sample weight. This temperature is particularly important because it gives information about the highest temperature that a polymer can be processed. Nevertheless, one should take in account that initial mass losses can be observed due to the presence of moisture in the sample (Machado et al., 2015). The onset temperature (T_{onset}) is calculated by extending the predegradation portion of the curve to the point of the interception with a line drawn as a tangent to the steepest portion of the mass curve occurring during degradation (Turi, 2012). As represented in Fig. 7.18 it refers to the temperature were oxidation just begins. Some features in the TGA curve may not be readily perceived and can be more easily detected by applying a first-order derivative in the thermogram. The derivative thermogravimetric (DTG) curve is the best indicator of the temperature at which the various stages of thermal decomposition take place and provides information about the decomposition rates. The maximum of the reaction rate ($T_p = \partial m / \partial T$) is obtained by the peak of the DTG and indicates the point of greatest rate of change on the weight loss curve (Lobo and Bonilla, 2003; Turi, 2012).

The residual mass ($M_{residual}$) obtained in the end of the thermogravimetric experiment is usually attributed to ashes resulting from the sample pyrolysis process.

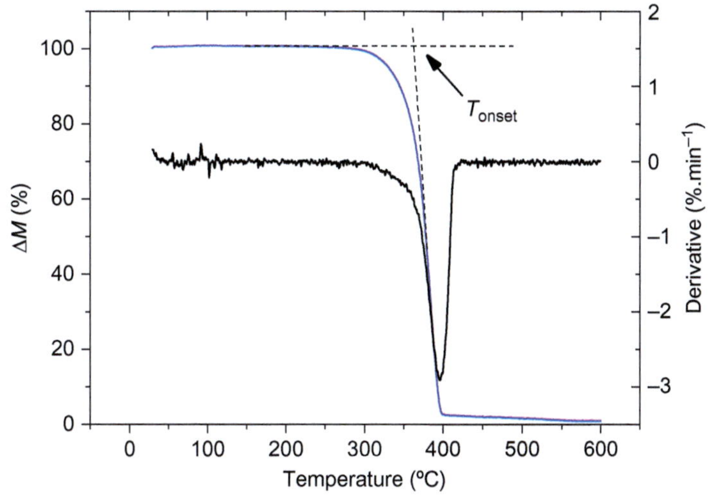

Fig. 7.18 TGA thermogram and derivative obtained for a poly(lactic acid) at a heating rate of 20°C/min under nitrogen atmosphere.

7.5.4 Thermal degradation kinetics

From the TGA data, the kinetics of the thermal degradation process can be studied. A typical model for the thermal decomposition rate ($-\frac{\partial(1-\alpha)}{\partial t}$) of a homogeneous system follows the general expression:

$$-\frac{\partial(1-\alpha)}{\partial t}=k(T)f(\alpha) \tag{7.26}$$

where, $f(\alpha)$ represents the net result of elementary steps, as the polymer thermal degradation is often a chain reaction, $k(T)$ is the rate constant and α is the of conversion of the sample under degradation, and is defined by:

$$\alpha=\frac{w_0-w_{(t)}}{w_0-w_\infty} \tag{7.27}$$

where w_0, w_∞, and $w_{(t)}$ are the weight of the sample before degradation, at a given time (t), and after complete degradation, respectively. The rate constant has an Arrhenius behavior with the absolute temperature:

$$k=Ae^{\left(\frac{-E_{act}}{RT}\right)} \tag{7.28}$$

where A is the preexponential factor, E_{act} is the activation energy of the degradation process, R is the gas constant, and T is the absolute temperature.

Substituting Eq. (7.28) in Eq. (7.26), one obtains:

$$-\frac{\partial(1-\alpha)}{\partial t} = Ae^{\left(\frac{-E_{act}}{RT}\right)} f(\alpha) \tag{7.29}$$

If the temperature of the sample is changed by a constant value of β, being $\beta = \partial T / \partial t$, the variation of the degree of decomposition can be analyzed as a function of temperature. Therefore the decomposition rate is given by:

$$-\frac{\partial(1-\alpha)}{\partial t} = \frac{A}{\beta} e^{\left(\frac{-E_{act}}{RT}\right)} f(\alpha) \tag{7.30}$$

Based in these mathematical expressions, several empirical models were developed to characterize and study the degradation kinetics for polymeric materials, the most used being the Ozawa–Flynn–Wall and Kissinger methods:

(a) *Ozawa–Flynn–Wall (OFW) model*: this isoconversional method is integral. Rearranging and integrating Eq. (7.30), the following can be obtained:

$$g(\alpha) = \int_{\alpha_o}^{\alpha_p} \frac{\partial \alpha}{f(\alpha)} = \frac{A}{\beta} \int_{\alpha_o}^{\alpha_p} e^{\left(\frac{-E_{act}}{RT}\right)} \partial T \tag{7.31}$$

where α_p is the maximum conversion. Defining $x = \frac{E_{act}}{RT}$ (Ou et al., 2010) and integrating the right-hand side of the Eq. (7.31):

$$\frac{A}{\beta} \int_{\alpha_0}^{\alpha_p} e^{\left(\frac{-E_{act}}{RT}\right)} \partial T = \frac{AE_{act}}{\beta R} p(x) \tag{7.32}$$

After taking the logarithms, we get:

$$\log(\beta) = \log \frac{AE_{act}}{g(\alpha)R} + \log(p(x)) \tag{7.33}$$

Doyle demonstrated that the log($p(x)$) for polymer systems, obeys to the following expression (Ou et al., 2010; de Britto and Campana-Filho, 2007; Doyle, 1962):

$$\log(p(x)) = -2.315 - 0.4567x \tag{7.34}$$

Replacing in Eq. (7.33), the general expression for the OFW can be obtained:

$$\log(\beta) = \log \frac{AE_{act}}{g(\alpha)R} - 2.315 - \frac{0.4567E_{act}}{RT} \tag{7.35}$$

The values of the activation energy over a wide range of decomposition can be obtained by plotting log(β) vs $1/T$, at a constant value of the conversion rate. The slope of each line is $-\frac{0.4567E_{act}}{RT}$.

(b) *Kissinger model*: this method relies on experiments performed at different heating rates, and is expressed by:

$$\ln\left(\frac{\beta}{T_p^2}\right) = \left\{\ln \frac{AR}{E_{act}} + \ln\left[n(1-\alpha_p)^{n-1}\right]\right\} - \frac{E_{act}}{RT_p} \tag{7.36}$$

where T_p is the temperature of the maximum reaction rate, and generally is obtained by the minimum of the derivative, according to Fig. 7.18. The plot of $\ln\left(\frac{\beta}{T_p^2}\right)$ vs $\frac{1}{T_p}$ will yield the straight line whose slope is $\frac{E_{act}}{R}$.

Both methods here described allow for the calculation of the thermal degradation activation energy of a polymer system without the knowledge of the thermal degradation reaction order.

7.6 Scanning electron microscopy

Scanning electron microscopy (SEM) is a very powerful and versatile technique used in materials science with a major impact on the applications of microscopy due to the variety of surfaces that can be observed using a relatively simple approach.

The SEM equipment uses a beam of high-energy electrons generated by an electron gun that is processed using magnetic lenses that are focused on the surface of the specimen and rastered across the sample surface (Facility, 2016). In this technique, the image is a result of the beam probe illuminating the sample one point at a time in a rectangular scanning pattern, with the strength of the signal generated from each point being a reflection of differences (eg, topographical or compositional) in the sample. There is a one-to-one relationship between the number of points on the specimen and points on a collected image screen. In general, an increase in the magnification leads to a decrease in the size of the scanned area. Fig. 7.19 presents a scheme of the general SEM layout and its function.

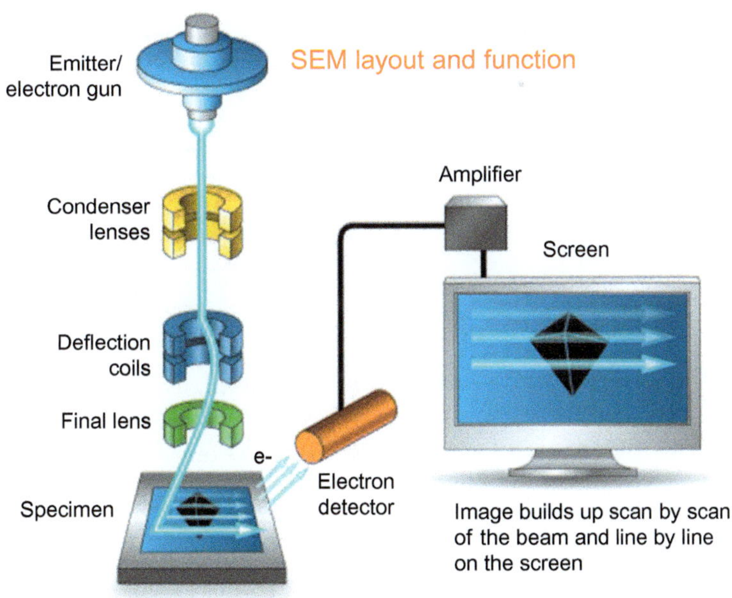

Fig. 7.19 Scanning electron microscope layout and function (Facility, 2016).

The interaction between the electrons and the sample produces various signals, including secondary electrons, backscattered electrons, characteristic X-rays, light (cathodoluminescence), specimen current, and transmitted electrons (Fig. 7.20). They provide information about sample morphology, topography, chemical composition, among other material information (Facility, 2016).

Backscattered electrons are promoted by elastic interaction with sample atoms, and are sent back almost in the same direction as the one they came from, and with a very little energy loss. Chemical elements with higher atomic number produce more backscattered electrons than the ones that have a low atomic number, which enables the differentiation of the chemical elements or phases present in a sample, according to their atomic number. Generally atoms with a higher atomic number appear as white and those with lower atomic number look black (Kuo, 2007).

Secondary electrons result from the inelastic interaction between the high-energy electrons produced by the beam with the valence electrons of atoms in the sample, which causes the ejection of the electrons from the atoms. Secondary electrons have lower energy, less than 50 eV, and are independent of the atomic number of the scattering electrons (unlike the situation for backscattered electrons). Images obtained with the detection of secondary electrons mostly represent the sample topography (Amelinckx et al., 2008; Smith, 1990).

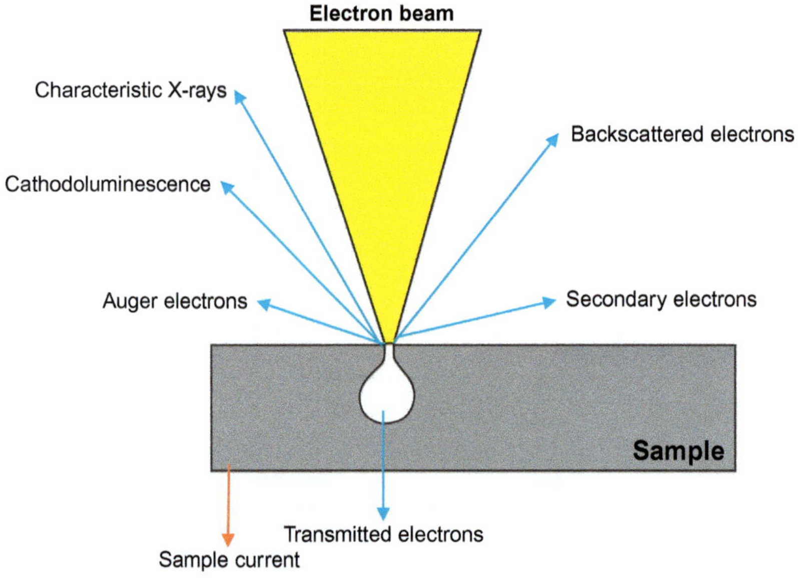

Fig. 7.20 Signals coming from the sample as a result of the interaction of an electron beam with a bulk sample.

The microscope electron beam is able to remove electrons from the various electronic layers of the atoms present in the observed sample. When an electron is ejected, it is replaced by another from an upper layer, and a photon with energy equal to the energy difference between the two layers is emitted, and the process will continue until the last layers of electrons have been replaced, and all characteristic rays of the atom will be emitted. The X-ray detector present in the SEM equipment is able to determine the quantity of photons energy that hits the detector, and a histogram can be drawn with the photons energy versus the number of photons received, and thanks to the database, the spectrum interpretation is facilitated, thereby making it possible to obtain the list of elements present in the sample (Kuo, 2007; Amelinckx et al., 2008).

7.6.1 Sample preparation for SEM analysis

The SEM experiment will only work if the sample is prepared in a proper manner. Metals do not require any particular preparation, as they already conduct electricity when they are bombarded with electrons, and current flows throughout the sample. However, ceramic and polymeric materials, especially biological samples, need an extra thin layer of a conductive material on the surface of the sample, in order to avoid electron charge that can lead to a local increase of temperature, interacting with the sample, and consequently to the loss of the original specimen morphology (Kuo, 2007).

The thin layer of conductive material, usually gold, gold-palladium alloy, or even amorphous carbon, is generally deposited by sputter coaters. Biological samples can absorb moisture from the environment and they need to be carefully stored in order to avoid adsorbed water molecules in the material. If present, these molecules will vaporize in a vacuum chamber, creating obstacles for the electron beams and obscuring the clarity of the image (Amelinckx et al., 2008; Hunter et al., 1993).

New SEM equipment no longer requires a full vacuum to operate; nevertheless, the image quality produced has a weaker resolution, but they still open up the possibility to observe the sample without an extra conductive layer external to the material, and consequently obtain a morphology close to the real sample (Kuo, 2007; Facility, 2016).

7.6.2 The applications of SEM

Since their invention in 1935, this powerful technique has opened up the possibility of observing an entire new world in scientific fields such as physics, engineering and biology, allowing scientists to access new, and useful information about materials' microscopic properties and correlate these to materials' macroscopic features.

The main application of SEM equipment is to observe sample morphology, porosity, crystal, and grain size orientation and some bonding differences, through contrast and using backscattered electrons (Fig. 7.20). Nevertheless, combined with Energy-Dispersive X-Ray Spectroscopy (EDS) it is a useful technique for the production of material elemental maps, accurately representing the distribution of chemical elements present within the samples. With this equipment it is possible to remove material from samples, cut pieces out or remove progressive slices from samples, using a focused ion beam.

With a cryo-scanning electron microscope, it is possible to freeze-dry a sample inside the equipment, coat it with a thin layer of conductive material, and observe the morphology when it is immersed in a liquid.

Bioinspired materials are often processed in the shape of micro and nanofibers by a number of techniques such as drawing, template synthesis, phase separation, selfassembly, and electrospinning. This fibrous shape has the ability to tailor fiber mats that resemble the native ECM, in terms of its nanostructure, biochemical cues, and morphology. This feature is of the outmost importance since the alignment of the substrate nanofibers seems to be directly related with oriented cell growth (Sundararaghavan et al., 2013).

Fiber alignment within the mats can be quantified through the analysis of sample morphology acquired by SEM. A method based in the analysis of the images by Fast Fourier Transform (FFT), which converts the information present in the original SEM image from the "real" space into mathematically defined "frequency" space was developed. The resulting FFT output image contains grayscale pixels that are distributed in a pattern that reflects the degree of fiber alignment present in the selected area (Alexander et al., 2006; Ayres et al., 2006). This procedure was developed for open source software Image J (Schneider et al., 2012) and allows the quantifying of the overall alignment of fibers, and the angular distribution (Valente et al., 2016), and the utter correlation with cell morphology when placed in the presence of such material morphologies.

Technological development today gives us fast, reliable and easy-to-operate equipment to obtain accurate material visual information, which is one of the most useful characterization techniques available.

An SEM virtual laboratory were one can simulate the equipment operation, acquiring expertise, and many other useful information is available on Australian Microscopy and Microanalysis Research facility (http://www.ammrf.org.au/myscope/sem/introduction) (Facility, 2016).

7.7 Cytotoxicity testing

A biomaterial is defined as a material that exists in contact with tissues of the human body without causing an unacceptable degree of harm to that body (Williams, 2008). In the development of biomaterials there are several parameters that need to be addressed before considering its potential application. Factors like biocompatibility, cell attachment and proliferation, and biodegradation are of great importance as they relate to the biological performance of a given material.

According to Williams (2008), biocompatibility is defined as "the ability of a biomaterial to perform its desired function with respect to a medical therapy, without eliciting any undesirable local or systemic effects in the recipient or beneficiary of that therapy, but generating the most appropriate beneficial cellular or tissue response in that specific situation, and optimizing the clinically relevant performance of that therapy." A broader definition is proposed by Vert et al. (2012) following the IUPAC (International Union of Pure and Applied Chemistry) recommendations in which, the biocompatibility of a given polymer is defined as the "ability to be in contact with a living system without producing an adverse effect." Nevertheless, one can easily figure out that evaluation of biocompatibility is a complex task generally involving animal experiments and long-term evaluation after implantation.

Among the biocompatibility tests, cytotoxicity is preferred and is routinely evaluated using in vitro methodologies as a preliminary screening for biocompatibility assessment. Despite presenting several disadvantages such as neglecting the diversity of medical devices, the variability of the environment of the body and the complexity of the interaction between the body and the biomaterial (Li et al., 2015), cytotoxicity testing is one of the most important methods for biological evaluation.

Cytotoxicity testing is simple, fast, and highly sensitive, representing an alternative to the use of animals while providing valuable initial indications to determine whether a biomaterial exhibits either cytotoxicity or cytocompatibility with living cells. Evaluation of cytotoxicity usually involves chemical substances that can be delivered to a cell culture in a defined dose. Consequently, the assessment of a biomaterial's cytotoxicity represents a challenge because biomaterials (and the resulting biomedical devices) are made of solid materials, creating extra difficulties or making it impossible to measure the specific dose of a substance of interest.

Biomaterials/devices are generally composed of relatively inert, high-molecular-weight materials and it is their leachable components (eg, contaminants, additives, fillers, and residual compounds derived from manufacturing) that usually present cytotoxicity. As a result, the rationale behind the in vitro testing of biomaterials is that cytotoxicity can be assessed by evaluating the impact of constituents that can be released from the biomaterial/device in in vivo conditions.

The Standard ISO 10993 describes a series of procedures for evaluating the biocompatibility of medical devices for testing solid samples. There are three main categories of tests stated in ISO 10993-5 (International Organization for Standardization, 2009), which relates to general tests for in vitro cytotoxicity: (i) test on extracts, (ii) test by direct contact, and (iii) test by indirect contact. These methods are designed to determine the biological response of mammalian cells following incubation of cultured cells in contact with extracts of the test sample or with a device/biomaterial. The following sections summarize essential ISO procedures for cytotoxicity testing (International Organization for Standardization, 2004, 2009).

7.7.1 Reference materials

Experimental controls namely, negative controls, blanks, and positive controls should be used in all biological evaluations to accurately validate a certain procedure and compare the results between materials. Some examples of materials that may be used as positive and negative controls for cytotoxicity assays are listed in Table 7.5.

7.7.2 Preparation of extracts

For the preparation of liquid extracts of a material, the extracting conditions should simulate the conditions of the intended clinical use. For this purpose, the extracting solutions (eg, culture medium with or without serum, water, physiological saline, freshly refined vegetable oil, ethanol/water, ethanol/saline, diluted polyethylene glycol 400, and dimethyl sulfoxide) should be chosen by taking into account the final application, should be compatible with the cell culture and not affect the extraction

Table 7.5 Materials that have been used as negative and positive controls for cytotoxicity assays according to ISO 10993-12 (International Organization for Standardization, 2004)

Material	Negative control	Positive control
High-density polyethylene	●	
Low-density polyethylene	●	
Silica-free polydimethylsiloxane	●	
Polyvinylchloride	●	
Polyetherurethane	●	
Polypropylene	●	
Aluminum oxide ceramic rods	●	
Stainless steel	●	
Commercially pure titanium alloys	●	
Polyvinylchloride with organotin additives		●
Polyurethane films containing zinc diethyldithiocarbamate		●
Polyurethane films containing zinc dibutyldithiocarbamate		●
Certain latex formulations		●
Solutions of zinc salts		●
Copper		●

temperature. Furthermore, the concentration of the extraction vehicle should be compatible with the culture system and not induce toxicity of the testing cells.

Having chosen the most adequate extracting vehicle, the extraction is often prepared at the highest temperature compatible with the physical characteristics of the extracting vehicle and sample (ie, without causing physical changes in the material) in order to maximize the amount of extractable substances as well as to simulate the highest temperature to which the biomaterial may be exposed. Moreover, the applied temperature should not exceed the glass transition temperature of the biomaterial or cause hydrolysis, as these can affect the amount and type of extractables (International Organization for Standardization, 2004).

Extraction conditions based on common practices are presented in Table 7.6. Nevertheless, other conditions that better simulate the end application and may occur during clinical use, such as prolonged or shortened extraction times, may be used. As for extracting conditions, and although most of extractions are performed under static conditions, these should be performed in conditions close to the end use that is, agitation should be considered when appropriate. Importantly, according to the ISO 10993-12 recommendations (International Organization for Standardization, 2004), the samples prepared for cytotoxicity testing should be properly sterilized to avoid contamination of the cell culture.

Table 7.6 Extraction conditions based on common practices (International Organization for Standardization, 2009)

Extraction time (h)	Extraction temperature (°C)
24 ± 2	37 ± 1
72 ± 2	50 ± 2
24 ± 2	70 ± 2
1 ± 0.2	121 ± 2

As noted earlier, extraction is a complex process influenced by parameters such as time, temperature, and extraction medium.

Another factor that needs to be considered during the extraction process is the surface-area-to-volume ratio (International Organization for Standardization, 2004). Before extraction and according to ISO 10993-12 recommendations, the materials should be cut into small pieces such as 10 mm × 50 mm or 5 mm × 25 mm to enhance submersion in the extracting medium. Table 7.7 presents the standard surface area and the corresponding volume of extracting solution needed, however if it is impossible to determine the surface area, a mass/volume of extracting solution should be used. Nevertheless, other surface-area-to-volume extraction ratios can be used if they simulate the clinical end use conditions.

Table 7.7 Standard surface areas and extraction solution volumes (International Organization for Standardization, 2004)

Thickness (mm)	Extraction ratio (surface area or mass/volume) ± 10%	Forms of material
<0.5	6 cm^2/mL	Film, sheet, and tubing wall
0.5–1.0	3 cm^2/mL	Tubing wall, slab, and molded items
>1.0	1.25 cm^2/mL	Larger molded items
Irregularly shaped solid devices	0.2 g/mL	Powder, pellets, foam, nonabsorbent, and molded items
Irregularly shaped porous devices (low-density materials)	0.1 g/mL	Membranes

7.7.3 *Preparation of material for direct contact assay*

For the direct contact tests, materials with at least one flat surface need to be used, although the materials can have various shapes, sizes, or physical states (eg, liquid, solid, and gel). An important factor to consider is that the sterility of the sample must be maintained throughout the test procedure as, for example, bacterial contamination can lead to false evaluation of cytotoxicity. In this regard, the effect of sterilization on the biomaterial/device should also be considered as it can alter the properties of the material. In the case of liquid samples, these can be tested either by direct deposition of the sample or by deposition in biologically inert absorbent matrices such as filter disks.

7.7.4 Assessment of cytotoxicity according to ISO standards

Cell cytotoxicity may be assessed either qualitatively or quantitatively by observing changes in cell morphology, as well as by assessing changes in viable cell populations. However, one should take into account that ISO 10993-5 recommends the use of quantitative assays over qualitative methods. In the qualitative evaluation, cell cytotoxicity can be determined microscopically with the optional use of cytochemical or vital stains by assessing changes in general morphology, vacuolization, cell detachment, cell lysis, and membrane integrity (Tables 7.8 and 7.9). Qualitative assessment of cytotoxicity may be measured or estimated using descriptive terms (eg, none, slight, mild, etc.) or semiquantitative numeric terms (eg, 0, 1, 2, etc.). ISO 10993-5 recommends that a grade higher than 2, based on Tables 7.8 and 7.9, is considered to come out from a cytotoxic effect.

Vital stains are useful to discriminate between live and dead or injured cells on the basis of membrane permeability whereas cytochemical stains are useful to identify specific cellular components (Rana, 2008). Examples of vital stains include neutral red, which is taken by the lysosomes of healthy viable cells, and trypan blue, which is taken up by dead cells as the dye only crosses the membrane of dead cells. The cytochemical staining depends on the chemical composition or the enzymatic activity of the stain component and, therefore, cytochemical stains are used to assess the presence/absence of specific organic compounds and their localization (Rana, 2008).

Table 7.8 Morphological qualitative graded scale for test on extracts assay (International Organization for Standardization, 2009)

Grade	Reactivity	Conditions of all cultures
0	None	Discrete intracytoplasmatic granules, no cell lysis, and no reduction of cell growth
1	Slight	Not more than 20 of the cells are round, loosely attached, and without intracytoplasmatic granules, or show changes in morphology; occasional lysed cells are present; only slight growth inhibition observable
2	Mild	Not more than 50% of the cells are round, devoid of intracytoplasmatic granules, no extensive cell lysis; not more than 50% growth inhibition observable
3	Moderate	Not more than 70% of the cell layers contain rounded cells or are lysed; cell layers not completely destroyed, but more than 50% growth inhibition observable
4	Severe	Nearly complete or complete destruction of the cell layers

The quantitative evaluation of cytotoxicity measures cell death, inhibition of cell growth, and cell proliferation by assessing the number of cells, amount of protein, release of enzymes, release of vital dye, reduction of vital dye, etc. One should take into account that according to the ISO 10993-5 recommendation, a reduction of cell viability of more than 30% may be attributed to a cytotoxic effect.

Table 7.9 Graded scale for direct and indirect contact tests (International Organization for Standardization, 2009)

Grade	Reactivity	Description of reactivity zone
0	None	No detectable zone around or under specimen
1	Slight	Some malformed or degenerated cells under specimen
2	Mild	Zone limited to area under specimen
3	Moderate	Zone extending specimen size up to 1.0 cm
4	Severe	Zone extending farther than 1.0 cm beyond specimen

7.7.4.1 Test on extracts

This test determines if a biomaterial extract (a solution containing the extractable compounds of a biomaterial) has potential to cause cell morphology changes and/or lysis and is generally suitable for detecting the toxicity of soluble substances of medical devices. This assay allows for both quantitative and qualitative assessment of cytotoxicity and is usually consistent with animal toxicity tests. In the standard assay (Fig. 7.21), a cell suspension is evenly distributed over the surface of a tissue culture disk and incubated at 37 ± 1°C with or without carbon dioxide depending of the culture conditions, and allowed to attach until reaching a near-confluent monolayer of cells. The culture medium is removed and replaced with fresh medium containing the extract sample, and a toxicity assay is performed usually for a period of 24–72 h. The toxic substances present in the extract will be evenly distributed within the culture medium, resulting in a consistent pattern throughout the plated cells. Cytotoxicity is then evaluated, for example, by measuring live and dead cells as previously described. Qualitative assessment of cytotoxicity based on morphological changes is recorded in a graded scale as the example provided in Table 7.8.

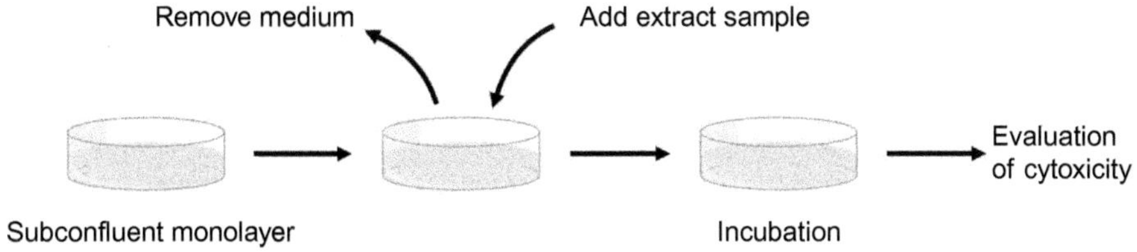

Fig. 7.21 Schematic representation of test on extracts assay.

7.7.4.2 Test by direct contact

Similarly, to the tests on extracts, the direct contact assays allows for both qualitative and quantitative assessment of cytotoxicity. This test determines if a material itself has potential to be cytotoxic and is the most sensitive, allowing the measurement of toxicity in biomaterials even at low levels. In this test, the cultured mammalian cells are in direct contact with the biomaterial (Fig. 7.22). This test is dependent on the diffusion of substances from the testing biomaterial into the culture medium and thus, extreme care should be put in sample handling to avoid disturbing the cell layer as this may induce a physical trauma to the cells and lead to a misinterpretation of cell death as cytotoxicity response. In the same way as in the extracts assay, a cell suspension is evenly distributed over the surface of a tissue culture disk and incubated at 37 ± 1°C with or without carbon dioxide depending of the culture conditions, and allowed to attach until reaching a near-confluent monolayer of cells. The culture medium is removed and replaced with fresh medium and the testing material sample is carefully placed in the center of the cell layer ensuring that at least one-tenth of the cell culture is covered by the sample. The cell cultures are then incubated for 24–48 h under the same conditions as the initial cell propagation, and the cell viability is assessed after discarding the supernatant culture medium, for example, through the use of vital stains. Qualitative assessment of cytotoxicity may be measured or estimated using descriptive terms (eg, none, slight, mild, etc.) or semiquantitative numeric terms (eg, 0, 1, 2, etc.) as described in Table 7.9.

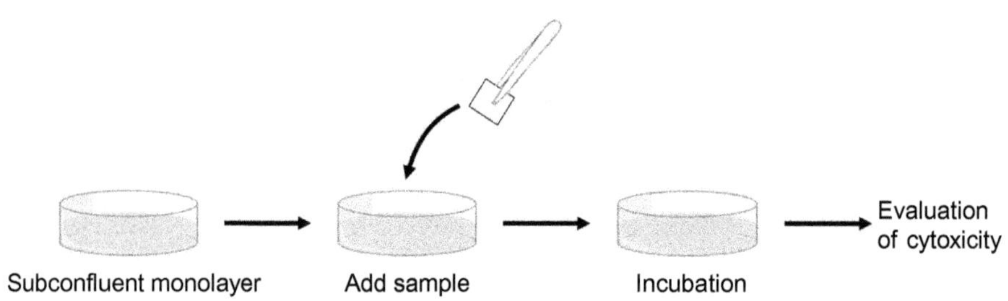

Fig. 7.22 Schematic representation of direct contact assay.

7.7.4.3 Test by indirect contact

This test determines if a material itself has potential to release agents that may be cytotoxic and is suitable for biomaterials with large toxicity. The indirect contact test includes the agar overlay assay and filter diffusion, giving a qualitative assessment of cytotoxicity (Table 7.9).

Agar diffusion assay

In contrast to placing the testing material directly on a monolayer of cells as in the direct contact test, the agar diffusion assays use a monolayer of cells with a semisolid agar or agarose overlay (3–4 mm) on which the material sample is placed (Fig. 7.23). Agarose is generally preferred since the gelling point is between 30°C and 34°C, whereas, the gelling point of agar is generally at 40–45°C, which contributes to a thermal shock during the overlay process. Like the direct contact test, this assay is based on the diffusion of substances into the culture medium. In the standard assay and as in the other cytotoxicity tests, a cell suspension is evenly distributed over the surface of a tissue culture disk and incubated at 37 ± 1 °C with or without carbon dioxide depending of the culture conditions, and allowed to attach until reaching a near-confluent monolayer of cells. The culture medium is removed and an appropriate volume of fresh medium containing serum with melted agar at a concentration of 0.5–2% is added. The agar/medium mixture should be in a liquid state and at a temperature compatible with cells to avoid cell damage that may be inadvertently misinterpreted as a cytotoxicity response.

After solidification of the agar layer the testing material sample is placed in the center ensuring that at least one-tenth of the cell layer surface is covered by the sample. The cell cultures are then incubated for 24–72 h under the same conditions as the initial cell propagation after which the testing material is carefully removed from the agar layer. If desired, vital dyes may be incorporated into the agar or agarose for analysis before and after incubation with the testing biomaterial. However, if the vital dye is added before incubation, care should be employed to protect the culture from light as the photoactivation of the stain can lead to cell damage.

Cytotoxicity is qualitatively evaluated using a semiquantitative graded scale (Table 7.9). Importantly, as the agar diffusion test is a barrier model, since agents must diffuse through the agar before coming into contact with the pleated cells, this assay is not appropriate for leachables (definition below) that cannot diffuse through the agar layer, or that may react with agar.

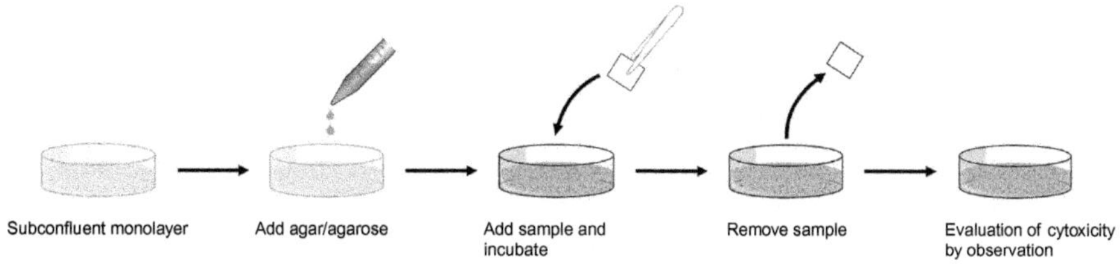

Fig. 7.23 Schematic representation of the agar diffusion assay.

Filter diffusion assay

The filter diffusion assay is another barrier model assay that gives a qualitative assessment of cytotoxicity. In the standard test, a surfactant-free filter with 0.45 μm of pore size is placed in a culture dish. A cell suspension is evenly distributed over the surface of the filter and incubated at 37 ± 1°C, with or without carbon dioxide depending of the culture conditions, and allowed to grow to near confluency at the end of the logarithmic phase of the growth curve. The medium is removed and the filters transferred with cell side down onto a layer of solidified agar as described for the agar diffusion assay (medium with agar at a concentration of 0.5–2%). The sample of the biomaterial to be tested is placed in the top of the filter, in the acellular side, with nonreactive rings delimitating the area in order to retain any liquids.

Following incubation under the same conditions of the initial cell propagation for $2\,h \pm 10\,min$, the material samples are carefully removed from the filter and the filter separated from the agar surface. Cells are stained with adequate dyes and qualitatively evaluated using a semiquantitative graded scale (Table 7.9).

Further considerations

According to ISO 10993 and as described earlier, cytotoxicity assessment is performed using a solution containing the compounds (extractables) that are released from the biomaterial under aggressive conditions, such as elevated temperature, extended contact time or aggressive solvent system. Under normal conditions of exposure, the compounds that migrate from the surface of a material to a drug product formulation as a result of direct contact with the formulation are defined as leachables. For example, considering a closed container system or a packaging material with a drug content, the extractables are the chemical species that migrate from the container into the contents when exposed to aggressive conditions and the leachables are the chemical species that make their way into the product under normal application conditions. Although leachables may be classified as a subset of the extractables, they can interact with the drug product originating new components. Therefore in the evaluation of cytotoxicity of biomedical devices containing active products/drug formulations, it is advised to conduct an examination of both the extractable and leachable substances.

References

Alexander, J.K., Fuss, B., Colello, R.J., 2006. Electric field-induced astrocyte alignment directs neurite outgrowth. Neuron Glia Biol. 2, 93–103.

Amelinckx, S., Van Dyck, D., Van Landuyt, J., Van Tendeloo, G., 2008. Electron Microscopy: Principles and Fundamentals. VCH Verlagsgesellschaft mbH, Weinheim.

American Society for Testing and Materials, 1965. Internal Friction, Damping, and Cyclic Plasticity. American Society for Testing and Materials, Philadelphia, PA.

Anand, L., Parks, D.M., 2004. Defect Free Fatigue: Supplementary Notes of Mechanics and Materials II. MIT-Open Courseware. Massachusetts Institute of Technology, Cambridge, MA.

Araujo, J., Padrão, J., Silva, J.P., Dourado, F., Correia, D.M., Botelho, G., Gomez Ribelles, J.L., Lanceros-Méndez, S., Sencadas, V., 2014. Processing and characterization of α-elastin electrospun membranes. Appl. Phys. A 115, 1291–1298.

Ashby, M.F., Jones, D.R.H., 2012. Fatigue failure. In: Ashby, M.F., Jones, D.R.H. (Eds.), Engineering Materials 1, fourth ed. Butterworth-Heinemann, Boston, MA (Chapter 17).

Ayres, C., Bowlin, G.L., Henderson, S.C., Taylor, L., Shultz, J., Alexander, J., Telemeco, T.A., Simpson, D.G., 2006. Modulation of anisotropy in electrospun tissue-engineering scaffolds: analysis of fiber alignment by the fast Fourier transform. Biomaterials 27, 5524–5534.

Bigi, A., Cojazzi, G., Panzavolta, S., Rubini, K., Roveri, N., 2001. Mechanical and thermal properties of gelatin films at different degrees of glutaraldehyde crosslinking. Biomaterials 22, 763–768.

Bower, D.I., 2002. An Introduction to Polymer Physics. Cambridge University Press, Cambridge.

Bower, D.I., Maddams, W.F., 1989. The Vibrational Spectroscopy of Polymers. Cambridge University Press, Cambridge.
Branciforti, M.C., Sencadas, V., Lanceros-Mendez, S., Gregorio Jr., R., 2007. New technique of processing highly oriented poly(vinylidene fluoride) films exclusively in the β phase. J. Polym. Sci. B Polym. Phys. 45, 2793–2801.
Campbell, D., Pethrick, R.A., White, J.R., 2000. Polymer Characterization: Physical Techniques, second ed. Stanley Thornes (Publishers) Ltd, Cheltenham.
de Britto, D., Campana-Filho, S.P., 2007. Kinetics of the thermal degradation of chitosan. Thermochim. Acta 465, 73–82.
Doyle, C.D., 1962. Estimating isothermal life from thermogravimetric data. J. Appl. Polym. Sci. 6, 639–642.
Erber, T., Guralnick, S.A., Michels, S.C., 1993. Hysteresis and fatigue. Ann. Phys. 224, 157–192.
Facility, A. M. A. M. R., 2016. MyScope: training for advanced research.
Frunz, G., Diaconescu, E.N., 2006. Hysteresis and mechanical fatigue. The Annals of the University "Dunarea de JOS" of Galati Fascicle VIII. Tribology 1, 61–66.
Gedde, U., 2001. Polymer Physics. Springer, Dordrecht.
Goodfellow, 2015. PHB physical properties. Available from: http://www.goodfellow.com/E/Polyhydroxybutyrate-Biopolymer.html (accessed 12/11/2015).
Hunter, E.E., Maloney, P., Bendayan, M., 1993. Practical Electron Microscopy: A Beginner's Illustrated Guide. Cambridge University Press, Cambridge.
Ince, A., Glinka, G., 2011. A modification of Morrow and Smith–Watson–Topper mean stress correction models. Fatigue Fract. Eng. Mater. Struct. 34, 854–867.
International Organization for Standardization, 2004. ISO 10993-12. Biological Evaluation of Medical Devices—Part 12: Sample Preparation and Reference Materials. British Standards Institution, London.
International Organization for Standardization, 2009. ISO 10993-5. Biological Evaluation of Medical Devices—Part 5: Tests for in Vitro Cytotoxicity. International Organization for Standardization, Geneva.
Kämpf, G., 1986. Characterization of Plastics by Physical Methods: Experimental Techniques and Practical Application. Hanser Publishers, Munich.
Kanchanomai, C., Mutoh, Y., 2004. Low-cycle fatigue prediction model for pb-free solder 96.5Sn-3.5Ag. J. Electron. Mater. 33, 329–333.
Kuo, J., 2007. Electron Microscopy: Methods and Protocols. Humana Press, Totowa, NJ.
Li, W., Zhou, J., Xu, Y., 2015. Study of the cytotoxicity testing of medical devices. Biomed. Rep. 3, 617–620.
Lobo, H., Bonilla, J.V., 2003. Handbook of Plastics Analysis. Taylor & Francis, New York.
Machado, R., da Costa, A., Sencadas, V., Garcia-Arévalo, C., Costa, C.M., Padrão, J., Gomes, A., Lanceros-Méndez, S., Rodríguez-Cabello, J.C., Casal, M., 2013. Electrospun silk-elastin-like fibre mats for tissue engineering applications. Biomed. Mater. 8, 065009.
Machado, R., da Costa, A., Sencadas, V., Pereira, A.M., Collins, T., Rodríguez-Cabello, J.C., Lanceros-Méndez, S., Casal, M., 2015. Exploring the properties of genetically engineered silk-elastin-like protein films. Macromol. Biosci. 15, 1698–1709.
NETZSCH, 2015. Functional principle of a heat-flux DSC. Available from: https://www.netzsch-thermal-analysis.com/en/landing-pages/principle-of-a-heat-flux-dsc/ (accessed 9/11/2015).
Ou, C.-Y., Zhang, C.-H., Li, S.-D., Yang, L., Dong, J.-J., Mo, X.-L., Zeng, M.-T., 2010. Thermal degradation kinetics of chitosan–cobalt complex as studied by thermogravimetric analysis. Carbohydr. Polym. 82, 1284–1289.
Panadero, J.A., Vikingsson, L., Gomez Ribelles, J.L., Sencadas, V., Lanceros-Mendez, S., 2013. Fatigue prediction in fibrin poly-ε-caprolactone macroporous scaffolds. J. Mech. Behav. Biomed. Mater. 28, 55–61.

Panadero, J.A., Sencadas, V., Silva, S.C.M., Ribeiro, C., Correia, V., Gama, F.M., Gomez Ribelles, J.L., Lanceros-Mendez, S., 2015a. Mechanical fatigue performance of PCL-chondroprogenitor constructs after cell culture under bioreactor mechanical stimulus. J. Biomed. Mater. Res. B Appl. Biomater. 104, 330–338.
Panadero, J.A., Vikingsson, L., Gomez Ribelles, J.L., Lanceros-Mendez, S., Sencadas, V., 2015b. In vitro mechanical fatigue behavior of poly-ε-caprolactone macroporous scaffolds for cartilage tissue engineering: influence of pore filling by a poly(vinyl alcohol) gel. J. Biomed. Mater. Res. B Appl. Biomater. 103, 1037–1043.
Rana, S.V.S., 2008. Biotechniques Theory & Practice. Rastogi, New Delhi, India.
Schneider, C.A., Rasband, W.S., Eliceiri, K.W., 2012. NIH Image to ImageJ: 25 years of image analysis. Nat. Methods 9, 671–675.
Sencadas, V., Gregorio, R., Lanceros-Méndez, S., 2009. α to β phase transformation and microestructural changes of PVDF films induced by uniaxial stretch. J. Macromol. Sci. Part B Phys. 48, 514–525.
Smith, W.F., 1990. Principles of Materials Science and Engineering. McGraw-Hill, New York.
Sperling, L.H., 2006. Introduction to Physical Polymer Science. John Wiley & Sons, Hoboken, NJ.
Stuart, B.H., 2004. Introduction. Infrared Spectroscopy: Fundamentals and Applications. John Wiley and Sons, Chichester.
Sundararaghavan, H.G., Saunders, R.L., Hammer, D.A., Burdick, J.A., 2013. Fiber alignment directs cell motility over chemotactic gradients. Biotechnol. Bioeng. 110, 1249–1254.
Turi, E., 2012. Thermal Characterization of Polymeric Materials. Elsevier Science, New York.
Valente, T.A.M., Silva, D.M., Gomes, P.S., Fernandes, M.H., Santos, J.D., Sencadas, V., 2016. Effect of sterilization methods on electrospun poly(lactic acid) (PLA) fibre alignment for biomedical applications. ACS Appl. Mater. Interfaces 8, 3241–3249.
Vert, M., Doi, Y., Hellwich, K.-H., Hess, M., Hodge, P., Kubisa, P., Rinaudo, M., Schué, F., 2012. Terminology for biorelated polymers and applications (IUPAC Recommendations 2012). Pure Appl. Chem. 84, 377–410.
Williams, D.F., 2008. On the mechanisms of biocompatibility. Biomaterials 29, 2941–2953.
Zhang, J.-F., Sun, X., 2004. Mechanical properties of poly(lactic acid)/starch composites compatibilized by maleic anhydride. Biomacromolecules 5, 1446–1451.

Sources of further information

This chapter focuses on the main general techniques that are useful to characterize and understand the mechanical, chemical, and thermal properties of materials. Nevertheless, other characterization techniques can be used to assess a particular feature of the material under study, in order to correlate the properties of the material to its structure, and processing technique. The following books are a good source for general reading:

Hollinger, J.O. (Ed.), 2011. An Introduction to Biomaterials. CRC Press, Boca Raton, FL.
Ratner, B.D., Hoffman, A.S., Schoen, F.J., Lemons, J.E., 2004. Biomaterials Science: An Introduction to Materials in Medicine. Elsevier Academic Press, San Diego, CA.
Sperling, L.H., 2006. Introduction to Physical Polymer Science. Wiley and Sons, New Jersey.
von Recum, A.F. (Ed.), 1998. Handbook of Biomaterials Evaluation: Scientific, Technical and Clinical Testing of Implant Materials. In: Taylor & Francis, Philadelphia.

Imaging strategies for bioinspired materials

8

L. Moreira, N.M. Guimarães, N.F. Azevedo
University of Porto, Porto, Portugal

8.1 Introduction

Over the past few years, the application of bioinspired materials in clinical diagnosis and therapy has attracted a great deal of attention. Bioinspired materials can be applied for biological recognition and as tunable reporter molecules, or to generate new delivery systems. They can also be used in the development of theranostic agents that simultaneously deliver an imaging element and a therapeutic element within the same intake (Krasia-Christoforou and Georgiou, 2013).

Several imaging systems are used to diagnose and monitor disease progression, both in human patients and in animal models (Luo et al., 2011). The predominant modalities are magnetic resonance imaging (MRI), biophotonic imaging (BPI), positron or single photon emission computed tomography (PET/SPECT), X-ray computerized tomography (CT), and microtomography (micro-CT) (Luo et al., 2011; Qin et al., 2010). More recently, confocal laser endomicroscopy (CLE) has been introduced. These imaging techniques have different principles and properties, and operate with different radiations of the electromagnetic spectrum (Fig. 8.1).

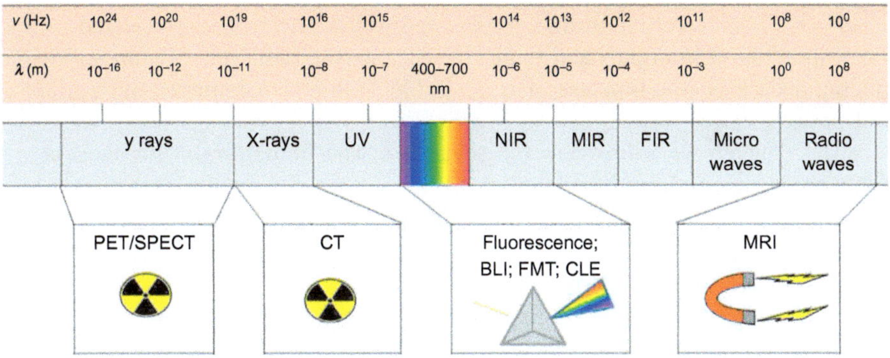

Fig. 8.1 Relation between different in vivo imaging modalities and the electromagnetic spectrum. PET and SPECT are based on the detection of high-energy photons (gamma rays), generated directly or indirectly by radionuclide decay. CT images detect the attenuation of X-rays when absorbed or scattered by biological tissues. BPI encompasses a large variety of modalities that detect wavelengths that range from the visible to near infrared. In MRI radio wave pulses "flip" the spin of the hydrogen nuclei into an excited state. The relaxation of the spin as it realigns with the magnetic field emits a pulse of radio waves that can be detected by specialized equipment.

Bioinspired Materials for Medical Applications. http://dx.doi.org/10.1016/B978-0-08-100741-9.00008-5

These powerful techniques are widely used in many chemical/biological applications, however each one presents particular limitations, such as insufficient spatial resolution and/or unsatisfactory sensitivity, fluorescent dye toxicity, need for labels (Liu et al., 2011), limited anatomical information (Qin et al., 2010), and radioactive risks (Luo et al., 2011). Also, some other requirements need to be satisfied, namely noninvasiveness (Liu et al., 2011), rapid detection (as short as a few minutes), real-time detection, and cost-effectiveness (Tallury et al., 2010). Multimodality settings that combine two or more imaging techniques are being proposed as solutions to overtake some of these drawbacks and requirements (Qin et al., 2010), but the development of new settings and the improvement of current methods is also needed. To better understand the power and limitations of each imaging technique, a comparison is shown in Table 8.1.

The specific visualization of tissues, cells (prokaryote or eukaryote) or molecules in live animals requires a suitable contrast level that is not always detectable by direct visualization or by applying free dyes. Design of ligands and delivery agents which carry a suitable contrast agent is expected to overcome visual limitations and improve image quality. The affinity of a ligand to its target allows the contrast agent to be selectively accumulated at the target site for a prolonged period of time. The limited number of receptors on the cell surface and the coexistence of the same receptors in cells present in different places remains a limitation (Lee et al., 2014). There are several types of ligands that can be used together with the different imaging modalities thus improving the final results.

An ideal imaging system would be capable of generating complete anatomical information associated with a high-contrast image, to be supported by specific and nontoxic target ligands for each kind of tissue, and to benefit a suitable probe's delivery system enabling to extend its blood half-life time and accumulation in the targets. The detection system is expected to have no limitation related to the penetration depth in organs and to be free of ionizing radiation. Noninvasiveness and rapid data acquisition are also desirable features to improve the patient's well-being.

In this chapter, we will review the advantages and limitations of the most commonly used targeting ligands and their application in the different imaging modalities. Subsequently, we will address the different imaging techniques and their most important advantages and limitations, while referring to examples of current applications and forthcoming developments.

8.2 Targeting ligands

Targeting ligands are molecules that target a specific site via direct ligand–receptor interaction. They can be categorized as amino acids (proteins and peptides), nucleic acids, carbohydrates, and vitamins. More recently, phages have also started to be explored as targeting ligands (Bannas et al., 2015; Farrar et al., 2014; Lee et al., 2014; Schmidt et al., 2004).

Table 8.1 Comparison between relevant characteristics of the different imaging modalities

Technique	Spatial resolution	Temporal resolution	Depth	Sensitivity	Radiation	Availability of specific contrast agents	Structures and biophysiologic functions targeted
PET	1–2 mm	Minutes–hours	Unlimited	10^{-14}–10^{-15} M	Ionizing (gamma rays)	High	Physiological; molecular
SPECT	0.5–1 mm	Minutes–hours	Unlimited	10^{-10}–10^{-14} M	Ionizing (gamma rays)	High	Physiological; molecular
CT	20–200 μm	Minutes	Unlimited	Not well characterized	Ionizing (X-rays)	Low	Anatomical; physiological
Fluorescence	1–3 mm	Millisecond–seconds	1 mm–2 cm	10^{-9}–10^{-12} M	Nonionizing (visible; NIR)	High	Physiological; molecular
BLI	1 mm	Minutes	<1.5 cm	10^{-10}–10^{-11} M	Nonionizing (visible)	High	Physiological; molecular
FMT	1 mm	Minutes–hours	<5 cm	Not well characterized	Nonionizing (visible)	High	Physiological; molecular
pCLE	[a]AR: 5–15 μm/ LR: 1–3.5 μm	Seconds	130 μm	Not well characterized	Nonionizing (visible)	Low	Physiological; molecular
MRI	10–100 μm	Minutes–hours	Unlimited	10^{-3}–10^{-5} M	Nonionizing (radio waves)	Low	Anatomical; physiological; molecular

Spatial resolution defines the smallest discernible detail in an image and strongly influences image quality. Temporal resolution is defined as the amount of time needed to acquire data for the exact same location. Penetration depth measures how deep an electromagnetic radiation can penetrate into a tissue. Sensitivity is the ability of a technique to respond to slight changes in the conditions of a system under analysis. The radiation wavelength is the base of each reporter system and can be strongly affected by scattering and absorption properties of each tissue. Low availability of specific contrast agents limits the range of application to each imaging modality. The ability to generate anatomical, physiological, and/or molecular information is also an important aspect to take into account when selecting a suitable imaging modality.

[a] *AR*, axial resolution; *LR*, lateral resolution.

In the amino acids category, antibodies are the most attractive proteins to be used as a targeting moiety due to their high specificity and the fact that they can be efficiently selected by phage display. On the other hand, antibodies present several disadvantages for preclinical and clinical application related to their high-molecular mass (150 kDa), such as the inability to target intracellular components, limited drug-administration routes, high production costs, slow clearance from circulation, and long retention in nontargeted tissues (Kaur et al., 2012; Mujić-Delić et al., 2014). In response to these disadvantages, some antibodies derivative ligands with great potential in imaging approaches have appeared. These include diabodies, minibodies, single-chain variable fragments, and nanobodies. Among these, nanobodies are the smallest available antigen-binding fragments (with only 15–18 kDa), and due to their small size they are expected to penetrate tissues faster than conventional antibodies. Furthermore, they are soluble in water, very stable and rapidly cleared from the circulation by kidneys (Bannas et al., 2015).

Peptides, in comparison to proteins, present advantages such as low toxicity and immunogenicity. Their small size improves pharmacokinetic characteristics and tissue distribution patterns, helps to obtain a more efficient conjugation to the imaging agent, and simplifies synthesis and production (Chen and Conti, 2010; Marr et al., 2011). Low bioavailability, which is related to the susceptibility of the peptides to protease activity, to the poor absorption of peptides by tissues, and also to the short circulation half-life in the blood stream, is the major limitation of these ligands (Ibraheem et al., 2014; Yu et al., 2014).

Nucleic acids may form aptamers, which consist of 15–40 base pairs and have a 3D configuration that offers a binding affinity to a specific target. Aptamers can be efficiently selected by a strategy named as systematic evolution of ligands by exponential enrichment (Farrar et al., 2014). They present similar advantages and disadvantages as those of peptides; for instance, they display low immunogenicity and are easy to manufacture due to their small size, but have limited stability in the blood stream due to the presence of nucleases (Lee et al., 2014). When injected in the blood stream, aptamers are also rapidly excreted via the urinary tract, but distribution can be improved by the addition of polymers such as polyethylene glycol (Delač et al., 2015).

The possibility of these ligands to be coupled with fluorescent or radionuclide labels, and be incorporated in nanoparticles, allows them to be used in any of the imaging modalities. Aptamers may be constituted of nucleic acids mimics, which are modified nucleic acids with improved biostability and excellent mismatch discrimination when hybridizing with DNA or RNA.

The most widely used nucleic acid mimics are peptide nucleic acids (PNA), locked nucleic acid (LNA), 2′-*O*-methyl-RNA (2′OMe), and phosphorothioate DNA (PS-DNA) (Cerqueira et al., 2008). PNAs are nucleic acid mimics where the phosphate deoxyribose or ribose backbones have been replaced by uncharged *N*-(2-aminoethyl) glycine linkages (Nielsen et al., 1991; Nielsen and Egholm, 1999). LNA is a RNA mimic with a bicyclic ribonucleoside, which is linked between the 2′-oxygen and the 4′-carbon atom with a methylene unit. LNAs show high-affinity recognition of single-stranded DNA or RNA (ssDNA or ssRNA), substantially increase helical thermostability and, moreover, are nuclease resistant (Veedu and Wengel, 2010).

Another widely used nucleic acid mimic is 2′-*O*-methyl-RNA (2′OMe), which displays nuclease resistance, higher affinity, and increased specificity towards RNA and DNA, and faster hybridization kinetics compared to DNA (Molenaar et al., 2001). In PS-DNAs a nonbridging oxygen is replaced by a sulfur atom in the phosphate backbone of an oligo. PS-DNAs have higher resistance towards inter- and intracellular phosphodiesterases, and when complexed with RNA are able to activate RNase H (Boczkowska et al., 2002). These nucleotide analogues and many others are being used not only in aptamers, but also as small antisense oligonucleotides (Blasberg, 2002; Schmidt et al., 2004).

Carbohydrates and vitamins are low-molecular ligands that recognize specific receptors on the cell surface (Lee et al., 2014). For instance, hyaluronic acid is a polymer of disaccharides composed of D-glucuronic acid and D-*N*-acetylglucosamine, which interacts with cluster determinant 44 receptors overexpressed on tumors. Acid folic is a vitamin that shows high affinity to the folate receptor that is also overexpressed on tumors. They have low-molecular weight, are relatively inexpensive to synthetize and results can be more reproducible due to the limited number of inherent structural diversities of the molecules.

Phages are highly specific agents that target and recognize specific cells. Recent developments have used in vivo phage display to yield disease-specific or organ-specific phage clones. For instance, two fluorescently labeled clones for in vivo imaging were developed to specifically target vascular cell adhesion molecule-1 (VCAM-1) expressing blood vessels, which can be used for imaging VCAM-1 expression in diseases such as atherosclerosis, and to target secreted protein acidic and rich in cysteine expressed in invasive cancers (Kelly et al., 2006). Rapid and economical biologic expansion (rather than the more time-consuming chemical synthesis); rapid, simple, and cheap screening process without the need for expensive equipment (Willats, 2002); and the availability of many types of phage clones and libraries (Smith and Petrenko, 1997) are important advantages related to other targeting ligands. On the other hand, after screening the potential phage clones require extensive validation, which is a time-consuming and costly process (Kelly et al., 2006).

An important aspect related to the described ligands is that their functionality implies their ability to reach their target and for that, many of them require suitable delivery systems. In fact, most of the described ligands are coupled to a delivery system or an imaging agent using a suitable bioconjugation method that must avoid the inactivation of their functions or decrease the steric hindrance between molecules (Tian et al., 2003). These methods include direct conjugation, linker chemistry between ligand and reporter agent, click chemistry, and physical interactions, such as ionic, hydrophobic, and host–guest (Lee et al., 2014).

The delivery system is one of the most important aspects to consider when molecules used as contrast agents or therapeutic drugs are injected into the blood stream. Encapsulation is a common strategy used for the protection of molecules against in vivo degradation, reduction of potentially toxic side effects that occur with the direct administration of the solution, to avoid repetitive bolus injections or the use of perfusion pumps and pharmacokinetic improvements (Vrignaud et al., 2011). Delivery systems currently under investigation are based on liposomes, smart polymers, viral nanoparticles (Portney and Ozkan, 2006), and dendrimers (Villaraza et al., 2010), but many other systems can be found in the literature.

All referred ligands and many different delivery systems can be combined with suitable imaging agents to generate probes to overcome the individual limitations of the currently available imaging modalities, to extend its application and respond to the requirements of in vivo imaging and diagnosis. Fig. 8.2 shows schematic representations of several probe configurations coupled to different delivery systems. The following sections will address the different imaging modalities, and also relate them to the types of targeting ligand that are generally used for their application.

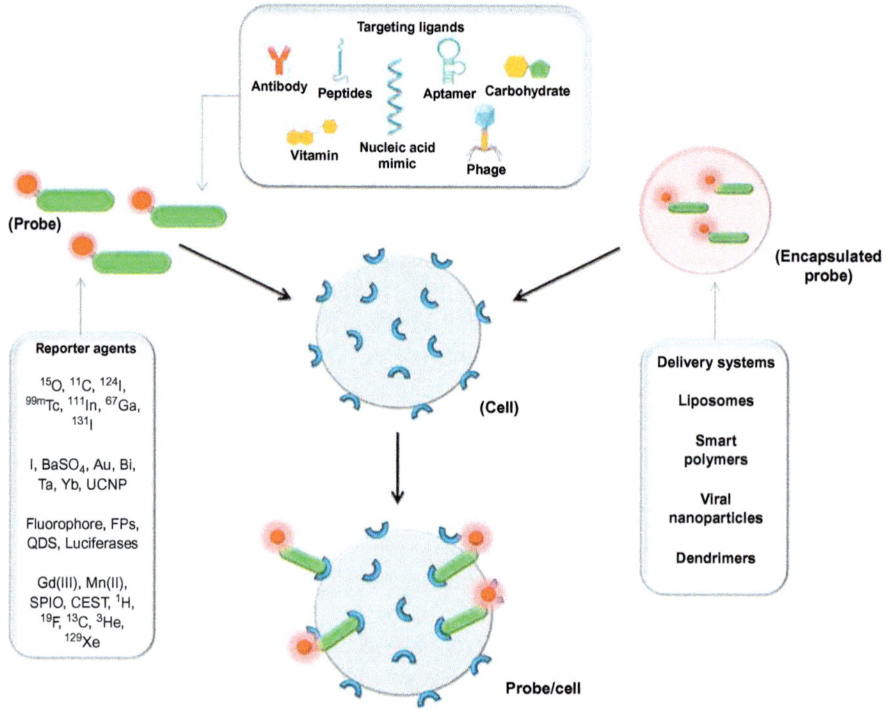

Fig. 8.2 Schematic representation of an imaging probe targeting a specific cell. Free probes or encapsulated probes target specific receptors on the cell surface. Probes are targeting ligands coupled to a suitable reporter agent and can be associated to different delivery systems to improve their pharmacokinetic features.

8.3 Positron emission tomography

Positron emission tomography (PET) is a quantitative and noninvasive technique that enables in vivo investigations of cellular and molecular processes (Dufort et al., 2010). This technique assesses the 3D spatial distribution of special tracers, incorporating positron emitting radioactive isotopes injected into the body (Hoff, 2005).

Table 8.2 Radionuclide's half-lives used as labels in PET and SPECT

PET		SPECT	
Radionuclide	**Half-life**	**Radionuclide**	**Half-life**
^{15}O	2 min	^{99m}Tc	6.02 h
^{13}N	10 min	^{86}Y	14.7 h
^{11}C	20 min	^{111}In	67.3 h
^{18}F	1.8 h	^{201}Tl	73 h
^{76}Br	16.2 h	^{67}Ga	78 h
^{124}I	4 days	^{131}I	8 days

Radionuclides used for SPECT analysis usually have longer half-lives than in PET.

The most commonly used isotopes are oxygen-15, nitrogen-13, carbon-11, fluorine-18, bromine-76, and iodine-124 (Table 8.2), which present radioactive half-lives in the range of 2 min to 4 days (Pien et al., 2005). As such, these radionuclides usually have to be produced on a daily basis or even 1 h before the intended use. The positron emitting radionuclide is first generated with a cyclotron and then reacts with a suitable precursor, which is a molecule that allows the incorporation of the radionuclide in a fast and efficient manner (Piel et al., 2014; Ziegler, 2005). Advantages of radionuclide-labeled substances include their very high specificity (molecular targeting), the possibility of using biologically active substances and the very low amounts applied, ranging from picomolar to nanomolar, which guarantees that the system under investigation is less disturbed by the applied radiotracers (Hoff, 2005; Ziegler, 2005).

Imaging of regional tracer concentrations is accomplished by the unique properties of positron decay and annihilation. Upon the decay of the radioactive label a positron is emitted from the atomic nucleus. The positron then travels a short distance through the tissue, typically ranging from 1 mm to 2 cm (mean range in water: 1.1 mm, 1.5 mm, 0.6 mm for ^{11}C, ^{13}N, ^{18}F, respectively) until it becomes thermalized by electrostatic interactions between the electrons and the atomic nuclei of the medium. After losing most of its kinetic energy, the positron can interact with a free electron to form a positronium. The positronium decays by annihilation, generating a pair of photons (gamma rays) that travel in nearly opposite directions with an energy of 511 keV each (Hoff, 2005; Piel et al., 2014; Ziegler, 2005). The opposed photons from positron decay can be detected by using pairs of collinearly aligned detectors. A pair of radiation detectors of a PET system is installed in a ring-like pattern, which allows measurement of radioactivity along lines through the organ of interest at a large number of angles and radial distances (line of response). This information about the approximate spatial location of the radionuclide is used in the reconstruction of tomographic images. Data gaps between imaging planes can be minimized by combining multiple and closely packed rings of detectors that enable simultaneous imaging of several image planes. Coincident events between rings of the camera are acquired and cross-data are generated, with spatial resolution of 1–2 mm for contemporary human PET scanners and <1 mm for small animal PET scanners (Piel et al., 2014; Wang et al., 2014; Ziegler, 2005).

The spatial resolution that can be achieved in a PET image is mainly limited by positron range and gamma ray noncollinearity. In addition, the width of the detection elements in the tomograph determines the width of the coincidence response function and image resolution (Ziegler, 2005). PET technique displays no limited tissue depth penetration, a temporal resolution from minutes to hours, and a sensitivity ranging from 10^{-14} to 10^{-15} M (Dufort et al., 2010). An absolute quantification of the measured activity can be obtained, usually in units of Becquerel per milliliter (Bq/mL), which corresponds to the concentration of the tracer in the tissue (Hoff, 2005; Piel et al., 2014). PET studies are commonly reinforced by CT or MRI images since PET tracers are very specific and anatomical information that can be found in PET images is limited (Ziegler, 2005).

Structures and biophysiologic functions targeted by these tracers include substrate (mainly glucose) metabolism, catecholamine transport, amino acid transport, protein synthesis (Ziegler, 2005), enzyme activity, and receptor density/affinity (Hoff, 2005). Time sequences can be acquired (4D PET) that build the basis for compartmental modeling aiming at measuring physiological constants such as metabolic or transport rates (Ziegler, 2005).

Most clinical PET studies are performed to determine the extent of a tumor and the location and number of metastases. For example, fluorine-18 labeled fluorodeoxyglucose (FDG), a sugar analogue, is widely used for tumor detection and staging, since tumor cells have an increased glucose uptake compared to normal tissue: a phenomenon known as the Warburg effect (Warburg, 1956). FDG is taken up by the cell in the same way as glucose, but is not further metabolized. This trapping effect is very useful for imaging purposes as a single scan at a given time after injection of the radiotracer will show activity concentrations that are proportional to FDG absorption. The most commonly employed PET protocol is the whole body scan. About 40 min after intravenous injection of approximately 400 MBq FDG, the patient is positioned on the scanner bed and acquisitions of 1–10 bed positions are performed. Total scanning time with modern systems is around 30 min for a 10 bed position whole body scan (Ziegler, 2005). Other clinical applications of FDG include brain scans for diagnosing Alzheimer's disease (Ziegler, 2005), pneumonia and tuberculosis diagnosis, osteomyelitis, and infections of the spine and bone (Israel and Keidar, 2011). FDG is also being employed in drug research (Piel et al., 2014).

Many different radiolabeled probes are under investigation to reinforce diagnosis in different fields of medicine and it is expected that PET provides the basis for monitoring disease progression and improve therapies in the future. Indeed, the recently developed dynamic PET (4D PET) has improved pharmacokinetics studies of antisense nucleic acids drugs by visualization of radiolabeled oligodeoxynucleotides distribution in animal bodies and quantifying the time required for drugs excretion. Moreover, radiolabeled nucleic acid mimics containing modified backbone nucleotides have been tested for therapeutic applications (Mukai et al., 2014).

8.4 Single photon emission computed tomography

Similarly to the PET technique, single photon emission computed tomography (SPECT) is an imaging procedure in which a radionuclide-labeled biomolecule is injected and monitored. Once the biochemical compound enters the bloodstream, it travels to body organs (brain, liver, kidney, heart, and the peripheral vascular system) and is absorbed by them according to each organ's affinity for the particular compound (Gullberg et al., 2010).

SPECT is based on photons (gamma rays) emitted as a consequence of isotope decay. Photons travel from the body to the detector and are recorded by a camera that provides a digital image of the radiotracer distribution in the body. Radionuclide labels commonly used are technetium-99m (^{99m}Tc), yttrium-86 (^{86}Y), indium-111 (^{111}In), thallium-201 (^{201}Tl), gallium-67 (^{67}Ga), and iodine-131 (^{131}I) (Table 8.2), which have longer radioactive half-lives relative to PET radiotracers (Fass, 2008; Schillaci et al., 2007; Hildebrandt and Gambhir, 2004).

SPECT's detection system may have up to three detectors and is based on gamma cameras and collimators (apertures that allow only particles traveling directly through the hole to be detected). The detector(s) rotate from 180 to 360 degrees allowing images of the distribution of the radiotracer from different projections to be recorded (Gullberg et al., 2010; Hildebrandt and Gambhir, 2004). This kind of detector makes SPECT less sensitive than PET (Ziegler, 2005). It displays a sensitivity ranging from 10^{-10} to 10^{-14} M, a spatial resolution from 0.5 to 1 mm and, similarly to PET, an unlimited depth tissue penetration (Dufort et al., 2010; Wang et al., 2014).

This technique allows conducting basic research studies on gene and immunotherapy, and cell trafficking. Diagnosis of infectious diseases is also under investigation to be performed by SPECT studies where radiolabeled nucleic acid mimics are used as probes (Chen et al., 2013). At the preclinical and clinical investigation level, it allows the study of autoimmune diseases, inflammations, and cancers (Hildebrandt and Gambhir, 2004). Clinical applications include cerebral perfusion studies to support dementia (including Alzheimer disease), cerebrovascular diseases, and epilepsy diagnostics (McArthur et al., 2011). A very useful advantage of SPECT applied in clinical and scientific research studies is the availability of many different biochemical compounds to target organs or specific regions of the animal/human body. Many of them are experimental molecules but they have a great potential to improve SPECT diagnosis.

A new approach is the so-called dynamic SPECT, a technique that uses tracers to obtain images that reflect the fundamental biophysiologic functions of perfusion and metabolism in body organs. This is achieved by quantifying the temporal changes of radionuclide concentrations in tomographic sections through angular sampling of projections. This technique, in conjunction with mathematical model-based analysis of regional kinetics of the radiotracer, allows the quantification of functional parameters, which are estimated using a time series of dynamic reconstructed images. The development and use of kinetic analysis in dynamic SPECT applications has been limited by low sensitivity, poor spatial resolution, and poor temporal resolution, which are consequences of the need to mechanically rotate the detector head for most of the studies (Gullberg et al., 2010).

8.5 X-ray computed tomography

CT is a 3D radiographic imaging technique where sequential radiographic projections of several angular positions around the body are acquired and an image is topographically formed. The cross-sectional field of view is reconstructed using established computational techniques based on radon projection theory. The reconstructed image is based on X-ray attenuation in tissues and organs and image intensity depends of the material property related to the object's electron density (atomic number and mass density). Due to calcium hydroxyapatite, the bone matrix is denser than the surrounding media, and as such the contrast between soft and mineralized tissue is naturally high (Burghardt et al., 2011; Lee et al., 2014).

Clinical contrast agents include low-molecular-weight iodine-based molecules and barium sulfate. Barium sulfate is restricted for use as a gastrointestinal contrast agent due to its toxicity. Limited iodine half-life in blood is driving research studies to use liposome or micelle to encapsulate the iodinated contrast agents. Polymer-based nanoparticles or dendrimers such as polyamidoamine conjugating iodinated compounds are also under investigation (Lee et al., 2014).

The development of CT contrast agents has been limited because X-ray imaging has low contrast sensitivity. Metal-based nanoparticles are being developed due to their high atomic weight, which increases X-ray attenuation compared to the conventional iodine moiety. Gold, bismuth, tantalum, and ytterbium have been studied as potential elements for the development of CT imaging agents. Upconversion nanoparticles, which use sequential absorption of lower energy photons to emit higher energy photons (Lin et al., 2012), have also attracted significant attention for use in X-ray/multimodality imaging. These are generally lanthanide doped rare-earth nanoparticles (such as Gd-, Yb-, and Lu-doped) having intrinsic upconversion luminescence properties (Toy et al., 2014). The difficulty in designing contrast agents and probes for this modality has limited this technology as a molecular imaging tool (Hildebrandt and Gambhir, 2004).

CT is a quantitative method showing a spatial resolution of 20–200 μm, with a data acquisition time of minutes and an unlimited depth tissue penetration. For rodents, a recent approach named micro-CT allows a spatial resolution ranging from 10 to 100 μm. In general, CT is a very sensitive technique for skeletal tissue visualization and bone diseases diagnosis (Dufort et al., 2010). Other body sections can be imaged by contrast agents administration such as vascular and cardiac structures, abdominal organs, or cerebral structures. The fat content of body and organs can also be quantified (Schambach et al., 2010). Another very useful application consists of chemical composition determination of urinary tract stones because X-rays show different attenuation with the material composition, which is important to manage patients with urolithiasis (Eliahou et al., 2010). Due to its limitation as a molecular imaging techinque, CT will remain, for the foreseeable future, a complementary tool to other imaging modalities, by providing anatomical information to complete, for instance, studies by PET.

8.6 Biophotonic imaging

BPI is a highly sensitive, noninvasive, nontoxic technique based on the detection of light that arises from either the excitation of a fluorescent protein (FP) or molecule or from an enzyme-catalyzed oxidation reaction (bioluminescence). Several factors influence the sensitivity of BPI, of which the most important are (a) inherent body or organ features that affect the propagation of light through tissue, (b) inherent background signals from living organisms, and (c) oxygen availability (Andreu et al., 2011; Hernandez et al., 2013; Richards-Kortum, 1996; Stringer and Moghissi, 2004). These factors will now be addressed in detail.

Tissues are a complex heterogeneous mixture of the many different molecular species that compose the cells, and this heterogeneity is the reason why tissues show distinct scattering and absorption properties depending on light wavelength (Stringer and Moghissi, 2004). When photons in the visible (400–760 nm) and infrared (IR) wavelengths interact with tissues, they are highly scattered because they cannot propagate along straight lines, thus resulting in photon diffusion. Endogenous chromophores such as myoglobin and mainly hemoglobin (nonfluorescent chromophore), absorb in the blue and green part of the visible spectrum (<600 nm), allowing light transmission of wavelengths longer than 600 nm, as red light, through several centimeters of tissue. Melanin is also a significant contributor to absorption in pigmented animals, meaning that signals within animals with dark fur will be much more attenuated than signals from nude animals or those with white fur (Andreu et al., 2011). Water is another endogenous chromophore that predominantly absorbs in the IR range (>1000 nm) (Richards-Kortum, 1996).

Autofluorescence is generally many orders of magnitude brighter than autoluminescence and, as such, living animals show high levels of background fluorescence compared with luminescence. Thus, luminescence imaging can be more sensitive than fluorescence imaging as a result of better signal-to-noise ratios (Hernandez et al., 2013). Tissue autofluorescence is produced by endogenous fluorophores such as keratin, porphyrins, reduced NADH, collagen, elastin, flavins, tryptophan, pyroxidine, tyrosine, and lipopigments (Stringer and Moghissi, 2004).

Oxygen is a cofactor required by all luciferases (the most commonly used enzymes to produce bioluminescence) and for the synthesis of most of the FPs discovered to date. Although luminescence can be detected in marine bioluminescent bacteria under oxygen concentrations as low as 10 nM, it has been suggested that luminescence-based BPI may be limited when used to image anaerobic environments, such as the necrotic cores of large tumors (Andreu et al., 2011).

To improve the sensitivity of BPI, the detection of the weak surface light signal can be performed by a high sensitivity photon detector, such as a cooled charge-coupled device (CCD) camera and photomultiplier tube. The external interference of ambient light should be avoided using a light-tight imaging chamber (Andreu et al., 2011; Qin et al., 2010). Planar optical imaging is the simplest direct method to implement and uses the photographic principle to obtain 2D transmitted and scattered light distribution on the surface. Corresponding imaging instrumentation is also relatively cheap. Limitations are related to photon attenuation due to the nonlinear relationship between the signal detected, its depth localization and the optical properties of the surrounding tissues. Nevertheless, it can provide relative quantification information depending on depth and sample-type. As mentioned above, photons propagating in the biological tissue are strongly scattered before either being totally absorbed by the tissue or escaping from the surface where they are captured, resulting in a very poor spatial resolution of planar optical imaging (Andreu et al., 2011; Qin et al., 2010).

8.6.1 Fluorescence imaging

Fluorophores linked to probes or FP inside the biological tissue absorb the radiation with a specific wavelength produced by an external light source and then reemit some photons at a longer wavelength (lower energy in relation to exciter radiation). The external excitation light source is indispensable in fluorescence imaging. Adequate fluorescent reporters require suitable excitation and emission wavelengths, photostability (a measure of the time that the reporter takes to lose 50% of its initial emission, under constant illumination), brightness and maturation speed (the time taken to the full formation of the fluorophore).

According to the mode of data acquisition (Fig. 8.3A and B), fluorescence imaging can be classified as reflectance imaging and transillumination imaging. In the reflectance imaging (or epi-illumination), the excitation light source and the detection instrumentation are placed on the same side, while in transillumination imaging the light source is located on the opposite side to the detector. Transillumination is capable of imaging signals located deeper within the tissue. The resulting signal is then captured in complete darkness, which may take from seconds to minutes depending on the strength and location of the signal and the sensitivity of the imaging system (Andreu et al., 2011; Qin et al., 2010). Recent evidence demonstrates that normalized transillumination presents significant advantages over nonnormalized ones and over planar reflectance (Qin et al., 2010).

Combining multispectral information and spectrum separation techniques, it is possible to obtain high sensitivity by removing autofluorescence and consequently increasing image contrast. This allows the autofluorescence limitation to be partially overcome, improving weak fluorescent signals and allowing the use of several kinds of fluorophores (Qin et al., 2010). These systems show a spatial resolution of 1–3 mm, sensitivity of 10^{-9}–10^{-12} M (Wang et al., 2014), and signals can be detected in a time window ranging from milliseconds to seconds (Dufort et al., 2010).

With visible wavelengths shorter than 650 nm, the detection is limited to a depth from 1 to 2 mm (Dufort et al., 2010), but for longer wavelengths (ranging from 650 to 900 nm) the tissues have lower absorbance and less light scattering (Filonov et al., 2011), and hence fluorophores operating in the NIR window can achieve 7–14 cm tissue penetration using sensitive photon collection systems (Tung, 2004).

Fluorescence molecular tomography (FMT) that involves the illumination of the sample at different points or projections to create a 3D image is already available. FMT has shown a spatial resolution of about 1 mm with tissue penetration depth of about 5 cm and a temporal resolution from minutes to hours. These improvements associated with the quantitative determination of biological parameters foresee a clinical use in the near future, for example for prostate imaging. Additionally, it is also a suitable method for quantifying protein levels and enzymatic activities (Dufort et al., 2010).

The green fluorescent protein from the jelly fish *Aequorea victoria* was the first FP to be reported but numerous other FPs in all the colors of the rainbow have been discovered since. In addition, near-infrared FPs systems are being developed using naturally occurring photosensory receptors named phytochromes as a basis (Filonov et al., 2011).

Another approach uses NIR cyanine dyes, which represent the most prominent class of NIR fluorochromes (Tung, 2004). Molecular imaging using FPs has been an important technique to quantitatively and noninvasively monitor biological processes including gene expression, angiogenesis, tumor growth, metastasis, and bacterial and viral infections (Filonov et al., 2011).

Another class of reporter particles, named quantum dots (QDs), has been studied mostly on mammalian cells. QDs are colloidal semiconductor nanocrystals with between 1 and 10 nm in diameter, which offer tunable fluorescence (including NIR) as a result of quantum-confinement effects that are related to the size and composition of the nanocrystal (Farkhani and Valizadeh, 2014; Tavares et al., 2011). Their advantages are related to their relatively small size, brightness, photostability, independence of emission from the excitation wavelength, and stability under different environments (Farkhani and Valizadeh, 2014). However, there are features undesirable for in vivo imaging applications, such as high background retention and nonspecific accumulation; incomplete removal from the body (Tavares et al., 2011). Despite the small size of QDs, the conjugation with targeting ligands increases its diameter, which should have a maximum of 5.5 nm for tumor targeting probes to allow efficient renal clearance. The charge surface is also a concern because highly charged QDs have a tendency to bind to serum proteins that increase their diameter (Choi et al., 2010).

8.6.2 Bioluminescence imaging

Bioluminescence imaging (BLI) is based on oxidation of a substrate (a luciferin) by an enzyme (a luciferase), which usually requires energy ($FMNH_2$ and ATP), Mg^{2+}, and oxygen to generate bioluminescent photons (Qin et al., 2010). There are five basic luciferin–luciferase systems (Table 8.3). The most widely studied are those belonging to luminous beetles in the families Lampyridae and Elateridae (mainly the firefly *Photinus pyralis* and the click beetle *Pyrophorus plagiophtalamus*), the sea pansy *Renilla reniformis*, the marine copepod *Gaussia princeps* and numerous luminous bacteria (terrestrial *Photorhabdus luminescens* and marine *Vibrio*) (Andreu et al., 2011).

The beetle luminescence reaction (the most efficient bioluminescent reaction) is catalyzed by a monomeric luciferase (Fluc) of approximately 62 kDa, encoded by the single gene *luc*, and using benzothiazoyl-thiazole as substrate and ATP, resulting in the production of oxyluciferin, AMP, CO_2, and the emission of light. The light generated by the firefly luciferase has a peak at 560 nm and is influenced by temperature, shifting to a peak of 610 nm at 37°C, and tends to be the reporter of choice for expression by eukaryotic cells. The click beetle reaction emits light in the range 546–593 nm. The genes required for luciferin production have not been completely elucidated and, therefore, exogenous luciferin has to be administered. Luciferin is assumed to be nontoxic when injected in animals and has been used in the muscle, the knee joint, vaginal tract, and in nasal and pulmonary studies (Andreu et al., 2011; Brock, 2012; Hernandez et al., 2013).

The sea pansy and copepod have monomeric luciferases (35 kDa and 19 kDa) that are encoded by the genes *rluc* and *gluc*, respectively. They oxidize imidazolopyrazine

Table 8.3 **Characteristics of the luciferases used in bioluminescence systems**

Luciferase origin	Organism (family)	Substrate	Co-substrate	Composition (mass, kDa)	Peak emission (nm)
Photinus pyralis	Firefly (Lampyridae)	Benzothiazoyl-thiazole	O_2; ATP	Monomer (62)	560 (610 at 37°C)
Pyrophorus plagiophthalamus	Click beetle (Elateridae)	Benzothiazoyl-thiazole	O_2; ATP	Monomer (62)	546–593
Renilla reniformis	Sea pansy (Renillidae)	Benzylimidazo-pyrazinone coelenterazine	O_2	Monomer (35)	480
Gaussia princeps	Copepod (Metridinidae)	Benzylimidazo-pyrazinone coelenterazine	O_2	Monomer (19)	480
Photorhabdus	Bacteria (Enterobacteriaceae)	Long-chain aliphatic aldehyde	O_2; FMNH2	Heterodimer (77)	490
Vibrio	Bacteria (Vibrionaceae)	Long-chain aliphatic aldehyde	O_2; FMNH2	Heterodimer (77)	490

The origin of each luciferase, substrates, and co-substrates required to signals generation, luciferase's mass and composition, and emission wavelength of each bioluminescence-based system are indicated.

substrates such as coelenterazine, producing CO_2, coelenteramide and blue light (480nm). Gluc appears to be strongly resistant to heat and extreme pH and has been shown to be secreted from both mammalian and bacterial cells. The requirement of coelenterazine, its low bioavailability, and high chemiluminescent (which reduces sensitivity by reducing the signal-to-noise ratio) are important limitations for in vivo applications. However, Gluc and Rluc have been studied in tumor cells (Andreu et al., 2011; Brock, 2012).

For the generation of bioluminescent bacteria generally a *lux* operon is used. The bacterial luciferase is a heterodimeric enzyme of 77kDa composed of α and β subunits encoded by the *luxA* and *luxB* genes, respectively. The reaction involves the oxidation of a long-chain aldehyde and reduced flavin mononucleotide ($FMNH_2$), resulting in the production of oxidized flavin (FMN) and a long-chain fatty acid, while bioluminescent photons are emitted at 490nm. A significant advantage of the *lux* operon in comparison with the other luminescence systems is the presence of three genes, namely the *luxC*, *luxD*, and *luxE*, which encode the subunits of a multienzyme complex responsible for regeneration of the aldehyde substrate from the fatty acid produced by the reaction. Thus, no exogenous substrate is needed (Andreu et al., 2011; Brock, 2012).

The bioluminescent signal on the external surface of organisms can be directly collected by a CCD camera without external excitation light source (Fig. 8.3C). Compared with fluorescence imaging, bioluminescent signals are low, but provide superior signal-to-noise ratios and excellent sensitivity because of the very low autoluminescence levels (Hernandez et al., 2013). BLI-based systems already achieved a sensitivity from 10^{-10} to 10^{-11}M (lower than fluorescent systems) (Wang et al., 2014) and spatial resolution of approximately 1mm. The signal can be detected in a few minutes (Dufort et al., 2010) but depth penetration is still poor (<1.5cm).

Unlike for fluorescence imaging, bioluminescence tomography systems are not currently available because the absence of an external excitation source makes it difficult to reconstruct the 3D tissue image (Andreu et al., 2011; Qin et al., 2010). Bioluminescence systems are being used to monitor different biological processes such as tumor volume, transcriptional activation during tumor development/therapy, immune cell infiltration into the tumor environment, gene expression, and disease progression caused by pathogenic bacteria (eg, *Listeria monocytogenes* and *Mycobacterium tuberculosis*) and fungi (eg, *Candida albicans* and *Aspergillus fumigatus*) (Brock, 2012; Hernandez et al., 2013; Maguire et al., 2013).

8.6.3 Confocal laser endomicroscopy

CLE is in essence a fluorescence imaging technique, but it uses invasive equipment that implies a very high spatial resolution in comparison with other techniques (Fig. 8.3D). On the other hand it is still mostly employed in the gastrointestinal tract. It is based on detection of reflected laser light after tissue illumination by a low power laser. The returned light is refocused onto the detection system by the same lens (Neumann et al., 2010). The imaging laser and light collection pathway are in the same focal plane (confocal) (Dunbar and Canto, 2010). CLE can be used as a tool for real-time microscopic gastrointestinal imaging and provides high-resolution images, enabling optical biopsies and in vivo histology (Neumann et al., 2010). Gastrointestinal mucosa images allow visualization of gastric pits, colonic crypts, capillaries, and individual epithelial and blood cells, but not of the gastrointestinal tract deeper structures (Dunbar and Canto, 2010).

There are two confocal endomicroscopy systems available: a confocal endoscope (eCLE) and a probe-based confocal endomicroscope (pCLE). eCLE enables standard resolution white-light endoscopic imaging, while pCLE can be performed with both standard and high-resolution endoscopes. Axial and lateral resolutions for eCLE are 7 μm and 0.7 μm, respectively, and the imaging depth can reach up to 250 μm. pCLE shows different resolution and imaging depth depending on the selected settings. Axial resolution ranges from 5 to 15 μm, lateral resolution ranges from 1 to 3.5 μm and tissue depth penetration can reach 130 μm (Dunbar and Canto, 2010). Images can be acquired within a few seconds of contrast agent administration (Abbaci et al., 2014).

Multiphoton endoscopic devices, which can distinguish different types of gastrointestinal tissue without the application of fluorescent dyes are being developed (Dunbar and Canto, 2010), however for high-resolution image generation, exogenous fluorescence agents have to be applied. Fluorescein sodium, acriflavine hydrochloride, and cresyl violet are routinely used dyes. Fluorescein is considered a nontoxic dye (very few cases showing toxicity have been reported) and highlights the interstitial space. Despite its nontoxicity, patients will show yellow skin, eyes, and urine for several hours after the procedure. Acriflavine is used typically at low concentrations (0.05% weight/volume in saline) because it accumulates in the nuclei with potential mutagenic risk, but it has been successfully used for the detection of *Helicobacter pylori* in vivo. It stains superficial epithelial cells, nuclei, and weakly the cytoplasm. Cresyl violet dyes the cytoplasm and hence nuclear morphology can be inferred. It is also useful as a surface chromoendoscopy agent. Near-infrared approaches are also available (Dunbar and Canto, 2010; Neumann et al., 2010).

Fluorescein has been conjugated with short peptides and antibodies to identify colonic neoplasia (Abbaci et al., 2014; Dunbar and Canto, 2010). Similarly to PET, fluorescently labeled deoxyglucose has been used to detect oral neoplasia and an analogue of choline is under investigation to target cancerous lesions (Abbaci et al., 2014). Fontenete et al. (2015, 2016) successfully detected *Helicobacter pylori* in the gastric mucosa of mice using RNA mimics molecular probes labeled with fluorescein. These works pave the way for genetic sequence-based identification and location of microorganisms within the human body.

Confocal endomicroscopy imaging provides a significant reduction of repeated and random biopsies (Abbaci et al., 2014). However, besides the invasiveness character of endoscopy technique and the limited section of body that can be visualized, other limitations can be found. One is related with the maximal depth of imaging that basically restricts the examination to the epithelium. Low dye concentrations in the tissue due to limited diffusion of the dye into the tissue sublayers increases the difficulties in discriminating details at greater depths. Lack of nuclear cell staining with low toxicity is also a huge limitation (Abbaci et al., 2014; Dunbar and Canto, 2010). Certain sections of the body can be challenging to image with eCLA because the distal tip has limited bendability and the pCLE's probe can be damaged when the accessory channel is retroflexed (Dunbar and Canto, 2010). In a molecular imaging context, endomicroscopy is also limited by restricted availability of molecular probes, as would be expected since it is a very recent technology.

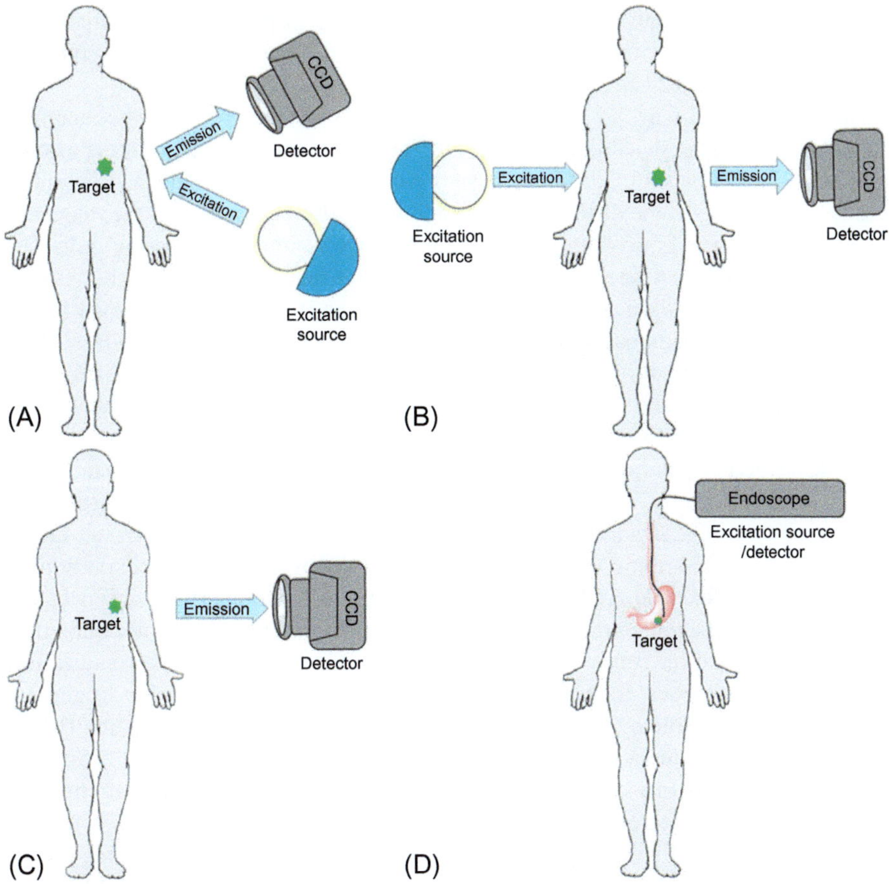

Fig. 8.3 Optical imaging modes. (A) In fluorescence reflectance imaging, the excitation source and the detector are placed on the same side; (B) in fluorescence transillumination, the fluorescence signal is also generated after excitation of the reporter molecule by an excitation source placed on the opposite side of the detector; (C) BLI signals are generated by chemical reactions and the light is captured by the detector; and (D) endomicroscopy is an invasive technique that allows body cavities to be imaged through the insertion of a probe containing both an excitation source and detector.

8.7 Magnetic resonance imaging

MRI is a quantitative technique that uses radiofrequency pulses and strong magnetic fields to align the spin of hydrogen nuclei in tissues and allows signals from changes in nuclear magnetic moments to be obtained (Dufort et al., 2010; Hildebrandt and Gambhir, 2004; Pien et al., 2005). First a pulse of radio waves is applied, which “flips” the spin of the hydrogen nuclei into an excited state. The relaxation of the spin of the hydrogen allows it to realign with the principal magnetic field, while a pulse of radio waves is emitted (Hildebrandt and Gambhir, 2004). More specifically, as the alignment and relaxation of protons occur in response to pulsed radio-frequencies, characteristic relaxation times can be measured, most notably T1 (the longitudinal relaxation time) and T2 (the transverse relaxation time) (Pien et al., 2005).

There are several ways to generate image contrast in order to delineate anatomy and pathology and the detection of the ^{1}H NMR signal of endogenous water is a common step. Thus, images of different tissues can be generated based on: (a) proton density, which reflects the different water content in different tissue; (b) the magnetic and physical properties of water because the relaxation times can vary by orders of magnitude in different tissues; (c) water diffusion rates that allow distinguishing flowing blood from static tissue; (d) transference of magnetization from the broad signal of water associated with macromolecules, or saturation of exchangeable N–H or O–H protons; (e) chemical shift differences mainly associated with mobile lipid protons versus water protons; and (f) the addition of an exogenous probe (Boros et al., 2015; Wozniak and Lim, 2006).

As described for the other techniques, exogenous probes are administered to generate image contrast. Contrast agents modulate the properties of the tissues and can enhance the signal without loss of resolution due to changes in tissue depth (Hildebrandt and Gambhir, 2004). They are detected by altering the relaxation of surrounding spin-excited protons through magnetic interactions (Rosenblum et al., 2010). Relaxation agents are paramagnetic or superparamagnetic compounds that shorten the relaxation times of water molecules. Chemical exchange saturation transfer (CEST) probes are based on the presence of exchangeable hydrogen atoms. The exchangeable hydrogen resonances of these probes are magnetically saturated by a radiofrequency pulse and, then, chemical exchange with hydrogen of the bulk water leads to a decrease of the bulk water signal. Relaxation agents and CEST probes are detected indirectly by their effect on bulk water. Other probes can be detected directly due to their different magnetic resonance frequency (other ^{1}H resonances, ^{19}F-based probes, hyperpolarized ^{13}C, ^{3}He, or ^{129}Xe-based probes) (Boros et al., 2015).

Clinically, the only approved probes are relaxation agents based on discrete Gd(III) (paramagnetic ions) or Mn(II) complexes or (superparamagnetic) iron oxide nanoparticles. Hydrophilic Gd(III) complexes are by far the most widely used while the Mn(II) and iron oxide-based probes are being discontinued. Hyperpolarized ^{13}C, ^{3}He, and ^{129}Xe-based and CEST probes have been used in clinical trials (Boros et al., 2015; Hildebrandt and Gambhir, 2004). There are essential requisites for clinical probe design, namely the compound must be safe, completely excreted (if Gd-containing), produced by a standard (reproducible) method, highly soluble for formulation, and must provide diagnostic quality images in a short time frame after administration (Boros et al., 2015). A particular group of particles are being widely studied and modified with respect to the above requisites, aiming to improve their properties and applications, such as for liver imaging and cell tracking (Frangioni and Hajjar, 2004; Rosenblum et al., 2010). These particles are superparamagnetic iron oxide (SPIO) particles that are composed of an iron oxide core of magnetite or maghemite with a hydrophilic coating for stabilization and dispersion in aqueous media allowing cell-labeling and oral-administration. They are categorized as USPIO (ultrasmall SPIO), SPIO (small size), and mRNA (micron-sized iron oxide nanoparticles) and their sizes are 20–40 nm, 60–150 nm, and micrometer-size, respectively (Rosenblum et al., 2010).

MRI can image deep into the tissue (no depth limitation); there is no ionizing radiation (CT and SPECT/PET); it provides 3D images with submillimeter spatial resolution (10–100 μm), much higher than the resolution offered by optical techniques; it is characterized by far more parameters (in comparison to CT), including proton density, relaxation times, flow, diffusion, and susceptibility, among others; and it provides excellent soft-tissue contrast. There are also multiple types of contrast agents available and the imaging is not operator dependent (Boros et al., 2015; Dufort et al., 2010; Hildebrandt and Gambhir, 2004; Pien et al., 2005; Wang et al., 2014).

The major drawbacks to MRI as a molecular imaging tool are related to relatively long imaging times (minutes to hours); contrast agents must be injected or used as cellular labels and the required amounts can be toxic; most of the contrast agents have large sizes, and are thus harder to deliver to cells, particularly when injected into the blood stream; the effective reporter signal amplification scheme is difficult to perform for cell trafficking and molecular imaging in addition to the lack of optimization; sensitivity is relatively poor (10^{-3}–10^{-5} M) because it needs large amounts of a molecular-probe accumulated at a target site to obtain a measurable signal. Compared to CT, MRI has lower resolution and requires more time for data acquisition (Dufort et al., 2010; Hildebrandt and Gambhir, 2004; Pien et al., 2005; Wang et al., 2014).

Due to its superior soft-tissue contrast (compared to CT), MRI is the modality of choice for imaging the brain, in addition to specific applications in musculoskeletal and gastrointestinal systems. It is also performed for numerous assessments such as tissue perfusion, water diffusion, tumor permeability, and blood oxygenation level-dependent functional MRI studies (Pien et al., 2005). Serum albumin-targeted probes are being used to image the blood pool, a complex with substantial liver clearance can be used to image the hepatobiliary tree, and many other probes have been used to identify vascular irregularities, detect and delineate tumor boundaries, and characterize blood flow (Boros et al., 2015). Despite the difficulties, MRI has shown promising results in stem cell and lymphocyte trafficking studies, pharmacological research for a variety of disorders (Hildebrandt and Gambhir, 2004), degenerative joint diseases, stroke, diseases of the airways (Beckmann et al., 2004), and in infectious diseases diagnosis, such as *Mycobacterium tuberculosis* (Santy et al., 2011). Developments in MRI are mostly aimed at increasing the probe's relaxivity, keeping the dosage non-toxic for the patient or decreasing the probe's size to enable delivery into the cells.

8.8 Conclusion and future perspectives

Herein we have focused on six imaging methods that have been extensively used for a variety of purposes. As an emergent area, molecular imaging techniques have been widely applied in basic research, preclinical imaging, drug development, tumor progression monitoring, and treatment evaluation, to name but a few. Molecular imaging-based techniques have been reinforced by the incredible advances in molecule design and new detection systems combined with corresponding algorithms (Qin et al., 2010).

MRI and CT are two techniques largely applied in the diagnosis of pathologic diseases. MRI is routinely employed in preclinical and clinical research allowing direct visualization of tissues and organs. This technique appears to be more advantageous than CT when we aim to image soft tissues, being nowadays the key technique in oncology research to develop and validate new animal models of cancer and monitor the effects of therapy in these models (Santy et al., 2011). The movement of flowing blood also enables static tissue to be distinguished from nonstatic. On the other hand, CT is particularly interesting when the aim is to visualize injured dense tissue, as those commonly observed in spinal and bone diseases. Nonetheless, the use of these two techniques for molecular imaging is not considered due to their low sensitivity. To improve results, high amounts of probe (for MRI) or high-molecular-weight material (for the CT) would be required, leading in both cases to an increase of the toxicity. Lack of adequate probes, together with the deep penetration of sensing radiation and lack of sensitivity have limited the application of these techniques for infectious diseases diagnosis.

Optical imaging is an inexpensive, easy-to-use, nonionizing, and nontoxic tool that can provide rapid semiqualitative (2D), quantitative (3D), and functional information ranging from micro to macroscale (Andreu et al., 2011; Dufort et al., 2010). Light absorption and scattering appear as the main reasons for low-depth penetration of electromagnetic signals. New developments on reporter molecules have enhanced the spatial resolution using the near infrared based approach, since longer wavelength suffers lower absorbance and light scattering. The same area has provided wavelength tunable nanoparticles, such as QDs, capable of emitting light from visible to NIR. BPI seems to be inappropriate when deep tissue and cell visualization is required. The low-depth penetration and poor spatial resolution hamper its use for pathologic diseases diagnosis. However, infectious diseases can be better understood with this technique, because it can provide new data about microorganism behavior and the niches exploited by them in vivo. Therefore fluorescent and bioluminescent imaging techniques are particularly advantageous for research. Another advantage is the improvement of research studies, due to the fact that BPI can reduce and refine the use of animals. FMT has also shown potential for clinical applications (Dufort et al., 2010). CLE is an optical imaging modality that has great potential for application in routine clinical diagnosis. It has mainly been used for gastrointestinal visualization, but several adaptations to imaging other organs have been developed. Beyond the fact that it is an invasive technique, other disadvantages are related with poor depth tissue penetration and lack of contrast agents. However, it is a powerful technique for detecting neoplastic formation in the gastrointestinal tract and is expected to be a helpful tool for infectious disease diagnosis.

PET and SPECT systems enable molecular and cell/tissue 3D visualization to be widely applied in clinical diagnosis and research studies. Studies supported by these techniques should allow the development of new therapies, such as immuno- and gene therapies, cell trafficking, infectious diseases, and cancer. PET and SPECT are very sensitive techniques that allow sections of a body to be imaged independently of physical properties and, therefore, there seems to be no limit to the range of applications. The reasons for this versatility are related to the availability of many different probes and of reporter molecules to target each kind of molecule. Both modalities allow more comprehensive knowledge to be gained regarding animal physiology by means of dynamic studies (4D) that consist of the in vivo measurement of parameters such as metabolic and transport rates. The drawbacks of these techniques are related to the temporal and spatial resolution limitations, employment of ionizing gamma rays, lack of anatomical information and the elevated cost of the detections systems.

As described so far, all the techniques present advantages and limitations, and no modality can image all of the anatomical structure and functional processes of live, higher-order organisms (Qin et al., 2010). To overcome the individual limitations of each system, strategies that combine two or more modalities have been proposed. For instance MRI and CT provide anatomical information that can complete the functional information generated by PET, SPECT, and optical imaging. Multimodality approaches can open new frontiers in the study of cancer in small animals that provide efficient evaluation of new treatments (Dufort et al., 2010) and can reduce the amount of animals required for research studies by multidata acquisition. The complexity of infection processes can be better understood using optical imaging to monitor in vivo pathogen dynamics and, at the same time, obtain information about host gene expression and host physiologic and anatomic changes, during the infection progress, by combination with other modalities (Andreu et al., 2011). This may also be a particularly interesting technique for monitoring the way the human body accepts an implant made out with bioinspired materials.

Molecular imaging will be improved through the development of new biomedical probes, reporter molecules and delivery systems supported by bioinspired materials, together with the development of new imaging systems and algorithms. As the technology progresses, imaging systems are expected to bring extraordinary advances in spatial and temporal resolution, tissue penetration, sensitivity, throughput, and cost-effectiveness.

Acknowledgments

This work was financially supported by: Project POCI-01-0145-FEDER-006939 (Laboratory for Process Engineering, Environment, Biotechnology and Energy—LEPABE) funded by FEDER funds through COMPETE2020—Programa Operacional Competitividade e Internacionalização (POCI)—and by national funds through FCT—Fundação para a Ciência e a Tecnologia; Project PEst-C/EQB/UI0511, NORTE-07-0124-FEDER-000025—RL2_Environment&Health and Project "DNA mimics" PIC/IC/82815/2007; and Postdoctoral Fellowship [SFRH/BPD/78846/2011].

The complete affiliation for all authors is as follows: Laboratory for Process Engineering, Environment, Biotechnology and Energy (LEPABE), Department of Chemical Engineering, Faculty of Engineering, of the University of Porto, Porto, Portugal. N.M. Guimarães is also affiliated to IPATIMUP, Institute of Molecular Pathology and Immunology of the University of Porto, Porto, Portugal and i3S, Instituto de Investigação e Inovação em Saúde, Universidade do Porto, Porto, Portugal.

References

Abbaci, M., Breuskin, I., Casiraghi, O., Leeuw, F., Ferchiou, M., Temamc, S., Laplace-Builhé, C., 2014. Confocal laser endomicroscopy for non-invasive head and neck cancer imaging: a comprehensive review. Oral Oncol. 50, 711–716.

Andreu, N., Zelmer, A., Wiles, S., 2011. Noninvasive biophotonic imaging for studies of infectious disease. FEMS Microbiol. Rev. 35, 360–394.

Bannas, P., Lenz, A., Kunick, V., Well, L., Fumey, W., Rissiek, B., Haag, F., Schmid, J., Schütze, K., Eichhoff, A., Trepel, Martin, Adam, G., Ittrich, H., Koch-Nolte, F., 2015. Molecular imaging of tumors with nanobodies and antibodies: timing and dosage are crucial factors for improved in vivo detection. Contrast Media Mol. Imaging 10, 367–378.

Beckmann, N., Laurent, D., Tigani, B., Panizzutti, R., Rudin, M., 2004. Magnetic resonance imaging in drug discovery: lessons from disease areas. Drug Discov. Today 9 (1), 35–42.

Blasberg, R., 2002. PET imaging of gene expression. Eur. J. Cancer 38, 2137–2146.

Boczkowska, M., Guga, P., Stec, W.J., 2002. Stereodefined phosphorothioate analogues of DNA: relative thermodynamic stability of the model PS-DNA/DNA and PS-DNA/RNA complexes. Biochemistry 41, 12483–12487.

Boros, E., Gale, E.M., Caravan, P., 2015. MR imaging probes: design and applications. Dalton Trans. 44, 4804–4818.

Brock, M., 2012. Application of bioluminescence imaging for in vivo monitoring of fungal infections. Int. J. Microbiol. 2012, 1–9.

Burghardt, A.J., Link, T.M., Majumdar, S., 2011. High-resolution computed tomography for clinical imaging of bone microarchitecture. Clin. Orthop. Relat. Res. 469, 2179–2193.

Cerqueira, L., Azevedo, N.F., Almeida, C., Jardim, T., Keevil, C.W., Vieira, M.J., 2008. DNA mimics for the rapid identification of microorganisms by fluorescence in situ hybridization (FISH). Int. J. Mol. Sci. 9, 1944–1960.

Chen, K., Conti, P.S., 2010. Target-specific delivery of peptide-based probes for PET imaging. Adv. Drug Deliv. Rev. 62, 1005–1022.

Chen, L., Wang, Y., Cheng, D., Liu, X., Dou, S., Liu, G., Hnatowich, D.J., Rusckowski, M., 2013. ^{99m}Tc-MORF oligomers specific for bacterial ribosomal RNA as potential specific infection imaging agents. Bioorg. Med. Chem. 21, 6523–6530.

Choi, H.S., Liu, W., Liu, F., Nasr, K., Misra, P., Bawendi, M.G., Frangioni, J.V., 2010. Design considerations for tumor-targeted nanoparticles. Nat. Nanotechnol. 5, 42–47.

Delač, M., Motaln, H., Ulrich, H., Lah, T.T., 2015. Aptamer for imaging and therapeutic targeting of brain tumor glioblasto. Cytometry A 87A, 806–816.

Dufort, S., Sancey, L., Wenk, C., Josserand, V., Coll, J.L., 2010. Optical small animal imaging in the drug discovery process. Biochim. Biophys. Acta 1798, 2266–2273.

Dunbar, K.B., Canto, M.I., 2010. Confocal endomicroscopy. Tech. Gastrointest. Endosc. 12, 90–99.

Eliahou, R., Hidas, G., Duvdevani, M., Sosna, J., 2010. Determination of renal stone composition with dual-energy computed tomography: an emerging application. Semin. Ultrasound CT 31, 315–320.

Farkhani, S.M., Valizadeh, A., 2014. Review: three synthesis methods of CdX (X = Se, S or Te) quantum dots. IET Nanobiotechnol. 8 (2), 59–76.

Farrar, C.T., William, C.M., Hudry, E., Hashimoto, T., Hyman, B.T., 2014. RNA aptamer probes as optical imaging agents for the detection of amyloid plaques. PLoS One 9 (2), 1–8.

Fass, L., 2008. Imaging and cancer: a review. Mol. Oncol. 2, 115–152.

Filonov, G.S., Piatkevich, K.D., Ting, L., Zhang, J., Kim, K., Verkhusha, V.V., 2011. Bright and stable near-infrared fluorescent protein for in vivo imaging. Nat. Biotechnol. 29 (8), 757–761.

Fontenete, S., Leite, M., Guimarães, N., Madureira, P., Ferreira, R.M., Figueiredo, C., Wengel, J., Azevedo, N.F., 2015. Towards fluorescence in vivo hybridization (FIVH). Detection of *H. pylori* in gastric mucosa using advanced LNA probes. PLoS One 10 (4), e0125494.

Fontenete, S., Leite, M., Cappoen, D., Santos, R., Ginneken, C.V., Figueiredo, C., Wengel, J., Cos, P., Azevedo, N.F., 2016. Fluorescence in vivo hybridization (FIVH) for detection of *Helicobacter pylori* infection in a C57BL/6 mouse model. PLoS One 11 (2), e0148353.

Frangioni, J.V., Hajjar, R.J., 2004. In vivo tracking of stem cells for clinical trials in cardiovascular disease. Circulation 110, 3378–3383.

Gullberg, G.T., Reutter, B.W., Sitek, A., Maltz, J.S., Budinger, T.F., 2010. Dynamic single photon emission computed tomography—basic principles and cardiac applications. Phys. Med. Biol. 55, R111–R191.

Hernandez, R., Orbay, H., Cai, W., 2013. Molecular imaging strategies for in vivo tracking of MicroRNAs: a comprehensive review. Curr. Med. Chem. 20 (29), 3594–3603.

Hildebrandt, I.J., Gambhir, S.S., 2004. Molecular imaging applications for immunology. Clin. Immunol. 111, 210–224.

Hoff, J., 2005. Principles of quantitative positron emission tomography (Review). Amino Acids 29, 341–353.

Ibraheem, D., Elaissari, A., Fessi, H., 2014. Administration strategies for proteins and peptides. Int. J. Pharm. 477, 578–589.

Israel, O., Keidar, Z., 2011. PET/CT imaging in infectious conditions. Ann. N. Y. Acad. Sci. 1228, 150–166.

Kaur, S., Venktaraman, G., Jain, M., Senapati, S., Garg, P.K., Batra, S.K., 2012. Recent trends in antibody-based oncologic imaging. Cancer Lett. 315, 97–111.

Kelly, K.A., Waterman, P., Weissleder, R., 2006. In vivo imaging of molecularly targeted phage. Neoplasia 8 (12), 1011–1018.

Krasia-Christoforou, T., Georgiou, T.K., 2013. Polymeric theranostics: using polymer-based systems for simultaneous imaging and therapy. J. Mater. Chem. B 1, 3002–3025.

Lee, S.Y., Jeon, S.I., Jung, S., Chung, I.J., Ahn, C., 2014. Targeted multimodal imaging modalities. Adv. Drug Deliv. Rev. 76, 60–78.

Lin, M., Zhao, Y., Wang, S., Liu, M., Duan, Z., Chen, Y., Li, F., Xu, F., Lu, T., 2012. Recent advances in synthesis and surface modification of lanthanide-doped upconversion nanoparticles for biomedical application. Biotechnol. Adv. 30, 1551–1561.

Liu, R., Liu, J., Zhou, X., Jiang, G., 2011. Applications of Raman-based techniques to on-site and in-vivo analysis. Trends Anal. Chem. 30 (9), 1462–1476.

Luo, S., Zhang, E., Su, Y., Cheng, T., Shi, C., 2011. A review of NIR dyes in cancer targeting and imaging. Biomaterials 32, 7127–7138.

Maguire, C.A., Bovenberg, M.S., Crommentuijn, M.H.W., Niers, J.M., Kerami, M., Teng, J., Sena-Esteves, M., Badr, C.E., Tannous, B.A., 2013. Triple bioluminescence imaging for in vivo monitoring of cellular processes. Mol. Ther. Nucleic Acids 2, 1–9.

Marr, A., Markert, A., Annette Altmann, A., Askoxylakis, V., Haberkorn, U., 2011. Biotechnology techniques for the development of new tumor specific peptides. Methods 55, 215–222.

McArthur, C., Jampana, R., Patterson, J., Hadley, D., 2011. Applications of cerebral SPECT. Clin. Radiol. 66, 651–661.

Molenaar, C., Marras, S.A., Slats, J.C.M., Truffert, J.C., Lemaître, M., Raap, A.K., Dirks, R.W., Tanke, H.J., 2001. Linear 2′ *O*-methyl RNA probes for the visualization of RNA in living cells. Nucleic Acids Res. 29 (17), e89.

Mujić-Delić, A., Wit, R.H., Verkaar, F., Smit, M.J., 2014. GPCR-targeting nanobodies: attractive research tools, diagnostics, and therapeutics. Trends Pharmacol. Sci. 35 (5), 247–255.

Mukai, H., Ozaki, D., Cui, Y., Kuboyama, T., Yamato-Nagata, H., Onoe, K., Takahashi, M., Wada, Y., Imanishi, T., Kodama, T., Obika, S., Suzuki, M., Doi, H., Watanabe, Y., 2014. Quantitative evaluation of the improvement in the pharmacokinetics of a nucleic acid drug delivery system by dynamic PET imaging with ^{18}F-incorporated oligodeoxynucleotides. J. Control. Release 180, 92–99.

Neumann, H., Kiesslich, R., Wallace, M.B., Neurath, M.F., 2010. Confocal laser endomicroscopy: technical advances and clinical applications. Gastroenterology 139 (2), 388–392.

Nielsen, P.E., Egholm, M., 1999. An introduction to peptide nucleic acid. Curr. Issues Mol. Biol. 1 (2), 89–104.

Nielsen, P.E., Egholm, M., Berg, R.H., Buchardt, O., 1991. Sequence-selective recognition of DNA by strand displacement with a thymine-substituted polyamide. Science 254, 1497–1500.

Piel, M., Vernaleken, I., Rösch, F., 2014. Positron emission tomography in CNS drug discovery and drug monitoring. J. Med. Chem. 57, 9232–9258.

Pien, H.H., Fischman, A.J., Thrall, J.H., Sorensen, A.G., 2005. Using imaging biomarkers to accelerate drug development and clinical trials. Drug Discov. Today 10 (4), 259–266.

Portney, N.G., Ozkan, M., 2006. Nano-oncology: drug delivery, imaging, and sensing. Anal. Bioanal. Chem. 384, 620–630.

Qin, C., Zhu, S., Tian, J., 2010. New optical molecular imaging systems. Curr. Pharm. Biotechnol. 11, 620–627.

Richards-Kortum, R., 1996. Quantitative optical spectroscopy for tissue diagnosis. Annu. Rev. Phys. Chem. 47, 555–606.

Rosenblum, L.T., Kosaka, N., Mitsunaga, M., Choyke, P.L., Kobayashi, H., 2010. In vivo molecular imaging using nanomaterials: general in vivo characteristics of nano-sized reagents and applications for cancer diagnosis (Review). Mol. Membr. Biol. 27 (7), 274–285.

Santy, K., Nan, P., Chantana, Y., Laurent, D., Nadal, D., Richner, B., 2011. The diagnosis of brain tuberculoma by ^{1}H-magnetic resonance spectroscopy. Eur. J. Pediatr. 170, 379–387.

Schambach, S.J., Bag, S., Schilling, L., Groden, C., Brockmann, M.A., 2010. Application of micro-CT in small animal imaging. Methods 50, 2–13.

Schillaci, O., Filippi, L., Danieli, R., Simonetti, G., 2007. Single-photon emission computed tomography/computed tomography in abdominal diseases. Semin. Nucl. Med. 37, 48–61.

Schmidt, K.S., Borkowski, S., Kurreck, J., Stephens, A.W., Bald, R., Hecht, M., Friebe, M., Dinkelborg, L., Erdmann, V.A., 2004. Application of locked nucleic acids to improve aptamer in vivo stability and targeting function. Nucleic Acids Res. 32 (19), 5757–5765.

Smith, G.P., Petrenko, V.A., 1997. Phage display. Chem. Rev. 97, 391–410.

Stringer, M., Moghissi, K., 2004. Photodiagnosis and fluorescence imaging in clinical practice. Photodiagnosis Photodyn. Ther. 1, 9–12.

Tallury, P., Malhotra, A., Byrne, L.M., Santra, S., 2010. Nanobioimaging and sensing of infectious diseases. Adv. Drug Deliv. Rev. 62, 424–437.

Tavares, A.J., Chong, L., Petryayeva, E., Algar, W.R., Krull, U.J., 2011. Quantum dots as contrast agents for in vivo tumor imaging: progress and issues. Anal. Bioanal. Chem. 399, 2331–2342.

Tian, X., Aruva, M.R., Rao, P.S., Qin, W., Read, P., Sauter, E.R., Thakur, M.L., Wickstrom, E., 2003. Imaging oncogene expression. Ann. N. Y. Acad. Sci. 1002, 165–188.

Toy, R., Bauer, L., Hoimes, C., Ghaghada, K.B., Karathanasis, E., 2014. Targeted nanotechnology for cancer imaging. Adv. Drug Deliv. Rev. 76, 79–97.

Tung, C., 2004. Fluorescent peptide probes for in vivo diagnostic imaging. Biopolymers (Peptide Science) 76, 391–403.

Veedu, R.N., Wengel, J., 2010. Locked nucleic acids: promising nucleic acid analogs for therapeutic applications. Chem. Biodivers. 7 (3), 536–542.
Villaraza, A.J.L., Bumb, A., Brechbiel, M.W., 2010. Macromolecules, dendrimers, and nanomaterials in magnetic resonance imaging: the interplay between size, function, and pharmacokinetics. Chem. Rev. 110, 2921–2959.
Vrignaud, S., Benoit, J., Saulnier, P., 2011. Strategies for the nanoencapsulation of hydrophilic molecules in polymer-based nanoparticles. Biomaterials 32, 8593–8604.
Wang, D., Lin, B., Ai, H., 2014. Theranostic nanoparticles for cancer and cardiovascular applications. Pharm. Res. 31, 1390–1406.
Warburg, O., 1956. On the origin of cancer cells. Science 123, 309–314.
Willats, W.G.T., 2002. Phage display: practicalities and prospects. Plant Mol. Biol. 50, 837–854.
Wozniak, J.R., Lim, K.O., 2006. Advances in white matter imaging: a review of in vivo magnetic resonance methodologies and their applicability to the study of development and aging. Neurosci. Biobehav. Rev. 30, 762–774.
Yu, Y., Wang, Q., Liu, Y., Xie, Y., 2014. Molecular basis for the targeted binding of RGD-containing peptide to integrin $\alpha_V\beta_3$. Biomaterials 35, 1667–1675.
Ziegler, S.I., 2005. Positron emission tomography: principles, technology, and recent developments. Nucl. Phys. A 752, 679c–687c.

Injectable hydrogels as a delivery system for bone regeneration

9

I. Pereira, C. Rodrigues, A. Rodrigues, M. Oliveira, M. Gama
University of Minho, Braga, Portugal

9.1 Introduction

9.1.1 Bone biology

Bone is a dynamic and highly vascularized tissue that has been most appropriately referred to as the ultimate smart material for its scar-less regenerative capacity (Pirraco et al., 2010). Bone is composed of inorganic salts and an organic matrix. The organic fraction consists mainly of type I collagen fibers (around 90%) and various protein/carbohydrate complexes such as glycosaminoglycans, proteoglycans, glycoproteins, and growth factors. The inorganic part of bone consists predominantly of phosphate and calcium ions; however, significant amounts of bicarbonate, sodium, potassium, citrate, magnesium, carbonate, fluorite, zinc, barium, and strontium are also present. Calcium and phosphate ions nucleate to form the hydroxyapatite (HAP) crystals. The bone functional characteristics are defined by the collagen and mineral components. The mineral components are responsible for the matrix compression strength, whereas the collagen fibers determine the elasticity and toughness of the tissue (Florencio-Silva et al., 2015).

To carry out the diverse functions of bone formation, resorption and repair of mineral homeostasis, bone cells assume specialized forms distinguished by morphology, function, and characteristic location. Osteoblasts, osteocytes, and osteoclasts are the three main cell types that can be found in bone tissue, each one having defined functions, crucial for bone homeostasis (Fig. 9.1; Buckwalter et al., 1995; Pirraco et al., 2010). Osteoblasts are derived from mesenchymal stem cells and are responsible for bone formation, producing the organic material of the bony matrix by a process called ossification, or osteogenesis. They are responding cells, specialized to secrete the unique collagen-rich extracellular matrix (ECM), enabling mineralization of the bone tissue. An osteocyte is a mature cell that sits in bone lacunae, communicates with other osteocytes through long cellular processes, senses mechanical stress, and sends signals for bone remodeling due to mechanical stress. Finally, osteoclasts are macrophage-like cells that degrade the bone. They tunnel through bone and are usually followed close behind by osteoblasts. Bone is in a constant state of remodeling in healthy individuals (Buckwalter et al., 1995).

Bioinspired Materials for Medical Applications. http://dx.doi.org/10.1016/B978-0-08-100741-9.00009-7

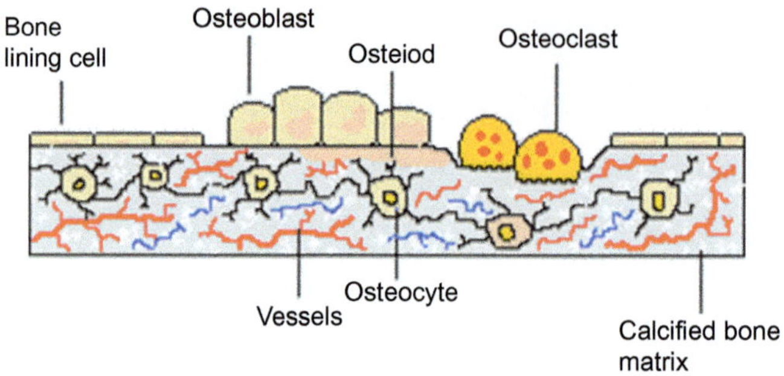

Fig. 9.1 Components of the bone tissue.

9.1.2 The need for bone grafts

Ageing and degenerative diseases are responsible for the loss and injury of biological tissues, which results in reduced quality of life and morbidity for patients, as well as a heavy burden for health systems. These are the main factors driving the need for bone graft substitutes (BGSs), which has dramatically increased in the last decade. A wide range of materials are considered, from ceramics to polymers, from cements to injectable solutions. Every year, roughly 2 million patients worldwide undergo a bone grafting procedure to repair bone defects stemming from a disease or a traumatic event, such as large bone tumors, defects, fractures, and nonunions (Greenwald et al., 2001).

To address the need for intervention in these cases, many materials are currently in use to repair or replace bone. Autografts and allogenic grafts are routinely used in the clinic. The autograft (a bone graft harvested from the patient) provides not only a scaffold but also a certain number of osteoblasts, bearing the best osteogenic effect. Therefore it is considered the gold standard for bone defect repair (Bauer and Muschler, 2000). However, both the need of a second surgery and morbidity at the extraction site have been incentives to search for alternative treatments (Younger and Chapman, 1989). Bone allograft is another way of providing a scaffold for bone regeneration, obtained from human cadavers or living donors, which bypasses the problems associated with harvesting and quantity of graft material. Nevertheless, it may represent a high risk of disease transmission and some medical ethics issues may also limit the clinical application of allogeneic bone graft (De Long et al., 2007). These limitations have spurred the search for the optimal artificial bone substitute material to overcome some of these current issues (Kregar-Velikonja et al., 2012). Furthermore, the ease of use of the product and patient recovery is of particular concern to the surgeon who is responsible for the bone-grafting procedure.

The lack of effective treatments for the identified clinical needs motivates the current trend in the development of synthetic graft substitutes. Numerous synthetic bone substitutes (SBSs) are commercially available and are presented in block or particulate form, with relatively few nonsetting BGSs being injected to a defect and shaped in situ (Bhandari, 2012). A BGSs should be osteoinductive (promote the differentiation of primitive, undifferentiated, and pluripotent cells to an osteoblastic lineage), should exhibit osteoconductivity (the process by which bone cells grow in the surface of a foreign material), should be capable of osseointegration (material's integration by bone tissue without the formation of fibrous tissue at the bone–material interface) (Stevens, 2008), and, finally, should gather physicochemical and mechanical properties similar to native bone tissue. Furthermore, it should be biocompatible and resorbable. To date, no synthetic material meets all these requirements.

The synthetic products target the fast-growing global orthobiologics market, which is predicted to reach $9.6 billion in 2016 and will be worth $15.3billion by 2022 (compound annual growth rate (CAGR) of 12%). The largest sector in orthobiologics, in 2010, was the BGS segment, accounting for 41.6% of the global market (PRNewswire, 2012). BGS will remain the largest segment of the orthobiologics market and is foreseen to continue very attractive and growing worldwide. Globally, this market was valued at $1.9 billion in 2010 and is expected to reach $3.3 billion in 2017 with a CAGR of 8.3%. The high number of surgical procedures performed yearly and the increased preference for SBSs as replacements or complementary to autograft/allografts justify the orthobiologic market's growing trend (PRNewswire, 2012).

To summarize, the large increase in active elderly people has dramatically raised the need for load-bearing BGS. Strategies applied in the last 4 decades towards this goal have failed (Bohner, 2010a). Therefore it is imperative to develop superior/advanced biomaterials and therapeutics for osteoregenerative medicine. The challenge lies in the difficulty in accomplishing the functional sophistication of viable synthetic tissue regeneration scaffolds (e.g., physical properties enabling easy surgical handling and stable graft fixation, structural and biomechanical properties facilitating its tissue integration, biocompatibility ensuring long-term safety) within an easy-to-fabricate biomaterial that can be reproducibly manufactured at low cost.

9.2 SBSs based on ceramics

Several synthetic materials for bone substitution have been developed and characterized during the last few decades. Different approaches have been used for the design of bone substitute materials. Most are formulated as granules of different sizes or porous blocks (or sponges). The aim of this section is to provide an overview of the currently available ceramic bone substitutes.

Ceramics are the best-studied bone substitute materials due to their chemical and structural similarity to the mineral phase of bone tissue. Ceramic-based materials began to gain extreme popularity for biomedical applications in the late 1960s. The huge advance in knowledge and technology during the last 40 years has caused ceramics to be universally appreciated in terms of biocompatibility, osteoconductivity and bioactivity, and nowadays they are used in several applications in orthopaedic and craniofacial surgery (Bohner, 2010a; El-Ghannam, 2005). Ceramic-based products include materials, such as calcium phosphate (CaP), calcium sulfate (CaS), and bioactive glass (BG), used alone or in combination with other grafts. Among these materials, those based on CaP are the most attractive (Heini and Berlemann, 2001; Schnürer et al., 2003; Vaccaro and Madigan, 2002). Currently, the most common types of CaP ceramics used as SBS are porous HAP, β-tricalcium phosphate (β-TCP), their derivatives or a combination of both, such as biphasic calcium phosphate (BCP) (Dorozhkin, 2010; Navarro et al., 2008). CaPs are bioactive, biodegradable, and osteoconductive. In spite of these positive attributes, inherent brittleness and relatively slow degradation limit their clinical application as SBS materials. Moreover, they have no osteogenic or osteoinductive properties (Eniwumide et al., 2007; Gupta et al., 2015).

HAP-, β-TCP-, and BCP-based products are available in granular or powder form, as well as in compact and porous form (blocks). Nevertheless, as typical ceramics, they are hard and rigid, and therefore are not easy to handle and to fit into the surgical sites, leaving empty spaces between bone tissues and the filling material. In fact, with ceramic granular bone substitutes it is very difficult to fill the defect cavities, namely in a bleeding situation, because the granules can be washed out by the blood stream and, consequently, migration of granular particles to the surrounding tissues occurs, which can cause adverse events. Also, sedimentation of the granules is yet another issue and, as a result, the distribution of the granules in the defect cavity is very irregular (Bohner, 2010a; Bongio et al., 2010; Navarro et al., 2008). In the case of ceramic blocks, they cannot be shaped intraoperatively, which means that they can only be worked into different forms to a limited extent. Moreover, they usually exhibit poor mechanical properties (Bohner et al., 2005; Chow, 2009).

The limitations previously described suggest the need for various handling requirements to promote a reliable and safe clinical application. In fact, easy handling is of paramount importance for the commercial success of bone substitute materials. Thus, the current challenge to potentiate the clinical application of the ceramic-based SBS lies on the development of injectable bone substitutes (IBSs), in which a binder or gel is added to the granules.

9.3 Ceramic-based IBSs commercially available

The development of IBSs has garnered great importance in the field of bone regeneration therapies, as a unique therapeutic method to reach areas of the body using minimally invasive procedures, and showing the ability to conform to any shape irrespective of the defect geometry. Furthermore, IBSs can be used as a filler to reinforce the mechanical properties of diseased/injured bone and as a competent carrier of cells and therapeutic agents, such as drugs and growth factors (Ifkovits and Burdick, 2007; Kretlow et al., 2007; Temenoff and Mikos, 2000).

With respect to ceramic-based IBSs, research and the market have mainly focused on CaP cements and polymeric solutions with granules incorporated to obtain pastes/putties. These systems can be applied to the bone defects using a syringe (Bohner, 2010b; Bongio et al., 2010, 2012).

9.3.1 CaP bone cements

CaP cements are essentially mixtures of CaP powders and aqueous solutions. The powder and the liquid are mixed in an appropriate ratio prior to implantation to form a paste that subsequently hardens at body temperature within several minutes. Once injected, the CaP paste forms a low-crystallinity HAP that can be absorbed over time (Bohner, 2010b; Khan et al., 2008; Navarro et al., 2008). Some commercial CaP cements available on the market are listed in Table 9.1.

Table 9.1 Commercial CaP cements and their clinical application

Commercial cement	Company	Application
Norian SRS	Synthes Inc.	Bone fractures
ChronOs inject	Synthes Inc.	Bone remodeling and cyst treatment
HydroSet	Stryker Inc.	Bone void filler
BoneSource	Stryker Inc.	Bone void filler for trauma and reconstructive surgery
Calcibon	Biomet Inc.	Bone fractures
Callos	Skeletal Kinetics LLC	Bone void filler

A very important handling property of cements is their hardening rate, in addition to the denominated setting rate. This feature can directly affect the clinical procedure, because a too early setting reaction limits the period during which the surgeon can apply the cement, whereas a too late setting reaction prevents the surgeon from closing the defect and therefore increases the overall procedure duration (Bohner, 2010a).

Only a few drawbacks are associated with CaP cements, such as: (i) a lack of paste cohesion may prevent setting and lead to negative in vivo reactions due to the release and migration of microparticles to the surrounding tissues (Bohner, 2010a,b); (ii) inadequate hydraulic properties, that is, inability to flow easily under pressure through a cannula attached to the syringe (Bohner, 2010b; Low et al., 2010); and (iii) an absence of adequate porosity, which compromises cell ingrowth (Gauthier et al., 1998).

Most of the presently available CaP cements are in the form of a powder and a liquid that are mixed immediately before use. In the clinical scenario, the ability of the surgeon to properly mix and inject the cement in the defect within the prescribed time is a crucial factor. In this context, premixed cements have been described. However, these premixed formulations tend to have poor mechanical properties and have a relatively short shelf-life (Carey et al., 2005; Xu et al., 2007).

9.3.2 Injectable polymer–ceramic composites

Polymers are increasingly gaining interest in terms of the development of injectable matrices for tissue engineering and regenerative medicine applications. Polymer injectable formulations, such as polymeric viscous solutions or hydrogels, provide the ability to conform to the cavity in which they are placed; therefore they can fill irregular defects (Liu and Ma, 2004).

The polymeric materials used in the biomedical field and particularly in bone regeneration applications may be of natural or synthetic origin. These, in turn, can be divided further into degradable and nondegradable. Natural polymers can be considered as the first biodegradable biomaterials used clinically. They can mimic the endogenous ECM, playing critical biological functions, for example, display cell adhesion motifs or antimicrobial properties. On the other hand, the surrounding tissues can recognize and metabolize their degradation products through common pathways. Some of the most commonly used materials include chitosan, collagen, hyaluronic acid (HA), alginate, cellulose, gelatin, and starch. However, some natural polymers can cause immunological responses, present variability among different supply sources, and may offer inferior mechanical properties to synthetic polymers (Laurencin et al., 2014; Nair and Laurencin, 2007; Yannas, 2004). In turn, synthetic polymers present certain properties (e.g., porosity, degradation time, and mechanical characteristics) that can be tailored for specific applications. They are often cheaper than biologic scaffolds, can be produced in large amounts with uniform and reliable properties and have a long shelf-life. Despite these advantages, they can lead to toxicity or chronic inflammation and exhibit a lack of bioactivity (Gunatillake et al., 2006; Liu et al., 2013; Ma, 2004; Okamoto and John, 2013).

Polymer/ceramic composites have attracted much attention. In this approach, hydrosoluble polymers, such as hydroxypropylmethylcellulose (HPMC) and collagen, are considered to be merely carriers for ceramic granules, in which particles are suspended in physiological fluids containing the polymer. Then, the viscous solution allows the injectability of the granules without phase separation (Bohner, 2010b). Moreover, the combination of polymers and ceramic phases enhances the morphological and functional properties of the scaffolds: ceramic granules support bone healing by osteoconduction, while the polymer provides intergranular spaces for bone ingrowth and ensures the attachment of granules in the bone defect (Daculsi et al., 2010, 2011).

Usually, ceramic-only scaffolds are prepared via high temperature sintering to ensure strength and stability, crippling the incorporation of biochemical agents, such as drugs and/or growth factors, and hampering replication of any biomimetic process, such as co-deposition and co-precipitation, that occurs in the physiological environment during natural bone regeneration (Sarkar and Lee, 2015). Their combination with hydrosoluble polymers can overcome such limitation.

Some of pastes/putties based on granular ceramic–polymer conjugation available on the market are listed in Table 9.2.

Regarding the application procedure, the IBS products may be divided into two main classes: the premixed (ready-to-use) and in situ mixing formulations (the mixture occurs immediately before surgery). Premixed products provide some advantages, namely simple application, because they do not require any mixing on transfer into an appropriate delivery system (ready-to-use formulations). However, they present limitations in clinical practice, including the low versatility, since the mixture composition is already predefined. For example, these products do not have the ability to incorporate other bioactive agents (osteogenic factors, cells) (Bohner, 2010b). In addition, premixed formulations are presented in the form of "viscous

Table 9.2 Injectable bone substitutes based on granular ceramic–polymer conjugation

Company	Product	Composition	Commercial form
ApaTech (UK)	Actifuse	HAP, polymer and aqueous solution	Premixed
Biomatlante (France)	In'Oss	BCP granules (60% HAP, 40% β-TCP; 80–200 m) and 2% HPMC	Premixed
DePuy Spine (USA)	Healos Fx	HAP (20–30%) and collagen	In situ mixing
Therics (USA)	Therigraft Putty	β-TCP granules and polymer	Premixed
Integra LifeSciences (USA)	Integra Mozaik Putty	β-TCP granules and collagen	Premixed

pastes," which hinders the adjustment of its viscosity to targeted therapeutic procedures for each clinical condition.

In situ mixing formulations combine the powder(s) with the polymeric solution(s) just before use. This approach is more cumbersome, but also more versatile than the premixed products since it allows the addition of various components (drugs, cells). Moreover, it is generally easier to process the liquid and the solid components individually. For instance, polymers and ceramics may require different sterilization methods, thus this kind of products overcome technical issues related to premixed ones (Bohner, 2010a).

Although current pastes and putties based on polymers have shown good biocompatibility and convenient rheological properties for injection, they are nonhardening (Table 9.2), which impairs the composite mechanical stability, so that the viscous suspension shows a tendency to flow after implantation in vivo (Fatimi et al., 2008). Moreover, some pastes/putties, particularly premixed formulations, are brittle and create string-like fragments, failing to fill the defect correctly. Therefore self-hardening composites have been investigated for the development of a new generation of IBSs. Hydrogels have been appointed as the best candidates to produce such formulations. In the next section the potential of hydrogels for the development of new ceramic-based IBSs is discussed.

9.4 IBSs based on hydrogels

Hydrogels are 3D, crosslinked networks of hydrophilic polymers swollen with a large amount of water or biological fluids without dissolving. These can be produced through chemical or physical crosslinking of polymers. The chemically crosslinked hydrogels can be further divided into several types, according to the kind of reaction or catalyst used: radical polymerization, chemical reaction of complementary groups, high-energy irradiation, and enzyme catalysed. Within the physically crosslinked hydrogels, we can find those stabilized through ionic interactions, crosslinked from amphiphilic blocks and graft copolymers. Hydrogel properties depend on the chemical composition, crosslinking density, and hydrophobicity (Geckil et al., 2010; Hoare and Kohane, 2008). Hydrogels can be formed from both natural and synthetic polymers, with advantages and disadvantages for each case, as well as from hybrid combinations, which can mitigate some disadvantages of the individual components (Kim et al., 2011; Zhu and Marchant, 2011).

Generally, hydrogels are biocompatible, biodegradable, and mimic many of the properties of the native ECM, namely high water content and viscoelastic mechanical properties, functional activity as provisional artificial support for cells and lack of mechanical strength. They display porosity and interconnectivity, enabling the transport of nutrients, gas diffusion, and removal of metabolic wastes; they can also perform as carriers of growth factors or cells and as drug-delivery systems. Moreover, hydrogels can be injectable, enabling less invasive clinical procedures, and can conform to the shape of the surface to which they are applied (Drury and Mooney, 2003; Geckil et al., 2010; Hoare and Kohane, 2008).

The first goal when incorporating ceramics into a hydrogel is to ensure the granules' cohesiveness during injection and after implantation into the bone defect. Hydrogels can also serve as space-holders to prevent granule packing and allow easier bone ingrowth (Fellah et al., 2006; Trojani et al., 2006). In recent years, the ability of different types of injectable hydrogels to homogeneously incorporate various types of ceramics has been demonstrated (Table 9.3). For instance, Morais et al. (2013a) developed an alginate-based hydrogel able to envelope and aggregate granules with 500–1000 μm, allowing a good handling and facile injectability. However, most reports use hydrogels as an injectable carrier of nanoceramics (Table 9.3). The crosslinking density of hydrogels is the main responsible for the maintenance of the granules' cohesiveness and prevention of their washout in the biological fluids.

However, an equilibrium between crosslinking density, mechanical properties, and hydrogel degradation should be found in order to achieve a better in vivo bone ingrowth. For instance, HPMC is currently used as a carrier of BCP granules (MBCP Gel and In'Oss) (Daculsi et al., 2011; Seris et al., 2013). However, the viscous suspension shows a tendency to flow after implantation in vivo. The long-term flow was suppressed by using a silated HPMC (Si-HPMC), which resulted in a crosslinked hydrogel. The strength of the crosslinked Si-HPMC hydrogel was sufficient to maintain the BCP granules in the bone defects (Fellah et al., 2006), since the use of silane improved the rheological and mechanical stability of the composite (Fatimi et al., 2008). On the other hand, because of the higher density after reticulation, cell colonization followed by bone tissue ingrowth was delayed over time with Si-HPMC, as compared to the HPMC without gelation (Daculsi et al., 2010, 2011).

Besides acting as binders for ceramic particles and providing injectability, hydrogels within these composites can contribute to obtain suitable scaffolds able to mimic the natural functions/structure of the bone. For example, the ceramics mimic bone's inorganic phase, providing mechanical properties (stiffness and mechanical strength) and nanotopographic features, while hydrogel provides toughness and elasticity, as the bone

ECM, and creates intergranular spaces for fluid penetration, cell colonization and bone ingrowth. The interconnected pore structure, typical of hydrogels, is maintained intact after incorporation of ceramics, without significant changes in pore size (Dhivya et al., 2015; Fu et al., 2009, 2012; Gaharwar et al., 2011; Gao et al., 2013; Liu et al., 2015; Moreira et al., 2016; Ni et al., 2012; Niranjan et al., 2013; Sadat-Shojai et al., 2015).

Moreover, by combining the advantages of hydrogels and ceramics, synergetic effects are generated which, in the ideal case, are able to counteract individual material's disadvantages. For instance, the combination of bioactive properties of ceramics with the elastomeric properties of hydrogels, results in composites with higher extensibilities, fracture stresses, compressive strengths, and toughness (Gaharwar et al., 2011; Gao et al., 2013; Han et al., 2013; Killion et al., 2013, 2014a,b; Nguyen et al., 2014). Killion et al. (2013) and Ni et al. (2014) by incorporation of BG and acellular bone matrix granules, were able to overcome the inherent brittleness typically associated with this kind of granules. The improved mechanical strength of the composites has been attributed to two factors: physical interaction between polymer–ceramic and reduction in swelling degree (Gaharwar et al., 2011; Killion et al., 2013, 2014a,b). Besides the space-filling effect, ceramic particles can act as physical crosslinking points that reinforce the hydrogel and, consequently, reduce the degree to which it swells. However, high loadings of ceramics can disturb the crosslinked structure of hydrogel and negatively affect mechanical performance (Han et al., 2013; Killion et al., 2014b).

9.4.1 In situ gelation hydrogels for IBSs

One of the major advantages in using hydrogels to develop IBS is its ability to gel in situ in response to external physical or chemical stimuli, as temperature, pH, or light (stimuli-responsive hydrogel). Thus, the in situ forming hydrogels with ceramics incorporated can be administered as flowable viscous liquids (sol state) into the bone defect and then turn into standing hydrogels (gel state). The mechanical stability and integrity are achieved by subsequent triggered network formation (He et al., 2008). Therefore in situ gelation hydrogels facilitate the mixing/manipulation of granules and their injectability using minimally invasive methods, are able to mold perfectly to the shape of bone defects, are suitable for delivery of cells and other bioactive agents, and can be prepared during surgery, under aseptic conditions. Since injectable and in situ crosslinking hydrogels can overcome the main drawbacks inherent in current IBS (cements, pastes, putties), they have been intensively studied. Table 9.3 summarizes the different in situ gelation systems investigated to incorporate diverse ceramics.

Thermosensitive hydrogels constitute an interesting system, since they avoid using any noxious substances as initiators of sol–gel transition (such as the pH adjustments, oxidants, or UV light) owing to the sensitivity to the temperature. Currently, reported thermogelling systems include chitosan in presence of β-glycerophosphate, which is responsible for the chitosan solubility at neutral pH and room temperature (Chen et al., 2012a,b; Couto et al., 2009; Dhivya et al., 2015; Gao et al., 2013; Huang et al., 2011a,b,c; Moreira et al., 2016) and poly(ethylene glycol)–poly(ε-caprolactone)–poly(ethylene glycol) (PEG–PCL–PEG) (Fu et al., 2009, 2012; Ni et al., 2012, 2014). These hydrogels undergo sol–gel transition at body temperature.

Other authors have been testing photo-crosslinked hydrogels based on PEG (Gaharwar et al., 2011; Killion et al., 2013, 2014a,b) and gelatin derivatives (Sadat-Shojai et al., 2015) (Table 9.3). The incorporation of di(meth)acrylate groups into the PEG chains and methacrylate groups into gelatin allows the formation of hydrogel network upon UV light. Photopolymerization has several advantages over conventional polymerization techniques, such as spatial and temporal control over polymerization, fast curing rates (less than a second to a few minutes) at room or physiological temperatures, and minimal heat production (Nguyen and West, 2002). Furthermore, it can be carried out in the presence of cells and proteins/drugs without compromising its viability/bioactivity (Killion et al., 2014a,b; Sadat-Shojai et al., 2015).

Chemical and ionic crosslinking hydrogels can also be formed in situ. As these types of hydrogels are generally composed by two components (polymer and crosslinking agent, or polymers modified with chemically complementary groups) they can easily be mixed by the surgeon under aseptic conditions and injected. In other words, initially there are two solutions and the ceramics can be dispersed in one or in both solutions; such solutions can be loaded into interconnected syringes (Martínez-Álvarez et al., 2013; Stenfelt et al., 2014) or into the separate chambers of a dual syringe system (Cardoso et al., 2014; Hulsart-Billström et al., 2011) for mixing and posterior injection. Such devices are available for this purpose and commercialized, for example, by MEDMIX and Nordson Corporation.

After mixing the formulation, the crosslinking process starts, the mixed solution becomes more viscous over time as it gels. The gelation process will finish in situ. Authors have reported gelling times from seconds to several minutes for this kind of composite hydrogels (Table 9.3). Surgeons generally advise 5–30 min as a suitable gelation time (Tan et al., 2009). This type of hydrogel can also be used as ready-to-use injectable formulations (as pastes or putties), however its properties can change over time.

In a subcutaneous assay, Stenfelt et al. (2014) evaluated the effect of the crosslinking period on mechanical and biological properties of HA-based hydrogel crosslinked via hydrazone linkage, loaded with HAP and BMP-2 (bone morphometric protein-2). Three preincubation times that resulted in slightly (1 min), moderately (5 h) and fully cured (3 days) hydrogels at the time of their injection were compared. It was observed that longer preincubation times gave rise to an increase in bone volume, corresponding to a lower bone density, and changed BMP-2 release profiles, as well as its activity. The extrusion of 3 days incubated hydrogels through the needle, during injection, created thin string-like fragments, which fused together to form a compact scaffold, providing increased mechanical stability to these hydrogels. The authors suggested the use of different preincubations times according to the clinical requirements.

Alginate has been used to prepare in situ crosslinking hydrogels incorporating various types of ceramics in the presence of calcium ions (Table 9.3). Such ions can be provided by an extraneous calcium solution (Liu et al., 2015; Morais et al., 2013a,b; Tan et al., 2009, 2010) or from the dissolution of the ceramics (Cardoso et al., 2014; Han et al., 2013) in the presence of D-gluconic acid δ-lactone, which accelerates the release of calcium from ceramics. Amosi et al. (2012) developed a ionic crosslinking hydrogel based on synthetic acidic peptide Pro-Asp-(Phe-Asp)$_5$-Pro (P_{FD}-5) whose gelation is triggered by calcium ions. The authors reported an improvement in bone regeneration, due to its ability to maintain the calcium ions at the defect, where they are utilized in the new bone formation and control their availability and release.

pH-sensitive hydrogels have also been reported for the development of new IBS, particularly Si-HPMC (Fellah et al., 2006; Sohier et al., 2010; Struillou et al., 2011; Trojani et al., 2006; Table 9.3). Dissolution of Si-HPMC takes place in a strong basic medium. Hydrogel formation occurred by adding an acidic buffer to achieve both final physiological osmotic pressure and pH.

9.4.2 IBSs based on hydrogels with additional bioactivity

Hydrogels can also modulate cell colonization, as well as the healing process, since they can act as scaffolds and carriers of bioactive agents and cells. This is mainly the case of in situ crosslinking hydrogels. Although ceramic particles provide osteoconductivity to the composite, the hydrogel may incorporate other biomaterials/particles allowing the development of IBSs with improved cell adhesion, osteoinductivity, and osteointegration, as well as with antimicrobial properties (Table 9.3).

One strategy to improve the hydrogel's cell adhesion relies on the use of a naturally derived polymer with cell adhesion sites, particularly ECM components (proteins/peptides, HA). For instance, in order to improve cell adhesion and protein adsorption in an alginate hydrogel, Morais et al. (2013a,b) associated chitosan or hyaluronate to alginate. Besides providing cell adhesion cues, natural polymers display other biological functions. HA, for example, is a nonsulfated glycosaminoglycan present in ECM, which is involved in many biological processes, such as the embryonic development, morphogenesis, tissue organization, wound healing, cell signaling (Burdick and Prestwich, 2011), and inhibition of osteoclast differentiation (Chang et al., 2007). Many chemical modifications have been introduced on the HA chain in order to form crosslinking-based hydrogels, and it has been demonstrated that its bioactivity can be conserved (Burdick and Prestwich, 2011; Collins and Birkinshaw, 2013).

The incorporation of BMP-2 into composite hydrogels has been carried out in order to improve osteoinduction (Table 9.3). Hydrogels can often be combined with proteins without inducing denaturation, providing protection from degradation and allowing for prolonged release. Besides HAP, BG, and other ceramic materials, especially nanosized particles, are known to be specifically prone to protein adsorption, and may thus perform as carriers of therapeutic proteins (Utech and Boccaccini, 2016).

Successful outcomes have been reported in preclinical assays, resulting from combination of injectable hydrogel with nanoHAP and BMP-2. Martínez-Sanz et al. (2012) studied a HA-based hydrogel-containing nanoHAP and BMP-2 to achieve mandibular bone augmentation in rats, using a minimally invasive method. The hydrogel worked not only as a ceramic and BMP-2 carrier, but also as an expander that defines the space to be substituted by newly formed bone. The conventional approaches used for mandibular bone augmentation involve screws, plates, incisions, dissections, graft exposure, and sutures. In this study, the authors mixed the components of the hydrogel with BMP-2 and nanoHAP into syringes; the composite was injected subperiosteally through needles 25-gauge into the innate mandibular diastema. The injection procedure was quick, bloodless, and resulted in fast healing with no sign of inflammation, distress, or discomfort. After 8 weeks, newly formed bone was observed and the bone volume was dependent on the concentration of BMP-2 incorporated within the hydrogel.

Martínez-Álvarez et al. (2013) used HA-based hydrogel commercially available (AuxiGel) containing nanoHAP and BMP-2 (250 μg/mL) to develop a new technique to treat congenital cleft palate, named injection/adhesion technique, which consists in two steps: (i) injection of the composite at the cleft palate margins, and (ii) direct closure of the cleft. Cleft lip and palate remains the most prevalent major facial malformation. It has major clinical implications, requiring multidisciplinary treatment throughout childhood and the current treatments (e.g., palatoplasty) display adverse effects, such as impaired mid-facial growth, with alveolar arch collapse, midface retrusion, and malocclusion. The composite hydrogel was injected into the dogs' cleft palate margins, using a needle 18-gauge. The procedure took about 30 min and was bloodless. After 4 weeks, the tested formulation had caused the cleft palate margins to reach the midline and a direct closure was carried out by the surgeon. The observed bone augmentation was primarily attributed to the swelling of the hydrogel by the hydrolytic cleavage of some of its crosslinks and by the underlying bone formation later on. In comparison with two-flap palatoplasty, the new technique based on injectable composite hydrogel was easier, reduced trauma and pain, and overlapping or bending of palatal bone did not occur (Martínez-Álvarez et al., 2013).

9.5 Regulation of medical devices: Europe versus United States

Medical devices are used for the diagnosis, monitoring, and treatment of almost every disease or condition. Due to their central role in clinical practice, medical devices require certification and registration prior to their placement on the market. Since IBSs are categorized as medical devices, they must meet certain legal requirements to be allowed to go to the market, in compliance with national and international regulations.

Recommendations and assurance of efficacy and safety that medical devices have to meet prior to marketing differ between Europe Union and United States. While the United States utilizes a centralized approach through the regulatory agency Food and Drug Administration (FDA), the European CE (*Conformité Européene*) marking process is much more decentralized, based on independent public or private organizations, designated as notified bodies. These two distinctive regulatory structures have led to a noteworthy impact in timelines and costs between Europe and United States approval process. This section describes the regulatory path of medical devices in Europe and United States, highlighting their main differences. The second part is intended to explore how these differences have been reflected specifically in the regulatory process of IBSs.

Regulatory systems for medical devices have an important role in supporting market access to technological innovations, while also ensuring the patients protection. To achieve these goals, the United States and Europe use a combination of premarket

Table 9.3 Examples of injectable bone substitutes based on in situ gelation hydrogels

Network formation	Hydrogel components	Ceramic filler	Other bioactive agents	Additional information	References
Thermally induced crosslinking	• Chitosan • β-Glycerophosphate	NanoHAP	Zinc sulfate	• Gelation in situ at body temperature in 10 min • Zinc ions provide antimicrobial activity • Accelerates bone formation in vivo (critical-sized bone defects in rat tibia)	Dhivya et al. (2015)
		HAP: $d=55\,nm$	• Dexamethasone • BMP-2	• Dexamethasone and BMP-2 loaded on the HAP through the soak-absorbed method	Gao et al. (2013)
		BG: $d=40–100\,nm$		• Gelation temperature around 37°C: it decreases with increasing of BG content • Composites, even with 40% of BG, workable in the liquid state • BG nanoparticles form well dispersed agglomerates, between 5 and 10 μm in size	Couto et al. (2009)
		BG: $d=87\pm5\,nm$	Collagen	• Injectable by an insulin syringe with ultrafine 6 mm needle • Show proper viscous behavior and flow smoothly and evenly through the needle opening	Moreira et al. (2016)
		NanoHAPC	MSC	• Injectable by a syringe with a 26-gauge needle • Gelation around 31°C • NanoHAPC uniformly disperse in the chitosan matrix • Strong and stable composite, partially thermoreversible • Show some features of natural bone both in main composition and hierarchical structure • Able to load MSC homogeneously and provide a biocompatible environment for MSC survival in vivo • MSC improve the biocompatibility and enhance new bone formation in vivo (cancellous bone defects in rabbit femurs)	Huang et al. (2009, 2011a,b,c); Chen et al. (2012a,b)

Continued

Table 9.3 Continued

Network formation	Hydrogel components	Ceramic filler	Other bioactive agents	Additional information	References
	• PEG–PCL–PEG	Acellular bone matrix: the shape and size of granules were irregular (1–20 μm)		• Composite sterilization by ^{60}Co gamma rays • Gelation in situ at body temperature in a few minutes • Reinforced hydrogel due to hydrogen bonds between polymer and acellular bone matrix • Present mild cytotoxicity to MSC (in vitro) and good biocompatibility in subcutaneous assays (mice) • Display enhanced bone regeneration guidance in rabbit calvarial defects	Ni et al. (2012, 2014)
		HAP: d=20–40 nm, l=80–120 nm	• Collagen	• Composite sterilization by ^{60}Co gamma rays • Gelation at body temperature • Hydrogen-bond formation between polymer and HAP • Enhanced cell-material interaction due to collagen • Good degradability and biocompatibility • Good performance in guided bone regeneration (rabbit calvarial defect)	Fu et al. (2009, 2012)
Photo-crosslinking	• PEG diacrylate • Photoinitiator: Irgacure 2959	HAP: d=20–70 nm		• Relative low viscosities of the precursor solutions • Strong physical crosslinking between PEG diacrylate and HAP	Gaharwar et al. (2011)
	• PEG dimethacrylate • Photoinitiator: Irgacure 2959	BG: d<45 μm		• Photopolymerization time: 10 min • Physical crosslinking between PEG dimethacrylate and BG • Do not display the inherent brittleness typically associated with BG • Suitable for cancellous bone defects, or low load bearing orthopaedic applications such as bone defect filler and coating-agent onto metallic bioimplants	Killion et al. (2013)

		HAP: $d < 45\ \mu m$	• Dexamethasone • Vancomycin	• Strong physical crosslinking between PEG dimethacrylate and HAP • Suitable for cancellous bone defects, or low load bearing defects • Vancomycin provides antimicrobial activity	Killion et al. (2014a)
		β-TCP powder	Vancomycin	• Photopolymerization time: 10 min • Physical crosslinking between PEG dimethacrylate and β-TCP • Incorporation of β-TCP accelerates vancomycin release profile • Suitable for cancellous bone defects, or low load bearing orthopaedic applications such as bone defect filler	Killion et al. (2014b)
	• Gelatin methacrylate • Photoinitiator: Irgacure 2959	HAP: $d \approx 60\ nm$		• Mechanical strength • Encapsulated preosteoblasts readily elongated, proliferated, and formed a 3D interconnected network • Suitable for low load-bearing applications	Sadat-Shojai et al. (2015)
Hydrazone crosslinking	• Aldehyde–HA • Hydrazide–polyvinyl alcohol	• Clods of HAP: $d > 100\ \mu m$ • HAP: $d = 1$–$50\ \mu m$ • NanoHAP: $d \approx 20\ nm$ • β-TCP: $d \approx 45\ nm$	BMP-2	• A dual compartment syringe system (MiniMix) was used • The hydrogel containing nanoHAP and BMP-2 induced ectopic bone formation with a higher density compared with the other groups	Hulsart-Billström et al. (2011)
		HAP: $d \approx 3.39\ \mu m$	BMP-2	• Injectable by a syringe with a 21-gauge needle • Evaluation of biological effects in hydrogels with different crosslinking duration	Stenfelt et al. (2014)
	• Aldehyde–HA • Hydrazide–HA	HAP: $d \approx 30\ nm$	BMP-2	• Gelling time: 1 min • Injected after 1 h, using 25-gauge needle • Successful bone mandibular augmentation (rats) • The increase of bone volume depends on BMP-2 concentration	Martínez-Sanz et al. (2012)

Continued

Table 9.3 Continued

Network formation	Hydrogel components	Ceramic filler	Other bioactive agents	Additional information	References
Chemical crosslinking	• AuxiGel (HA-based hydrogel)	HAP: $d \approx 30\,nm$	BMP-2	• Hydrogel components mixture using two interconnected syringes • Gelling time: 1 min • Composite injected after 3 h • Successful development of a minimally invasive procedure to treat congenital cleft palate (facial malformation)	Martínez-Álvarez et al. (2013)
Ionic crosslinking	• Alginate • Calcium chloride	Glass-reinforced HAP: $d = 500–1000\,\mu m$	• HA • Cerium(III) nitrate	• Polyelectrolyte complex formation between HA and alginate using cations as intermediate agents • Injectable using low extrusion forces • Cerium ions enhance antimicrobial activity	Morais et al. (2013a,b)
		Glass-reinforced HAP: $d = 500–1000\,\mu m$	• Chitosan	• Polyelectrolyte complex formation between chitosan and alginate • Injectable with low extrusion forces	Morais et al. (2013a)
	• Alginate • Calcium sulfate	NanoHAPC		• Promote proliferation and differentiation of MSC	Liu et al. (2015)
	• Alginate • Calcium sulfate • Trisodium phosphate	HAPC: $d = 50 \pm 6.6\,\mu m$		• Trisodium phosphate avoids an abrupt gelation process: the gelling time increases with increasing of sodium (3–47 min) • Injectability of the system tunable • Good degradability and biocompatibility	Tan et al. (2009, 2010)
	• Alginate • D-Gluconic acid δ-lactone	CaS: $d = 100–150\,\mu m$		• Gelling time can be controlled, from about 30 s to 10 min, by varying the amounts of CS and D-gluconic acid δ-lactone • Not suitable for load-bearing applications	Han et al. (2013)

	• Alginate • Glycerol • D-Gluconic acid δ-lactone	Crystalline CaP nanoparticles: (i) Monetite (ii) HAP (VPP132, AAP biomaterials)		• Dual syringe system (MEDMIX, L-system, 2.5 mm chamber, mixing tip 25 mm) used • Gelling time controlled from seconds to 10 min by varying the solubility of the CaP phase (HAP vs monetite) or the amount of D-gluconic acid δ-lactone • Composite display biocompatibility (subcutaneous assay) and osteocompatibility (rabbit femoral condyle) • Composites disintegrate upon implantation in subcutaneous or bone tissue • Not suitable for load-bearing conditions	Cardoso et al. (2014)
	• P_{FD}-5 • Calcium chloride	Two types of 150–500 μm β-TCP particles: (i) Nonporous (TCP DENTAL, Kasios) (ii) 65% porous (Cerasorb M, Curasan AG)		• Peptide hydrogel itself induce better bone regeneration in comparison to nontreated defects • The hydrogel and the ceramics act synergistically to enhance bone regeneration (rat femur defect) • Superior in vivo regeneration with hydrogels loaded with porous β-TCP • Hydrogel accelerates β-TCP dissolution and acts as a reservoir for calcium and phosphate ions	Amosi et al. (2012)
pH induced crosslinking	Si-HPMC	BCP: d=40–80 μm	MSC	• Sol–gel transition in about 30 min • Injectable using a syringe with a 18-gauge needle • Good biocompatibility (subcutaneous and intramuscular assays) • Support bone healing process (critically sized femoral defect in rabbits)	Fellah et al. (2006); Trojani et al. (2006)
Enzyme induced crosslinking	• TTeC • Horseradish peroxidase • Hydrogen peroxide	BCP: d=60–100 nm		• Gelling times within a few seconds • Strong physical interactions between chitosan and BCP surface	Nguyen et al. (2014)

Abbreviations: *HAPC,* hydroxyapatite/collagen; *MSC,* mesenchymal stem cells; *TTeC,* tyramine-tetronic-grafted chitosan copolymer.

testing and postmarket vigilance strategies; however, there are fundamental contrasts in their approaches, especially in terms of the clinical data required for premarket approval (Chai, 2000; Hines et al., 2010; Sweet et al., 2011).

9.5.1 Europe

In the European Union the legal core framework of medical devices consists of three main directives, which define the safety and performance requirements:

- Directive 90/385/EEC on active implantable medical devices (AIMDD) (1990)
- Directive 93/42/EEC on medical devices (MDD) (1993)
- Directive 98/79/EC on in vitro diagnostic medical devices (IVDMD) (1998).

It should be noted that these directives have been supplemented over time by several modifying and implementing directives, including the last technical revision brought about by Directive 2007/47/EC.

Medical devices are categorized into four classes (I, IIa, IIb, and III), according to classification rules listed in Directive 93/42/ECC (European Commission, 2012), on the basis of increasing risks associated with their intended use. The classification criteria take into consideration the following parameters:

- Intended purpose of the device
- The duration of contact with the patient
- The degree of invasiveness
- The part of the body affected by the use of the device.

Initial consideration of these factors gives a basis for further classification (which can be made by the manufacturer himself) and also determines the relevant conformity assessment procedure that must be followed by the manufacturer.[1] Table 9.4 presents the classification of medical devices according to the European regulation—Directive 93/42/ECC (European Commission, 2012).

As presented in Table 9.4, and exception made for sterile and/or measuring devices, for low risk devices (Class I) the manufacturer is allowed to self-declare conformity with the essential requirements. For medium- to high-risk devices (Classes IIa, IIb, III), the manufacturer must call on a third party to assess conformity (called a notified body). Notified bodies are European-accredited private organizations that operate independently of each other. They are responsible for undertaking the certification process of a new medical device, including the evaluation and assessment of the submitted data by manufacturers (European Commission, 2016). Currently, in the European Union, there are 74 notified bodies authorized in 25 countries to approve medical devices (Davis et al., 2011). On the other hand, postmarket surveillance functions are under the responsibility of a member state via the competent authority. Indeed, each member state is responsible for overseeing medical devices legislation. For example, in Portugal these functions are assumed by Infarmed and in the United Kingdom it is the Medicines and Health Regulatory Authority (MHRA).

[1] Manufacturer means a body responsible for the design, manufacture, packaging, and labeling of the device.

Table 9.4 Classification of medical devices in Europe

Classification	Description	Premarket requirements
Class I—low risk	Noninvasive devices that do not interact with the body; simple in design and manufacture	• Manufacturers ensure and formally declare, via a written statement, that the products meet the essential requirements of the directive • If the device includes sterile products or has a measuring function, the involvement of a notified body is needed
Class II IIa—low/medium risk	Include short- or long-term use of devices posing relatively low risk to the human body. Generally invasive but limited to natural orifices; if hazardous to a patient then it becomes a Class IIb	• A notified body must assess conformity procedure. In general, manufacturers are required to submit a dossier of relevant supporting literature (clinical and nonclinical data) to validate safety and performance requirements
IIb—medium risk	Include invasive devices that pose a relatively high risk for human body, such as respirators, dialyzers, etc.	
Class III—high risk	These devices include long-term, surgically invasive devices that may endanger the patient's life	• A notified body must assess conformity procedure. Clinical studies (focused on demonstrating safety) generally are recommended for this class of devices

Specifically for Class III devices, the assessment of conformity relies in most cases on the submission of clinical data. Nevertheless, according to European directives, manufacturers just have to demonstrate the safety and performance of devices, while evidence of effectiveness is not required at the stage of certification by a notified body. Also, specific requirements for the clinical evaluation of most devices are not available in the guidance. In fact, in most cases, the submission of robust clinical data is limited, and often the evidence submitted is from laboratory testing, literature reviews, or small clinical trials. Typically, this means nonrandomized and feasibility studies involving less than 100 patients for which the primary objective is to demonstrate safety (Fraser et al., 2011).

In the absence of such specific requirements, the manufacturer must decide which data are sufficient for CE marking (i.e., number of subjects, type of study design, primary and secondary endpoints, type and schedule of assessments, minimum patient follow-up period, among others). The notified body may be consulted prior to initiating the clinical trial to verify whether or not the protocol is designed to yield adequate data for CE marking. This dynamic led to a lack of uniform evidence requirements among notified bodies, which allow a high degree of variation and regulatory unpredictability to be applied to similar devices.

An important aspect related to the conformity assessment, is the compilation of technical documentation, also designated the CE technical dossier. The purpose of the technical file of a medical device, in the scope required by the medical devices directive, is to provide the evidence that the manufacturer meets essential requirements concerning the device in question. Although there is no template standard for the technical documentation, basically for all classes of devices it should include:

- Information on medical device classification
- General description of the device including planned variants, its operation, and intended use
- Design drawings, diagrams, or description of the production process
- Descriptions and explanations necessary to understand drawings and diagrams and operation of a medical device
- Results of physicochemical, microbiological, or other research recommended by the notified body for the given device
- Risk analysis
- Preclinical evaluation
- Clinical evaluation
- Methods of sterilization and validation report
- Labels and instructions for use
- List of harmonized standards, applied in full or in part, as well as descriptions of the solutions adopted in order to meet the essential requirements if harmonized standards have not been fully applied
- Checklist of conformity with essential requirements
- Declaration of conformity.

The designated notified body regulates CE marking and the final result of all the certification process (Fig. 9.2) is the achievement of a certificate of conformity that enables the manufacturer to apply a "CE marking" to the product. A CE mark is a guarantee of medical device certification and registration and enables access to the entire EU market (European Commission, 2012).

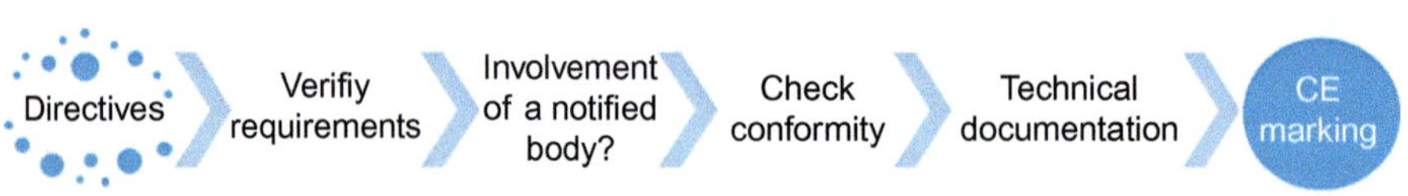

Fig. 9.2 Regulatory process for medical devices certification in Europe.

9.5.2 United States

Unlike Europe, all the aspects of registration and market approval of medical devices in the United States are under the responsibility of a single and centralized body: the Center for Devices and Radiological Health (CDRH) of the FDA. The FDA assigns medical devices to one of three regulatory classes (Classes I, II, and III) based on their intended use, whether the device is invasive or implantable, and the risk posed by the device to the user. Regulatory control increases from Class I to Class III and the manufacturer can use the FDA's classification database to determine the classification of the medical device. As presented in Table 9.5, and similar to Europe, the device classification defines the regulatory path and premarket requirements (FDA, 2014).

Table 9.5 Classification of medical devices in the United States

Classification	Description	Premarket requirements
Class I (lowest risk)	Medical devices present a simple design and manufacture and have a history of safe use.	• Most Class I devices are generally exempt from premarket notification and good manufacturing practices regulation, although their manufacturers are subject to general controls, such as device registration and listing with the FDA and labelling regulations
Class II (moderate risk)	These devices are more complex and are associated with a higher level of risk than Class I technologies	• Most Class II are devices required to clear premarket notification 510(k) requirements, which means the demonstration of substantial equivalence to another legally US marketed device • In rare cases, clinical studies are required for a 510(k) submission. In addition, other requirements may be imposed (special controls), such as special labelling requirements and mandatory postmarket surveillance
Class III (high risk)	Devices belonging to this category, usually support or sustain human life, are of substantial importance in preventing impairment of human health, or present a potential, unreasonable risk of illness or injury to the patient	• These technologies are generally required to undergo the most formal review process for devices: premarket authorization (PMA), in which a device must demonstrate safety and effectiveness through the submission of clinical studies

Since general controls are enough to assure safety and effectiveness for the most Class I devices, an FDA formal review is not required before their market introduction (Kramer et al., 2012). On the other hand, Class II devices usually are required to clear the 510(k) review, which implies that the medical device manufacturer must provide data to demonstrate that the new device is "substantially equivalent" to one legally in commercial distribution in the United States, also designated as predicate device. Substantial equivalence is established with respect to intended use, design, energy used or delivered, materials, chemical composition, manufacturing process, performance, safety, effectiveness, labelling, biocompatibility, standards, and other characteristics, as applicable. Typically, substantial equivalence can be demonstrated on the basis of bench and animal tests, although approximately 10% of 510(k) applications include clinical data (Kramer et al., 2012).

Due to the level of risk associated with Class III devices, FDA has determined that general and special controls alone are insufficient to assure its safety and effectiveness. Therefore these devices require a premarket authorization (PMA) application in order to obtain marketing clearance. Approval of the PMA requires direct evidence of safety and effectiveness in the target population, which includes the submission of preclinical and clinical studies to support claims made for the device (FDA, 2008). According to FDA, novel devices without a predicate are automatically classified as Class III, regardless of their risk profile (Kramer et al., 2012).

Comparing to Europe, the approval process for high-risk medical devices in the United States is very different, especially in terms of the scope and size of clinical trials required. As already described in the previous section, to receive approval to market a high-risk device in Europe, the manufacturer must only demonstrate that the device is safe and that it performs in a manner consistent with the manufacturer's intended use. To receive approval to market a Class III high-risk device in the United States, the manufacturer must demonstrate that the device is reasonably safe and effective, which usually requires more clinical data. Indeed, clinical development of a new Class III device is divided into pilot and pivotal trial phases. These phases typically involve prospective, randomized controlled investigations involving a considerable number of patients (Feigal et al., 2003). These differences reflect the reason why many companies obtain approval in Europe first, often many years earlier in comparison to the US market (The Boston Consulting Group, 2012; Sorrel, 2006).

In conclusion, according to FDA, there are five main steps prior to marketing a medical device in the Unites States (Fig. 9.3).

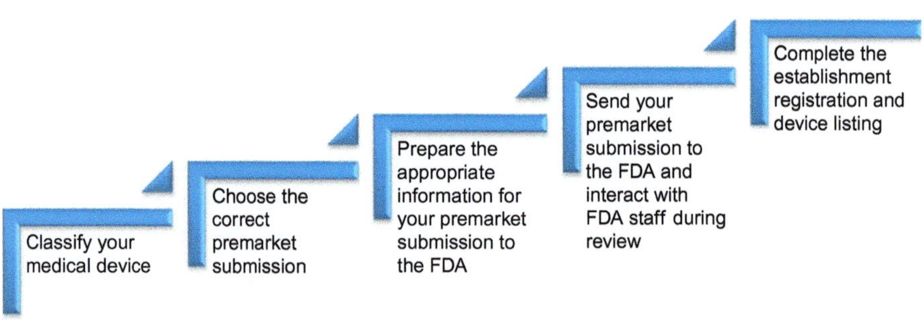

Fig. 9.3 Regulatory process for medical devices certification in the United States.

9.6 Regulatory perspective on IBSs

Bone substitutes belong to different classes (varying with composition, form, and bioactive compounds). Therefore each of these products has a distinct regulatory classification and, as such, requires a different regulatory path for approval before marketing. Specifically the main objective of this section is to provide an overview of the regulatory path for IBSs in Europe and the United States (Table 9.6).

Table 9.6 Regulatory requirements of injectable bone substitutes in Europe and the United States

Injectable bone substitutes	Europe	United States
Classification	Due to their implantable and biodegradable performance, IBS are classified as Class III devices according to the Medical Device Directive 93/42/EEC	• According to FDA, resorbable calcium salt bone void filler are Class II medical devices. Include granules, preformed block, or putty/paste intended to set ex vivo or in vivo
Premarket requirements	Conformance to the essential requirement needs to be demonstrated. Specifically, clinical studies are typically required to demonstrate the safety and performance of the device, and the risks associated with its use under normal conditions need to be minimized and acceptable in relation to the benefits to the patients As part of the regulatory approval, biocompatibility data in accordance with ISO 10993-1:2009 is required. Tests need to be performed under good laboratory practice (GLP) and generally include cytotoxicity, sensitization, irritation, systemic toxicity, pyrogenicity, genotoxicity and implantation	• Require 510(k) clearance by FDA. Therefore substantial equivalence can be demonstrated when the device has the same intended use and technological characteristics and thus is as safe and effective as the predicate device. Material characteristics, such as design, chemical composition, manufacturing process, performance, safety, biocompatibility and labelling have to be considered, whereas clinical studies are not a requisite • Thus, a manufacturer who intends to market a IBS should (i) conform to the general controls of the Federal Food, Drug & Cosmetic Act (the Act), including the premarket notification requirements described in 21 CFR 807 Subpart E, (ii) address the specific risks to health associated with the resorbable calcium salt bone void filler device, and (iii) obtain a substantial equivalence determination from FDA prior to marketing the device

Despite the regulatory differences between Europe and the United States, in general scarce information is currently available about the safety and performance of new injectable BGS. In the United States most IBSs are cleared through a less stringent process in which the new product must be shown to be equivalent to an already approved device. The concept of "substantial similarity to an already marketed device" is not objective enough, and in practice it allows a large variance in the approach taken to validate different products. Actually, these premarketing procedures can increase the risk that later studies may demonstrate that the device has no benefits or identify important adverse events that did not emerge at the time of market authorization. Nevertheless, in the United States concerns about the current system being suboptimal, which might lead to numerous device recalls and serious adverse events, have been raised. Complications have been reported from the off-label and misuse of BGS. Because products are commonly used off-label without formal data, invariably, there is an incomplete understanding of mechanism, tissue response, and proper application before patients are exposed.

9.7 Future trends/conclusions

The use of injectable bone systems in bone tissue engineering is experiencing a strong growth, and continued advances in biomaterial development and design are required to apply injectable strategies to bone regeneration. Furthermore, there is a clear trend towards a specialization of the products; indeed, companies are now designing biodegradable injectable products for specific clinical indications. To achieve these goals, an important trend in the future will be the improvement of the biological properties of IBSs, the aim being to transform a bone defect into new mature bone as fast as possible. This implies that the focus will be set on resorbable materials that possess an open-porous structure allowing cells to invade the structure. In this context, hydrogel–ceramics composites are strong candidates for bone substitutes, since these systems have the potential to embrace the role of drug-delivery systems, but also play a role in the regeneration process combining intrinsic osteogenic properties, the ability to support cells, and, potentially, gene therapeutics.

In particular, in situ gelation hydrogels have been proposed as the best candidates for the new generation of IBS, mainly due to their ability to undergo sol–gel transition in response to external physical or chemical *stimuli*. As this chapter highlights, hydrogels sensitive to, for example, temperature, pH, enzymes or UV light have been proposed for delivery of different types of ceramics (HAP, CaP, BCP, β-TCP, BG, hydroxyapatite/collagen, and acellular bone matrix particles) using minimally invasive methods. These kinds of systems (i) are able to better fill the bone defects with granules homogeneously dispersed in the matrix, improving the granules cohesiveness in the defect (in comparison to current commercial pastes and putties, these systems perform much better in this regard); (ii) facilitate the utilization of different sterilization processes, since each component of the IBS formulation can be sterilized in separate compartments; and (iii) allow the homogeneous mixture of cells and other sensitive bioactive agents with short shelf-life prior to administration. The incorporation of cells is of course not possible in ready-to-use formulations. However, further development of suitable syringes is required, since the injection device should be customized for each type of in situ gelation hydrogel, taking into consideration that incorporation of cells and other bioactive agents should be easily done by the surgeon under aseptic conditions prior to administration.

Different kinds of bone fracture and disease require different mechanical and biological properties. In order to satisfy the growing demand for products tailored for specific therapeutics, future research should explore the association and controlled release of antitumor, proangiogenic, antiosteoporotic, and analgesic drugs, as well as alternatives to BMP-2. The development of IBS-based in hydrogels for osteomyelitis (bone infections) should be also considered.

As this chapter highlights, medical devices must pass through rigorous mechanisms, for regulatory evidence. In fact, regulatory systems must provide guidelines to market for important innovation while also ensuring safeguard of public health. Certified effectiveness is perhaps the greatest challenge currently facing both the United States and European medical devices regulation. In this context, regulatory certification of an IBS as a medical device involves a meticulous developmental path from early concept to introduction into clinical practice. This review outlines that process and highlights some of the differences in the clinical and regulatory environments in the United States and Europe. Although each system has strengths and weaknesses, features of both environments require review to face the main challenges to effective medical device regulation.

References

Amosi, N., et al., 2012. Acidic peptide hydrogel scaffolds enhance calcium phosphate mineral turnover into bone tissue. Acta Biomater. 8 (7), 2466–2475. http://dx.doi.org/10.1016/j.actbio.2012.04.003.

Bauer, T., Muschler, G., 2000. Bone graft materials. An overview of the basic science. Clin. Orthop. Relat. Res. 371, 10–27. Available at: http://www.ncbi.nlm.nih.gov/pubmed/10693546.

Bhandari, M., 2012. Orthopedic medicine. In: Evidence-based orthopedics. Wiley-Blackwell/BMJ Books, Chichester, pp. 37–100. Available at: http://sgh.org.sa/Portals/0/Articles/Evidence-based Orthopedics.pdf [accessed 08.01.16].

Bohner, M., 2010a. Design of ceramic-based cements and putties for bone graft substitution. Eur. Cell. Mater. 20, 1–12.

Bohner, M., 2010b. Resorbable biomaterials as bone graft substitutes. Mater. Today 13 (1-2), 24–30.

Bohner, M., et al., 2005. Synthesis and characterization of porous beta-tricalcium phosphate blocks. Biomaterials 26 (31), 6099–6105. Available at: http://www.sciencedirect.com/science/article/pii/S0142961205002619.

Bongio, M., et al., 2010. Development of bone substitute materials: from "biocompatible" to "instructive". J. Mater. Chem. 20 (40), 8747.

Bongio, M., et al., 2012. Preclinical evaluation of injectable bone substitute materials. J. Tissue Eng. Regen. Med. http://dx.doi.org/10.1002/term.1637. Available at: http://www.ncbi.nlm.nih.gov/pubmed/23135814.

Buckwalter, J., et al., 1995. Bone biology. J. Bone Joint Surg. 77 (8), 1276–1289. Available at: http://www.academia.dk/BiologiskAntropologi/Osteologi/PDF/BoneBiology_1995.pdf (accessed 08.01.16).

Burdick, J., Prestwich, G., 2011. Hyaluronic acid hydrogels for biomedical applications. Adv. Mater. 23, 41–56.

Cardoso, D., et al., 2014. Gelation and biocompatibility of injectable alginate-calcium phosphate gels for bone regeneration. J. Biomed. Mater. Res. A 102 (3), 808–817. http://dx.doi.org/10.1002/jbm.a.34754.

Carey, L., et al., 2005. Premixed rapid-setting calcium phosphate composites for bone repair. Biomaterials 26 (24), 5002–5014. Available at: http://www.sciencedirect.com/science/article/pii/S0142961205000414.

Chai, J.Y., 2000. Medical device regulation in the United States and the European Union: a comparative study. Food Drug Law J. 55 (1), 57–80. Available at: http://www.ncbi.nlm.nih.gov/pubmed/12296349 (accessed 04.01.16).

Chang, E.-J., et al., 2007. Hyaluronan inhibits osteoclast differentiation via Toll-like receptor 4. J. Cell Sci. 120, 166–176.

Chen, Y., et al., 2012a. In vitro biocompatibility and osteoblast differentiation of an injectable chitosan/nano-hydroxyapatite/collagen scaffold. J. Nanomater. 2012, 1–6 (accessed 04.01.16).

Chen, Y., et al., 2012b. Noninvasive evaluation of injectable chitosan/nano-hydroxyapatite/collagen scaffold via ultrasound. J. Nanomater. 2012, 1–7 (accessed 04.01.16).

Chow, L., 2009. Next generation calcium phosphate-based biomaterials. Dent. Mater. J. 28 (1), 1–10.

Collins, M., Birkinshaw, C., 2013. Hyaluronic acid based scaffolds for tissue engineering—a review. Carbohydr. Polym. 92 (2), 1262–1279. http://dx.doi.org/10.1016/j.carbpol.2012.10.028.

Couto, D., Hong, Z., Mano, J., 2009. Development of bioactive and biodegradable chitosan-based injectable systems containing bioactive glass nanoparticles. Acta Biomater. 5 (1), 115–123. Available at: http://www.ncbi.nlm.nih.gov/pubmed/18835230 (accessed 05.01.16).

Daculsi, G., et al., 2010. Developments in injectable multiphasic biomaterials. The performance of microporous biphasic calcium phosphate granules and hydrogels. J. Mater. Sci. Mater. Med. 21 (3), 855–861. Available at: http://www.ncbi.nlm.nih.gov/pubmed/19882306.

Daculsi, G., et al., 2011. Scaffold effects of microporous biphasic calcium phosphate granules and role of HPMC hydrogels in injectable multiphasic bone substitute developments. Bioceram. Dev. Appl. 1, 1–4. Available at: http://www.omicsonline.com/open-access/scaffold-effects-of-microporous-biphasic-calcium-phosphate-granules-and-role-of-hpmc-hydrogels-in-injectable-multiphasic-bone-substitute-developments-2090-5025.110176.pdf (accessed 04.01.16).

Davis, S., Gilbertson, E., Goodall, S., 2011. EU medical device approval safety assessment: a comparative analysis of medical device recalls, 2005–2009. Available at: https://www.bcgperspectives.com/content/articles/medical_devices_technology_public_sector_eu_medical_device_approval_safety_assessment/ (accessed 05.01.16).

De Long, W., et al., 2007. Bone grafts and bone graft substitutes in orthopaedic trauma surgery. A critical analysis. J. Bone Joint Surg. 89 (3), 649–658. Available at: http://www.ncbi.nlm.nih.gov/pubmed/17332116.

Dhivya, S., et al., 2015. Nanohydroxyapatite-reinforced chitosan composite hydrogel for bone tissue repair in vitro and in vivo. J. Nanobiotechnol. 13, 40. Available at: http://www.pubmedcentral.nih.gov/articlerender.fcgi?artid=4464993&tool=pmcentrez&rendertype=abstract.

Dorozhkin, S., 2010. Bioceramics of calcium orthophosphates. Biomaterials 31 (7), 1465–1485. Available at: http://www.ncbi.nlm.nih.gov/pubmed/19969343 (accessed 28.10.15).
Drury, J., Mooney, D., 2003. Hydrogels for tissue engineering: scaffold design variables and applications. Biomaterials 24 (24), 4337–4351.
El-Ghannam, A., 2005. Bone reconstruction: from bioceramics to tissue engineering. Expert Rev. Med. Devices 2 (1), 87–101. Available at: http://www.ncbi.nlm.nih.gov/pubmed/16293032.
Eniwumide, J., et al., 2007. Ectopic bone formation in bone marrow stem cell seeded calcium phosphate scaffolds as compared to autograft and (cell seeded) allograft. Eur. Cell. Mater. 14, 30–38.
European Commission, 2012. Guidance relating to the application of the Council Directive 93/42/EEC on medical devices. MEDDEV 2. 4/1 Rev. 9 June 2010. Available at: http://ec.europa.eu/consumers/sectors/medical-devices/files/meddev/2_4_1_rev_9_classification_en.pdf (accessed 05.01.16).
European Commission, 2016. Nando (New Approach Notified and Designated Organisations) information system. Available at: http://ec.europa.eu/growth/tools-databases/nando/index.cfm (accessed 05.01.16).
Fatimi, A., et al., 2008. The rheological properties of silated hydroxypropylmethylcellulose tissue engineering matrices. Biomaterials 29, 533–543. Available at: http://www.ncbi.nlm.nih.gov/pubmed/17996292.
FDA, 2008. Guidance for industry and FDA staff: modifications to devices subject to premarket approval (PMA)—the PMA supplement decision-making process. Available at: http://www.fda.gov/downloads/MedicalDevices/DeviceRegulationandGuidance/GuidanceDocuments/ucm089360 (accessed 05.01.16).
FDA, 2014. Classify your medical device. Available at: http://www.fda.gov/MedicalDevices/DeviceRegulationandGuidance/Overview/ClassifyYourDevice/ (accessed 04.01.16).
Feigal, D., Gardner, S., McClellan, M., 2003. Ensuring safe and effective medical devices. N. Engl. J. Med. 348 (3), 191–192. Available at: http://www.ncbi.nlm.nih.gov/pubmed/12529457 (accessed 04.01.16).
Fellah, B.H., et al., 2006. Bone repair using a new injectable self-crosslinkable bone substitute. J. Orthop. Res. 24 (4), 628–635. Available at: http://www.ncbi.nlm.nih.gov/pubmed/16514642.
Florencio-Silva, R., et al., 2015. Biology of bone tissue: structure, function, and factors that influence bone cells. BioMed Res. Int. 2015, 1–17. http://dx.doi.org/10.1155/2015/421746.
Fraser, A., et al., 2011. Commentary: international collaboration needed on device clinical standards. BMJ 342 (may13_2), d2952. Available at: http://www.bmj.com/content/342/bmj.d2952 (accessed 04.01.16).
Fu, S., et al., 2009. Injectable biodegradable thermosensitive hydrogel composite for orthopedic tissue engineering. 1. Preparation and characterization of nanohydroxyapatite/poly(ethylene glycol)–poly(ε-caprolactone)–poly(ethylene glycol) hydrogel nanocomposites. J. Phys. Chem. B 113 (52), 16518–16525.
Fu, S., et al., 2012. Injectable and thermo-sensitive PEG–PCL–PEG copolymer/collagen/n-HA hydrogel composite for guided bone regeneration. Biomaterials 33 (19), 4801–4809.
Gaharwar, A., et al., 2011. Highly extensible, tough, and elastomeric nanocomposite hydrogels from poly(ethylene glycol) and hydroxyapatite nanoparticles. Biomacromolecules 12 (5), 1641–1650. http://dx.doi.org/10.1021/bm200027z.
Gao, C., et al., 2013. Development and characterization of injectable chitosan-based hydrogels containing dexamethasone/rhBMP-2 loaded hydroxyapatite nanoparticles. Mater. Lett. 93, 312–315. http://dx.doi.org/10.1016/j.matlet.2012.11.106.

Gauthier, O., et al., 1998. Macroporous biphasic calcium phosphate ceramics: influence of macropore diameter and macroporosity percentage on bone ingrowth. Biomaterials 19 (1-3), 133–139.

Geckil, H., et al., 2010. Engineering hydrogels as extracellular matrix mimics. Nanomedicine 5 (3), 469–484. Available at: http://www.pubmedcentral.nih.gov/articlerender.fcgi?artid=2892416&tool=pmcentrez&rendertype=abstract.

Greenwald, A., et al., 2001. Bone-graft substitutes: facts, fictions, and applications. J. Bone Joint Surg. Am. 83-A Suppl, 98–103. Available at: http://www.ncbi.nlm.nih.gov/pubmed/11712842 (accessed 01.10.15).

Gunatillake, P., Mayadunne, R., Adhikari, R., 2006. Recent developments in biodegradable synthetic polymers. Biotechnol. Annu. Rev. 12, 301–347.

Gupta, A., et al., 2015. Bone graft substitutes for spine fusion: a brief review. World J. Orthop. 6 (6), 449–456. Available at: http://www.ncbi.nlm.nih.gov/pubmed/26191491.

Han, Y., et al., 2013. The calcium silicate/alginate composite: preparation and evaluation of its behavior as bioactive injectable hydrogels. Acta Biomater. 9 (11), 9107–9117. http://dx.doi.org/10.1016/j.actbio.2013.06.022. Available at: http://www.ncbi.nlm.nih.gov/pubmed/23796407.

He, C., Kim, S., Lee, D., 2008. In situ gelling stimuli-sensitive block copolymer hydrogels for drug delivery. J. Control. Release 127 (3), 189–207. Available at: http://www.sciencedirect.com/science/article/pii/S0168365908000436.

Heini, P., Berlemann, U., 2001. Bone substitutes in vertebroplasty. Eur. Spine J. 10 (SUPPL. 2), 205–213.

Hines, J., et al., 2010. Left to their own devices: breakdowns in United States medical device premarket review. PLoS Med. 7 (7), 1–8.

Hoare, T., Kohane, D., 2008. Hydrogels in drug delivery: progress and challenges. Polymer 49 (8), 1993–2007. Available at: http://www.sciencedirect.com/science/article/pii/S0032386108000487.

Huang, Z., et al., 2009. A bone-like nano-hydroxyapatite/collagen loaded injectable scaffold. Biomed. Mater. 4 (5), 055005. Available at: http://www.ncbi.nlm.nih.gov/pubmed/19776494.

Huang, Z., et al., 2011a. Biomimetic properties of an injectable chitosan/nano-hydroxyapatite/collagen composite. Mater. Sci. Eng. C 31 (3), 683–687. Available at: http://www.sciencedirect.com/science/article/pii/S0928493111000075.

Huang, Z., et al., 2011b. In situ-forming chitosan/nano-hydroxyapatite/collagen gel for the delivery of bone marrow mesenchymal stem cells. Carbohydr. Polym. 85 (1), 261–267.

Huang, Z., et al., 2011c. In vivo bone regeneration with injectable chitosan/hydroxyapatite/collagen composites and mesenchymal stem cells. Front. Mater. Sci. 5, 301–310. Available at: http://www.scopus.com/inward/record.url?eid=2-s2.0-80052510649&partnerID=40&md5=4d5b96772b03bf35c584485ff52655dd.

Hulsart-Billström, G., et al., 2011. Calcium phosphates compounds in conjunction with hydrogel as carrier for BMP-2: a study on ectopic bone formation in rats. Acta Biomater. 7 (8), 3042–3049.

Ifkovits, J., Burdick, J., 2007. Review: photopolymerizable and degradable biomaterials for tissue engineering applications. Tissue Eng. 13 (10), 2369–2385.

Khan, Y., et al., 2008. Tissue engineering of bone: material and matrix considerations. J. Bone Joint Surg. Am. 90 (Suppl. 1), 36–42. Available at: http://jbjs.org/content/90/Supplement_1/36.abstract.

Killion, J., et al., 2013. Hydrogel/bioactive glass composites for bone regeneration applications: synthesis and characterisation. Mater. Sci. Eng. C 33 (7), 4203–4212. Available at: http://www.ncbi.nlm.nih.gov/pubmed/23910334 (accessed 05.01.16).

Killion, J., et al., 2014a. Fabrication and in vitro biological evaluation of photopolymerisable hydroxyapatite hydrogel composites for bone regeneration. J. Biomater. Appl. 28 (8), 1274–1283. Available at: http://www.ncbi.nlm.nih.gov/pubmed/24114559.

Killion, J., et al., 2014b. Compressive strength and bioactivity properties of photopolymerizable hybrid composite hydrogels for bone tissue engineering. Int. J. Polym. Mater. 63 (13), 641–650. http://dx.doi.org/10.1080/00914037.2013.854238 (accessed 05.01.16).

Kim, M., et al., 2011. Polymeric scaffolds for regenerative medicine. Polym. Rev. 51 (1), 23–52. http://dx.doi.org/10.1080/15583724.2010.537800.

Kramer, D., Xu, S., Kesselheim, A., 2012. Regulation of medical devices in the United States and European Union. N. Engl. J. Med. 366 (9), 848–855. http://dx.doi.org/10.1056/NEJMhle1113918.

Kregar-Velikonja, N., Krečič stres, H., Maličev, E., Gantar, D., Krkovič, M., Senekovič, V., Rode, M., Kneževič, M., Vunjak-Novakovic, G., Fröhlich, M., 2012. Autologous cell therapies for bone tissue regeneration. In: Tal, H. (Ed.), Bone Regeneration. InTech. pp. 33–58. Available at: http://www.intechopen.com/books/bone-regeneration/autologous-cell-therapies-for-bone-tissue-regeneration (accessed 05.01.16).

Kretlow, J., Klouda, L., Mikos, A., 2007. Injectable matrices and scaffolds for drug delivery in tissue engineering. Adv. Drug Deliv. Rev. 59 (4-5), 263–273.

Laurencin, C., Khan, Y., Veronick, J., 2014. Bone graft substitutes: past, present, and future. In: Laurencin, C.T., Jiang, T. (Eds.), Bone Graft Substitutes and Bone Regenerative Engineering. second ed.. ASTM International, West Conshohocken, PA, pp. 1–9. Available at: http://www.astm.org/DIGITAL_LIBRARY/MNL/PAGES/MONO62013002501.htm (accessed 04.01.16).

Liu, X., Ma, P., 2004. Polymeric scaffolds for bone tissue engineering. Ann. Biomed. Eng. 32 (3), 477–486.

Liu, Y., Lim, J., Teoh, S.H., 2013. Review: development of clinically relevant scaffolds for vascularised bone tissue engineering. Biotechnol. Adv. 31 (5), 688–705. http://dx.doi.org/10.1016/j.biotechadv.2012.10.003.

Liu, X., et al., 2015. The preparation and in vitro evaluations of a nanoscaled injectable bone repair material. J. Nanomater. 2015, 1–8 (accessed 05.01.16).

Low, K., et al., 2010. Calcium phosphate-based composites as injectable bone substitute materials. J. Biomed. Mater. Res. B Appl. Biomater. 94 (1), 273–286.

Ma, P., 2004. Scaffolds for tissue fabrication. Mater. Today 7 (5), 30–40.

Martínez-Álvarez, C., et al., 2013. Injection and adhesion palatoplasty: a preliminary study in a canine model. J. Surg. Res. 183 (2), 654–662. Available at: http://www.sciencedirect.com/science/article/pii/S0022480413002072.

Martínez-Sanz, E., et al., 2012. Minimally invasive mandibular bone augmentation using injectable hydrogels. J. Tissue Eng. Regen. Med. 6 (Suppl. 3), s15–s23. Available at: http://www.ncbi.nlm.nih.gov/pubmed/22941759.

Morais, D., et al., 2013a. Development and characterization of novel alginate-based hydrogels as vehicles for bone substitutes. Carbohydr. Polym. 95 (1), 134–142. Available at: http://www.ncbi.nlm.nih.gov/pubmed/23618249.

Morais, D., et al., 2013b. Biological evaluation of alginate-based hydrogels, with antimicrobial features by Ce(III) incorporation, as vehicles for a bone substitute. J. Mater. Sci. Mater. Med. 24 (9), 2145–2155. Available at: http://www.ncbi.nlm.nih.gov/pubmed/23756964.

Moreira, C., et al., 2016. Thermogelling chitosan-collagen-bioactive glass nanoparticle hybrids as potential injectable systems for tissue engineering. Mater. Sci. Eng. C 58, 1207–1216. Available at: http://www.ncbi.nlm.nih.gov/pubmed/26478423 (accessed 02.11.15).

Nair, L., Laurencin, C., 2007. Biodegradable polymers as biomaterials. Prog. Polym. Sci. 32 (8-9), 762–798.

Navarro, M., et al., 2008. Biomaterials in orthopaedics. J. R. Soc. Interface 5 (27), 1137–1158.

Nguyen, K., West, J., 2002. Photopolymerizable hydrogels for tissue engineering applications. Biomaterials 23 (22), 4307–4314.

Nguyen, T., et al., 2014. Enzyme-mediated in situ preparation of biocompatible hydrogel composites from chitosan derivative and biphasic calcium phosphate nanoparticles for bone regeneration. Adv. Nat. Sci. Nanosci. Nanotechnol. 5 (1), 015012. Available at: http://m.iopscience.iop.org/article/10.1088/2043-6262/5/1/015012/pdf (accessed 05.01.16).

Ni, P.-Y., et al., 2012. Synthesis and characterization of injectable, thermosensitive, and biocompatible acellular bone matrix/poly(ethylene glycol)–poly (ε-caprolactone)–poly(ethylene glycol) hydrogel composite. J. Biomed. Mater. Res. A 100 (1), 171–179. Available at: http://www.ncbi.nlm.nih.gov/pubmed/22009709 (accessed 05.01.16).

Ni, P., et al., 2014. Injectable thermosensitive PEG–PCL–PEG hydrogel/acellular bone matrix composite for bone regeneration in cranial defects. Biomaterials 35 (1), 236–248. Available at: http://www.ncbi.nlm.nih.gov/pubmed/24138826 (accessed 05.01.16).

Niranjan, R., et al., 2013. A novel injectable temperature-sensitive zinc doped chitosan/β-glycerophosphate hydrogel for bone tissue engineering. Int. J. Biol. Macromol. 54, 24–29. Available at: http://www.ncbi.nlm.nih.gov/pubmed/23201776 (accessed 02.11.15).

Okamoto, M., John, B., 2013. Synthetic biopolymer nanocomposites for tissue engineering scaffolds. Prog. Polym. Sci. 38 (10-11), 1487–1503. http://dx.doi.org/10.1016/j.progpolymsci.2013.06.001.

Pirraco, R., Marques, A., Reis, R., 2010. Cell interactions in bone tissue engineering. J. Cell. Mol. Med. 14 (1-2), 93–102. http://dx.doi.org/10.1111/j.1582-4934.2009.01005.x.

PRNewswire, 2012. Orthobiologics: global market prospects 2012–2022. Available at: http://www.prnewswire.com/news-releases/orthobiologics-global-market-prospects-2012-2022-149794185.html (accessed 05.01.16).

Sadat-Shojai, M., Khorasani, M.-T., Jamshidi, A., 2015. 3-Dimensional cell-laden nano-hydroxyapatite/protein hydrogels for bone regeneration applications. Mater. Sci. Eng. C 49, 835–843. Available at: http://www.ncbi.nlm.nih.gov/pubmed/25687015 (accessed 15.12.15).

Sarkar, S., Lee, B., 2015. Hard tissue regeneration using bone substitutes: an update on innovations in materials. Korean J. Intern. Med. 30 (3), 279–293. Available at: http://www.pubmedcentral.nih.gov/articlerender.fcgi?artid=4438282&tool=pmcentrez&rendertype=abstract.

Schnürer, S., et al., 2003. Bone substitutes. Orthopade 32, 2–10. Available at: http://www.ncbi.nlm.nih.gov/pubmed/12557080.

Seris, E., et al., 2013. Bone regeneration at the expense of bioceramic/hydrogel composite: clinical evidence. IRBM 34 (4-5), 342–345. Available at: http://www.sciencedirect.com/science/article/pii/S1959031813000845.

Sohier, J., et al., 2010. Hydrogel/calcium phosphate composites require specific properties for three-dimensional culture of human bone mesenchymal cells. Acta Biomater. 6 (8), 2932–2939.

Sorrel, S., 2006. Medical device development: U.S. and EU differences. Available at: http://www.appliedclinicaltrialsonline.com/medical-device-development-us-and-eu-differences (accessed 04.01.16).

Stenfelt, S., et al., 2014. Pre-incubation of chemically crosslinked hyaluronan-based hydrogels, loaded with BMP-2 and hydroxyapatite, and its effect on ectopic bone formation. J. Mater. Sci. Mater. Med. 25 (4), 1013–1023. Available at: http://www.ncbi.nlm.nih.gov/pubmed/24477873.

Stevens, M., 2008. Biomaterials for bone tissue engineering. Mater. Today 11 (5), 18–25. http://dx.doi.org/10.1016/S1369-7021(08)70086-5.

Struillou, X., et al., 2011. Treatment of periodontal defects in dogs using an injectable composite hydrogel/biphasic calcium phosphate. J. Mater. Sci. Mater. Med. 22 (7), 1707–1717. Available at: http://www.ncbi.nlm.nih.gov/pubmed/21611794 (accessed 05.01.16).

Sweet, B., Schwemm, A., Parsons, D., 2011. Review of the processes for FDA oversight of drugs, medical devices, and combination products. J. Manag. Care Pharm. 17 (1), 40–50. Available at: http://www.ncbi.nlm.nih.gov/pubmed/21204589 (accessed 05.01.16).

Tan, R., et al., 2009. Preparation and characterization of an injectable composite. J. Mater. Sci. Mater. Med. 20 (6), 1245–1253. Available at: http://www.ncbi.nlm.nih.gov/pubmed/19267262.

Tan, R., et al., 2010. In vitro and in vivo degradation of an injectable bone repair composite. Polym. Degrad. Stab. 95 (9), 1736–1742. http://dx.doi.org/10.1016/j.polymdegradstab.2010.05.015.

Temenoff, J., Mikos, A., 2000. Injectable biodegradable materials for orthopedic tissue engineering. Biomaterials 21 (23), 2405–2412. Available at: http://ac.els-cdn.com/S0142961200001083/1-s2.0-S0142961200001083-main.pdf?_tid=d318cbc4-b3a7-11e5-85da-00000aacb35e&acdnat=1451997088_1a0d55ba35a44d685f6c4f658767f0ff (accessed 05.01.16).

The Boston Consulting Group, 2012. Regulation and access to innovative medical technologies: a comparison of the FDA and EU approval processes and their impact on patients and industry. Available at: http://archive.eucomed.org/uploads/Modules/Publications/2012_bcg_report_regulation_and_access_to_innovative_medical_technologies.pdf (accessed 07.01.16).

Trojani, C., et al., 2006. Ectopic bone formation using an injectable biphasic calcium phosphate/Si-HPMC hydrogel composite loaded with undifferentiated bone marrow stromal cells. Biomaterials 27 (17), 3256–3264.

Utech, S., Boccaccini, A., 2016. A review of hydrogel-based composites for biomedical applications: enhancement of hydrogel properties by addition of rigid inorganic fillers. J. Mater. Sci. 51 (1), 271–310. Available at: http://download.springer.com/static/pdf/9/art%253A10.1007%252Fs10853-015-9382-5.pdf?originUrl=http%3A%2F%2Flink.springer.com%2Farticle%2F10.1007%2Fs10853-015-9382-5&token2=exp=1452004175~acl=%2Fstatic%2Fpdf%2F9%2Fart%25253A10.1007%25252Fs10853-015-9382-5 (accessed 05.01.16).

Vaccaro, A.R., Madigan, L., 2002. Spinal applications of bioabsorbable implants. J. Neurosurg. 97 (4 Suppl.), 407–412.

Xu, H., Carey, L., Simon, C., 2007. Premixed macroporous calcium phosphate cement scaffold. J. Mater. Sci. Mater. Med. 18 (April 2006), 1345–1353.

Yannas, I., 2004. Classes of materials used in medicine: natural materials. In: Ratner, B.D., et al. (Eds.), An Introduction to Materials in Medicine. Elsevier Academic Press, San Diego, CA. Available at: http://www.efn.uncor.edu/escuelas/biomedica/Plandeestudios/materias completas/biomateriales/Biomaterials Science - An Introduction to Materials in Medici.pdf (accessed 06.01.16).

Younger, E., Chapman, M., 1989. Morbidity at bone graft donor sites. J. Orthop. Trauma 3 (3), 192–195. Available at: http://www.ncbi.nlm.nih.gov/pubmed/2809818 (accessed 10.01.16).

Zhu, J., Marchant, R., 2011. Design properties of hydrogel tissue-engineering scaffolds. Expert Rev. Med. Devices 8 (5), 607–626.

Therapeutic proteins in bioactive materials for wound healing

10

J. Leppiniemi, V.P. Hytönen
University of Tampere, Tampere, Finland

10.1 Introduction

10.1.1 Wounds

A wound is a defect or a break in the skin that results from physical or thermal damage, or as a result of the presence of an underlying medical or physical condition (Lazarus et al., 1994). According to the repair process, wounds can be classified as acute or chronic wounds. Acute wounds usually heal completely with minimal scarring. Depending on the thickness of the wound, the complete closing of acute wounds typically takes 10–21 days (Percival, 2002). After closure, the remodeling of the scar takes place over months or years (Harding et al., 2002). Chronic wounds instead, fail to produce anatomic and functional integrity of the injured site within 12 weeks of initial injury (Sen et al., 2009; Boateng et al., 2008). Usually chronic wounds remain in an inflammatory phase of healing, which disrupts the normal balance between deposition and degradation of extracellular matrix (ECM) components (McCarty and Percival, 2013).

Chronicity may result from repeated tissue injuries or underlying physiological conditions such as diabetes, malignancies, obesity and infections that challenge healing (Boateng et al., 2008). The modern western lifestyle, as well as an increase in the numbers of elderly with diseases such as diabetes and cardiovascular diseases, has resulted in a significant increase in the appearance of chronic wounds that are diagnosed at an alarming rate. Chronic wounds are estimated to affect about 1% of the European population and nearly 2% of the healthcare budgets are devoted to their treatment (Schreml et al., 2010). Thus, new advanced wound-care solutions are needed to save healthcare costs, and, more importantly, to improve patients' well-being, for example by avoiding leg amputation.

10.1.2 Wound healing

Wound healing is a complex phenomenon where angiogenesis, ie,, formation of new blood vessels plays an essential role (Bates and Jones, 2003). The wound healing process can be divided into three main phases: inflammatory phase, proliferation phase, and maturation and remodeling phase (Witte and Barbul, 1997), as discussed in the following text (Fig. 10.1).

The *inflammation phase* (~0–6 days postwounding) involves increased vascular permeability and chemotaxis of cells from the surrounding tissues into the wound. Release of cytokines and growth factors takes place and cell migration is activated

Bioinspired Materials for Medical Applications. http://dx.doi.org/10.1016/B978-0-08-100741-9.00010-3

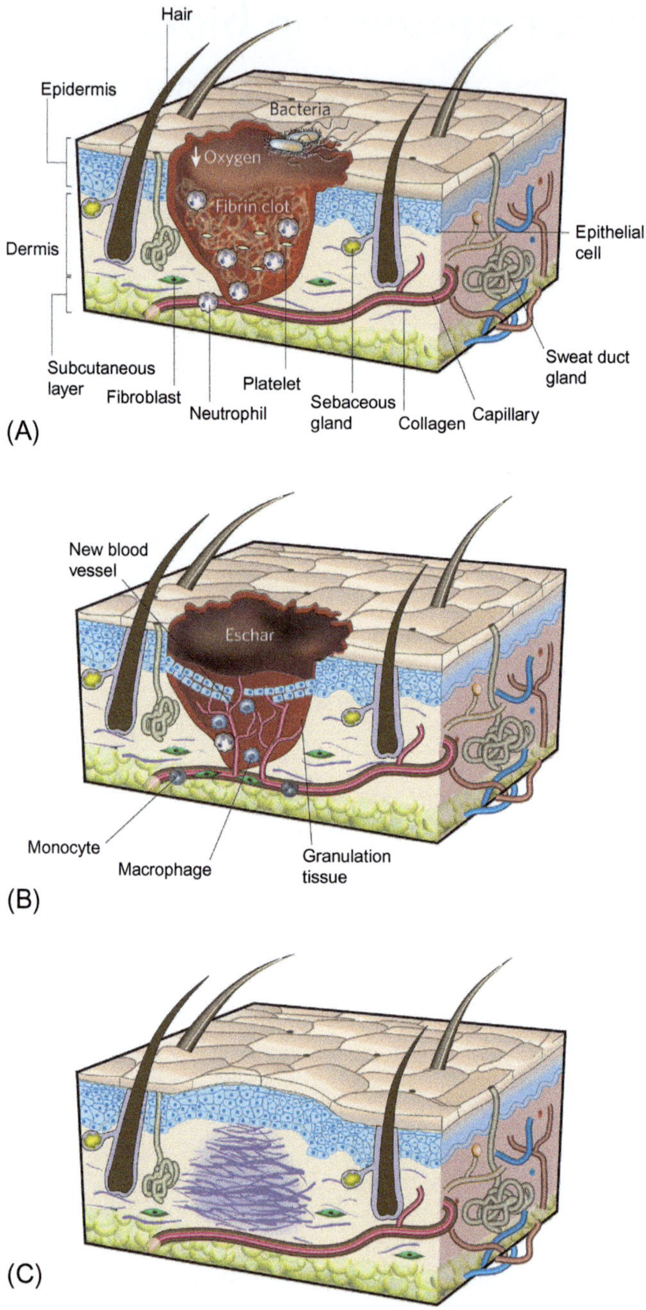

Fig. 10.1 Main stages of wound healing. (A) Inflammatory phase. (B) Proliferation phase. (C) Maturation and remodeling phase.
Reprinted by permission from Macmillan Publishers Ltd: [Nature]. Gurtner, G.C., Werner, S., Barrandon, Y., Longaker, M.T., 2008. Wound repair and regeneration. Nature, 453(7193), 314–321. Copyright (2008).

(Witte and Barbul, 1997). The exposure of extracellular proteins triggers platelets to release cytokines and growth factors, including platelet-derived growth factor (PDGF), transforming growth factor β (TGF-β), platelet-activating factor (PAF), fibronectin and serotonin. A fibrin clot is formed and it provides scaffold for invading cells (Kurkinen et al., 1980). The first cells migrating into the wound are neutrophils, followed by macrophages, fibroblasts and lymphocytes. Chemotaxis is followed by functional activation of the cells (Witte and Barbul, 1997).

Proliferation phase. The primary cells proliferating in this phase (~4–15 days postwounding) are fibroblasts and endothelial cells. Endothelial cells form new capillaries through a process called angiogenesis. Fibroblasts require activation to start proliferation and factors such as PDGF and epidermal growth factor (EGF) are involved in fibroblast activation. One important part of the proliferation phase is the reepithelialization and wound closure (Witte and Barbul, 1997).

Maturation and remodeling phase. The remodeling phase (~8–16 days postwounding) is manifested by deposition of collagen in the wound. The amount and quality of the deposited matrix determines the strength of the scar. The main source of collagen is fibroblasts (Witte and Barbul, 1997).

10.2 Therapeutic proteins and their role in wound healing

A number of studies have reported the use of therapeutic proteins to improve wound healing. The majority of those studies focus on the use of growth factors. However, there are also other classes of proteins potentially suitable for improving the wound-healing process. Table 10.1 lists examples of therapeutic proteins studied and the mechanisms by which they might contribute to the wound-healing process.

10.2.1 Growth factors

Growth factors are important players in normal tissue-healing processes. Their binding to specific cell-surface receptors or ECM protein receptors stimulates cellular signal transduction pathways, which eventually leads to activation of transcription factors that regulate the transcription of proteins controlling events such as cell migration, survival, adhesion, proliferation, growth and differentiation (Goldman, 2004). These responses are thus heavily involved in angiogenesis and wound healing (Grazul-Bilska et al. 2003). Because of their critical role, the secretion of growth factors has to be spatially and temporally tightly controlled.

The EGF family includes several members. The main members involved in wound healing are EGF, heparin binding EGF (HB-EGF) and transforming growth factor-alpha (TGF-α). When these ligands bind to the EGF receptor (EGFR), which is a tyrosine kinase transmembrane protein, this process results in dimerization of the receptor and its autophosphorylation, and tyrosine phosphorylation of downstream signaling proteins. Signaling pathways will be activated and important steps in reepithelialization, such as keratinocyte migration and proliferation, will be promoted (Barrientos et al., 2008).

Table 10.1 Examples of therapeutic proteins studied to promote wound healing and their main functions in wound healing

Protein	The main function in wound healing	References
Growth factors		
Epidermal growth factor (EGF)	Promotes reepithelialization.	Barrientos et al. (2008)
Platelet-derived growth factor (PDGF)	Induces migration of several cells to the wound site. Stimulates macrophages to produce and secrete TGF-β. Affects blood vessel maturation. Induces the production of VEGF and insulin-like growth factor (IGF). Enhances fibroblast proliferation and production of ECM.	Barrientos et al. (2008)
Basic fibroblast growth factor (bFGF)	Stimulates granulation tissue formation, reepithelialization, matrix formation, and remodeling.	Barrientos et al. (2008), Demidova-Rice et al. (2012)
Transforming growth factor-beta (TGF-β)	Increases expression of ECM proteins and integrins. Increases granulation tissue formation.	Barrientos et al. (2008)
Vascular endothelial growth factor (VEGF-A)	Stimulates granulation tissue formation. Promotes vascular endothelial cell survival, migration, proliferation, and differentiation. Induces angiogenesis.	Barrientos et al. (2008)
Adhesion-promoting factors		
Collagen	Gives structural support. Functions as signaling molecule. Inactivates proteases. Protects exogenously added growth factors.	Demidova-Rice et al. (2012)
Fibronectin	Acts as a biological glue mediating interaction between cells and other ECM proteins. Forms a pericellular structure for collagen matrix deposition. Serves as a reservoir for growth factors increasing their local bioavailability and activity.	(Sawicka et al., 2015)

Table 10.1 Continued

Protein	The main function in wound healing	References
Laminin	Forms basement membrane together with other molecules. Promotes reepithelialization and angiogenesis.	Iorio et al. (2014)
Vitronectin	Supports a thrombus formation. Affects the stability of vessel occlusion and inflammation and immune responses.	Leavesley et al. (2013)
Fibrin	Participates in the clotting of blood.	Demidova-Rice et al. (2012)
Other therapeutic proteins		
Granulocyte macrophage-colony stimulating factor (GM-CSF)	Induces differentiation of myofibroblasts. Causes local recruitment of inflammatory cells. Mediates epidermal cell proliferation and induces keratinocyte proliferation.	Hu et al. (2011)

The PDGF family includes homo- and heterodimeric growth factors such as PDGF-AA, PDGF-AB, PDGF-BB, PDGF-CC and PDGF-DD (Barrientos et al., 2008). These ligands bind to a complementary family of receptor tyrosine kinases such as PDGFR-$\alpha\alpha$, PDGFR-$\alpha\beta$ and PDGFR-$\beta\beta$. Ligand binding is followed by homodimerization or heterodimerization of PDGFR and their phosphorylation, which activates several signaling pathways. PDGF is released by platelets, macrophages, keratinocytes, fibroblasts, and endothelial cells. It is one of the first factors that are produced in tissue after injury and it induces cellular responses during all phases of the healing process (Demidova-Rice et al., 2012). PDGF induces neutrophils, macrophages, fibroblasts and smooth muscle cells to migrate to the wound site. PDGF also stimulates macrophages to produce and secrete TGF-β and thereby increases granulation tissue formation. PDGF has an important role in blood vessel maturation by recruiting pericytes to capillaries and thus increasing their structural integrity. In addition, production of PDGF induces the production of vascular endothelial growth factor (VEGF) and insulin-like growth factor (IGF). Additionally, PDGF plays a role in reepithelialization and it enhances the proliferation of fibroblast and thus ECM production (Barrientos et al., 2008).

Currently, PDGF is the only growth factor approved for clinical use for the treatment of wounds, specifically for the treatment of diabetic neuropathic ulcers. A recombinant human PDGF, rhPDGF-BB is supplied in a gel form with sodium carboxymethyl cellulose (Regranex®, becaplermin) (Goldman, 2004). The gel is applied topically once a day and the wound is dressed after the application. A large number of patients do not respond to the treatment, probably because the growth factor is rapidly degraded in the proteolytic wound environment resulting in insufficient concentration and endurance of the PDGF in the chronic wound bed (Demidova-Rice et al., 2012). However, a postmarket epidemiologic study revealed that diabetic patients that used three or more tubes of Regranex® had a fivefold increased risk of death due to cancer compared to patients who did not use it. Therefore FDA recommends the use of Regranex® only when the benefits can be expected to outweigh the potential risks (Gainza et al., 2015).

The *fibroblast growth factor* (FGF) family includes 23 members, of which FGF-2, FGF-7 and FGF-10 are the most important members involved in wound healing. FGFs are produced by keratinocytes, fibroblasts, endothelial cells, smooth muscle cells, chondrocytes and mast cells. They bind to FGF receptors (FGFR), which are tyrosine kinase transmembrane proteins. FGF must bind proteoglycan, such as heparin, to activate its receptor. The binding induces receptor dimerization and transphosphorylation and activation of downstream signaling pathways. FGF-2, also known as basic FGF (bFGF), affects reepithelialization, angiogenesis, and granulation tissue formation (Barrientos et al., 2008). FGF-2 also stimulates production of ECM-degrading enzymes, thus contributing to matrix synthesis and remodeling, which are crucial for the normal wound healing (Demidova-Rice et al., 2012).

The TGF-β family includes TGF-β1–3, bone morphogenetic proteins (BMP) and activins. TGF-β1–3 is the main form found in mammals. TGF-β1 is mainly involved in cutaneous wound healing and it plays an important role in inflammation, angiogenesis, reepithelialization and connective tissue regeneration. The expression of TGF-β1 is increased upon injury, it facilitates the recruitment of inflammatory cells and increases the expression of genes associated with ECM and integrin formation, which helps to initiate granulation tissue formation (Barrientos et al., 2008).

The VEGF family includes VEGF-A, VEGF-B, VEGF-C, VEGF-D, VEGF-E and placental growth factor, of which the VEGF-A is the most comprehensively studied in the context of wound healing (Barrientos et al., 2008). VEGF-A is heparin binding glycoprotein, which functions by binding to cell-surface tyrosine kinase receptors VEGFR1 and VEGFR2 (Demidova-Rice et al., 2012). After injury, activated platelets release VEGF-A and during wound healing, macrophages release VEGF-A and TNF-α, which induces VEGF-A expression in keratinocytes and fibroblasts. Also other cytokines and growth factors act as inducers of VEGF-A production. However, hypoxia in the acute wound is the major stimulus for VEGF-A production in monocytes, fibroblasts, keratinocytes, myocytes and endothelial cells. VEGF-A promotes the early events in angiogenesis, especially vascular endothelial cell survival, migration, proliferation and differentiation. This will result in reformation of microcirculation and increased oxygen tension at the wound site (Barrientos et al., 2008). Thus, VEGF-A is considered the most potent angiogenic factor (Dvorak, 2000).

As described above, growth factors have essential roles in wound healing. However, in some diseases or after trauma, the production of growth factors may be distorted. For example, in chronic wounds the level of growth factors has been proven to decrease due to increased levels of proteases, which delays the normal healing process (Barrientos et al., 2008). Therapeutic systems releasing growth factors have been extensively studied in vivo in order to stimulate the healing of chronic wounds, but their clinical use has been very limited because of the high costs of treatments and safety-issues, which may result from nonoptimized delivery of growth factors at enormously higher levels than normally observed in physiological conditions. Additionally, the proteases such as matrix metalloproteinases and plasmin present in chronic wounds can destroy delivered growth factors (Briquez et al., 2015). Therefore there is an unmet medical need for novel elegant systems capable of protecting and releasing growth factors in a controlled fashion.

10.2.2 Adhesion-promoting factors

The ECM surrounds most of the cells in our body and it provides structural scaffold for the cells and molecules that regulate cell signaling. ECM is composed of fibrous proteins such as collagens and elastin, glycoproteins, proteoglycans and glycosaminoglycans (GAGs) such as hyaluronan. In addition to giving structural support, the ECM also undergoes important changes after injury that are essential for directing cell behavior during the wound-healing process. The ECM may facilitate healing directly by modulating cell adhesion, migration, proliferation, metabolism, differentiation and survival, or indirectly by modulating secretion/activation of extracellular proteases, or by modulating the activity and bioavailability of growth factors (Ghatak et al., 2015). In addition to ECM components, other adhesion-promoting factors in the wound include fibrin, which is involved in blood clotting.

Collagens are the main class of fibrous proteins composing the healthy dermal ECM (Briquez et al., 2015). Collagens give the structural integrity for the tissue and they function as signaling molecules via the interactions with their cellular receptors, particularly integrins. Collagens are classified into fibrillary collagens such as collagen I, II and III, whereas collagens IV and V are network-forming (Demidova-Rice et al., 2012). Collagen I is mostly used in wound-healing products, although some dressings obtained from natural matrices contain other collagens as well (Ruszczak, 2003). In wound-healing products collagen may be in the form of a sponge produced from lyophilized matrices, as skin substitutes containing dermal and/or epidermal cells, collagen-based matrices with synthetic backings or in combination with oxidized regenerated cellulose. Collagen-based materials may effectively control wound exudate, inactivate proteases and protect exogenously added growth factors (Demidova-Rice et al., 2012).

Collagen-based materials were proposed for growth factor delivery already in 1989 (Stompro et al., 1989). Several methods can be used to load growth factors into the collagen scaffolds, such as simply rehydrating the collagen sponge with a solution of biologically active molecules, addition of heparin-like moieties into a collagen scaffold or covalently cross-linking growth factors into the scaffold. In addition, affinity interactions have been used. For example, Stompro et al. used avidin–biotin interaction by attaching biotinylated EGF or biotinylated heparin binding growth factor 2 (HBGF2) to biotinylated collagen with the help of tetravalent avidin (Stompro et al., 1989). In vitro experiments demonstrated that biotinylated growth factors retained their activity and were available for cells, but the effectiveness of this method for the delivery of EGF into the wound is not known (Demidova-Rice et al., 2012). More recently, EGF have been fused with a collagen-binding domain (CBD) derived from fibronectin. This fusion protein, FNCBD-EGF had high affinity towards collagens I, II, III and IV, and in vivo experiments revealed that FNCBD-EGF applied with collagen sponge improved wound epithelialization (Ishikawa et al., 2001) and induced granulation tissue formation (Ishikawa et al., 2003).

Fibronectin is an adhesive ECM glycoprotein. The amount of fibronectin found in ECM is highest during dynamic remodeling conditions such as wound healing, development and the progression of diseases such as cancer and atherosclerosis. After acute injury, fibronectin is deposited to the wound from the blood plasma in fibrin clot, whereas later in the healing phase it is deposited by activated tissue cells such as epidermal cells, fibroblasts, and endothelial cells. Within ECM, fibronectin has a fibrillar structure and it is organized as an extensive network of elongated branching fibrils. Because of its structure, fibronectin reinforces perimatrix formation by acting as a biological glue mediating interaction between cells and other ECM proteins, and as a pericellular structure for collagen matrix deposition. Fibronectin has multiple binding sites for growth factors, and therefore it may serve as a reservoir for growth factors increasing their local bioavailability. Fibronectin has been studied as a delivery matrix for growth factors as it can influence on growth factor stability and activity, and growth factors can modulate fibronectin activity (Sawicka et al., 2015).

Laminins are large molecules that assemble with collagen IV, nidogens, agrin and perlecan into a structured region of the ECM, named basement membrane. During homeostasis, the basement membrane acts as an attachment substrate for epithelial and endothelial cell sheets separating those cells from the interstitial matrix. Laminins also have an important role in reepithelialization and angiogenesis of wound healing. Laminins provide a substrate for epithelial keratinocytes for moving to cover the wound and reestablish an intact epithelial barrier. Laminins are also involved in blood vessel growth and maturation (Iorio et al., 2014).

Vitronectin is an ECM glycoprotein detected in most tissues, particularly after trauma or stress, and it is synthesized mostly in the liver by hepatocytes. Vitronectin is present in plasma in micromolar concentrations wherein it circulates in a complex with fibrinogen and with PAI-1, which prevents unintended coagulation and fibrinolysis. When the clotting and coagulation cascades become activated upon tissue injury, plasma vitronectin undergoes rapid conformational changes leading to selfassembly into fibrils and exposes GAG-binding motifs. This dramatically increases the local concentrations of available binding sites and precipitating interactions that support the assembly of the thrombus. Vitronectin also affects the stability of vessel occlusion, inflammation and immune responses (Leavesley et al., 2013).

Fibrin is a fibrous protein that is formed from fibrinogen by the cleavage of thrombin, which causes polymerization to a 3D fibrin network. Fibrin is involved in the clotting of blood and it is a major component of the natural wound matrix that is formed immediately after injury (Demidova-Rice et al., 2012). Fibrin-based materials have FDA approval for their use as hemostatic agents such as sealant of colostomy closures and for skin graft attachment (Spotnitz, 2014). In addition, several studies have been conducted to use fibrin for drug and growth factor delivery. The release rate of growth factors from the fibrin matrix has been altered by blending fibrin with natural polysaccharides, such as GAGs. Also growth factors can be modified, for example, FGF-10 was modified with a fibrin-binding site of an α2-plasmin inhibitor, which allowed FGF-10 to interact with fibrin in the presence of factor XIII, from where it (FGF-10) was released in vivo after fibrin degradation by the cells residing within the wound (Demidova-Rice et al., 2012). Furthermore, fibrin(ogen) possess a natural affinity for many growth factors and the fibrin matrix has been shown to be efficient in delivering low doses of FGF-2 and placenta growth factor-2 (PlGF-2) into the wound of diabetic mice (Martino et al., 2013). Interestingly, when the growth-factor binding domain of fibrin(ogen) was isolated and incorporated into a synthetic matrix based on polyethylene glycol (PEG), these matrices sequestered growth factors similarly to fibrin. Treatment of the wounds of diabetic mice by delivering FGF-2 and PlGF-2 through these synthetic matrices performed well, delivering the same growth factors as found within natural fibrin (Martino et al., 2013).

Some of the described adhesion-promoting factors directly interact with growth factors. For example, fibronectin, fibrinogen, and vitronectin have specific growth factor-binding domains. Collagens have also been reported to directly interact with some growth factors such as hepatocyte growth factor (HGF), although their specific growth factor-binding sites have not yet been fully characterized (Mitchell et al., 2016). The ECM glycoproteins have different affinities for growth factors, which enable the spatio-temporal control of growth factor release in the wound microenvironment. In addition to growth factor-binding domains, the ECM glycoproteins also contain cell-adhesion sites, in particular, integrin-binding domains. The spatial proximity of growth factors and integrin-binding sites allows molecules to form clusters at the cell surface, which may strongly modulate growth factor signaling and mediate synergetic effects (Mitchell et al., 2016). For example, simultaneous binding of $\alpha_5\beta_1$ integrin to the domains 9 and 10 of fibronectin ($FNIII_{9-10}$) and VEGF-A to the neighboring domains ($FNIII_{12-14}$), greatly enhances VEGF-A effects on endothelial cell responses, including receptor phosphorylation (Wijelath et al., 2006).

10.2.3 Other therapeutic proteins

Other important proteins involved in wound healing include signaling proteins such as cytokines and chemokines. For example, the granulocyte macrophage-colony stimulating factor (GM-CSF) is a cytokine that is secreted into the wound by keratinocytes or macrophages shortly after injury. In vivo studies have indicated that GM-CSF induces differentiation of myofibroblasts, causes local recruitment of inflammatory cells, mediates epidermal cell proliferation and induces proliferation of keratinocytes. Several animal and clinical studies have been conducted to study the effect of GM-CSF on wound healing when applied topically, within a hydrogel or as injections to the wound or into subcutaneous tissue. Although the results have mostly been promising, there has been some diversity depending on the type of wound treated and whether GM-CSF has been applied alone or together with a growth factor. Therefore more evidence for the performance of GM-CSF is still needed before translation to generalized use (Hu et al., 2011). GM-CSF is one of the promising wound-therapy molecules that may benefit from advanced delivery systems.

10.3 Delivery of therapeutic proteins for wound

Growth factors are very promising molecules to aid wound healing, but their clinical use has been limited because of safety-issues and the high cost of treatments. These may result from nonoptimized delivery systems that require the dosing of growth factors at enormously higher concentrations than normally needed in wound healing due to the rapid degradation of the growth factors by proteases present in the healing site (Briquez et al., 2015). The balance between growth factor release and retention is critical for the efficacy of growth factor-based treatments (King and Krebsbach, 2012). Thus, improved systems for the controlled delivery of therapeutic proteins are needed, which are able to protect growth factors from protease cleavage. The aim in designing delivery systems is to obtain sustained delivery of optimal doses of therapeutic proteins to the wound, extend their presence at the site of injury by minimizing their systemic diffusion, and to prevent immune responses (Lee et al., 2011; Gainza et al., 2015). These functions resemble the natural role of ECM under physiological conditions (Briquez et al., 2015).

The dose and duration of growth factor delivery must be thoroughly controlled to ensure safety and efficacy of treatment (Martino et al., 2015). Especially the concentration of growth factors at the microenvironmental level need to be well controlled, as, for instance, the same total dose of released VEGF in vivo has shown a therapeutic or toxic effect depending on whether VEGF is distributed homogenously in the tissue or not (Banfi et al., 2005). For example, clinical trials of VEGF gene therapy have failed in the context of wound healing, possibly because it is challenging to achieve the required well-balanced expression levels in vivo (Sacchi et al., 2014). By the direct delivery of recombinant VEGFs to the wound, more homogenous microenvironmental distribution could be achieved. However, released VEGFs have short half-lives in vivo, because of wound proteases (Martino et al., 2015). Therefore the delivery system should be able to protect VEGF from wound proteases until the delivery, and sustained VEGF stimulation should last for at least 4 weeks to stabilize newly induced vessels (Sacchi et al., 2014). Certain intrinsic properties of the growth factors, such as low protein stability, short circulating half-life, rapid rate of cellular internalization, and localized tissue activity, make their utilization challenging (Mitchell et al., 2016).

10.3.1 *Incorporation of therapeutic proteins to scaffold material*

Both synthetic and natural scaffold materials have been studied as delivery systems for therapeutic proteins. There are excellent articles and reviews describing the properties of these materials and reporting the results of clinical trials (Lee et al., 2011; Demidova-Rice et al., 2012; Gainza et al., 2015). Here we describe approaches to incorporate therapeutic proteins to such scaffold materials. Therapeutic proteins may be adsorbed or encapsulated on matrix material or the interaction may be based on covalent bonding or noncovalent interaction such as affinity interaction (Fig. 10.2, Table 10.2).

Adsorption. The simplest strategy to incorporate therapeutic agents into scaffold materials is by adsorption/physisorption. For example, growth factors can be deposited on the material surface trough diffusion, flow, or thermal convection. Proteins

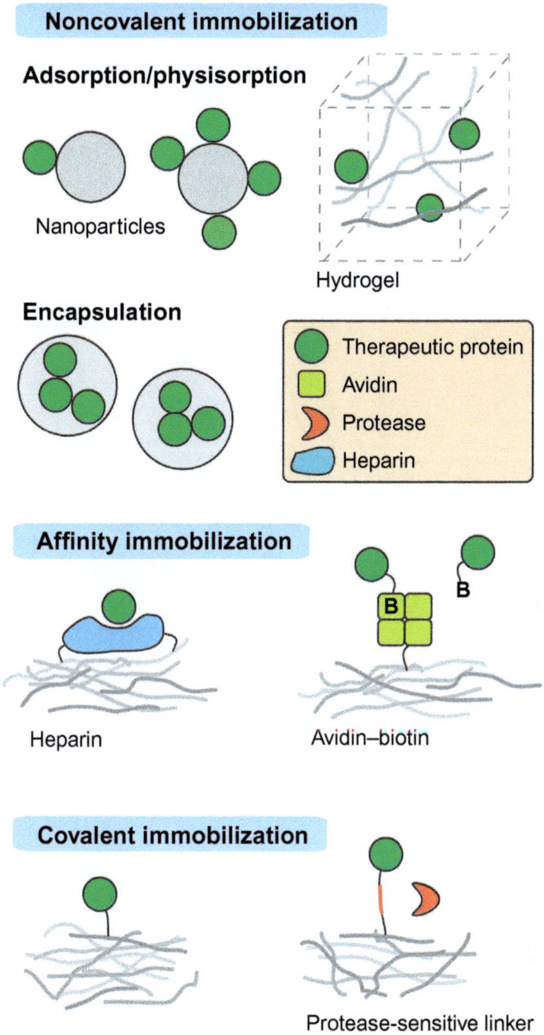

Fig. 10.2 Delivery systems for therapeutic proteins. Noncovalent delivery systems include adsorption and encapsulation. By using pairs of interacting molecules, it is possible to implement affinity-based immobilization. Heparin-growth factor and avidin–biotin are shown here as examples. When covalent immobilization is used, the release of the therapeutic protein is dependent on the degradation of the matrix/scaffold. Alternatively, it is possible to use protease cleavable linker for the protein deposition in order to release the growth factor in response to specific proteases.

then bind via a thermodynamically favorable adsorption involving noncovalent intermolecular interactions such as electrostatic interactions, hydrophobic interactions, hydrogen bonding and Van der Waals forces. The physicochemical properties, such as the isoelectric point, and biological properties of the therapeutic protein need to be considered when designing scaffolds for controlled delivery to retain the bioactivity of

Table 10.2 Main approaches for the incorporation of the therapeutic proteins onto matrices; classified by the type of interaction

Interaction type	Therapeutic protein	Matrix material	Release	References
Noncovalent interaction				
Adsorption			Release via diffusion, convective fluid flow or their combination.	Lee et al. (2011), King and Krebsbach (2012)
Electrostatic interaction	Bone morphogenetic protein-2 (BMP-2) and VEGF	Hyaluronic acid (HA) hydrogel	Release rate may be adjusted by the degradation rate of the polymer. Fast degrading hydrogels released growth factors rapidly, 100% was released within 7 days along with the hydrogel degradation. Slowly degrading hydrogels had a high burst release, which was followed by release at nanogram levels per week. The release of VEGF was faster than BMP-2, ~95% of VEGF and ~80% of BMP-2 was released during 50 days.	Patterson et al. (2010)
Encapsulation				
Physical encapsulation	VEGF-A, PDGF	Poly(lactide-*co*-glycolide), PLGA microspheres	Sustained release in vitro over a few tens of days. Release rate may be adjusted by the degradation rate of the polymer and altering the amount of growth factor applied.	Richardson et al. (2001)

Ionic interaction				
Polyion complexation	Basic fibroblast growth factor (bFGF)	Gelatin microspheres	In vitro data not available. Microspheres within collagen sponge was implanted into rat's wound and sutured to the wound edge. The sustained release of bFGF from microspheres suppressed the infection, and accelerated new capillary formation and tissue regeneration when compared to the single application of bFGF or the control group.	Kawai et al. (2005)
Affinity interaction				
Heparin-binding domain of fibrinogen incorporated into fibrin-mimetic synthetic PEG-matrix. Protease cleavable site was incorporated to enable release by plasmin	PlGF-2 and FGF-2	Polyethylene glycol (PEG)	PlGF-2 and FGF-2 showed good retention within the PEG matrix, with ~55% and 35% released in vitro after day 7, respectively. After degradation by plasmin, growth factors were completely released. In vivo in diabetic mice the synthetic PEG-matrix performed as well as fibrin for the delivery of FGF-2 and PlGF-2.	Martino et al. (2013)

Continued

Table 10.2 Continued

Interaction type	Therapeutic protein	Matrix material	Release	References
Fusion of an ECM-binding domain (PlGF-$2_{123-144}$) on growth factor	VEGF-A and PDGF-BB	Fibrin	VEGF-A and PDGF-BB showed good retention within the fibrin matrix, with ~25% and 25% released in vitro after day 7, respectively.	Martino et al. (2014)
Covalent interaction				
Chemical crosslink			Release rate depends on matrix degradation rate.	Briquez et al. (2015)
Factor XIIIa substrate sequence of α2-plasmin inhibitor (α2PI_{1-8}, NQEQVSPL=TG) fused to N-terminus of fusion protein allowing factor XIIIa-mediated covalent linkage to fibrin matrix during fibrinogen polymerization	Bifunctional fusion protein, TG-$FNIII_{10}$-VEGF-A_{165}, TG-VEGF-A_{165}	Fibrin	Protein released in a cell-dependent manner as cells degraded the fibrin matrix. Fusion proteins containing TG-sequence exhibited substantially slower in vitro release kinetics compared to native $FNIII_{10}$-VEGF-A_{165} and VEGF-A_{165}.	Traub et al. (2013)

One or a few examples of scaffold materials used and therapeutic proteins involved in each interaction type are specified.

the protein and to enhance its retention at the target site. The adsorbed mass of therapeutic protein can be controlled by scaffold material properties such as surface wettability, roughness, porosity, surface area, surface charge, charge density and functional groups of material. Also the pH and ionic strength of the solution and other proteins in the media may influence the adsorbed amount of growth factors. In addition, adjacent proteins also effect the conformation and orientation of growth factor adsorption onto biomaterials. Parameters affecting adsorption are usually protein-specific. Generally, increasing the electrostatic attraction between protein and scaffold also increases the protein adsorption onto the scaffold (King and Krebsbach, 2012).

The release of adsorbed agents from the biomaterial matrix occurs via diffusion, convective fluid flow or scaffold degradation, or by a combination of those. The kinetics of the release can be controlled by the types of noncovalent interactions between protein and scaffold, the scaffold environment and the scaffold degradation rate. An increased amount of electrostatic interactions between proteins and scaffold may decrease the initial burst release, which may be harmful or even toxic, and result in longer retention of protein within the scaffold. Protein diffusion from a hydrogel network may be controlled by hydrogel mesh size, which in turn may be controlled by the polymer concentration in the hydrogel network, the cross-linking density and solubility of the polymer chains (King and Krebsbach, 2012). However, modification of the physical properties of the scaffold material to obtain an optimal, sustained release profile may be challenging, as, usually, cells are supposed to colonize the biomaterial matrix and remodel it. Therefore other methods to control and to slow down the release of growth factors have been studied by modifying biomaterial matrix and/or therapeutic proteins to introduce covalent or affinity interactions between them.

Affinity interaction. The specific affinity interactions can be used for the incorporation of therapeutic proteins to scaffolds. The ligand specific to the protein of interest is coupled to the scaffold, for example covalently. The affinity of the protein towards the ligand drives the delivery and release (Reed and Wu, 2014). Therapeutic proteins may naturally have affinity towards specific sites in the ECM. For example, fibronectin, fibrinogen, tenascin C and vitronectin have specific growth factor-binding domains. Collagens have also been reported to directly interact with some growth factors such as HGF, although their specific growth factor-binding epitopes have not yet been fully characterized (Mitchell et al., 2016). Most angiogenic growth factors will first interact with ECM before finding their cell-surface receptor or co-receptor (Martino et al., 2015). For instance, VEGF-A_{165}, FGF-2 and PDGF-BB interact with heparin sulfate proteoglycans within the ECM (Capila and Linhardt, 2002; Macri et al., 2007). Heparin is a highly sulfated GAG that has acidic sulfate and carboxylic acid moieties, which can interact electrostatically with basic heparin-binding domains of growth factors (Reed and Wu, 2014). To take advantage of these affinity interactions, the biomaterial matrices have been modified with heparin or heparin sulfate-mimetic molecules. For example, synthetic hydrogel films based on cross-linked GAGs that were covalently linked with heparin and a derivative of chondroitin sulfate, were capable of successfully controlling the delivery of FGF-2 in wound to *db/db* diabetic mice and showed acceleration of vascularization (Liu et al., 2007).

Therapeutic proteins may also be engineered to enhance their affinity for a biomaterial matrix or for the endogenous ECM. For example, Martino et al. screened several growth factors for their affinity towards six ECM proteins fibronectin, vitronectin, tenascin C, osteopontin, fibrinogen and collagen I. They found that PlGF-2 exhibited the strongest affinity towards all ECM proteins tested, because of a heparin-binding sequence (PlGF-$2_{123-144}$) near the C-terminus of the protein. They fused this heparin-binding sequence to VEGF-A, PDGF-BB and bone morphogenetic protein-2 (BMP-2). The engineered fusion proteins sustained their ability to activate their receptors and they had high affinity (K_D in nanomolar range) towards the ECM proteins and heparin sulfate. For example, the fusion proteins could be strongly retained in the fibrin matrix that mimics a clot and they could be released by fibrin-dissolving protease, plasmin. In in vivo skin wound-healing experiments using diabetic mouse, the delivery of PDGF-BB and VEGF-A either topically or within the fibrin matrix revealed that wounds treated with PlGF-$2_{123-144}$-fused PDGF-BB and VEGF-A led to significantly faster wound closure and more extensive granulation tissue formation compared to nonmodified growth factors. Also the angiogenesis within granulation tissue was much more pronounced with affinity engineered PDGF-BB and VEGF-A (Martino et al., 2014).

Covalent interaction. In order to control the release and prevent the free diffusion of growth factors from the matrix, a covalent linkage of growth factors to the matrix material may be used. The conjugation chemistry has to be carefully considered when designing the proper functional groups for the target protein and scaffold material. The conjugation chemistry should yield sufficient conjugation efficiency and the conjugated protein should remain bioactive. It is important that the binding of growth factor with cells will not be disturbed. The linker spacing and arm length need to be optimized to retain the activity of the proteins. Usually the longer linker gives the growth factor a greater degree of mobility to retain its bioactivity and binding affinity towards the target. If using cleavable linkers, the linker must allow protease intrusion. The covalent immobilization of therapeutic protein prevents its internalization by cells until the scaffold is degraded thus increasing the protein's active lifetime. However, some signaling molecules need to be internalized for the downstream signaling activation. On the other hand, in some cases the prolonged presence of the growth factor may be detrimental and lead to tissue overgrowth (Reed and Wu, 2014).

Chemical conjugation methods include homo- and heterobifunctional cross-linkers and click-chemistry reactions, but their use has been limited with growth factors because of the possibility of denaturation and the compromised bioactivity. To circumvent this limitation, therapeutic proteins may be covalently immobilized on scaffold materials through peptide sequences that act as substrates for specific proteases. Upon cleavage by protease, the growth factor is released on cell demand, as cells produce proteases to assist ECM breakdown and remodeling. This allows sustained release of therapeutic protein and its internalization by cells. The release rate of the protease-cleavable growth factor depends on protease concentration and bulk scaffold degradation followed by diffusion (Reed and Wu, 2014).

For example, the protease sensitive factor XIIIa substrate sequence of α2-plasmin inhibitor ($\alpha 2PI_{1-8}$, NQEQVSPL (TG, transglutaminase substrate)) has been fused to N-terminus of VEGF-A_{165} (TG-VEGF-A_{165}) to covalently cross-link growth factor into fibrin matrix during fibrinogen polymerization (Briquez et al., 2015). Also bifunctional proteins containing a fibrin-binding domain, 10th type III domain of fibronectin ($FNIII_{10}$) fused to VEGF-A_{165} that contained a TG-sequence has been generated (TG-$FNIII_{10}$-VEGF-A_{165}). The fusion protein containing the TG-sequence exhibited substantially slower in vitro release kinetics when compared to native $FNIII_{10}$-VEGF-A_{165} and VEGF-A_{165}, which demonstrated that covalently bound fusion proteins were released in a cell-dependent manner when cells invaded within the fibrin matrix and released or activated proteases such as matrix metalloproteinases and plasmin, which degraded the fibrin matrix. In vivo experiments focusing on wound tissue treated with fibrin gel containing TG-$FNIII_{10}$-VEGF-A_{165} and TG-VEGF-A_{165} showed pronounced vascular response as well as increased cell proliferation and increased density of capillaries when compared to wounds treated with fibrin alone or soluble VEGF in fibrin. Thus, covalent binding of growth factors may lead to sustained release of low concentrations of VEGF, which is favorable for the induction of blood vessels (Traub et al., 2013).

10.3.2 Systemic delivery of therapeutic proteins

In systemic delivery of drugs the major problem is that only a small proportion of the administered drug reaches its intended target site. In addition, large molecules such as antibodies and other proteins may suffer from poor penetration to tissues and therefore they do not always reach the target cells (AlDeghaither et al., 2015). Because of these problems the systemic administration of therapeutic proteins has been rejected (Järvinen et al., 2015).

The angiogenic blood vessels express specific molecular markers, which are not found in the preexisting blood vessels in the body. Järvinen et al. have identified a 9-amino acid peptide (CARSKNKDC), called CAR that is capable of specifically recognizing and targeting angiogenic blood vessels in skin wounds and in other regenerative tissues. They developed a systemically administered CAR-decorin fusion protein. Decorin is a proteoglycan that is able to prevent scar formation and fibrosis and simultaneously promote tissue regeneration. Fusion with CAR-peptide greatly increased the accumulation of intravenously injected decorin to the skin wound of mice when compared to nonmodified decorin. In addition, the CAR-decorin fusion protein was able to promote wound healing and suppress scar formation at doses at which nonmodified decorin was inactive (Järvinen and Ruoslahti, 2010, 2011). CAR-decorin promises a lot, but clinical trials are needed to show its efficiency in the treatment of human skin wounds.

10.3.3 Gene therapy

Gene therapy has been an important research topic and applications for gene therapy in the management of wounds have been described. However, according to ClinicalTrials.gov no open clinical studies focusing on gene therapy for wound healing exist at the moment (ClinicalTrials.gov, accessed 2/2016). For example, clinical trials of VEGF gene therapy has failed, possibly because achieving homogenous expression levels in vivo with gene-therapy vectors is challenging (Sacchi et al., 2014). In this review we focus on a small number of recent studies.

Topical gene therapy for the modulation of wound-healing pathways with the help of transcutaneous siRNA has been found to improve healing of cutaneous pathologies. Layliev et al. (2011) utilized this method to silence SMAD3, and they found this beneficial for wound closure in mice. Another approach by Randeria et al. utilized topically administered spherical nucleic acids to cause knockdown of ganglioside-monosialic acid 3 (GM3) synthase. This protein is a mediator of impaired wound healing in type 2 diabetic mice (Randeria et al., 2015). The third example covered here is based on biodegradable cationic poly(β-amino esters) (PBAE) nanoparticles (Park et al., 2012). In this study, specific modification of the PBAE termini significantly improved the efficiency of gene delivery in vitro and in vivo, simultaneously reducing the cytotoxicity. The authors demonstrated that PBAE nanoparticles can be used for intradermal delivery of therapeutic genes for wound healing in an animal skin wound model. They targeted the approach to a protein Sonic hedgehog, which is a prototypical morphogen with angiogenic potential. This study revealed that wound closure was accelerated in mice receiving the PBAE/SHH gene therapy as compared to control group.

10.4 How does the release kinetics affect the activity of therapeutic proteins?

In order to support formation of a vascular network, Richardson et al. incorporated PDGF and VEGF into scaffolds made of poly(lactide-*co*-glycolide), PLGA (Richardson et al., 2001). They used two approaches; first they simply mixed lyophilized VEGF with polymer particles before processing the polymer into a porous scaffold, and in the second approach they preencapsulated PDGF into PLGA microspheres, which were then processed to scaffolds. This scaffold enabled sustained release of the growth factors in vitro over a few tens of days. The magnitude of the release rate may be adjusted by altering the amount of growth factor incorporated and the kinetics may be altered by varying the degradation rate of PLGA. The performance of the scaffold was evaluated by implanting the scaffold into the subcutaneous tissue of Lewis rats. As compared to bolus injections of the growth factors resulting in a negligible increase in blood vessel formation, the scaffold-embedded growth factors provided significantly improved formation of blood vessels. Importantly, a clear difference was observed between scaffolds containing only either PDFG or VEGF or both of them. In line with these results, sustained release of VEGF from the fibrous poly(L-lactic acid) scaffold was found to increase the number of branching points of the capillary-like network formed by HUVEC cells as compared to bolus treatment with VEGF (Chung et al., 2015).

Interferon alpha-2b (IFNα-2b) is used as a therapeutic protein to treat leukemia, multiple myeloma, carcinoma, hepatitis B and hepatitis VC. The use of IFNα-2b requires frequent injections due to the short half-life of the protein, resulting in fluctuation in serum concentration. Li et al. produced microspheres containing solidified IFNα-2b prepared by lyophilization of the protein with gelatin and $ZnSO_4$

(Li et al., 2011). Solidified IFNα-2b was then encapsulated into microspheres made of PEGT/PBT–PLGA (poly(ethylene glycal/butylenes terephthalate)–poly(D,L-lactide-*co*-glycolide)). The protein was found to release from the microspheres following zero-order kinetics. These particles were administered to rats and a steady release of IFNα-2b was observed for 13 days.

A strong affinity towards the matrix and resulting slower release kinetics was found to be important for the activity of VEGF-A and PDGF-BB in vivo. As already briefly discussed in Section 10.3.1, the PlGF-2 has strong affinity towards several ECM proteins, because of its heparin-binding sequence (PlGF-$2_{123-144}$). The fusion of this sequence to VEGF-A and PDGF-BB meant they were well retained in the fibrin matrix and the in vitro release of fusion proteins was very slow. The release reached a plateau after 1 or 2 days, and less than 25% of the loaded amount was released over 7 days. The release of nonmodified VEGF-A and PDGF-BB instead, was fast and reached a plateau over 2 days when >90% of the loaded amount was released. However, the release of fusion proteins was increased by fibrin-dissolving protease, plasmin whereas over 80% of the loaded VEGF-A/PlGF-$2_{123-144}$ was released over 5 days in the presence of plasmin. In vivo experiments with diabetic mice revealed that the delivery of the growth factor either topically or within the fibrin matrix had different outcomes: wounds treated with PlGF-$2_{123-144}$-fused PDGF-BB and VEGF-A led to significantly faster wound closure, and more granulation tissue as well as angiogenesis formation as compared to nonmodified growth factors (Martino et al., 2014).

One potential methodology available for immobilization and controlled release of therapeutic molecules is avidin–biotin technology. Avidin–biotin interaction is widely utilized in biotechnology (Laitinen et al., 2007) and the fact that makes it even more intriguing for the development of novel wound healing approaches is that biotin can be attached to almost all biomolecules using a range of chemistries, typically without disturbing the biological activity of the target molecule. In this context, avidin would offer a generic docking platform for biotinylated therapeutic molecules. We have demonstrated functional avidin immobilization on various materials, including gold (Vikholm-Lundin et al., 2012), polythiophene (Albers et al., 2012), poly(methyl methacrylate) (Heikkinen et al., 2011a) and on cellulose acetate (Heikkinen et al., 2011b). The availability of avidin variants (Laitinen et al., 2006) enables one to tailor the binding strength and thereby the release of the biotinylated molecules from the immobilized layer.

10.5 Conclusions

Wound healing is a complex process, which involves collaboration between several different cell types, signaling molecules and ECM components. To find better treatment for chronic wounds, new delivery systems for the therapeutic proteins are presently being studied. As chronic wounds contain a lot of proteases, topically applied or injected growth factors become rapidly degraded before they have fulfilled their tasks. Therefore successful delivery methods should be capable of retaining therapeutic proteins in an active state, and releasing them in a controlled way, when needed. Several promising delivery systems have been developed, where the therapeutic proteins are retained within the scaffold material by adsorption, via affinity interaction or covalent bonding, possibly utilizing protease-cleavable bonds. The delivery of multiple therapeutic proteins simultaneously or sequentially may be needed to obtain an efficient tissue repair and regeneration of the most demanding chronic wounds. The challenge is first to understand the biology of the wound healing—what are the optimal concentrations for each specific growth factor detected by different cells at the specific time points (Briquez et al., 2015). The translation into clinical applications requires innovations in material science and at a molecular level. We should aim for safe and powerful, but at the same time feasible products, which requires both innovation and novel knowledge.

Acknowledgments

Academy of Finland is acknowledged for the financial support of this work (projects 279442 and 290506). We thank Dr. Olli Laitinen and Dr. Inger Vikholm-Lundin for helpful comments concerning the manuscript draft.

References

Albers, W.M., Pelto, J.M., Suspène, C., Määttä, J.A., Yassar, A., Hytönen, V.P., Vikholm-Lundin, I., Tappura, K., 2012. Structural and functional characteristics of chimeric avidins physically adsorbed onto functionalized polythiophene thin films. ACS Appl. Mater. Interfaces 4 (8), 4067–4077.

AlDeghaither, D., Smaglo, B.G., Weiner, L.M., 2015. Beyond peptides and mAbs-current status and future perspectives for biotherapeutics with novel constructs. J. Clin. Pharmacol. 55 (Suppl. 3), S4–S20.

Banfi, A., Von Degenfeld, G., Blau, H.M., 2005. Critical role of microenvironmental factors in angiogenesis. Curr. Atheroscler. Rep. 7 (3), 227–234.

Barrientos, S., Stojadinovic, O., Golinko, M.S., Brem, H., Tomic-Canic, M., 2008. Growth factors and cytokines in wound healing. Wound Repair Regen. 16 (5), 585–601.

Bates, D.O., Jones, R.O., 2003. The role of vascular endothelial growth factor in wound healing. Int. J. Low. Extrem. Wounds 2 (2), 107–120.

Boateng, J.S., Matthews, K.H., Stevens, H.N., Eccleston, G.M., 2008. Wound healing dressings and drug delivery systems: a review. J. Pharm. Sci. 97 (8), 2892–2923.

Briquez, P.S., Hubbell, J.A., Martino, M.M., 2015. Extracellular matrix-inspired growth factor delivery systems for skin wound healing. Adv. Wound Care 4 (8), 479–489.

Capila, I., Linhardt, R.J., 2002. Heparin-protein interactions. Angew. Chem. 41 (3), 391–412.

Chung, H.J., Kim, J.T., Kim, H.J., Kyung, H.W., Katila, P., Lee, J.H., Yang, T.H., Yang, Y.I., Lee, S.J., 2015. Epicardial delivery of VEGF and cardiac stem cells guided by 3-dimensional PLLA mat enhancing cardiac regeneration and angiogenesis in acute myocardial infarction. J. Control. Release 205, 218–230.

ClinicalTrials.gov, 2016. Available from: https://clinicaltrials.gov/ (accessed 2/2016).

Demidova-Rice, T.N., Hamblin, M.R., Herman, I.M., 2012. Acute and impaired wound healing: pathophysiology and current methods for drug delivery, part 2: role of growth factors in normal and pathological wound healing: therapeutic potential and methods of delivery. Adv. Skin Wound Care 25 (8), 349–370.

Dvorak, H.F., 2000. VPF/VEGF and the angiogenic response. Semin. Perinatol. 24 (1), 75–78.

Gainza, G., Villullas, S., Pedraz, J.L., Hernandez, R.M., Igartua, M., 2015. Advances in drug delivery systems (DDSs) to release growth factors for wound healing and skin regeneration. Nanomedicine 11 (6), 1551–1573.

Ghatak, S., Maytin, E.V., Mack, J.A., Hascall, V.C., Atanelishvili, I., Moreno Rodriguez, R., Markwald, R.R., Misra, S., 2015. Roles of proteoglycans and glycosaminoglycans in wound healing and fibrosis. Int. J. Cell Biol. 2015, 834893.

Goldman, R., 2004. Growth factors and chronic wound healing: past, present, and future. Adv. Skin Wound Care 17 (1), 24–35.

Grazul-Bilska, A.T., Johnson, M.L., Bilski, J.J., Redmer, D.A., Reynolds, L.P., Abdullah, A., Abdullah, K.M., 2003. Wound healing: the role of growth factors. Drugs Today 39 (10), 787–800.

Harding, K.G., Morris, H.L., Patel, G.K., 2002. Healing chronic wounds. Br. Med. J. 324 (7330), 160–163.

Heikkinen, J.J., Kivimäki, L., Määttä, J.A.E., Mäkelä, I., Hakalahti, L., Takkinen, K., Kulomaa, M.S., Hytönen, V.P., Hormi, O.E.O., 2011a. Versatile bio-ink for covalent immobilization of chimeric avidin on sol–gel substrates. Colloids Surf. B: Biointerfaces 87 (2), 409–414.

Heikkinen, J.J., Riihimäki, T.A., Määttä, J.A.E., Suomela, S.E., Kantomaa, J., Kulomaa, M.S., Hytönen, V.P., Hormi, O.E.O., 2011b. Covalent biofunctionalization of cellulose acetate with thermostable chimeric avidin. ACS Appl. Mater. Interfaces 3 (7), 2240–2245.

Hu, X., Sun, H., Han, C., Wang, X., Yu, W., 2011. Topically applied rhGM-CSF for the wound healing: a systematic review. Burns 37 (5), 729–741.

Iorio, V., Troughton, L.D., Hamill, K.J., 2014. Laminins: roles and utility in wound repair. Adv. Wound Care 4 (4), 250–263.

Ishikawa, T., Terai, H., Kitajima, T., 2001. Production of a biologically active epidermal growth factor fusion protein with high collagen affinity. J. Biochem. 129 (4), 627–633.

Ishikawa, T., Terai, H., Yamamoto, T., Harada, K., Kitajima, T., 2003. Delivery of a growth factor fusion protein having collagen-binding activity to wound tissues. Artif. Organs 27 (2), 147–154.

Järvinen, T.A.H., Ruoslahti, E., 2010. Target-seeking antifibrotic compound enhances wound healing and suppresses scar formation in mice. Proc. Natl. Acad. Sci. 107 (50), 21671–21676.

Järvinen, T.A.H., Ruoslahti, E., 2011. Targeted antiscarring therapy for tissue injuries. Adv. Wound Care 2 (2), 50–54.

Järvinen, T.A., May, U., Prince, S., 2015. Systemically administered, target organ-specific therapies for regenerative medicine. Int. J. Mol. Sci. 16 (10), 23556–23571.

Kawai, K., Suzuki, S., Tabata, Y., Nishimura, Y., 2005. Accelerated wound healing through the incorporation of basic fibroblast growth factor-impregnated gelatin microspheres into artificial dermis using a pressure-induced decubitus ulcer model in genetically diabetic mice. Br. J. Plast. Surg. 58 (8), 1115–1123.

King, W.J., Krebsbach, P.H., 2012. Growth factor delivery: how surface interactions modulate release in vitro and in vivo. Adv. Drug Deliv. Rev. 64 (12), 1239–1256.

Kurkinen, M., Vaheri, A., Roberts, P.J., Stenman, S., 1980. Sequential appearance of fibronectin and collagen in experimental granulation tissue. Lab. Investig. 43 (1), 47–51.

Laitinen, O.H., Hytönen, V.P., Nordlund, H.R., Kulomaa, M.S., 2006. Genetically engineered avidins and streptavidins. Cell. Mol. Life Sci. 63 (24), 2992–3017.

Laitinen, O.H., Nordlund, H.R., Hytönen, V.P., Kulomaa, M.S., 2007. Brave new (strept)avidins in biotechnology. Trends Biotechnol. 25 (6), 269–277.
Layliev, J., Wilson, S., Warren, S.M., Saadeh, P.B., 2011. Improving wound healing with topical gene therapy. Adv. Wound Care 1 (5), 218–223.
Lazarus, G.S., Cooper, D.M., Knighton, D.R., Margolis, D.J., Pecoraro, R.E., Rodeheaver, G., Robson, M.C., 1994. Definitions and guidelines for assessment of wounds and evaluation of healing. Arch. Dermatol. 130 (4), 489–493.
Leavesley, D.I., Kashyap, A.S., Croll, T., Sivaramakrishnan, M., Shokoohmand, A., Hollier, B.G., Upton, Z., 2013. Vitronectin-master controller or micromanager? IUBMB Life 65 (10), 807–818.
Lee, K., Silva, E.A., Mooney, D.J., 2011. Growth factor delivery-based tissue engineering: general approaches and a review of recent developments. J. R. Soc. Interface 8 (55), 153–170.
Li, Z., Li, L., Liu, Y., Zhang, H., Li, X., Luo, F., Mei, X., 2011. Development of interferon alpha-2b microspheres with constant release. Int. J. Pharm. 410 (1-2), 48–53.
Liu, Y., Cai, S., Shu, X.Z., Shelby, J., Prestwich, G.D., 2007. Release of basic fibroblast growth factor from a crosslinked glycosaminoglycan hydrogel promotes wound healing. Wound Repair Regen. 15 (2), 245–251.
Macri, L., Silverstein, D., Clark, R.A.F., 2007. Growth factor binding to the pericellular matrix and its importance in tissue engineering. Adv. Drug Deliv. Rev. 59 (13), 1366–1381.
Martino, M.M., Briquez, P.S., Ranga, A., Lutolf, M.P., Hubbell, J.A., 2013. Heparin-binding domain of fibrin(ogen) binds growth factors and promotes tissue repair when incorporated within a synthetic matrix. Proc. Natl. Acad. Sci. 110 (12), 4563–4568.
Martino, M.M., Briquez, P.S., Guc, E., Tortelli, F., Kilarski, W.W., Metzger, S., Rice, J.J., Kuhn, G.A., Muller, R., Swartz, M.A., Hubbell, J.A., 2014. Growth factors engineered for super-affinity to the extracellular matrix enhance tissue healing. Science 343 (6173), 885–888.
Martino, M.M., Brkic, S., Bovo, E., Burger, M., Schaefer, D.J., Wolff, T., Gurke, L., Briquez, P.S., Larsson, H.M., Gianni-Barrera, R., Hubbell, J.A., Banfi, A., 2015. Extracellular matrix and growth factor engineering for controlled angiogenesis in regenerative medicine. Front. Bioeng. Biotechnol. 3, 45.
McCarty, S.M., Percival, S.L., 2013. Proteases and delayed wound healing. Adv. Wound Care 2 (8), 438–447.
Mitchell, A.C., Briquez, P.S., Hubbell, J.A., Cochran, J.R., 2016. Engineering growth factors for regenerative medicine applications. Acta Biomater. 30, 1–12.
Park, H., Lee, J., Kim, M., Kang, T.J., Jeong, Y., Um, S.H., Cho, S., 2012. Sonic hedgehog intradermal gene therapy using a biodegradable poly(β-amino esters) nanoparticle to enhance wound healing. Biomaterials 33 (35), 9148–9156.
Patterson, J., Siew, R., Herring, S.W., Lin, A.S.P., Guldberg, R., Stayton, P.S., 2010. Hyaluronic acid hydrogels with controlled degradation properties for oriented bone regeneration. Biomaterials 31 (26), 6772–6781.
Percival, N.J., 2002. Classification of wounds and their management. Surgery 20 (5), 114–117.
Randeria, P.S., Seeger, M.A., Wang, X.Q., Wilson, H., Shipp, D., Mirkin, C.A., Paller, A.S., 2015. siRNA-based spherical nucleic acids reverse impaired wound healing in diabetic mice by ganglioside GM3 synthase knockdown. Proc. Natl. Acad. Sci. 112 (18), 5573–5578.
Reed, S., Wu, B., 2014. Sustained growth factor delivery in tissue engineering applications. Ann. Biomed. Eng. 42 (7), 1528–1536.
Richardson, T.P., Peters, M.C., Ennett, A.B., Mooney, D.J., 2001. Polymeric system for dual growth factor delivery. Nat. Biotechnol. 19 (11), 1029–1034.
Ruszczak, Z., 2003. Effect of collagen matrices on dermal wound healing. Adv. Drug Deliv. Rev. 55 (12), 1595–1611.

Sacchi, V., Mittermayr, R., Hartinger, J., Martino, M.M., Lorentz, K.M., Wolbank, S., Hofmann, A., Largo, R.A., Marschall, J.S., Groppa, E., Gianni-Barrera, R., Ehrbar, M., Hubbell, J.A., Redl, H., Banfi, A., 2014. Long-lasting fibrin matrices ensure stable and functional angiogenesis by highly tunable, sustained delivery of recombinant VEGF164. Proc. Natl. Acad. Sci. 111 (19), 6952–6957.

Sawicka, K.M., Seeliger, M., Musaev, T., Macri, L.K., Clark, R.A.F., 2015. Fibronectin interaction and enhancement of growth factors: importance for wound healing. Adv. Wound Care 4 (8), 469–478.

Schreml, S., Szeimies, R., Prantl, L., Landthaler, M., Babilas, P., 2010. Wound healing in the 21st century. J. Am. Acad. Dermatol. 63 (5), 866–881.

Sen, C.K., Gordillo, G.M., Roy, S., Kirsner, R., Lambert, L., Hunt, T.K., Gottrup, F., Gurtner, G.C., Longaker, M.T., 2009. Human skin wounds: a major and snowballing threat to public health and the economy. Wound Repair Regen. 17 (6), 763–771.

Spotnitz, W.D., 2014. Fibrin sealant: the only approved hemostat, sealant, and adhesive—a laboratory and clinical perspective. ISRN Surg. 2014, 203943.

Stompro, B.E., Hansbrough, J.F., Boyce, S.T., 1989. Attachment of peptide growth factors to implantable collagen. J. Surg. Res. 46 (5), 413–421.

Traub, S., Morgner, J., Martino, M.M., Honing, S., Swartz, M.A., Wickstrom, S.A., Hubbell, J.A., Eming, S.A., 2013. The promotion of endothelial cell attachment and spreading using FNIII10 fused to VEGF-A165. Biomaterials 34 (24), 5958–5968.

Vikholm-Lundin, I., Auer, S., Paakkunainen, M., Määttä, J.A.E., Munter, T., Leppiniemi, J., Hytönen, V.P., Tappura, K., 2012. Cysteine-tagged chimeric avidin forms high binding capacity layers directly on gold. Sensors Actuators B Chem. 171–172, 440–448.

Wijelath, E.S., Rahman, S., Namekata, M., Murray, J., Nishimura, T., Mostafavi-Pour, Z., Patel, Y., Suda, Y., Humphries, M.J., Sobel, M., 2006. Heparin-II domain of fibronectin is a vascular endothelial growth factor-binding domain: enhancement of VEGF biological activity by a singular growth factor/matrix protein synergism. Circ. Res. 99 (8), 853–860.

Witte, M.B., Barbul, A., 1997. General principles of wound healing. Surg. Clin. N. Am. 77 (3), 509–528.

Smart devices: Micro- and nanosensors

11

A.C. Peixoto, A.F. Silva
University of Minho, Braga, Portugal

11.1 Introduction

It is incredible how technology has evolved and how we today are able to witness its impact on our lives. At the same time, we can foresee the impact that future developments will have. In the field of health care, over the last 2 decades we have witnessed a tremendous evolution with the emergence of a variety of technologies and devices that have transformed medicine and health care in general.

We currently have the ability to master the microscale and are on the verge of mastering the nanoscale. The miniaturization of devices and the inclusion of smart-features opened new possibilities not only in diagnosis and treatment, but also in continuous monitoring and health selfassessment.

The present chapter presents an overview regarding smart devices that take full advantage of and potential from micro- and nanosensors. From an introduction to the main concepts behind micro- and nanosensors to the identification of the current limitations and future trends, a few examples of smart devices are shown.

It is important to start with the definition of the main concepts regarding smart devices based on micro- and nanosensors, namely the definition of sensor, the meaning of the smart capability and the size features that define micro- and nanoscale.

11.1.1 Sensors

This chapter requires the prior understanding of the concept of a sensor. Although this concept might seem trivial, its definition is still somehow controversial when confronted with another concept, the transducer.

11.1.2 Sensor concept

One can define a sensor as a device/component capable of quantifying a physical quantity (Sinclair, 2001). However, one can still state that this is a barely rudimentary definition of a sensor, without any technical insight. Thus, another possible definition would be to consider a sensor as a component capable of detecting a given variation in input energy and converting it to another or the same type of energy as output (Patranabis, 2003). This definition matches the transducer definition as a component capable of translating a form of energy into another form. It is with this scenario that both concepts become blurry.

Bioinspired Materials for Medical Applications. http://dx.doi.org/10.1016/B978-0-08-100741-9.00011-5

Nonetheless, other definitions for transducers can be found, such as considering it as an element that uses its transduction property to convert a measurand[1] into a usable output. Here the term usable is used as a reference to all the remaining apparatus and mechanisms required for that conversion. However, for many, this arrangement is called instrumentation.

For the purpose of the present chapter, the sensor is considered as a component capable of performing the sensing task, thus enabling the quantification of a given measurand (outputs information). This implies that the transducer must be the element capable of converting a given energy form into another, which makes all sensors transducers. Nonetheless, similarly it also makes all actuators (the opposite of sensor) transducers as well.

Despite being transducer, sensor or actuator, all these components interact with different energy forms, including mechanical, thermal, electrical, acoustic, optical or electromagnetic, among others. In Section 11.3, the sensing principles for some of the energy forms listed before are described in detail.

If one considers the acoustic energy form, a sensor for this example would be a microphone, which is able to detect acoustic wave inputs and provide an electrical signal output in accordance. In contrast, a sound speaker works as an actuator. This concept is generalized in Fig. 11.1.

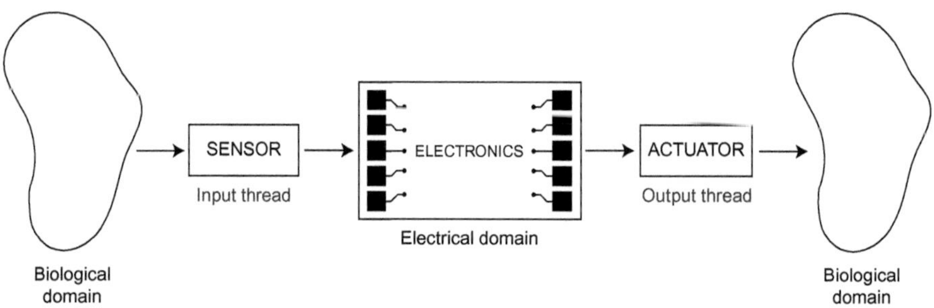

Fig. 11.1 General schematic for illustration of the transducers, sensors and actuators concept.

11.2 Static and dynamic characteristics

Depending on the purpose of the application, sensors' characteristics can be divided into two categories: static and dynamic. It is the full understanding of the sensor characteristics that allows its performance to be assessed.

Like any other similar types of device, precision, accuracy and repeatability are inherent properties.

Static characteristics consider quantities that do not show variation in a given interval of time during which the instrument is used, or variation that is slow as compared with the duration of the time interval. Within static conditions, sensitivity, range and linearity are the key factors (Fig. 11.2).

[1] A physical quantity which is measured.

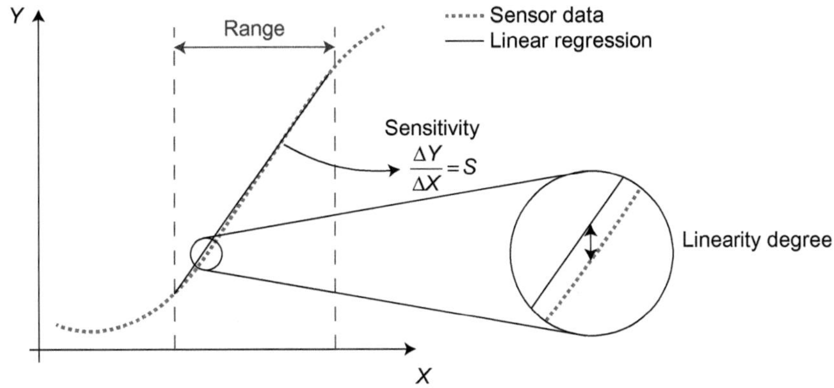

Fig. 11.2 Illustration of sensor's sensitivity, range and linearity characteristics.

The sensitivity (*S*) of a given sensor relates an output variation (ΔY) in respect to the sensor's input variation (ΔX), in the following way:

$$S(X_i) = \frac{\Delta Y}{X_i - X_0} \tag{11.1}$$

Eq. (11.1) shows the possibility of the sensitivity to change with the X_i input value. If the sensitivity is constant regardless of X_i, the sensor is considered to have a linear behavior (preferred behavior). Although most sensors have a constant sensitivity, this is only true as long as the X_i is within the sensor's operation range. Nonetheless, one seeks for a high-sensitivity sensor despite the input value, external disturbances and sensor's lifespan.

The operating window of the sensor is another key characteristic. It defines the range in which the sensor's input can change. On other words, it defines the minimum and maximum acceptable input/output values. Related to range, there is span, which instead of providing a range defines the variation window.

As already stated, desirably, one seeks to have a linear transfer function defined by:

$$Y(X) = SX + b \tag{11.2}$$

where *Y* is the output signal, *X* the input and *S* the sensor's sensitivity. The *b* parameter exists as many sensors, despite no input signal, might not respond with a null output. It is this baseline's offset that sets the value *b*.

In addition to the static characteristics, there are dynamic ones. These are related with the sensor's response to a time-related input. As sensors perform the transduction between a domain under analysis and a processable domain, the understanding of the dynamic characteristic of a sensor becomes fundamental.

The domain under analysis, if one considers for example a healthcare application, can most likely be a dynamic system itself. Automatically, the sensor selection needs to assess its dynamic behavior in order to select the most suitable sensor, capable of responding in an acceptable time frame. On the other hand, the sensor is connected downstream to a set of instrumentation circuits. In order to ensure that no bottleneck exists in such acquisition circuits, it is necessary to know beforehand how the sensor responds.

In the dynamic characteristics context, it is crucial to provide the transfer function for the sensor's response. Moreover, in dynamic systems, the responses may have different behaviors, which can be related to the mathematical orders. Fig. 11.3 illustrates the differences of orders for the same type of system. To understand how the components change the systems, it is advisable to explore the specific literature in the field (Nise, 2011).

Sometimes, the concept of resolution is mistaken for the concept of sensitivity. The resolution states the minimum input value change that can be quantified. This parameter might not be related with the sensor itself, but with the remaining apparatus connected to the sensor. Indeed, many sensors are analogic, meaning that they sense continuously within the defined range. However, as the signal is digitized through electronic components (analog-to-digital converters—ADCs) for processing in microcontrollers, it becomes digital, and thus dependent on the resolution of the system itself.

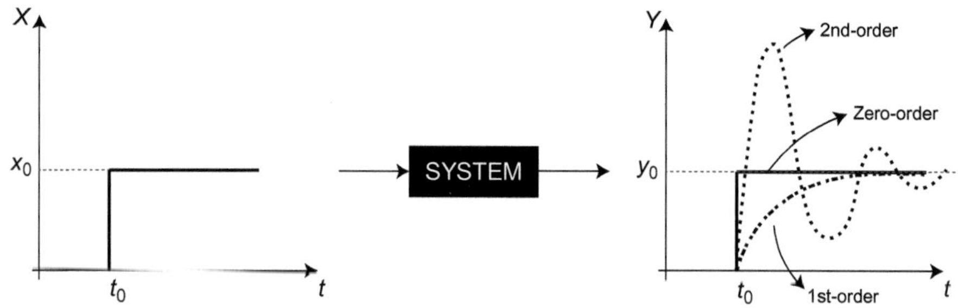

Fig. 11.3 Systems' dynamic responses according to their orders.

Hysteresis (Fig. 11.4) is another parameter commonly evaluated in sensors. Depending on how the sensor is approached, within its range, upward or downward input variation might result in different output signals. It is this difference that defines the hysteresis of the sensor.

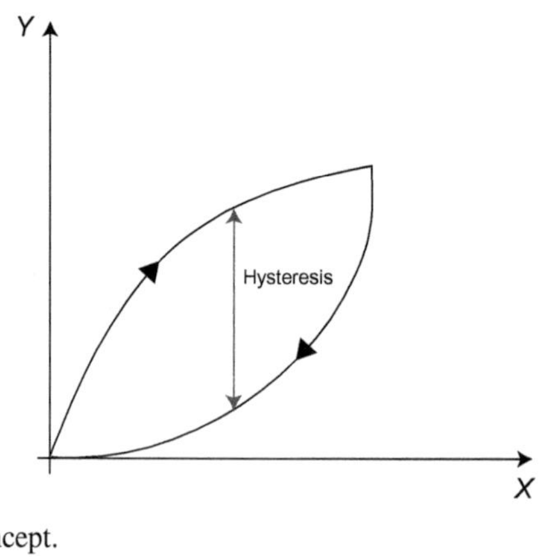

Fig. 11.4 Hysteresis concept.

As referred to in the concept of hysteresis, when the upward and downward terms are added, the sensor is being evaluated from a dynamic perspective.

The described characteristics are common performance indicators listed in the datasheet of sensors or in the performance analysis of sensors presented in research publications.

11.2.1 Smart devices

A sensor itself is not a standalone device. Instead, it is integrated in a system that acquires the sensor's output signal. It is what happens from this point onward that will define the smartness features of a given sensor.

An electrical sensor converts an input quantity into an electrical output that can be acquired by an acquisition circuit or device. As a user, one can read the value directly from an instrumentation device and relate it back to the quantity of interest (Fig. 11.5).

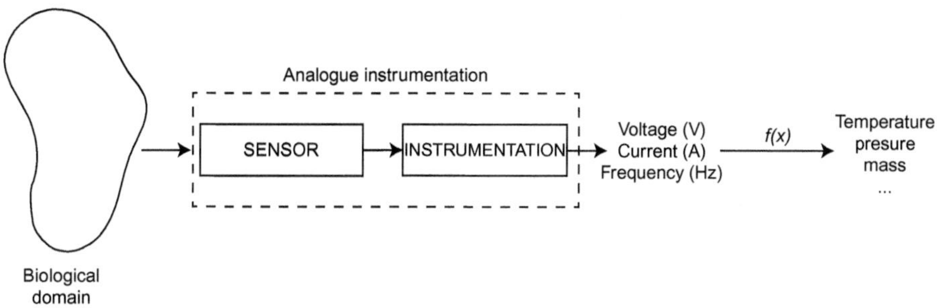

Fig. 11.5 Simplest sensor application scenario.

This is the simplest scenario, which can evolve into a scenario where the sensor output is acquired by a processing unit (as a simple microcontroller) (Fig. 11.6). In this scenario, the user might be able to directly see the output in the format of interest and, moreover, might have the system automatized to monitor and record the sensor's output signal. From this point, the user can process the signal or define thresholds or other processing or triggering mechanisms that result in outcomes. These outcomes may be simple alarms that, for example in the case of a temperature sensor, may tell the user that the temperature went beyond a defined threshold. In this situation, we have a smart system, a system capable of detecting a scenario.

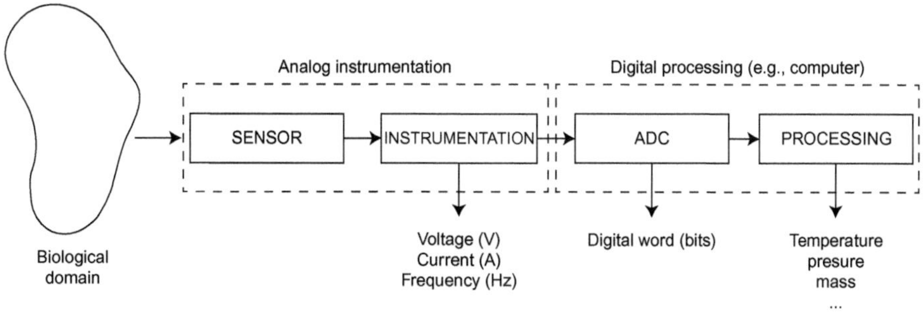

Fig. 11.6 The simple sensor-based device architecture.

However, it is important to underline that smartness is not associated to the sensor itself, but to the system as a whole. That is why we call it a smart-device. The device includes the sensor plus other components as the acquisition circuit (instrumentation amplifiers, filters and interface circuitry), the processing circuit (microprocessors) and several display components (from simple light-emitting diodes (LEDs), to more complex components as screens) for outcomes display.

Add-on components can also be included as wireless communication boards. This enables the processing and/or outcomes display to be performed far from the sensing site, e.g., remotely (Fig. 11.7). Other examples of add-on components include power supply through batteries or based on more recent inductive wireless technologies.

As communications platforms are added, many sensors and sensor systems may communicate to a single central unit or even broadcast through the internet platform (Fig. 11.8), providing centralized data access.

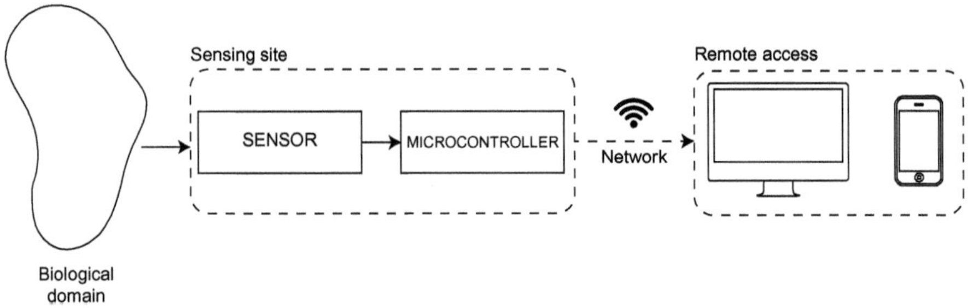

Fig. 11.7 Remote access.

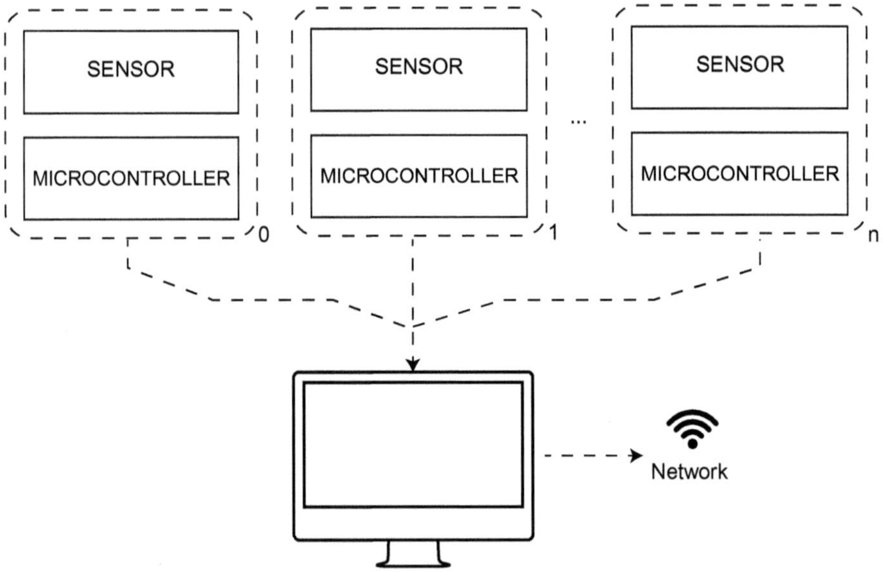

Fig. 11.8 The network of sensors.

This is an example of many monitoring systems available nowadays, such as the health monitoring home kits similar to the one illustrated in Fig. 11.9. Different sensors for different purposes perform their task and concentrate their data into a single processing unit that then displays all the information.

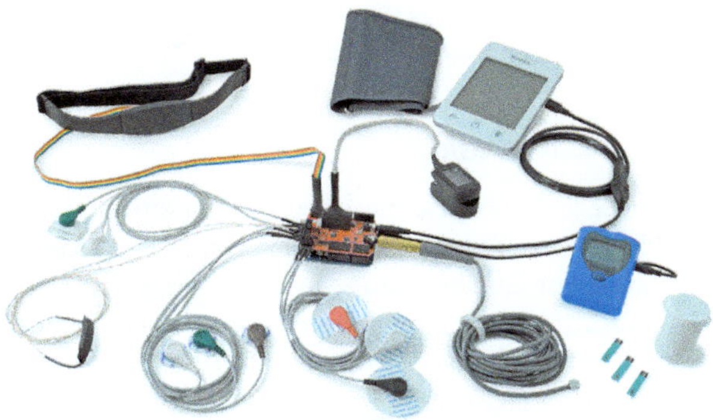

Fig. 11.9 e-Health Sensor Platform V2.0 for Arduino and Raspberry Pi with a variety of sensors connected to the same microcontroller, namely pulse and oxygen in blood, electrocardiogram (ECG), airflow, body temperature, blood pressure, patient position and falls, galvanic skin response, glucometer and electromyography sensor.
Reprinted from Libelium—www.libelium.com.

So far the smart-devices' architecture has been discussed. However, for a few applications, the smartness of the devices has been extended, making them intelligent. Though smart devices provide usable information and enable the triggering of alarms, they are not capable of actuating back over the system. Intelligent devices are able to, based on the acquired data and the decision algorithms that are embedded into the system, actuate back on the system in order to restore the input signal to the desired range (Fig. 11.10).

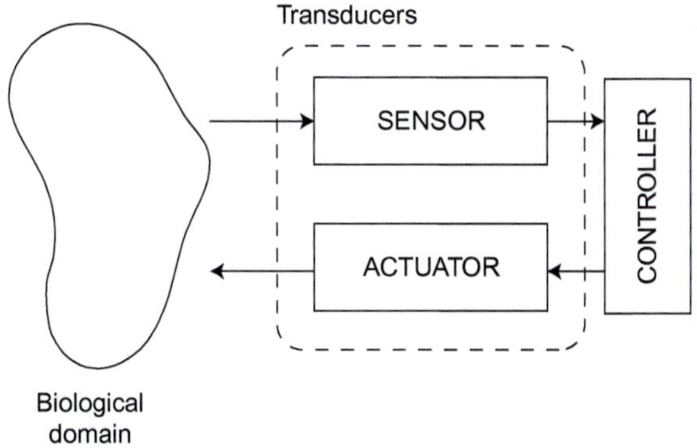

Fig. 11.10 The intelligent system diagram (close-loop).

This approach is called the close loop. Examples of well-established intelligent devices in the medical area are the cardiac pacemakers. Through a set of electrodes, the pacemaker is able to detect abnormalities in the heart electrical signal and artificially stimulate the heart to suppress such anomalies. Another example, not yet fully realized, is the implantable insulin pump (Spaan et al., 2014).

Despite the interest and the impact of intelligent solutions that are rather close to full autonomous operation, this requires the full understating of the biological system, which is not transferrable to all possible applications.

11.2.2 Micro- and nanoscale

Sensors, like many other technologies, have been taking advantage of the evolution of microfabrication processes. The ability to miniaturize devices has opened up the opportunity for making them implantable in ways that would not have been imaginable a few decades ago. However, miniaturization is not confined to the downsizing of the sensor. All of the other components required to work with the sensor need to be miniaturized as well, and engineered into a single device that would enable access to many measurement sites and signals. Driven by the semiconductor industry, through lithographic and thin-film deposition processes, we witnessed the evolution from macroscale into the microdimensions, and now we are looking at the opening of the nanoscale world (Son et al., 2011).

Fig. 11.11 shows the range of dimensions of several elements in the human body. As the sensors downsize, it becomes possible to gain access to the complexities of the smaller elements, enabling the understanding of physiological phenomena at a fundamental level (Rolfe, 2012). This is what is expected with the evolution of these devices. It is stated that a microscale device is defined by size-characteristics within the 1 mm–100 nm range, while nanoscale represents features sub-100 nm.

Moreover, the ability to access such structures at this scale has benefited research into sensory systems, which is key in biomimicry and biomimetics (Müller and Kuc, 2007).

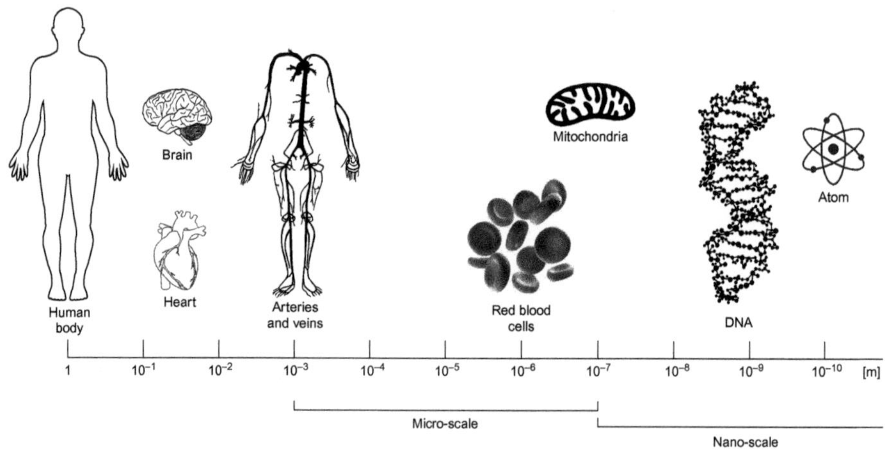

Fig. 11.11 Dimensions range for several elements of the human body.

Driven by these challenges, there is no doubt that the ability to downscale components and devices has an enormous impact on science due to the technical challenges that such downscaling implies (Kobel and Reymond, 2011). At the miniaturization level we can achieve today, it is no longer a question of simply linearly sizing down components. There is a need to revise the manufacturing processes as, at the micro- and nanolevel, tolerances barely match the normal standards. Moreover, at the microlevel, mechanical, thermal and optical effects do not behave as in the macrosize level. This drives a review of the manufacturing process in order to work at such small sizes. Moreover, to cope with the different effects, the design of the devices themselves needs to be adjusted.

Although much of this miniaturization was driven by transistor size reduction, as new processes and design methodologies became available, they quickly led to the development of new components, nowadays known as MEMS (microelectromechanical systems). MEMS sensors can now be found in any electronic device that we own, from our mobile phones, automobiles, to home appliances. However, evolution has not stopped at MEMS, and after breaking through the 100 nm critical barrier, the nanoworld has come within our reach, and NEMS (nanoelectromechanical systems) have emerged.

In this perspective, MEMS and NEMS offer unique characteristics for new functionalities and performance enhancements in sensing components. Nonetheless, as there were challenges at the microlevel, so are there challenges when trying to scale down MEMS into NEMS, as not all the microfabrication techniques developed so far are capable of making nanostructures (Cui and Gu, 2006). Moreover, as the size decreases, one should not forget that these components/devices need to interface with the real world, which becomes more difficult to do as their size continues to decrease. Examples of such difficulties are poor signal-to-noise ratio, low levels of signal, surrounding parasitics, variabilities, among others (Ionescu, 2009). Moreover, on a micro- and nanoscale other factors come into play, such as adhesion, friction, lubrication and surface contamination (Bhushan, 2011). These factors may not be an issue on the same magnitude with bulk-size materials/systems, but at this scale, they can cause significant problems. Thus, the overall performance of micro- and nanostructures is dependent on the structure's careful design.

11.3 Design of micro- and nanosensors for medical applications

Previously a few factors that influence the design of micro- and nanosensors were outlined. It is clear that not all of these issues affect the sensors to the same magnitude, as it all depends on the sensor's purpose and on the transduction principle. Therefore the design process will play a relevant role in ensuring the minimization of these effects. From an engineering perspective, the design process may be simplified with the definition of subfactors, in an attempt to address them individually. Olson (2009) proposed a categorization based on signal, environmental, medical and economic factors, as illustrated in Fig. 11.12. The signal category considers all the technical aspects related with the sensor performance, which were already discussed.

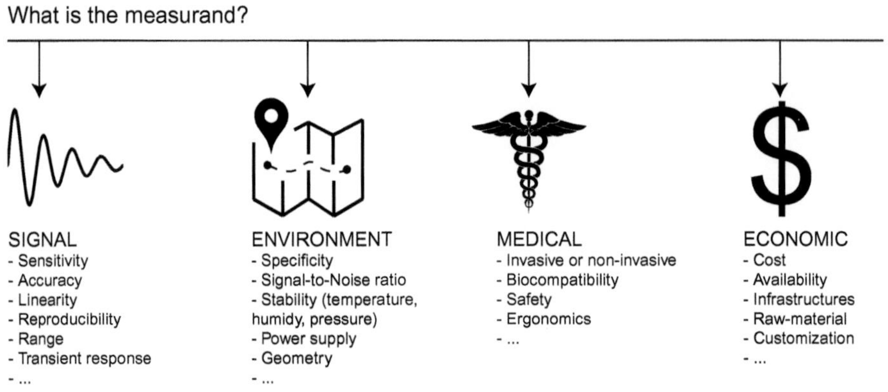

Fig. 11.12 Design process for medical devices.
Adapted from Olson, W.H., 2009. Basic concepts of medical instrumentation. In: Webster, J.G. (Ed.), Medical Instrumentation: Application and Design, fourth ed. John Wiley & Sons, Hoboken, pp. 1–44.

The environmental set of properties is related to the performance sensor in a given environment and not directly to the performance as a sensing device. This category is viewed as how the sensor behaves in the place/situation in which it is operating.

The medical factors are related to the health impact of the sensor. Questions such as "Is it biocompatible?," "Does it trigger any immunologic response?," "Is it safe for the subject?," among others, enable the assessment of the sensor performance in this criterion.

Finally, there are the economic factors, related to the burden of developing, manufacturing and usage of the sensor. Thus, for the economical assessment of the sensor design, its entire lifecycle is considered.

Although treated differently, all these categories are connected. From a researcher perspective, there is the temptation to give more weight to the signal, environmental and medical factors than to the economic ones. However, from the design perspective, the decisions taken in each of the categories will most likely have an influence on the others. It is the designer's role to identify the best balance between all the decisions taken.

As a result of this interconnection between the factors, the design process is highly cyclic and interactive, rarely following a linear and direct approach. However, the factors discussed so far are only related to the early phase of the design process.

Medical devices rely on knowledge from different sciences, from materials to electronics, mechanics or health among others. This wide scope forces the teaming up of different specialties from physicians to engineers (Santos and Tavares, 2013). As designs are driven by a current medical need, there may be a lack of information regarding requirements and specifications (Santos et al., 2012).

Fig. 11.13 illustrates a generic lifecycle for medical devices that goes beyond the design phase. This figure illustrates all the steps a medical device undergoes and how they interact. Although as researchers we may just focus on the device development phase, the understanding of the entire cycle and its interconnections drives research towards higher performance devices (Santos, 2012).

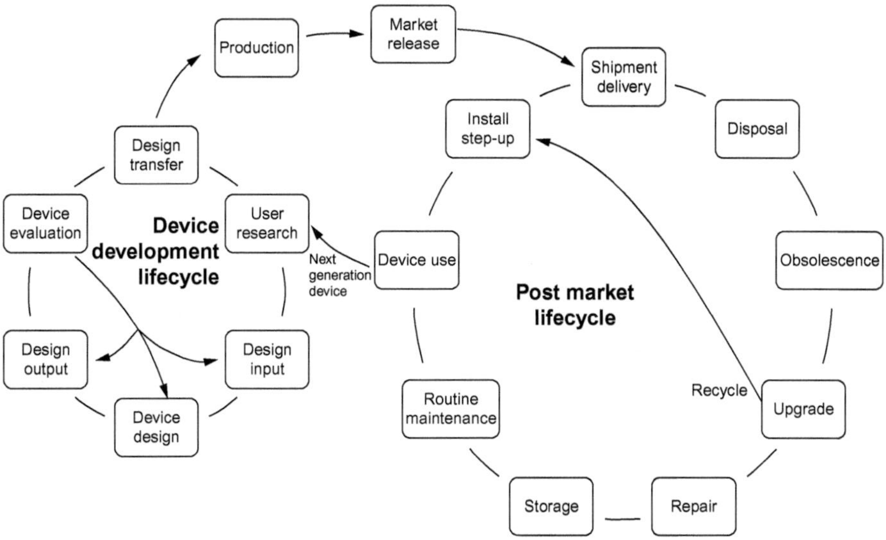

Fig. 11.13 Typical lifecycle of a medical device.
Reprinted from Santos, I., 2012. Product Development Methodologies—The Case of Medical Devices. University of Porto, Porto. [Internet]. Available from: http://hdl.handle.net/10216/76244; https://repositorio-aberto.up.pt.

The ability to materialize a device design is highly dependent on the availability of materials and processes to shape such devices in order to meet the requirements. This listing of materials and processes leads to a variety of possible designs, the performance of which depends upon their combination. Thus, the optimized design results from the thorough selection of materials and processes that fulfills as much as possible the design requirements. This selection efficiency is dependent on the clear understanding of the functional requirements of each component of the device and on their interface between each other and with the real world. This makes the selection process at the micro- and nanoscale a challenge, due to the multifunctional roles of the several components (Prashant Reddy and Gupta, 2010).

Over the years, Ashby has been one of the most prominent names in the field of materials research, with even a selection method being given his name. The key to this method is the ability to translate requirements into materials and processes attributes. The attributes in this context can take different expressions, from numeric as Young modulus, Boolean as recyclability or process compatibility, or ranking (from poor to very good) as in the case of resistance to corrosion. The translation between the application requirements and the materials and processes attributes, a key step in Ashby's method, is performed through (Ashby et al., 2004):

- Translation of design requirements into specifications
- Screening out materials that do not meet the defined requirements
- Ranking the selection materials and processes, pointing out the ones with larger potential
- Use of external supporting data about the top results for final selection criteria.

Although this method was developed initially for macroscale structures, it has become common to see it applied to micro- and nanosensors (Quinn et al., 2006). Though, as these devices range in sizes at the sub-100 μm level, many are based on a silicon material system. Nonetheless, new materials and techniques driven by the ability to perform precision engineering are being explored and developed (Qian and Zhao, 2002). Today, materials from different types, from metals to ceramics, polymers or composites, may have suitable attributes to be applied into micro- and nanosensors.

Within the selection process, the properties of micro- and nanoscale structures tend to be a function of length, as well as of the processing techniques employed, such as that most mechanical properties are scale dependent (Bhushan, 2011). However, in some cases, it is still possible to build a bridge between micro- and bulk properties. In a comparison between studies from Sharpe and Ashby (Prashant Reddy and Gupta, 2010), it is possible to consider the values from Table 11.1 as initial design value approximations based on the bulk material properties.

Table 11.1 Recommended initial design values of material properties

Property	Recommendation
Density, ρ (kg m^{-3})	$\rho_{\mu}=\rho_{bulk}$ (approx.)
Young's modulus, E (GPa)	$0.8E_{bulk} \leq E_{\mu} \leq E_{bulk}$
Poisson's ratio, ν (−)	0.25
Fracture strength, σ_F (MPa)	$\sigma_{F,\mu}=\alpha_{F,bulk}$ (approx.)
Linear expansion coefficient, α (K^{-1})	$\alpha_{\mu}=\alpha_{bulk}$ (approx.)
Specific heat, C_p (J kg^{-1} K^{-1})	$C_{p,\mu}=C_{p,bulk}$
Intrinsic loss coefficient, η_i	$10^{-2}<\eta_i$ (polymers) $10^{-5}<\eta_i$ (metals) $10^{-7}<\eta_i<10^{-4}$ (ceramics)
Residual stress, σ_R (MPa)	-1 GPa $<\sigma_R<1$ GPa

Reprinted from Prashant Reddy, G., Gupta, N., 2010. Material selection for microelectronic heat sinks: an application of the Ashby approach. Mater. Des. 31 (1), 113–117. Elsevier Ltd.; Available from: http://linkinghub.elsevier.com/retrieve/pii/S0261306909003549.

As a result of this design methodology, one ends up with a structure that meets the requirements and is satisfactory from the scientific perspective. However, most likely it will be based on nonconventional material, whose fabrication may not be feasible from an economical perspective (Baltes et al., n.d.). This leads the design to a paradox. The solution to overcome this is to take advantage of microfabrication technologies and to satellite the design around it. Microfabrication processes are proven to be reliable nowadays. The main available and compatible microfabrication processes are related with bulk micromachining and lithography, and thin-film deposition (both chemical and physical methods) (Srikar and Spearing, 2003). These have been the key technologies that have driven us to the microfabrication world.

This set of processes basically aims to machine the bulk material using either a top-down approach or a bottom-up approach through shaping and patterning techniques. These techniques enable the fabrication of micro- and nanostructures as bridges, cantilevers, frames, masses, flexible membranes, motion mechanisms, among others (Gopel et al., 1994). Microfabrication has brought value advantages including low size, low cost, performance enhancement (at the sensitivity, response time and resolution level). Moreover, these technologies allow the integration of electronics for sensor output signal processing within the same device. Still, microfabrication techniques are sensitive to physical phenomena with special magnitude at micro- and nanolevel, as already mentioned.

11.4 Types of sensors

As previously seen, a sensor is a device capable of converting one type of energy into electrical energy and this will allow, with the aid of the acquisition and processing instrumentation, the measurement to be displayed to the user.

11.4.1 Direct versus indirect sensing

In general terms, sensors can be grouped according to whether they can directly or indirectly convert a measurand into an electrical signal. In a direct sensor, the measurand is already of an electric nature or can directly convert a different type of energy into electricity (Fig. 11.14A). A commonly used example of direct sensing is the physiological electrodes that convert bioelectricity into electron-based electricity.

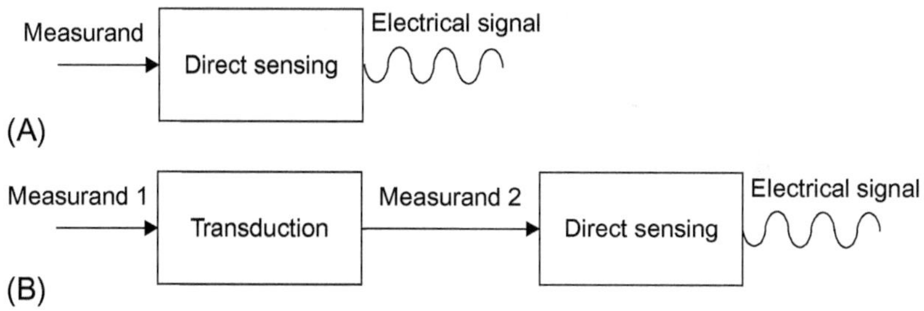

Fig. 11.14 Type of sensor according to sensing principle. (A) Direct sensor. (B) Indirect sensor.

Despite the existence of these kinds of sensors, there are a vast number of measurands that cannot be converted directly into electricity. In this case, an indirect conversion is necessary, where the sensor converts the measurand into another type of energy before transforming it into electricity (Fig. 11.14B). Indirect sensors can have one or more transduction stages according to the needs of the sensor.

The idea of indirect sensing can be more clearly understood when thinking of commercial thermometers used to measure body temperature. These devices rely on a two-step measuring process. In the first step, the temperature at the tip of the thermometer influences the resistivity of a sensor inside the thermometer. An electronic circuit inside the device detects the present resistivity and converts this value into an electrical signal that can be processed and shown in the display as the recorded temperature. In this sensor, a variation of temperature changes the resistivity, which in turn produces an electrical signal.

11.4.2 Active versus passive

Sensors can also be classified as active and passive. A passive sensor does not need external energy for the acquisition of the electric signal, while an active sensor does.

An example of a passive sensor is the photodiode. This device can generate an electrical current when exposed to light.

A widely used example of an active sensor is the accelerometer used in cell phones. These sensors allow the detection of the orientation of the cell phone as well as the occurrence of vibration. The same type of sensors is used in biomedical applications for the detection of heart rate in patients (Hung et al., 2008).

11.4.3 Sensing principles

Besides these general categorizations, sensors can also be classified according to their sensing principle, which is related to the transducer that composes them. Underlying the sensing principles are the physical principles, such as electromagnetism, harmonic vibrations, piezoelectricity and others that allow the conversion of one type of energy into another. Some of these principles followed by some basic application examples will be described in the subsequent sections.

11.4.4 Electrical sensors

Electrical sensors have the ability to transform electric potentials, fields and charges into electrical signals. Since the source measurand is already of electrical nature, these sensors use the direct sensing principle.

A commonly used example is that of the physiological electrodes. These devices can convert electrical fields and potentials generated by the movement and concentration of ions in biological systems into electric signals that can be acquired by electronic instrumentation. The physical principle behind the functioning of such electrodes is the electric potential generated by a point charge. A charged particle creates an electric field, and therefore an electric potential in space.

Consider the example of a group of ions with a positive net charge moving in the vicinity of a metallic electrode. The movement of the ions will change the electric field and therefore, the electric potential felt by the nearby electrode. If there is a second electrode with a reference potential, the ions will cause a variation in the potential of the first electrode, generating an electrical signal that can be measured by external electronics (Fig. 11.15).

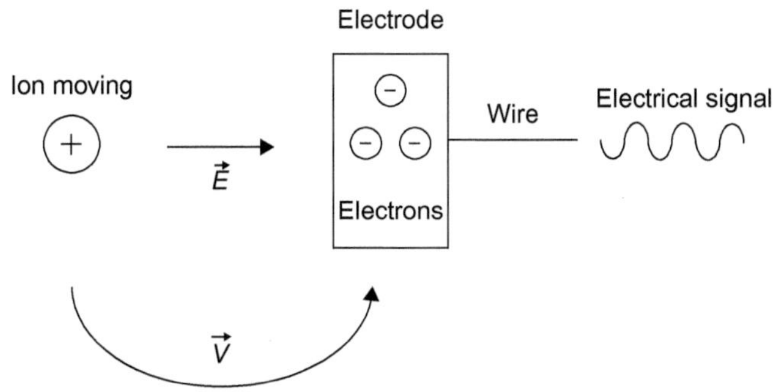

Fig. 11.15 Ions, electrons and electric potentials.

This kind of electrodes is used to measure many sources of electrical signals in the body, such as the heart electrical signal. In this example the myocardial depolarization and repolarization of heart cells can be measured through a system called electrocardiogram (ECG) with electrodes placed on the patient's skin (Thaler, 2007).

11.4.5 Mechanical sensors

Mechanical sensors target a large number of different measurands such as mass, force, pressure, strain, velocity, acceleration and weight, among others.

Practically, all motion-based sensors rely on Newton's laws of motion. Especially Newton's second law of motion is particularly useful since it relates force to mass and acceleration, and this can be used to transduce measurands.

Some mechanical sensors rely on the mechanical vibration of a microcantilever in order to detect attachment of mass to the structure. In microsensor applications, microcantilevers are structures made most often of silicon, despite it being possible to use other materials. The cantilever itself has dimensions in the microscale, as its length is in the order of 100–200 μm and its thickness is usually between 0.3 and 1 μm (Fraden, 2010). As a vibration is injected into the cantilever system, a shift in vibration means the presence of a mass attached to the cantilever. The detection can be performed by the bending or the frequency shift of the oscillating cantilever. The sensitivity of these sensors is based on the high area versus small volume of the sample, which amplifies surface stresses due to interaction with various substances. Microcantilever sensors can be used to determine other measurands such as acceleration and force. In these cases, the bending of the cantilever is observed instead of vibrations. For instance, accelerometers can precisely measure the bending of a cantilever to determine the acceleration that a certain sensor is experiencing. This latter example can be used to detect the physical vibrations in the chest of a patient and correlate them with heart function (Dinh, 2011).

Other mechanical sensors rely on the piezoresistive effect, which represents the variation of resistance of a given material when subjected to strain (Fraden, 2010). The change in resistance results from the mechanical deformation of the material and is the physical principle underlying the operation of many force and pressure sensors.

The variation in resistance occurs due to the variation in the geometry as well as the variation in the material's resistivity. One of the earliest applications of this physical effect to sensing was as a strain gauge (Beeby et al., 2004). This sensing element was composed of a stretchable foil underneath a series of metallic filaments. When a tension is applied at the two edges of the foil, the electrically conducting lines will stretch and change their resistance. The change in resistance can be related with the strain in the foil through the gauge factor.

Similarly to piezoresistive effect, there is the piezoelectric effect. When a crystalline material is subjected to stress, it generates an electrical field. Piezoelectric materials such as quartz, are made of atoms that have gained or lost electrons (ions), and hence accumulate an electric charge (Cady, 1964). Also, piezoelectric crystals are composed of alternating positive and negative ions, as seen in the example of Fig. 11.16. Positively charged silicon atoms (Si) are intercalated with three negatively charged oxygen atoms (O_2). In its resting state, no observable electric field can be detected at the perimeter of this cell due to charge symmetry. In turn, when subjected to either a compressive or tensional force, an electric field will be observed. This field is due to the relative position of the ions, which will generate an electric field observed at the edges (Fig. 11.16B and C).

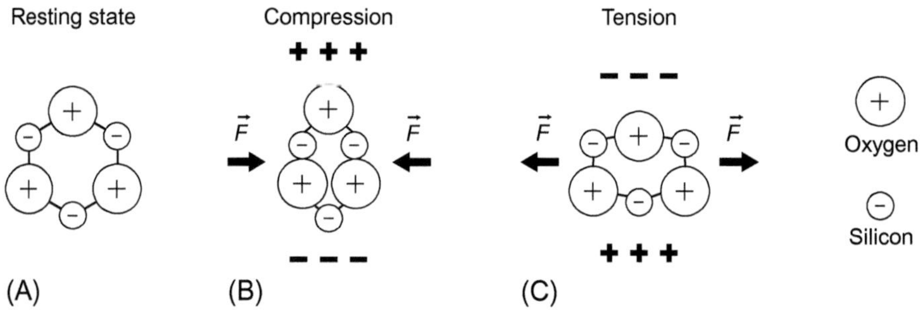

Fig. 11.16 Piezoelectric effect on quartz. Crystalline structure under (A) no stress, (B) compression, and (C) tension.
Adapted from Fraden, J., 2010. Handbook of Modern Sensors, fourth ed. Springer, New York, NY. [Internet]. Available from: http://link.springer.com/10.1007/978-1-4419-6466-3.

A simple sensor using this effect is the pressure sensor, where a force applied at the edges of a piezoelectric material will produce an electric potential. Usually metallic electrodes are attached to the piezoelectric material in order to conduct electric signals from the piezo material to the processing electronics. Besides being useful to measure the applied force, piezoelectric sensors are also used to measure other measurands such as pressure, acceleration, and temperature. Since this kind of sensor is very sensitive to small changes in displacement, it is also used to detect failures on biomechanical implants such as hip prosthesis and heart valve implants (Lanjef et al., 2006; Lanning and Shandas, 2003).

11.4.6 Optical sensors

Optical sensors have the capacity to detect and quantify various properties of light such as intensity, frequency, wavelength, and polarization. These sensors rely on light detectors that have the ability of converting light into electrical signals. These detectors are able to sense electromagnetic radiation from the infrared up to the ultraviolet wavelengths.

Many light detectors such as the photovoltaic and photoconductive, depend on the interaction between photons and the crystalline lattice of semiconductors. This interaction is known as the photoelectric effect, and was firstly proposed by Einstein in 1905. The photoelectric effect explains that when a photon hits the surface of a conductor it generates a free electron (Fig. 11.17). These free electrons will affect the material's electrical properties, therefore allowing the measurement of the properties of the incident light.

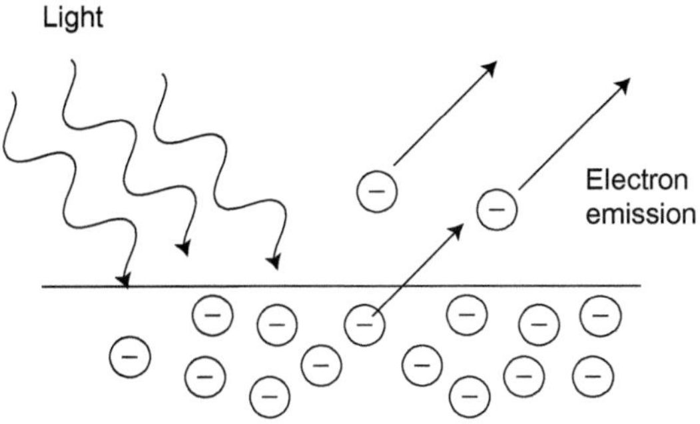

Fig. 11.17 Photoelectric effect.

A widely used tool for optical sensors is the photodiode. This device is capable of converting light into electric current and thus being able to sense light intensity. This device is composed of a p- and n-type semiconductor bonded together forming a diode. These devices are similar to semiconductor diodes, except that their packaging allows light to hit the pn-junction. When reversely biased, as light hits the semiconductor, free electrons will be generated and the current flowing in the circuit will increase quite noticeably. Even when there is no light, the circuit will generate a small current known as dark current. This current is independent of applied voltage and varies only with temperature. On the other hand, when light is shining over the semiconductor a significantly higher current will flow through the circuit and is generated by the photocurrent.

One example of an optical sensor used for medical applications is the pulse oximeter. This device is placed in a thin part of the patient's body such as a fingertip or earlobe. Two lights with different wavelengths are passed through the patient's body and absorbed in a photodetector on the other side. This system is able to detect the saturation of oxygen in the blood (Parker, 2004).

11.4.7 Chemical sensors

Chemical sensors respond to measurands through various chemicals and chemical reactions. They have the ability to identify and quantify liquid or gaseous chemical species. This class of sensors is currently used in many chemical analysis techniques, such as mass spectroscopy, chromatography, infrared technology and others (Fraden, 2010), due to the miniaturization of sensors. There are a variety of chemical sensors with various methods of transduction. The transduction methods of chemical sensors can be organized into three classes based on their modes of measurement: (i) electrical and electrochemical properties, (ii) changes in the physical properties, and (iii) optical absorption of the chemical analytes to be measured.

Electrochemical sensors are the most common approach, and operate by reacting with the chemical solutions and producing an electrical signal that is proportional to the analyte concentration (Chou, 1999). These types of sensors can be classified into three categories according to their operation mode (Fraden, 2010):

- Potentiometric, which relies on the measurement of voltage. To measure the concentration of analytes it is necessary for a combination of electric and ionic current to flow in a closed circuit. A practical application of this sensing principle will be given in the biosensors section.
- Amperometric, which relies on the measurement of current. These sensors have been shown to be effective in a broad range of applications, such as volatile organic compounds detection in soils and groundwater, detection of mines and analytes detection in blood (Brotherton and Wheeler, 2012; Guenther et al., 2012).
- Conductometric relies on the measurement of either conductivity or resistivity. This type of sensor comprises a capacitor that changes its capacitance when exposed to the desired analyte. The capacitance of the sensor changes due to a selectively absorbing material such as polymers or other insulators. These absorbing materials serve as the dielectric layer of the capacitor and their permittivity changes with exposure to the analyte. These sensors are commonly used to detect humidity as well as carbon dioxide and volatile organic compounds (Patel et al., 2003). In the humidity sensor case, the dielectric layer comprises a water-sensitive polymer (Lazarus and Fedder, 2011).

11.4.8 Biosensors

A biosensor can be best defined as a combination of a transducer and a bioreceptor (Fig. 11.18). A bioreceptor is a biomolecule that recognizes the target chemical substance, while the transducer converts the signal generated by the biomolecule into an electrical signal (Belluzo et al., 2007; Wilson, 2005).

This kind of sensor is derived from the development of the chemical sensors. The first biosensors were capable of reading the amount of oxygen in the blood. After this development, further improvements in this device made it able to sense other analytes in the body by adding enzymes to the oxygen electrode (Wilson, 2005). This represented the first biosensor and was called the enzyme electrode. In general, the main difference between biosensors, such as the enzyme electrode, and chemical sensors, such as the oxygen electrode, is that the first relies on biomolecules for the transducing process and the latter does not.

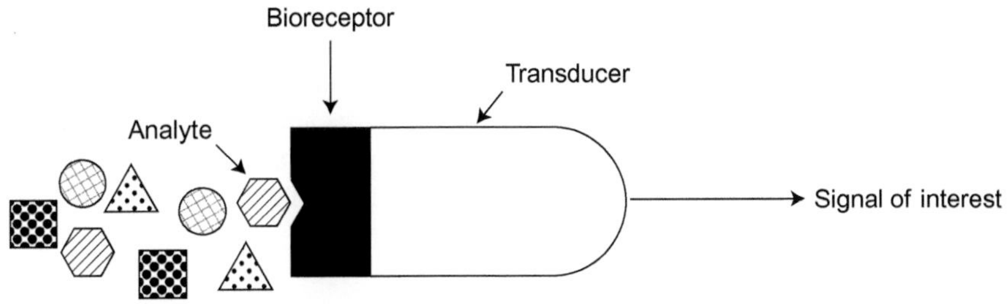

Fig. 11.18 Biosensors definition.
Adapted from Wilson, J., 2005. Sensor Technology Handbook. Elsevier/Newnes, Burlington, MA.

The enzyme electrode, as well as many other early biosensors, is based on the monitoring of electron-transfer processes, thus belonging to the amperometric category. In this type of biosensors the current acquired by the device is proportional to the analyte concentration. The electrical signal of these sensors is generated by the electron exchange between the biological system and the electrode. The first step happens when the analyte in the target solution undergoes redox reactions with the bioreceptor. The bioreceptor is a biomolecule responsible for selectively catalyzing the target analyte. The redox reaction promoted by the bioreceptor under certain conditions can generate an electron current in the nearby electrode. For this current to exist, it is necessary to apply a constant voltage between the electrode and the solution in order to supply electrons for the redox reactions taking place at the electrode. This mode of operation is known as chronoamperometry and represents the measurement of current in function of time while applying a constant potential at the electrode.

Many other types of biosensors have been developed using a large variety of different approaches, all of them being based on a biological element before a transducer. Many of the previous transducing principles can be combined with different types of bioreceptors (Belluzo et al., 2007).

11.5 Examples of medical micro- and nanodevices

With the introduction of the previous topics, it now becomes interesting to present and explore real medical devices based on micro- and nanosensors. These examples aim at supporting the importance and at highlighting new opportunities that micro- and nanosensor made possible in the diagnosis, monitoring and treatment of several diseases examples.

This section focuses first on implantable devices based on micro- and nanosensors. These are devices that were carefully designed and developed to be implanted inside the body. This implies that, besides the understanding of the most adequate sensing principle, for the target measurand the sensor should have the conditions in which the device will be implanted; therefore implantation method, compatibility with the surroundings of the implantation site, as well as physiological and anatomical singularities need to be considered from the design phase of the device.

11.5.1 Smart stent

An aortic aneurysm is today a common condition often related to cardiovascular diseases. This condition is identified as a swelling of the aortic artery section led by the local weakening of its walls and systemic pressure (Johnston et al., 1991) (Fig. 11.19A). Thus, one can easily understand the danger and the risk of fatality associated with a burst on the artery wall, leading to a massive loss of blood.

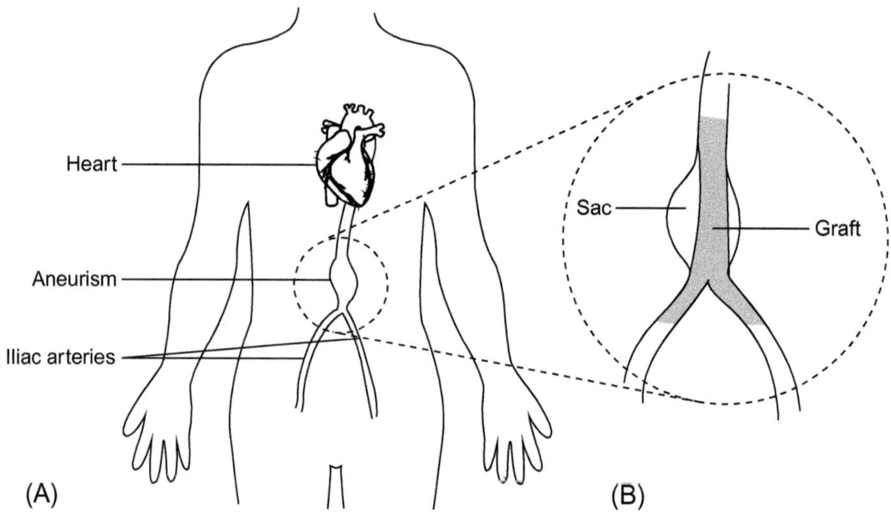

Fig. 11.19 Illustration of (A) aortic aneurism and (B) stent positioning.

Two approaches for the treatment of this condition are possible: either reconstruction of the aortic artery in open chest surgery, or an endovascular aneurism repair procedure. In medical procedures, the current trend is to minimize the open chest surgery and to prioritize minimally invasive methods whenever possible. The latter results in less physiological disturbance and faster recovery times.

In the endovascular aneurism repair, a stent is placed, via percutaneous pathways, inside the aneurism sac in order to exclude it from the systemic pressure that can lead to burst of the sac (Fig. 11.19B). Although this may be the preferred approach (when possible) and proven to be successful, it is not free from postoperative issues, namely stent displacement or endoleaks (Katzen and MacLean, 2006). It is the latter that served as a premise for the design of a smart stent graft (Sepulveda, 2013).

The current surveillance methods for detection of the postoperative issues are based on common imaging techniques such as ultrasounds, CT and MRI. Not only do these methods only provide visual information, they are highly expensive on a routine basis and are dependent on the trained eye of the technician. The proposed solution was to design a stent graft capable of monitoring the pressure inside the sac (sensing element) and transmitting the sensor's data (telemetry element), enabling the interrogation of the current pressure conditions inside the sac, which are related to the stent's performance.

The challenge of the design published in (Sepulveda, 2013) was to combine in a passive device a sensor capable of working within a pressure range of 20–250 mmHg, with a resolution of 1 mmHg, and a telemetry block capable of transmitting the pressure data. Moreover, all of these features are to be included in a device small and flexible enough to fit in the aneurism sac.

At the sensor level, the solution was to use a flexible pressure sensor based on aligned-CNTs/PDMS nanocomposites (carbon nanotubes (CNTs) embedded into polydimethylsiloxane (PDMS) elastomer). The pressure sensor was based on the capacitive principle (Fig. 11.20). The sensor design used a close box with air trapped inside (dielectric) at a specific pressure (P_0). As the outside pressure varies (P_{out}), the box deflects due to the pressure differential between the inside (reference pressure) and the outside domain.

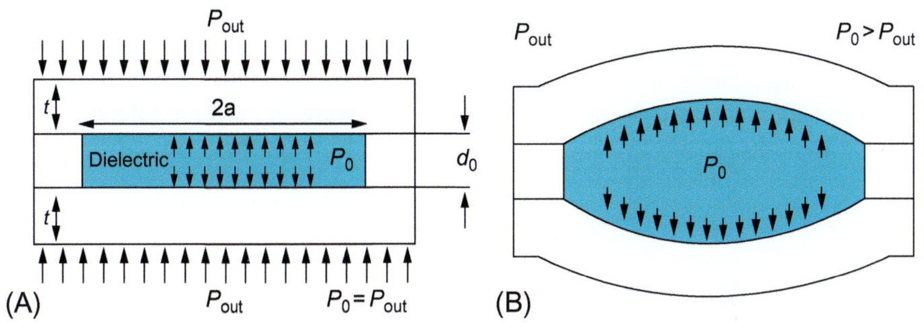

Fig. 11.20 (A) Cross section of the capacitive-based pressure sensor. (B) Cross section of the capacitive-based sensor when deflected.
Panel A: Reprinted from Sepúlveda, A.T., Villoria, R.G., De Viana, J.C., Pontes, A.J., Wardle, B.L., Rocha, L.A., 2012. Flexible pressure sensors: modeling and experimental characterization. Procedia Eng. 47, 1177–1180. Elsevier B.V.; Available from: http://linkinghub.elsevier.com/retrieve/pii/S1877705812044244.

Added to this deflection principle, two conductive plates as top and bottom membranes of the box lead to capacity changes as the space between them alters—the principle of a capacitive sensor (Oliveira et al., 2015).

The challenge was to fabricate the sensor (box) with two conductive membranes at each end, with air trapped between them (Fig. 11.21). This was solved using a nanocomposites of CNTs/PDMS (Sepúlveda et al., 2013a). Polydimethylsiloxane (PDMS) is a biocompatible silicone-based elastomer, with high degree of flexibility and elasticity, making it a suitable substrate for the stent application. However, it is not an electric

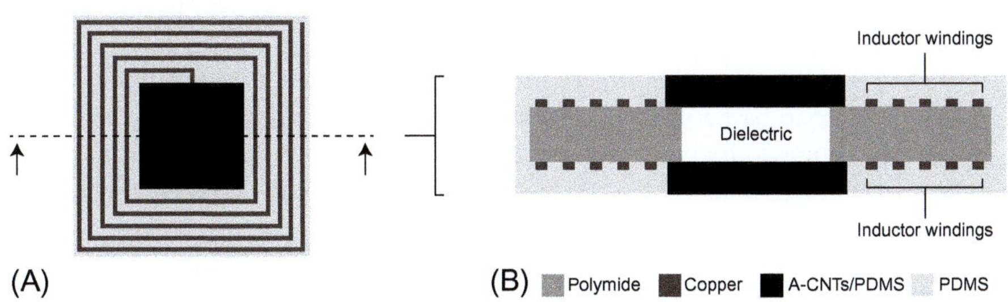

Fig. 11.21 Overview of the proposed pressure sensor's top structure (A) and cross section (B).

conductor. This was solved by embedding into the PDMS substrate, carbon nanotubes (CNTs) forests (Sepúlveda et al., 2013b). CNTs are one of today's most promising materials due to their electrical, mechanical and chemical properties (Malarkey and Parpura, 2010). By combining the two materials, it became possible to transform an inert material into a functional one, in this case to serve as the capacitor membrane plates.

The telemetry feature was based on LC[2] resonant network, C being the sensor's capacity. By adding an inductor, the LC response would change in accordance to the capacity change, which is driven by the pressure changes. In order to fabricate the inductor, a series of coils were printed on a flexible printed circuit, which serve as antenna to interrogate the sensor capacity. The readout system measures the oscillation frequency of the LC resonant circuit created by sensors and inductive coupling (Oliveira et al., 2015).

As a result (Fig. 11.22), the developed device is an excellent example of how a thorough design can result in a simple sensor device, without any active elements but still capable of measuring the aneurism's sac pressure and enabling the data to be accessed from the outside.

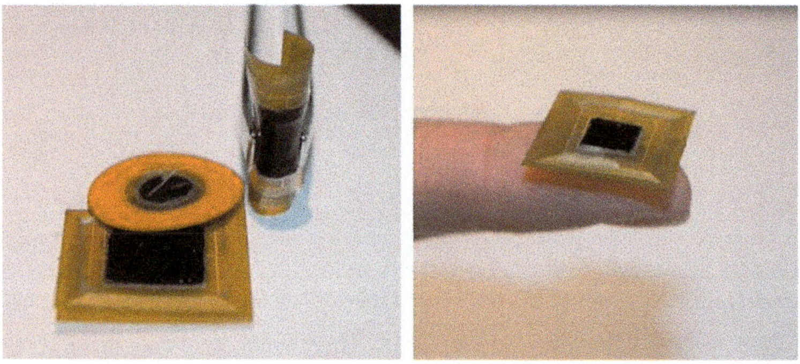

Fig. 11.22 Developed pressure sensor for stent graft.
Reprinted from Sepulveda, A., 2013. Use of Nanocomposites for Flexible Pressure Sensors. University of Minho, Portugal. Available from: http://hdl.handle.net/1822/34582; http://repositorium.sdum.uminho.pt/.

11.5.2 Optrodes

The ability to access deep areas of the brain and understand the neurophysiological events has always been considered the key to restore the system's lost functionalities (Normann, 2007). Microsystems technologies enabled this access through the development of microscale devices known as neuroprobes. The Michigan probe (Wise, 2009) and the Utah array (Sharma et al., 2011) are considered the two gold standards in microelectrode-based probes. It is currently possible to find 3D microelectrode arrays that comprise high aspect-ratio shafts and different penetrating length electrodes (from 3 to 4 mm) fabricated in bulk silicon substrate dicing saw technology

[2] Resonant circuit formed by an inductor (L) and a capacitor (C) in parallel. In the discussed device, the capacitor is structured by the two conductive layers of PDMS/CNTs nanocomposites, and the inductor results from the external windings.

to provide high-production and reproducibility (Goncalves et al., 2015). As a result, several applications for stimulation neuroprobes have been evaluated with satisfactory results (Benabid, 2003). However, external electromagnetic interference, signal artifacts and poor spatial selectivity (Cho et al., 2010; Im et al., 2011) are considered to be the main downside of this technology.

The optical stimulation neuroprobes are currently emerging as the new technological wave for neurosciences. Through optogenetics, neural cells become sensitive to light stimulation (Bernstein and Boyden, 2011), enabling excitatory and inhibitory actions in the neural circuitry, similarly to the electrical stimulation but more focal. As the result of this emerging field, micro- and nanofabrication technologies are being applied to fabricate the tools required for stimulation of the genetically altered neural cells.

Initially, optical fibers were used to guide the light from an external light source into the deep regions of the brain (Fig. 11.23A) in conjunction with neuroprobes for stimulation readout (Aravanis et al., 2007). However, this solution shows a few

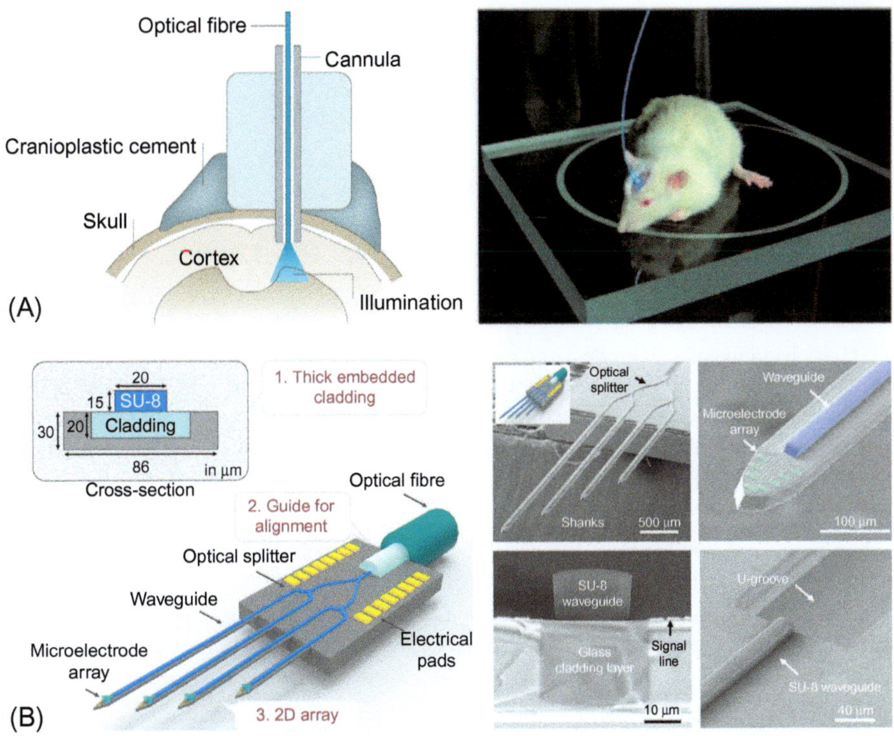

Fig. 11.23 Example of optrodes' structures. (A) Direct stimulation from an optical fiber. (B) Through an optical waveguide sourced.
Panel A: Reprinted from Zhang, F., Aravanis, A.M., Adamantidis, A., de Lecea, L., Deisseroth, K., 2007. Circuit-breakers: optical technologies for probing neural signals and systems. Nat. Rev. Neurosci. 8 (8), 577–581; Panel B: Reprinted from Son, Y., Lee, H.J., Kim, J., Shin, H., Choi, N., Lee, C.J., et al., 2015. In vivo optical modulation of neural signals using monolithically integrated two-dimensional neural probe arrays. Sci. Rep. 5 (October), 15466. Nature Publishing Group; Available from: http://www.nature.com/articles/srep15466.

limitations related to the possible injuries inferred to neurons during the fiber-guided insertion and low positioning accuracy on the stimulation sites (Cho et al., 2010). Alternatively (Cho et al., 2010), neuroprobes that directly integrate a single polymeric optical waveguide on its shank were developed (Fig. 11.23B) (Im et al., 2011), including with different stimulation depths (Zorzos et al., 2012), or high-density stimulation sites per array (Abaya et al., 2012).

Like the electrical-based neuroprobes, a second optical-enabled neuroprobe design emerged. Instead of using an optical fiber, which limits the test subject natural behavior (due to wiring and interfacing apparatus) (Kwon et al., 2013, 2014), microsize LEDs were employed, transferring the external light source directly into the stimulation sites.

The micro-LEDs enable spatial precision, cellular-scale delivery of photons, effective thermal management, reduced tissue damage and minimum inflammation during prolonged use (Kim et al., 2013). Fig. 11.24 shows an example of an array of 32-channel micro-LED-coupled optrode array (Kwon et al., 2015).

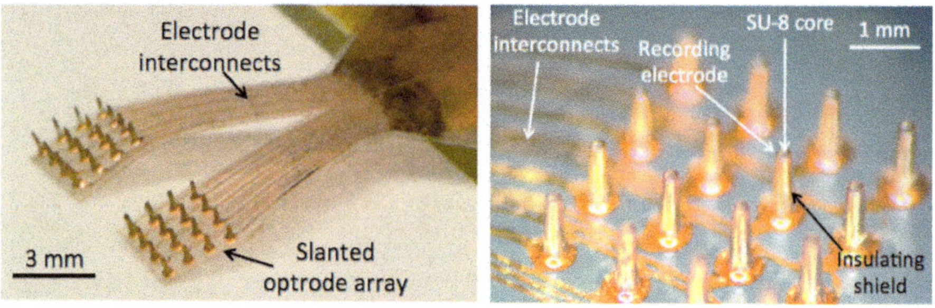

Fig. 11.24 Example of an optrode based on direct micro-LED stimulation.
Reprinted from Kwon, K.Y., Lee, H.-M., Ghovanloo, M., Weber, A., Li, W., 2015. Design, fabrication, and packaging of an integrated, wirelessly-powered optrode array for optogenetics application. Front. Syst. Neurosci. 9 (May), 69. Available from: http://www.pubmedcentral.nih.gov/articlerender.fcgi?artid=4422027&tool=pmcentrez&rendertype=abstract.

The identified downside of this LED-based design if the low light power emitted that may not be sufficient to stimulate the cells.

Despite the identified issues, the design and development of optical neuroprobes is still in its early stage, and many developments are expected in the next decade.

11.5.3 Organ-on-a-chip

Many micro- and nanodevices can play a significant role in medicine even when they are not implanted and are instead used externally as wearables or as laboratorial devices. In this section, a few devices are described as examples to demonstrate their impact and to highlight how micro- and nanofeatures were key to their performance.

Lab-on-a-chip is today a mature diagnosis technology (further discussion on the following chapter), although it still has many development opportunities. More recently, and deviating from the lab-on-a-chip, one can find the organ-on-a-chip. This type of device is a useful tool for laboratorial use, where a device mimics a tissue and its associated physiological processes (Dekker, 2013). Indeed, it can be looked upon as a combination of half tissue and half microelectronics. It goes beyond cell culture protocols and animal models. The premise for supporting its development is related to the capacity to mimic, in laboratorial environment, the physiological response of human tissues (and at macroscale, organs) when exposed to a variety of conditions.

Driven by the microfluidics development from the lab-on-a-chips, many organ-on-a-chips are currently being developed in many research groups, each using different instruments, cells and materials (Bhatia and Ingber, 2014). As a result, it is possible to find organ-on-chips dedicated to liver, lung, intestine, kidney, vasculature, bone narrow, brain, spleen, among others (Caplin et al., 2015). The developments aim at a multi-organ-on-chip (Fig. 11.25).

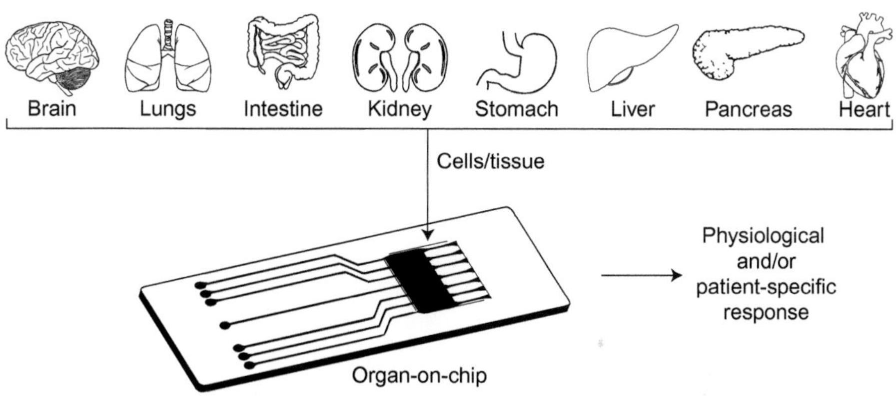

Fig. 11.25 Organ-on-chip principle.
Adapted from Luni, C., Serena, E., Elvassore, N., 2014. Human-on-chip for therapy development and fundamental science. Curr. Opin. Biotechnol. 25, 45–50. Elsevier Ltd; http://dx.doi.org/10.1016/j.copbio.2013.08.015.

The usability of such technology is easily understandable for the pharmaceutical industry, where drugs need to have their development times cut and side effects identified in a timely manner. There is a clear need for representative human models to minimize later drug failure (van de Stolpe and den Toonder, 2013) (Huh et al., 2010). The same principle in drug research may be imagined for cosmetics, food additives or environmental contaminants (Fig. 11.26) (van den Berg, 2014).

An impressive example of an organ-on-chip is the heart-on-chip (Dekker, 2013). In this example, heart muscle tissue is grown on top of electrode membranes that work

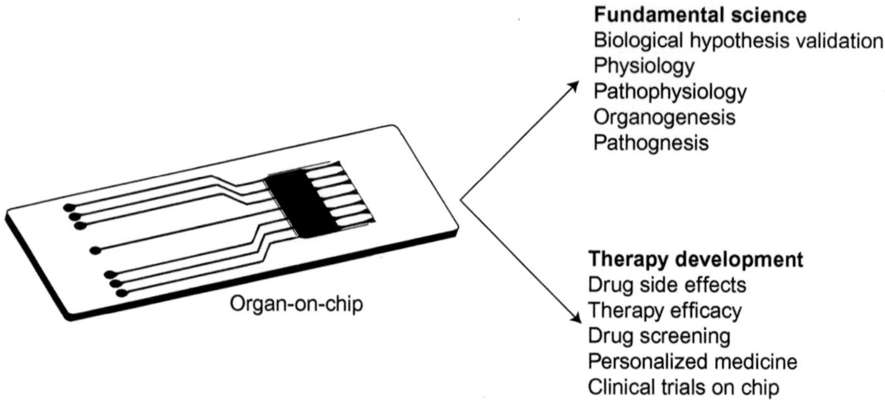

Fig. 11.26 Organ-on-chip applications.
Adapted from Luni, C., Serena, E., Elvassore, N., 2014. Human-on-chip for therapy development and fundamental science. Curr. Opin. Biotechnol. 25, 45–50. Elsevier Ltd; http://dx.doi.org/10.1016/j.copbio.2013.08.015.

as sensors for the electrical activity of the heart tissue. As the tissue is subjected to different drug compounds, its electrical activity is recorded and monitored, making it possible to identify the drug effects on the tissue. Moreover, the electrodes are placed on a membrane that, besides working as a support structure for the electrode and the tissue, have an additional feature, the ability to mimic the physical contraction of the muscle tissue. With the ability to stretch and contract the membrane, as it would on the muscle at different rates and strokes, and thus one is able to simulate different physiological conditions on the tissue and to evaluate its sensitivity to the drugs or other agents. The goal is to make the in vitro environment as close as possible to the in vivo conditions.

The developed heart-on-chip (Pakazad et al., 2014) was based on a stretchable microelectrode array (Pakazad et al., 2012) (Fig. 11.27) made by a PDMS membrane with TiN electrodes (12 μm in diameter) microfabricated on top of it. To promote the cell alignment and the adhesion to the PDMS membrane, microrecesses are patterned into the membrane, forcing the cells to lodge and to align in accordance with the recesses.

As a result and as a challenge related to having such a dynamic system with mechanical actuation, the sensors (electrodes) themselves placed on the membrane become sensitive to parasitic components induced by the mechanical behavior of the membrane (from the muscle contraction-like feature). To ensure the prolonged mechanical life and small inherent electrical noise, this device's design was carefully thought through, resulting in a dog-bone shape with the microfeatures and proper positioning of the interconnect nets (Pakazad et al., 2014).

The organs-on-chip enable health and disease models that represent and behave more closely to the human biological models (van de Stolpe and den Toonder, 2013), by mimicking the microenvironment of living cells at the tissue level (Agrawal, 2014).

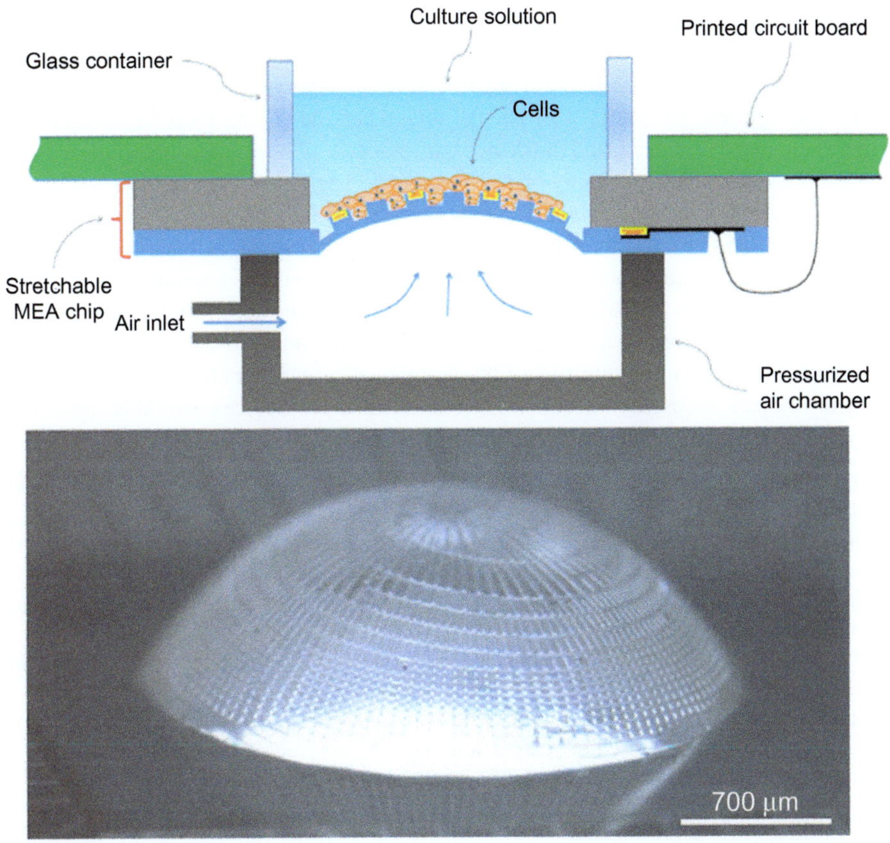

Fig. 11.27 Stretchable microelectrode array design used in a heart-on-a-chip device. Reprinted from Pakazad, S.K., Savov, A., Braam, S.R., Dekker, R., 2012. A platform for manufacturable stretchable micro-electrode arrays. Procedia Eng. 47, 817–820. Elsevier B.V.; http://dx.doi.org/10.1016/j.proeng.2012.09.272.

11.6 Future challenges

In the continuous research and development journey towards miniaturization, high performance and new sensing and treatments capabilities, many medical devices are today based on the ability to integrate micro- and nanosystems. Still, the process has its challenges, with solutions resulting from the evolution of small-size systems (micro- and nano) along the following paths (Deterre, 2012):

- The development of new types of measurements, opening the possibility to new physiological parameters
- The downsizing of components for a wider range of implantation sites
- The continuous sensor performance improvement (accuracy, precision, resolution, measurement rate, power consumption, among others).

Moreover, currently we are focused on devices with sensing features. However, as these devices evolve, there will be the opportunity to start actuating over the biological system. At that moment, allied to the sensors, developments regarding actuator's design and technology will join in. This will be the time when the control loop discussed early in the chapter will be closed, and the devices developed will be able to sense, take a decision and act in accordance directly on the biological system. MEMS already show some level of actuation, although it is still unclear how to apply it to a biological system. Other actuation technologies, as smart-materials also are not yet there, as their requirements in terms of actuation stimulus (power, temperature) or even their actuation performance at this scale-level may be still incompatible with the devices application. Nonetheless, research is being performed at a high pace on the micro- and nanoscale systems.

Despite this large momentum, and the amount of research and number of devices being developed in research groups, the amount of these devices available commercially is still limited. This is mainly caused by (Rajan, 2015):

- Stringent regulatory challenges as the healthcare industry is one of the most regulated industries in the world
- High-initial investments either for clinical trials, infrastructural requirements, or development costs
- Uneven technologies adoption due to the before mentioned issues, resulting in no world spread of technologies
- Stakeholders confidence in the devices, showing concerns about the performance and side effects
- Learning curve when new and disruptive devices appear, as the experience and practice of many professionals is a result of years of training
- Long time to market as a result of all the safety and regulatory process.

Still, in spite of the burdens related to market path, devices such as neuroprosthetics, smart-pills or artificial organs are considered, according to a study of Frost and Sullivan (Rajan, 2015), three examples of devices with micro- and nano size systems in their genesis for the top 10 technologies in 2015.

The ability to further design and develop medical devices, despite being based on or not micro- and nanosensors, is supported by the effective policies that target and attempt to facilitate the improvement of the individuals' health. It is this latter factor that serves as driver of the process. The development path is set to evolve along three main feeders (Nelson et al., 2011): (i) the scientific understanding; (ii) the new technologies; and (iii) the practice experience. As these elements come together, the required development platform becomes set by the science, technology and innovation research (Morlacchi and Nelson, 2011).

Acknowledgments

The authors acknowledge the funding by FCT with the reference project UID/EEA/04436/2013, by FEDER funds through the COMPETE 2020—Programa Operacional Competitividade e Internacionalização (POCI) with the reference project POCI-01-0145-FEDER-006941.

References

Abaya, T.V.F., Blair, S., Tathireddy, P., Rieth, L., Solzbacher, F., 2012. A 3D glass optrode array for optical neural stimulation. Biomed. Opt. Express 3 (12), 3087–3104.

Agrawal, S., 2014. Assessment of Cytostretch—A Heart-on-Chip Device. Delft University of Technology, Delft.

Aravanis, A.M., Wang, L.-P., Zhang, F., Meltzer, L.A., Mogri, M.Z., Schneider, M.B., et al., 2007. An optical neural interface: in vivo control of rodent motor cortex with integrated fiberoptic and optogenetic technology. J. Neural Eng. 4 (3), S143–S156.

Ashby, M.F., Bréchet, Y.J.M., Cebon, D., Salvo, L., 2004. Selection strategies for materials and processes. Mater. Des. 25 (1), 51–67. [Internet]. Available from: http://linkinghub.elsevier.com/retrieve/pii/S0261306903001596.

Baltes, H., Moser, D., Vlklein, F., 2008. Thermoelectric microsensors and microsystems. In: Bau, H.H., de Rooij, N.F., Kloeck, B. (Eds.), Sensors. Wiley-VCH Verlag GmbH, Weinheim, Germany, pp. 13–55. [Internet]. Available from: http://doi.wiley.com/10.1002/9783527620203.ch2.

Beeby, S., Ensell, G., Kraft, M., White, N., 2004. MEMS Mechanical Sensors. Artech House, Inc., Norwood, MA.

Belluzo, M.S., Ribone, M.É., Lagier, C.M., 2007. Assembling amperometric biosensors for clinical diagnostics. Sensors 8 (3), 1366–1399. [Internet]. Available from: http://www.mdpi.com/1424-8220/8/3/1366/.

Benabid, A.L., 2003. Deep brain stimulation for Parkinson's disease. Curr. Opin. Neurobiol. 13 (6), 696–706.

Bernstein, J., Boyden, E., 2011. Optogenetic tools for analyzing the neural circuits of behavior. Trends Cogn. Sci. 15 (12), 592–600.

Bhatia, S.N., Ingber, D.E., 2014. Microfluidic organs-on-chips. Nat. Biotechnol. 32 (8), 760–772. [Internet]. Nature Publishing Group; Available from: http://www.nature.com/doifinder/10.1038/nbt.2989.

Bhushan, B., 2011. MEMS/NEMS and BioMEMS/BioNEMS: materials, devices, and biomimetics. In: Bhushan, B. (Ed.), Nanotribology and Nanomechanics II. Springer, Berlin, Heidelberg, pp. 833–945. [Internet]. Available from: http://link.springer.com/10.1007/978-3-642-15263-4_23.

Brotherton, C.M., Wheeler, D.R. 2012. Development of Chemiresponsive sensors for detection of common homemade explosives.

Cady, W.G., 1964. Piezoelectricity: An Introduction to the Theory and Applications of Electromechanical Phenomena in Crystals. Dover Publications, New York, NY.

Caplin, J.D., Granados, N.G., James, M.R., Montazami, R., Hashemi, N., 2015. Microfluidic organ-on-a-chip technology for advancement of drug development and toxicology. Adv. Healthc. Mater. 4 (10), 1426–1450. [Internet]. Available from: http://www.ncbi.nlm.nih.gov/pubmed/25820344.

Cho, I.-J., Baac, H.W., Yoon, E., 2010. A 16-site neural probe integrated with a waveguide for optical stimulation. In: Proceedings of the IEEE International Conference on Micro Electro Mechanical Systems (MEMS). pp. 995–998.

Chou, J., 1999. Electrochemical Sensors. Hazardous Gas Monitors: A Practical Guide to Selection, Operation and Applications, first ed. McGraw-Hill, New York, NY.

Cui, Z., Gu, C., 2006. Nanofabrication challenges for NEMS. In: 2006 1st IEEE International Conference on Nano/Micro Engineered and Molecular Systems. pp. 607–610. [Internet]. Available from: http://ieeexplore.ieee.org/lpdocs/epic03/wrapper.htm?arnumber=4135028.

Dekker, R., 2013. Organ-on-a-chip: interfacing with living tissue. Maxwell Period. der Electrotech. Ver. 16 (3), 20–21.

Deterre, M., 2012. MEMS integration for smart medical devices: opportunities and challenges. In: Design, Test, Integration and Packaging of MEMS/MOEMS (DTIP), 2012 Symposium on. Cannes, France. pp. 253–257.

Dinh, A., 2011. Heart activity monitoring on smartphone. Int. Conf. Biomed. Eng. Technol. 11, 45–49.

Fraden, J., 2010. Handbook of Modern Sensors, fourth ed. Springer, New York, NY. [Internet]. Available from: http://link.springer.com/10.1007/978-1-4419-6466-3.

Goncalves, S.B., Peixoto, A.C., Silva, A.F., Correia, J.H., 2015. Fabrication and mechanical characterization of long and different penetrating length neural microelectrode arrays. J. Micromech. Microeng. 25 (5), 055014.

Gopel, W., Hesse, J., Zemel, J.N., 1994. Sensors: A Comprehensive Survey—Mechanical Sensors. Verlagsgesellschaft mbH, Weinheim, Germany 674 p.

Guenther, M., Gerlach, G., Wallmersperger, T., Avula, M.N., Cho, S.H., Xie, X., et al., 2012. Smart hydrogel-based biochemical microsensor array for medical diagnostics. Adv. Sci. Technol. 85 (2015), 47–52.

Huh, D., Matthews, B.D., Mammoto, A., Montoya-Zavala, M., Hsin, H.Y., Ingber, D.E., 2010. Reconstituting organ-level lung functions on a chip. Science 328 (5986), 1662–1668. [Internet]. Available from: http://www.sciencemag.org/cgi/doi/10.1126/science.1188302.

Hung, P.D., Bonnet, S., Guillemaud, R., Castelli, E., Yen, P.T.N., 2008. Estimation of respiratory waveform using an accelerometer. In: 2008 5th IEEE Int Symp Biomed Imaging From Nano to Macro, Proceedings, ISBI, pp. 1493–1496.

Im, M., Cho, I., Wu, F., Wise, K.D., Fellow, L., Yoon, E., 2011. A dual-shank neural probe integrated with double waveguides on each shank for optogenetic applications. In: 33rd Annual International Conference of the IEEE Engineering in Medicine and Biology Society, pp. 5480–5483.

Ionescu, A.M. 2009. Nano-electro-mechanical-systems: from ideas to reality check. New Dev Micro Electro Mech Syst Radio Freq Millim Wave Appl., pp. 89–96.

Johnston, K.W., Rutherford, R.B., Tilson, M.D., Shah, D.M., Hollier, L., Stanley, J.C., 1991. Suggested standards for reporting on arterial aneurysms. Subcommittee on Reporting Standards for Arterial Aneurysms, Ad Hoc Committee on Reporting Standards, Society for Vascular Surgery and North American Chapter, International Society for Cardiovascular. J. Vasc. Surg. 13 (3), 452–458. [Internet]. Available from: http://www.ncbi.nlm.nih.gov/pubmed/1999868.

Katzen, B.T., MacLean, A.A., 2006. Complications of endovascular repair of abdominal aortic aneurysms: a review. Cardiovasc. Intervent. Radiol. 29 (6), 935–946. [Internet]. Available from: http://www.ncbi.nlm.nih.gov/pubmed/16967225.

Kim, T., McCall, J.G., Jung, Y.H., Huang, X., Siuda, E.R., Li, Y., Kim, T., McCall, J.G., Jung, Y.H., Huang, X., Siuda, E.R., Li, Y., et al., 2013. Injectable, cellular-scale optoelectronics with applications for wireless optogenetics. Science 340 (6129), 211–216. [Internet]. Available from: http://www.ncbi.nlm.nih.gov/pubmed/23580530.

Kobel, P., Reymond, C., 2011. Miniaturization challenges and their impact on the micro-factory concept and manipulators. J. Jpn Soc. Precis. Eng. 77 (3), 263–268[Internet]. Available from: http://joi.jlc.jst.go.jp/JST.JSTAGE/jjspe/77.263?from=CrossRef.

Kwon, K.Y., Sirowatka, B., Weber, A., Li, Wen, Kwon, K.Y., Sirowatka, B., et al., 2013. Opto-uECoG array: a hybrid neural interface with transparent uECoG electrode array and integrated LEDs. IEEE Trans. Biomed. Circuits Syst. 7 (5), 593–600. [Internet]. Available from: http://ieeexplore.ieee.org/lpdocs/epic03/wrapper.htm?arnumber=6631491.

Kwon, K.Y., Lee, H.-M., Ghovanloo, M., Weber, A., Li, W., 2014. A wireless slanted optrode array with integrated micro leds for optogenetics. In: 2014 IEEE 27th International Conference on Micro Electro Mechanical Systems. IEEE, pp. 813–816.

Kwon, K.Y., Lee, H.-M., Ghovanloo, M., Weber, A., Li, W., 2015. Design, fabrication, and packaging of an integrated, wirelessly-powered optrode array for optogenetics application. Front. Syst. Neurosci. 9 (May), 69. [Internet]. Available from: http://www.pubmedcentral.nih.gov/articlerender.fcgi?artid=4422027&tool=pmcentrez&rendertype=abstract.

Lanjef, N., Chakrabartty, S., Elvin, N., Elvin, A., 2006. A sub-microwatt piezo-floating-gate sensor for long-term fatigue monitoring in biomechanical implants. In: Proceedings of the 28th IEEE EMBS Annual International Conference.

Lanning, C., Shandas, R., 2003. Development and validation of implantable sensors for monitoring function of prosthetic heart valves: in vitro studies. Med. Biol. Eng. Comput. 41 (4), 416–424.

Lazarus, N., Fedder, G.K., 2011. Integrated vertical parallel-plate capacitive humidity sensor. J. Micromech. Microeng. 21 (6), 065028.

Malarkey, E.B., Parpura, V., 2010. Carbon nanotubes in neuroscience. In: Czernicki, Z., Baethmann, A., Ito, U., Katayama, Y., Kuroiwa, T., Mendelow, D. (Eds.), Acta Neurochir. Suppl. 106 (8), 337–341. [Internet]. Vienna: Springer Vienna; Available from: http://www.springerlink.com/index/10.1007/978-3-211-98811-4.

Morlacchi, P., Nelson, R.R., 2011. How medical practice evolves: learning to treat failing hearts with an implantable device. Res. Policy 40 (4), 511–525. [Internet]. Elsevier B.V.; Available from: http://linkinghub.elsevier.com/retrieve/pii/S0048733311000023.

Müller, R., Kuc, R., 2007. Biosonar-inspired technology: goals, challenges and insights. Bioinspir. Biomim. 2 (4), S146–S161[Internet]. Available from: http://stacks.iop.org/1748-3190/2/i=4/a=S04?key=crossref.b84769ed578d93fd8e7929b532917e46.

Nelson, R.R., Buterbaugh, K., Perl, M., Gelijns, A., 2011. How medical know-how progresses. Res. Policy 40 (10), 1339–1344[Internet]. Elsevier B.V.; Available from: http://www.sciencedirect.com/science/article/pii/S0048733311001272.

Nise,N.S.,2011.ControlSystemsEngineering[Internet].sixthed.Wiley,Hoboken.926p.[Internet]. Available from: https://books.google.com/books?id=34zmCQAAQBAJ&pgis=1.

Normann, R.A., 2007. Technology insight: future neuroprosthetic therapies for disorders of the nervous system. Nat. Clin. Pract. Neurol. 3 (8), 444–452. Nature Publishing Group.

Oliveira, C.C., Sepulveda, A.T., Almeida, N., Wardle, B.L., da Silva, J.M., Rocha, L.A., 2015. Implantable flexible pressure measurement system based on inductive coupling. IEEE Trans. Biomed. Eng. 62 (2), 680–687. [Internet]. Available from: http://ieeexplore.ieee.org/lpdocs/epic03/wrapper.htm?arnumber=6933941.

Olson, W.H., 2009. Basic concepts of medical instrumentation. In: Webster, J.G. (Ed.), Medical Instrumentation: Application and Design. fourth ed.. John Wiley & Sons, Hoboken, pp. 1–44.

Pakazad, S.K., Savov, A., Braam, S.R., Dekker, R., 2012. A platform for manufacturable stretchable micro-electrode arrays. Procedia Eng. 47, 817–820. http://dx.doi.org/10.1016/j.proeng.2012.09.272 [Internet]. Elsevier B.V.

Pakazad, S.K., Savov, A., van de Stolpe, A., Dekker, R., 2014. A novel stretchable micro-electrode array (SMEA) design for directional stretching of cells. J. Micromech. Microeng. 24 (3), 034003. [Internet]. Available from: http://iopscience.iop.org/0960-1317/24/3/034003.

Parker, B. 2004. Universal Modular Pulse Oximeter Probe for use With Reusable and Disposable Patient Attachment Devices. U.S. Patent 6,721,585, filed August 17, 2001, and issued April 13, 2004.

Patel, S.V., Mlsna, T.E., Fruhberger, B., Klaassen, E., Cemalovic, S., Baselt, D.R., 2003. Chemicapacitive microsensors for volatile organic compound detection. Sensors Actuators B Chem. 96, 541–553.

Patranabis, D., 2003. Sensors and Transducers, second ed. Prentice-Hall, New Delhi.

Prashant Reddy, G., Gupta, N., 2010. Material selection for microelectronic heat sinks: an application of the Ashby approach. Mater. Des. 31 (1), 113–117. [Internet]. Elsevier Ltd; Available from: http://linkinghub.elsevier.com/retrieve/pii/S0261306909003549.

Qian, J., Zhao, Y.-P., 2002. Materials selection in mechanical design for microsensors and microactuators. Mater. Des. 23, 619–625.

Quinn, D.J., Spearing, S.M., Ashby, M.F., Fleck, N.A., 2006. A systematic approach to process selection in MEMS. J. Microelectromech. Syst. 15 (5), 1039–1050.

Rajan, B., 2015. Top medical device and imaging technologies in 2015 (Frost & Sullivan's Technical Insights).

Rolfe, P., 2012. Micro- and nanosensors for medical and biological measurement. Sens. Mater. 24 (6), 275–302.

Santos, I., 2012. Product development methodologies—the case of medical devices. University of Porto, Porto. [Internet]. Available from: http://hdl.handle.net/10216/76244.

Santos, I.C.T., Tavares, J.M.R.S., 2013. Additional peculiarities of medical devices that should be considered in their development process. Expert Rev. Med. Devices 10 (3), 411–420. [Internet]. Available from: http://www.ncbi.nlm.nih.gov/pubmed/23668711.

Santos, I.C., Gazelle, G.S., Rocha, L.A., Tavares, J.M.R., 2012. Medical device specificities: opportunities for a dedicated product development methodology. Expert Rev. Med. Devices 9 (3), 299–311. [Internet]. Available from: http://informahealthcare.com/doi/abs/10.1586/erd.12.3.

Sepulveda, A., 2013. Use of Nanocomposites for Flexible Pressure Sensors. University of Minho, Portugal. [Internet]. Available from: http://hdl.handle.net/1822/34582; http://repositorium.sdum.uminho.pt/.

Sepúlveda, A.T., Guzman de Villoria, R., Viana, J.C., Pontes, A., Wardle, B.L., Rocha, L.A., 2013a. Full elastic constitutive relation of non-isotropic aligned-CNT/PDMS flexible nanocomposites. Nanoscale 5, 4847–4854. [Internet]. Available from: http://www.ncbi.nlm.nih.gov/pubmed/23616092.

Sepúlveda, A.T., Guzman de Villoria, R., Viana, J.C., Pontes, A.J., Wardle, B.L., Rocha, L.A., 2013b. Full elastic constitutive relation of non-isotropic aligned-CNT/PDMS flexible nanocomposites. Nanoscale 5 (11), 4847. [Internet]. Available from: http://xlink.rsc.org/?DOI=c3nr00753g.

Sharma, A., Rieth, L., Tathireddy, P., Harrison, R., Oppermann, H., Klein, M., et al., 2011. Long term in vitro functional stability and recording longevity of fully integrated wireless neural interfaces based on the Utah Slant Electrode Array. J. Neural Eng. 8 (4), 045004.

Sinclair, I.R., 2001. Sensors and Transducers. third ed. Elsevier, Amsterdam.

Son, D., Park, S.Y., Kim, B., Koh, J.T., Kim, T.H., An, S., et al., 2011. Nanoneedle transistor-based sensors for the selective detection of intracellular calcium ions. ACS Nano 5 (5), 3888–3895.

Spaan, N.A., Teplova, A.E., Renard, E., Spaan, J.A.E., 2014. Implantable insulin pumps: an effective option with restricted dissemination. Lancet Diabetes Endocrinol. 2 (5), 358–360. [Internet]. Available from: http://linkinghub.elsevier.com/retrieve/pii/S221385871470035X.

Srikar, V.T., Spearing, S.M., 2003. Materials selection in micromechanical design: an application of the Ashby approach. J. Microelectromech. Syst. 12 (1), 3–10.

Thaler, M.S., 2007. The Only EKG Book You'll Ever Need. Plastic and Reconstructive Surgery. Lippincott Williams & Wilkins, Philadelphia, PA.

van de Stolpe, A., den Toonder, J., 2013. Workshop meeting report organs-on-chips: human disease models. Lab Chip 13 (18), 3449–3470. [Internet]. Available from: http://www.ncbi.nlm.nih.gov/pubmed/23645172.

van den Berg, A., 2014. Organ on Chip: Developing Tools for New, Better and Personalized Therapies, 2014, hDMT - Human Organ and Disease Model Technologies, Utrecht, NL.

Wilson, J., 2005. Sensor Technology Handbook. Newnes, Burlington, MA.

Wise, K.D., 2009. Wireless integrated microsystems: wearable and implantable devices for improved health care. In: Solid-State Sensors, Actuators and Microsystems, pp. 1–8.

Zorzos, A.N., Scholvin, J., Boyden, E.S., Fonstad, C.G., 2012. Three-dimensional multiwaveguide probe array for light delivery to distributed brain circuits. Opt. Lett. 37 (23), 4841–4843.

Smart devices: Lab-on-a-chip

12

S. Catarino, R. Lima*,†, G. Minas**
*University of Minho, Guimarães, Portugal, †Faculty of Engineering of the University of Porto, Porto, Portugal

12.1 Introduction to microfluidics and miniaturization

Microfluidics has played, over recent decades, a significant role in biomedical (Ruffien-Ciszak et al., 2008; Sackmann et al., 2014; Gupta et al., 2010; Foudeh et al., 2012), pharmaceutical (Postier et al., 2008; Foudeh et al., 2012), and environmental monitoring applications (Bridle et al., 2014; Mehta et al., 2006). Particularly, since the fluidic microsystems technologies for diagnosis applications tend to produce low-cost devices with low power consumption, they have an extremely enhanced potential for being used as point-of-care devices, for the detection and quantification of several biomolecules in physiological fluids, as well as for determining fluid properties (Kopp et al., 1997; Ribeiro et al., 2005; Urban, 2009). These miniaturized systems have been designed to operate as analytical devices able to perform all the required processes of a sample analysis: manipulation, transport, and control of fluid samples, as well as detection and readout electronics (Gupta et al., 2010; Tng et al., 2015; Ahn et al., 2004). When biological fluids are used they are called "lab-on-a-chip" systems. If the fluids are chemical they are called "micro total analysis systems." The lab-on-a-chip systems feature reduced size (devices present typical structural dimensions in the 10–100-mm range), high analytical performance (due to short diffusion distances and high surface-to-volume ratios), high system integration, improved potential for automation and control, and small volume of samples and reagents (and the consequent reduction of waste production), which are advantages over the conventional size systems and are a key to assure immediate, sensible, repeatable, and accurate results (Figeys and Pinto, 2000; Cardoso and Minas, 2011; Auroux et al., 2002; Haeberle and Zengerle, 2007; Whitesides, 2006; Squires and Quake, 2005; Lauks, 1998).

However, several challenges remain in the lab-on-a-chip systems miniaturization:

- Mixture, pumping, transport, separation, and control of fluids at the microscale level: these limitations are related, on one side, to the minimum sample volumes and flow rates in the biological analysis and, on the other side, to the microscale dimensions of the lab-on-a-chip systems. At the microscale level, the dominant physical and chemical effects are different from the ones at macroscale and, as a consequence, the microflow phenomena occurring at this level are complex and not well understood. Additionally, fluid handling is restricted to a laminar flow with a typical Reynolds number (Re) < 1, which limits the mixing of fluids and slows the response time of the device. Therefore significant research efforts are being developed on the design of micropumps and micromixers systems that can be incorporated on lab-on-a-chip devices to improve the transport and mixing of fluids (Cardoso and Minas, 2011;

Bioinspired Materials for Medical Applications. http://dx.doi.org/10.1016/B978-0-08-100741-9.00012-7

Haeberle and Zengerle, 2007), while addressing the non-Newtonian behavior of the majority of physiological fluids (Fung, 1997; Roselli and Diller, 2011). The differences in the fluids' behaviors need to be taken into account when designing lab-on-a-chip systems, since the flow scales are miniaturized to the micro- or nanoscale.

- Low-cost microfabrication techniques: the microfabrication techniques are still a challenge in the miniaturization of diagnostics devices, particularly when addressing low-cost techniques for different and innovative materials (Faustino et al., 2015; Pinto et al., 2014a; Cardoso and Minas, 2011; Koev et al., 2010; Abgrall and Gué, 2007).
- Integration of actuation and sensing technologies (optical, electrochemical, and acoustic) on a single chip: the detection and actuation schemes must be selected according to the optical, electrical, electrochemical, and physical properties of the analyte, the sample composition, and the detection limits. It is important to notice that the detection principles may not always be scaled down in a positive way that could lead to low signal-to-noise ratios. Additionally, particularly for disposable lab-on-a-chip devices, the fabrication and integration cost of the detection scheme is a very important factor, and can even limit the options for detection (Lee and Lee, 2004; Cardoso and Minas, 2011; Haeberle and Zengerle, 2007).

Thus, this chapter will approach the microtechnologies, microfluidics, miniaturization, and on-chip integration of lab-on-a-chip devices, focusing on the background and advantages of the different techniques, as well as their disadvantages and challenges for diagnosis applications. Additionally, the present section will include an overview of different diagnosis applications, including examples of analytical chemistry, particularly the detection of biomarkers for different diseases, evaluation of the red blood cells' (RBCs) deformability, and differential counting of lymphocytes for HIV (human immunodeficiency virus) diagnostics.

12.2 Microtechnologies in lab-on-a-chip devices

One of the main challenges of microtechnologies fabrication originates from the need to address the increasingly reduced dimensions in lab-on-a-chip devices, in order to create precise, accurate, and highly functional complex structures (such as tridimensional microchannels, functionalized surfaces, and microelectromechanical systems—MEMS). New materials and technologies have been studied and developed to obtain microdevices with enhanced features (Cardoso and Minas, 2011; Brecher et al., 2015). Silicon, glass, and polymers are the materials most often used to fabricate lab-on-a-chip devices but, recently, new research directions have been focusing on biomaterials and cells for lab-on-a-chip applications.

12.2.1 Silicon and glass technologies

In the 1990s photolithography and micromachining in silicon were the most popular microfabrication techniques, particularly for integration of microelectronics circuits and MEMS, especially due to silicon's well-known properties. Additionally, glass has also been widely reported because of its biocompatibility, resistance to some chemicals, and optical transparency, properties that make it suitable for many biological applications.

The first miniaturized analysis system was developed by Terry et al. (1979), based on the principles of gas chromatography. The main components of the system were fabricated in silicon using photolithography and chemical etching techniques, and the device was able to separate and analyze simple gas mixtures. A decade later, Manz et al. (1990) proposed a miniaturized total analysis system, able to automatically perform the sampling, transport, chromatographic separations, and detection of samples on a microscale. Since then, many authors have proposed micro total analysis systems, for different applications, exploring different microfabrication techniques. Different examples of microstructures in glass and silicon oxide are reported in literature (Whitesides et al., 2001; Wilding et al., 1994; Ziaie, 2004; Westin et al., 2000; Schena et al., 1995).

Silicon and glass microstructures fabrication can be performed using different techniques: surface micromachining, bulk micromachining, photolithography (Cardoso and Minas, 2011), electron-beam lithography (Broers et al., 1996), or X-ray lithography (Heuberger, 1988), among others. Surface micromachining consists of a microfabrication technique that produces tridimensional structures above the surface using a succession of thin-film deposition, patterning, and selective etching. For that, two materials (the sacrificial material and structural material) are deposited alternately on top of a substrate, requiring chemical etchants with high etch selectivity to remove the sacrificial material without affecting the structural material (French and Sarro, 1999; Linder et al., 1992; Bustjllo et al., 1998). Bulk micromachining is a fabrication technique where the structures are produced through a selective etching inside a substrate (Kovacs et al., 1998; French and Sarro, 1999; Aziz et al., 2008; Jansen et al., 1996; Ruan et al., 2007). Photolithography is a highly developed technology that begins with a mask production (typically a chromium pattern layer on a glass plate), followed by covering the substrate (such as silicon, glass, or gallium arsenide) with an ultraviolet light-sensitive polymer—photoresist. Ultraviolet light is then emitted through the mask onto the photoresist and it is developed, transferring the mask pattern to the photoresist layer above the substrate (Levinson, 2011; Fraden, 2004; Dresselhaus et al., 2010). Further descriptions of the referred techniques can be found in literature (Cardoso and Minas, 2011; Ziaie, 2004; Dresselhaus et al., 2010; Abgrall and Gué, 2007).

Although glass and silicon microtechnologies ensure high-precision structures, these materials are fragile and expensive for disposable devices, and the fabrication methods are complex, costly, and time-consuming, requiring the use of cleanroom facilities for the fabrication process (Faustino et al., 2015; Ziaie, 2004; Patel et al., 2008; Dresselhaus et al., 2010). Additionally, silicon is optically opaque and a semiconductor, which makes it inappropriate for some types of separation and detection mechanisms (with the risk of sample carry-over and cross-contamination) (Duffy et al., 1998). These limitations have led to an increase in research into low-cost alternative materials, such as polymers (Patel et al., 2008; Whitesides et al., 2001).

12.2.2 Polymer technologies

In the second half of the 1990s polymers were introduced and started slowly replacing silicon and glass in microfluidic structures fabrication, due to their low cost, wide range of mechanical and chemical properties, good biocompatibility, flexibility, and easy processing in the production of complex three-dimensional structures (Fujii, 2002; Becker, 2002; Becker and Gärtner, 2008; Whitesides, 2006; Duffy et al., 1998; Patel et al., 2008; Pinto et al., 2014b; Xia et al., 1997).

The most popular polymers used to fabricate lab-on-a-chip structures are poly(dimethylsiloxane) (PDMS), poly(methyl methacrylate) (PMMA), high-density polyethylene, low-density polyethylene, polyamide 6, and the epoxy-based photoresist SU-8 (Becker, 2002). Particularly, PDMS has been widely reported for microfluidic systems because it has many favorable properties for prototypes fabrication: the material is inexpensive, optically transparent to visible light, which makes it compatible with optical detection systems, and also biocompatible; its molding procedure is safe and easy to learn; and its flexibility allows the integration of elastomeric actuators and optical elements into devices.

The PDMS's excellent sealing properties make it very suitable for microfluidics and, since it can be easily bonded to itself, it allows the fabrication of multilayer structures (Wong and Ho, 2009; McDonald and Whitesides, 2002; Fiorini and Chiu, 2005; Becker, 2002; Duffy et al., 1998). The SU-8 has also gained importance mainly due to its use as a material for molds, but some authors have also used it for structures. It is an epoxy-based negative photoresist that features biocompatibility and it is mechanically and chemically stable (Dey et al., 2010; Lim et al., 2015; Lin et al., 2002). SU-8 photosensitivity allows its patterning by ultraviolet photolithography, permitting low-cost microstructures of almost any shape and size (planar, multilayer, and 3D microstructures) (Pinto et al., 2014b; Han et al., 2004; Rammohan et al., 2011). Since many polymers have been studied, different manufacturing processes have been developed and optimized.

Polymers fabrication processes are based on two major techniques: replication micromachining and direct micromachining (Duffy et al., 1998; Becker, 2002).

Replication micromachining processes lead to fast and cheap high-volume production of polymeric structures, when compared to those used in glass and silicon technologies (Duffy et al., 1998; Becker, 2002). These processes are based on the repetitive replication of a mold structure. Hot embossing or compression molding (Becker and Gärtner, 2008; Schift et al., 2000), injection molding (Edwards et al., 2002; Liou and Chen, 2006), and casting (Becker and Gärtner, 2008; Narasimhan and Papautsky, 2003) are the most common techniques in replication micromachining.

Hot embossing consists in three major steps: heating of the mold above the polymer glass transition temperature, pressing the mold to the polymer using a specific embossing pressure, and cooling the system to harden the polymer, resulting in an inverted replicate of the mold (Schift et al., 2000).

In injection molding, the molds that create the microstructures are heated to a temperature higher than the softening glass transition temperature of the polymers and, hence, the polymers can be injected into the molds (Edwards et al., 2002).

Casting is a technique in which a material is introduced into the mold in a liquid state, which later becomes solid using chemical processes to harden the polymer, and thus it acquires the shape of the mold (Narasimhan and Papautsky, 2003). Detailed descriptions of these techniques can be found in Narasimhan and Papautsky (2003) and Becker and Gärtner (2008).

Direct micromachining techniques produce the structures individually, increasing the time required to complete each device and, therefore, limiting the production volume. These techniques do not need previous master fabrication and are typically used for prototyping (Becker and Gärtner, 2008; Whitesides et al., 2001). The most common direct techniques are laser micromachining (Becker, 2002; Yuan and Das, 2007; Cheng et al., 2004), stereolithography (Becker and Gärtner, 2008; Sun et al., 2005a), and photopolymerization (soft lithography) (Pinto et al., 2014b; Williams and Wang, 2004; Becker and Gärtner, 2008).

Laser micromachining produces structures by applying a laser beam of ultraviolet or infrared radiation to the polymer, and the concentrated energy of the beam evaporates the material at the focal point. The precision of laser micromachining depends on the quality of the optical system, energy distribution of the beam, and laser wavelength (Yuan and Das, 2007).

Stereolithography is a technique for layer by layer structure fabrication, where a laser beam is focused to a free surface of a photosensitive liquid to induce polymerization of the liquid in that region and transform it to a polymerized solid (Sun et al., 2005a).

Photopolymerization is based on the removal of specific areas of a thin polymer film (with the ability to interact with energy radiation, such as ultraviolet light), accordingly to a mask design. The radiation may break chemical bonds or lead to other types of chemical change within the polymer material. The fabrication of microfluidic structures using soft lithography follows four main steps: pattern design, fabrication of the photomask and the master, fabrication of the polymeric stamp, and fabrication of micro- and nanostructures with the stamp by printing, molding, and embossing (Williams and Wang, 2004; Ziaie, 2004; Xia and Whitesides, 1998; Qin et al., 2010). The fabrication of a polymeric mold, as the PDMS, is illustrated in Fig. 12.1 (Kane, 1999).

Detailed descriptions of these and other techniques can be found in the literature (Narasimhan and Papautsky, 2003; Becker and Gärtner, 2008; Ziaie, 2004; Duffy et al., 1998; Whitesides et al., 2001; Patel et al., 2008; Pinto et al., 2014b; Qin et al., 2010; Becker, 2002; Pinho et al., 2013; Abdelgawad et al., 2008; McDonald and Whitesides, 2002; Abgrall and Gué, 2007).

12.2.3 Biomaterials for lab-on-a-chip devices

In recent years biomaterials have also been considered for lab-on-a-chip devices, to coat surfaces for functionalization with biological elements (such as deoxyribonucleic acid—DNA, enzymes, or antibodies) or even as the materials used for the device substrate.

The biomaterial films can be integrated into the microdevices by several deposition and patterning methods compatible with standard microfabrication technologies, including solution casting, spin casting, electrodeposition, microcontact printing,

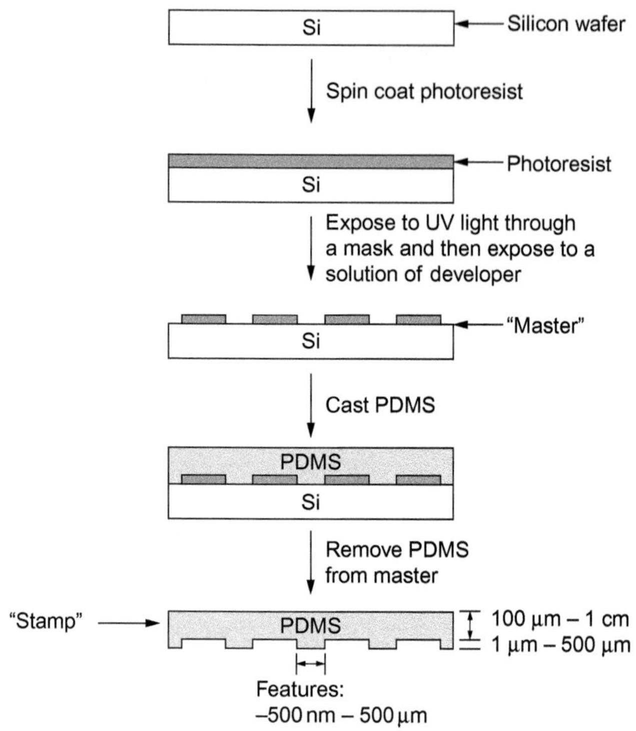

Fig. 12.1 Schematic illustration of the procedure used to fabricate a PDMS stamp from a master having relief structures in photoresist on its surface.
Reproduced from Kane, R., 1999. Patterning proteins and cells using soft lithography. Biomaterials 20 (23–24), 2363–2376. Available at: http://linkinghub.elsevier.com/retrieve/pii/S0142961299001659 with permission from Elsevier.

nanoimprinting, and photolithography (Koev et al., 2010; Wu et al., 2003; Park et al., 2007; Cheng and Pisano, 2008).

A wide variety of polymers, many of them biomaterials, have been used in microdevices: chitosan (Koev et al., 2010; Yi et al., 2005), alginate (Kim et al., 2008), cellulose (Suresha et al., 2008), collagen (Kim et al., 2007a), gelatin (Yang and Ou, 2005), polyethylene glycol (Revzin et al., 2001), polylysine (Cowan et al., 2001), or even spider silk (Bai et al., 2006). These materials have the functions of drug release, cell culture adhesion, structural support and actuation, scaffolding for tissue engineering, and biomolecules trapping (Koev et al., 2010).

In particular the natural polymer chitosan has emerged as a promising material for biological functionalization and improvement of specific biorecognition in MEMS and lab-on-a-chip device, since it is biocompatible and biodegradable, has unique chemical properties, and is easily deposited in thin-films (Koev et al., 2010; Yi et al., 2005; Wu et al., 2003). Chitosan has been reported for fabrication of nanowire and nanodot chitosan structures (Park et al., 2007), as well as films with controlled thickness (Zangmeister et al., 2006) and a variety of microscale geometries, such as released structures (Koev et al., 2007), out-of-plane surfaces (Dykstra et al., 2009), and sealed microchannels (Park et al., 2006). The primary role of chitosan in microdevices is to immobilize biomolecules, cells, or nanoparticles. A second role of chitosan is to enable the devices to perform advanced functions such as specific recognition of analytes and enzymatic conversions for sensor applications.

Chitosan films can also be modified with other substances (such as proteins and nanoparticles), in order to improve their mechanical properties (Zou et al., 2008; Lewandowski et al., 2008). Especially, nonmodified chitosan is characterized by low stiffness, which limits the possibility of using chitosan as a structural material. The previous examples presented chitosan as a coating layer but not as a structural material. However, Cheng et al. reported a cantilever fabricated using photolithographic techniques, made entirely of chitosan (Cheng and Pisano, 2008). The ability to produce devices entirely of chitosan can potentially decrease the fabrication complexity and consequently lower the cost of the entire process.

12.2.4 Integration of biologic sensing elements in lab-on-a-chip devices

Biosensors implemented in lab-on-a-chip devices require a biological surface for specific bonding of biological samples to the sensor. Different biological elements can be integrated into the surfaces: antibodies (natural or synthetic), antigens or proteins, among others, through a process of surface functionalization (Pinto et al., 2015; Ferreira and Sales, 2014). The functionalization of microstructure surfaces for posterior detection can be performed using different immobilization methods. Some examples of the reported immobilization methods will be described.

Pinto et al. reported the PDMS surface functionalization for the development of an immune-sensor for salivary cortisol analysis, using three different antibodies immobilization methods: immobilization by passive adsorption on pristine PDMS; silanization of PDMS surface with (3-aminopropyl)-triethoxysilane (APTES) to generate amino groups and posterior covalent immobilization of antibodies on APTES–PDMS using crosslinker glutaraldehyde (GA); coating the PDMS surface with BSA to block nonspecific protein adsorption, and then covalent bond of the protein A via GA (Pinto et al., 2015).

Shim et al. used a streptavidin/biotin system to investigate the adsorption behavior of proteins on the sides of single-walled carbon nanotubes, which were functionalized by coadsorption of a surfactant and poly(ethylene glycol) (Shim et al., 2002). Boozer et al. developed a surface plasmon resonance (SPR) sensor with a gold sensing surface lined by a high refractive index overlayer of tantalum pentoxide that works as a reference channel. The gold side of the chip is functionalized with a mixed self-assembled monolayer of polyethylene oxide (PEO) and biotin terminated thiols, for immobilization of biotinylated antibodies, whereas the tantalum pentoxide side is coated with PEO terminated silanes (Boozer et al., 2003). Lifson et al. reported an arrayed imaging reflectometry label-free biosensor that measures the light intensity of an angled beam reflected off a flat substrate that is composed of a protein-reactive film on a thermally grown silicon oxide layer. The authors used microgel nanoparticles as a simple and customizable construct to deposit antibodies on the biosensor surface (Lifson et al., 2015).

Sakudo et al. reported the functionalization of antibody-integrated magnetic beads for influenza A virus capture, using a combination of steps: introduction of amino groups in a surface of graphite-encapsulated magnetic beads; binding of antiinfluenza A virus hemagglutinin antibody via its surface sulfide groups to the amino groups on the beads via *N*-succinimidyl-3-(2-pyridyldithio)propionate (Sakudo et al., 2015).

Chitosan films can also be readily functionalized with proteins, enzymes, antibodies, and DNA, for selective coatings for biosensors. Different methods have been demonstrated for chitosan modification: physical interaction (eg, surface absorption, entrapment), chemical bonding, or covalent crosslink with each other (Koev et al., 2010).

Functionalized phospholipid polymer interfaces (2-methacryloyloxyethyl phosphorylcholine polymer biointerfaces) are also promising and useful for numerous applications to lab-on-a-chip devices in biomedicine, since these polymers can form cell membrane-like surfaces by surface chemistry and physics and thereby provide biointerfaces capable of suppressing protein adsorption and many subsequent biological responses in order to increase the specificity of the functionalized surfaces. These polymers can be incorporated with silane or hydrophobic moiety to construct stable interfaces on glass, quartz, PMMA, and PDMS, via a silane-coupling reaction or hydrophobic interactions (Xu et al., 2010).

Besides the functionalization of the biosensor surface, when micro- or nanoparticles are used (eg, magnetic particles), they also need to be functionalized. For instance, functional beads prepared by emulsion polymerization or dispersion polymerization offer a large specific surface for chemical binding. These small particles can be advantageously used as a "mobile substrate" for bioassays, or even for in vivo applications, as they can be easily recovered from dispersion (Gijs, 2004).

12.2.5 The lab-on-a-cell concept

Since the lab-on-a-chip technology has reached a mature state of research and development, a novel concept—lab-on-a-cell—is emerging: it relies on the use of a single cell as a minimal and highly confined experimental unit, or experimentation in the simple, but still unequalled, platform provided by nature itself (Zare and Kim, 2010; Le Gac and van den Berg, 2010; El-Ali et al., 2006).

A cell consists in a natural sophisticated laboratory, where thousands of reactions take place every second. When compared with a standard lab-on-a-chip, a lab-on-a-cell has some advantages: a cell performs much more functions than the ones that could be integrated into a lab-on-a-chip device; all the reactions are ruled by diffusion and molecular transport phenomena and occur at a millisecond timescale; the cells reactions are specific and produce pure and active compounds (Le Gac and van den Berg, 2010).

A nanofluidic system for single-cell analysis must include nanochannels or nanopumps for handling subcellular fluid volumes (El-Ali et al., 2006). These nanostructures can be manufactured using top-down or bottom-up approaches (Mijatovic et al., 2005), or using methods derived from soft lithography, such as micromolding in capillaries or nanoimprint lithography (Xia and Whitesides, 1998; Qin et al., 2010). Several authors developed nanosystems for manipulation of pico- or attoliters of fluids or detection of single cells or molecules (Hoang et al., 2009; Tas et al., 2002; Laforge et al., 2007).

Three types of lab-on-a-cell experimentation have been reported: (i) aimed at the elucidation of the cellular machinery (Takayama et al., 2001); (ii) the creation of novel production units (Khine et al., 2007); and (iii) the use of microfluidics for assisted reproduction technology (Wacogne et al., 2008; Le Gac and van den Berg, 2010). The unique flow properties found in microfluidic systems enable the precise temporal and spatial control of the cells environment, which allows innovative types of experimentation and improves the tests of cells sensitivity to chemicals in a concentration-dependent manner, all within a single assay (Keenan and Folch, 2008).

Cell experimentation has been studied at different complexity levels, from single cells to monolayers, microtissues or small organisms (Le Gac and van den Berg, 2010), and for different applications, from cell handling, sorting, treatment, and analysis (Andersson and Van den Berg, 2003; Chen and Cui, 2009; Kovac and Voldman, 2007; Quinto-Su et al., 2008). Lab-on-a-chip devices ensure ideal conditions for lab-on-a-cell experimentation since they can integrate in the device different micro- and nanofluidic tools and techniques for handling, characterization, and analysis of fluids.

Cell handling can be performed using mechanical, chemical, electrical, optical, or magnetic trapping techniques (Skelley et al., 2009; Dragavon et al., 2008; Théry and Bornens, 2006; Ozkan et al., 2003; Piggee, 2009; Saliba et al., 2010).

Cell characterization can be optical (performed by optical and fluorescent techniques, imaging with nanoparticles or thermal lens microscopy), biochemical (using ion-selective microelectrodes), or a combination of both (Lidke et al., 2004; Choi et al., 2009; Tamaki et al., 2002; Guenat et al., 2006; Cheng et al., 2006). The possibility to fabricate sensing structures at nanoscale, such as nanoelectrodes or nanowires, allows the possibility of subcellular and intracellular measurements (Tong et al., 2009).

After cell handling and cell characterization, a lab-on-a-cell system requires the access to the intracellular content, via crossing the cell membrane, which can be performed by an electric field, pore-inducing chemicals, or high-energy laser pulses (Wang et al., 2010; Olofsson et al., 2009). Fig. 12.2 presents an example of a lab-on-a-cell microfluidic device (Clausell-Tormos et al., 2008).

12.3 Manipulating and controlling microflows

In the fabrication of microfluidic structures for lab-on-a-chip applications, the integration of the fluidic, biological, and electronic modules in the same substrates must be assured. Additionally, those small and precise structures must guarantee the correct manipulation of micro- and nanoliter quantities of samples and reagents (Auroux et al., 2002; Kovarik and Jacobson, 2009). A fully automated system for fluids control (injection, transport, reaction, and measurement) is required for any

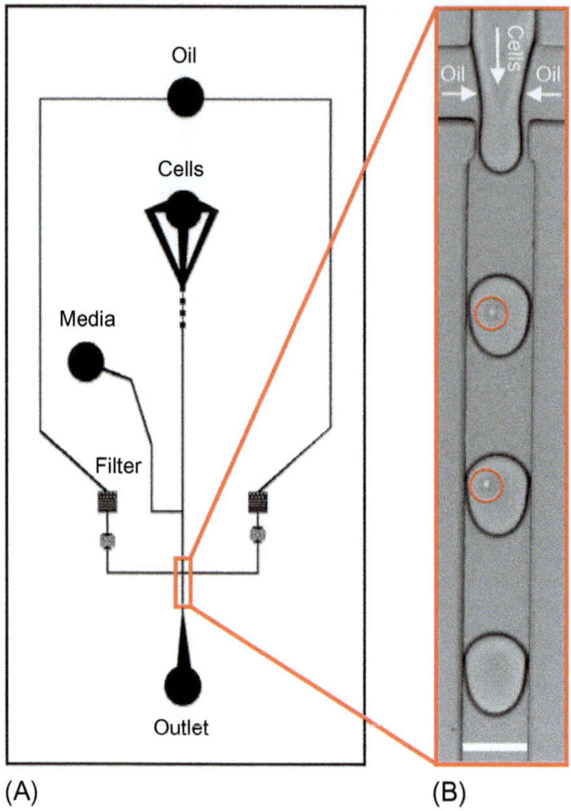

Fig. 12.2 Example of a microfluidic lab-on-a-cell platform. A droplet-based platform can be used for the isolation of individual cells within nanoliter-sized droplets that are created and trapped in a continuous oil stream. Cells are isolated in highly confined nanoreactors for the parallel experimentation of single cells. (A) Lab-on-a-cell platform. (B) Detail of isolated cells within the droplets.
Reproduced from Clausell-Tormos, J. et al., 2008. Droplet-based microfluidic platforms for the encapsulation and screening of mammalian cells and multicellular organisms. Chem. Biol. 15 (5), 427–437 with permission from Elsevier.

particular microdevice to be able to transport, separate, mix, and analyze the samples. However, the transport and mixing of fluids in a microdevice is a difficult task because the low Reynolds number—*Re* (in a miniaturized scale $Re < 1$) corresponds to a laminar flow regime. In this situation, there are no recirculation vortices, and transport and mixing occur mainly by diffusion, which can imply long transit times in the microchannels, mainly when large molecules with low diffusivity are present.

Therefore the implementation of additional transport and mixing techniques is essential (Kovarik and Jacobson, 2009). The control of fluids at microscale can be performed through passive (geometrical) or active (such as optical tweezers, magnetic or acoustic) techniques.

12.3.1 Pumping and mixing

The mixing and transport of fluids in a microchannel is a slow process due to the absence of recirculation regions (vortices), and to overcome this absence it is essential to assure the automation of the devices. The transport and mixing of fluids can be improved through passive or active techniques, using, for instance, mechanical actuators or tridimensional microstructures, fully integrated in the microdevices (Suh and Kang, 2010; Lee et al., 2011).

Passive techniques do not include external forces or mobile parts. Transport and mixing are only promoted by diffusion as a function of the structure geometry and typology. The most common passive techniques are geometrical obstacles, pillars and passive pressure valves that create pumping and recirculation regions (Chung et al., 2004; Kamholz and Yager, 2001; Squires and Quake, 2005; Khosravi Parsa et al., 2014; Rodrigues et al., 2015). Passive structures allow low cost and simple integration in the lab-on-a-chip devices. However, the complex typology of the microchannels increases the fabrication complexity. Furthermore, the microchannels must be long enough to assure uniform mixing, which might imply excessive long channels, mainly when the molecules in the fluids have low diffusivity.

Active techniques improve pumping and mixing using mobile parts or external mechanical, electrical, magnetic, or acoustic forces. Active structures are based on MEMS devices, and allow the creation of actuation systems for the transport of fluids in microchannels. Micropumps and microvalves are examples of these structures (Rife et al., 2000; Bradley et al., 1995), that can achieve proper flow rates, with values that can achieve 1 mm/s in $1.6 \times 1.6\,\text{mm}^2$ channels, as determined by Rife et al. (2000), or 1.15 mm/s in $1 \times 1\,\text{mm}^2$ channels, as obtained by Bradley et al. (1995).

Several authors have studied the use of electric fields to create electroosmotic and electrophoretic forces to conduct molecules through microfluidic channels (Auroux et al., 2002; Wang et al., 2000; Borowsky et al., 2008; Kawai et al., 2010), as well as magnetic fields to transport fluidic samples with magnetic micro- or nanoparticles (Khoo and Liu, 2000; Gijs, 2004). Therefore successful active structures are widely documented and assure effective mixing, pumping, and transport of fluids, with high flow rates. However, these types of active techniques require complex fabrication, control and integration processes, as well as high maintaining costs, increasing the cost of the device.

The use of acoustic waves has been proposed as an alternative or complement to promote mixing and transport in microfluidic systems, using piezoelectric transducers (Nyborg, 1953, 1958; Rife et al., 2000; Frampton et al., 2004; Riley, 1998). Acoustic techniques require external actuation. However, they overcome the limitations of active techniques, since acoustic actuators present high mixing efficiency, do not require mobile parts, and ensure easy integration on chip, while maintaining low manufacturing and maintenance cost, and economical viable performance. The acoustic waves propagate into the fluid and generate pressure gradients, inducing an acoustic driving force that promotes movement and agitation. The acoustic flows overcome the viscous forces associated with the micro- and nanochannels (Frampton et al., 2003). Over recent years, many authors reported the development of several experiments and models for describing the piezoelectric effect, the fluid flow, and the acoustic streaming generation. Fig. 12.3 shows different acoustic streaming patterns to promote mixing in fluidic devices (Catarino et al., 2014).

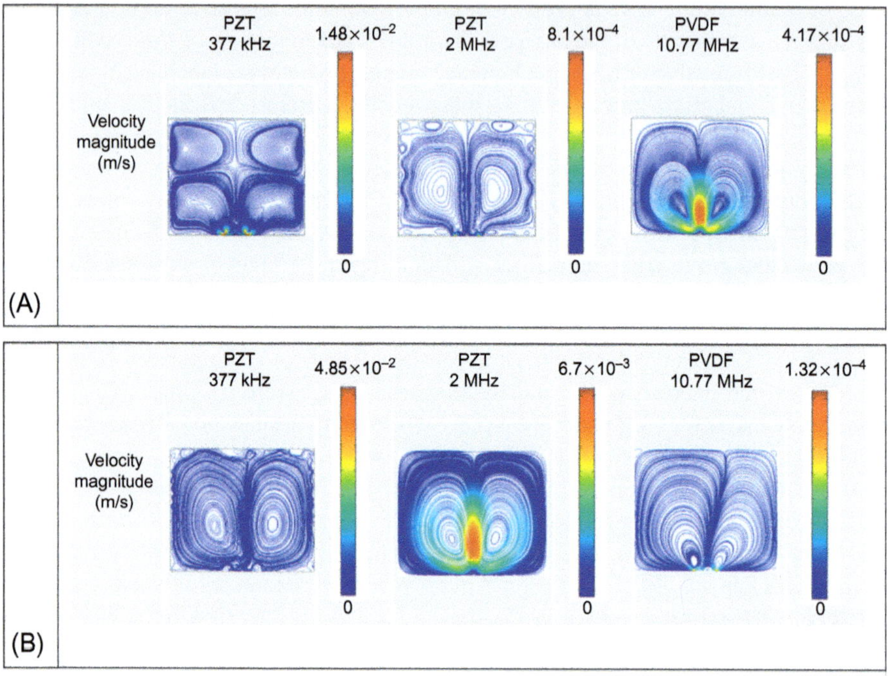

Fig. 12.3 Example of global flow velocity (m/s) and streamlines in cuvettes, actuated by PZT (lead zirconate titanate) and PVDF (poly(vinylidene fluoride)) transducers placed underneath, driven by a 24 Vpp sinusoidal voltage, after simulation of acoustic streaming. (A) 2.4 mm width × 2 mm height cuvette; (B) 8 mm width × 7 mm height cuvette.
Reproduced from Catarino, S.O. et al., 2014. Piezoelectric actuators for acoustic mixing in microfluidic devices—numerical prediction and experimental validation of heat and mass transport. Sens. Actuators B 205, 206–214. Available at: http://www.sciencedirect.com/science/article/pii/S0925400514009988 (accessed 02.09.14.) with permission from -Elsevier.

Further information can be found in Antil and Glowinski (2010), Gantner et al. (2007), Nguyen and Truong (2003), Nguyen and White (1999), Hamilton and Blackstock (1998), and Catarino et al. (2014).

12.3.2 Separation of species

Besides pumping and mixing, lab-on-a-chip devices can include tools for automatic separation of species (molecules, cells, among others). Different physical principles have been implemented to develop efficient cell separation mechanisms, providing powerful cell separation capability with high precision, high throughput, and continuous processing, which include: hydrodynamic inertial force, acoustic force, dielectrophoretic force, magnetic force, optical tweezer, microfiltration, and separation using surface properties (Lee et al., 2016).

Magnetic separation can be achieved through a magnetophoresis process, using different types of magnetic particles (Pamme and Manz, 2004; Gijs, 2004; Do and Ahn, 2008; Pushkarsky et al., 2014). In a continuous flow, magnetic particles are deflected from the direction of laminar flow by a perpendicular magnetic field depending on their magnetic susceptibility, size, and flow rate (Pamme and Manz, 2004; Gijs, 2004). Through this process, only the target molecules or cells are bonded to the magnetic beads and, therefore, the magnetic sorting process is highly specific (Gijs, 2004).

Magnetophoresis has a wide range of applications since magnetic particles are commonly used in bioanalysis as a support material for different biological samples: antigens, antibodies, DNA, and cells (Pamme and Manz, 2004; Cabrera et al., 2015; Do and Ahn, 2008; Pushkarsky et al., 2014). Fig. 12.4 shows an example of a microfluidic platform with magnetic separation of particles (Afshar et al., 2011).

Sorting and separation of cells can also be achieved by optical manipulation techniques. These methods use focused laser beams that provide high-precision trapping and sorting, by promoting radiation pressure forces on the particles (Lee et al., 2016; Khan et al., 2015; Chung et al., 2013). Acoustic forces, promoted by ultrasonic standing waves, have also been used for noncontact cells or particle manipulation. Particle manipulation techniques based on surface acoustic waves (SAWs) appear effective for lab-on-a-chip devices because they are noninvasive, compatible with soft lithography micromachining, have high-energy density, and work for nearly any microscale particles (Lee et al., 2016; Destgeer et al., 2013; Li et al., 2015; Wang and Zhe, 2011).

Dielectrophoresis is the electrokinetic motion of particles that occurs when a polarizable particle is placed in nonuniform electric fields, and the particle motion is influenced by the ambient electric field and by the properties of the dielectric particles or solutions (Lee et al., 2016; Song et al., 2012; Alshareef et al., 2013). Separation of particles and cells can also be achieved by microfiltration, which uses the size of micropores and the gap between microposts for the separation of particles and cells (Lee et al., 2016; Kang et al., 2014; Rodrigues et al., 2015).

12.3.3 Smart materials for controlling fluids

The implementation of different actuation systems in lab-on-a-chip devices requires smart materials to successfully perform the pumping, mixing, or separation actuation, while assuring an easy integration in the lab-on-a-chip devices. This section will focus on some examples of innovative materials to promote the control of fluids in a lab-on-a-chip: PVDF (poly(vinylidene fluoride)), modified chitosan and magnetic particles.

In particular, acoustic actuation systems require the availability of an acoustic-wave source that can be integrated within the microfluidic device and, therefore, different electroactive materials have been considered for integration in lab-on-a-chip devices. Lead zirconate titanate—PZT ceramic and quartz crystal are piezoelectric materials with high piezoelectric coefficients and well characterized. However, in the last years, an effort is being made to replace them with other piezoelectric materials that can achieve similar performance with easier integration in lab-on-a-chip systems (Catarino et al., 2014; Cardoso et al., 2011, 2014; Rife et al., 2000; Yaralioglu et al., 2004).

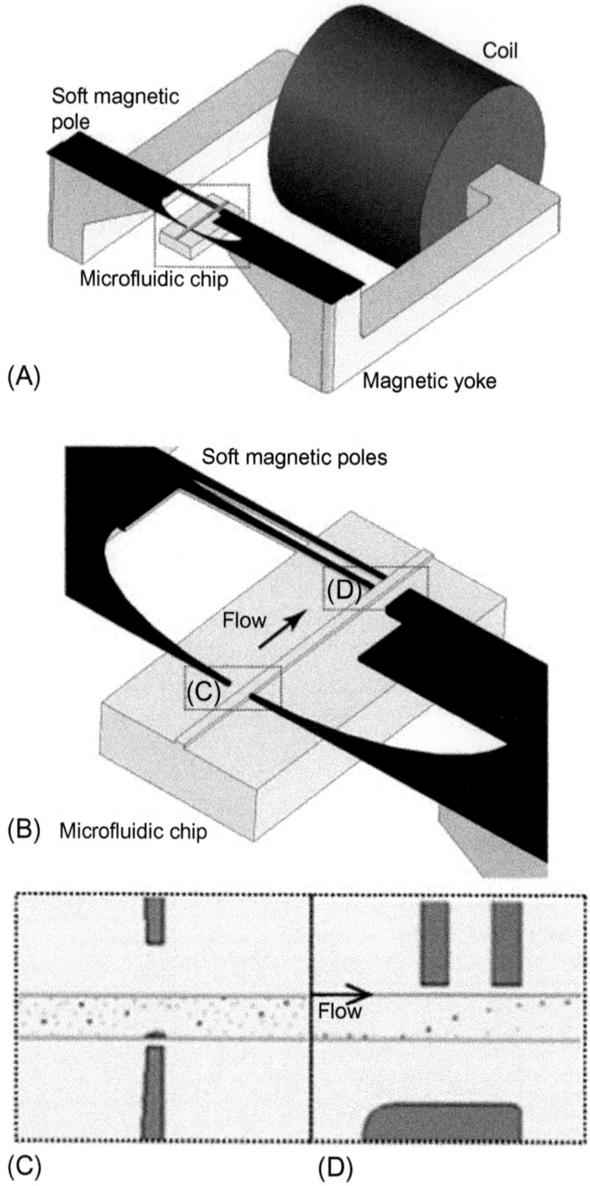

Fig. 12.4 (A) Magnetic actuation system comprising an electromagnet (coil), a magnetic yoke, and soft-magnetic poles, integrated with the microfluidic chip; (B) enhanced view of the microchip showing the magnetic pole arrangement and the microfluidic channel; (C) schematic view of the magnetic plug formation/release section for particle dosing and focusing; and (D) schematic view of the separation zone with two sharp and one broad tip. Beads in the flow are deviated in the field gradient towards the narrow tips.
Reproduced from Afshar, R. et al., 2011. Magnetic particle dosing and size separation in a microfluidic channel. Sens. Actuators B 154 (1), 73–80. Available at: http://linkinghub.elsevier.com/retrieve/pii/S0925400509006777 with permission from Elsevier.

One promising candidate is the PVDF in the β phase and its copolymers. They are the polymers with the best piezoelectric response and also show good mechanical, acoustic, thermal, and piezoelectric properties when processed in the β phase (Cardoso et al., 2014). PVDF is easily processed in thin-films with an easy control and low cost and, therefore, shows good potential for microprocessing and incorporation in microfluidic devices (Cardoso et al., 2011). It is also transparent, which is an interesting feature for lab-on-a-chip applications where optical measures are required (Cardoso et al., 2010; Sencadas et al., 2006; Brown and Mason, 1996).

Chitosan modified with cellulose has been used to produce electroactive actuator films, since cellulose exhibits a piezoelectricity effect, which is conferred to the chitosan–cellulose composite (Kim et al., 2007b). Chitosan modified with polyaniline has also been demonstrated as an actuator that allows two actuation modes (Spinks et al., 2007).

Magnetic actuation uses micro- or nanoparticles for the formation of magnetic fields and selective separation of species. Different types of magnetic beads can be used, from inorganic to biomaterials micro- and nanoparticles (Gijs, 2004). Polystyrene-coated magnetic particles are known for their excellent size distribution, but due to their hydrophobic surface, it needs chemical modification.

Magnetic silica particles are very efficient in adsorbing proteins and DNA on their surface, but are hardly available with a small size distribution. Magnetic polysaccharide particles combine biocompatibility with availability in a size range below 300 nm, but the particles are irregular in shape and sensitive to mechanical stress. Magnetic poly-(lactic acid) particles play an important role in in vivo applications, since they are biodegradable and their degradation time within the blood can be adjusted by their molecular weight and exact chemical composition (Gijs, 2004). Thereby, the selection of the particles must result from a balance between their advantageous and disadvantageous features.

12.4 Detection techniques in lab-on-a-chip devices

The physical and chemical measurement principles of different sensors were approached in the previous chapter (micro-/nanosensors). Therefore this chapter presents the challenges associated with the integration of the main detection techniques (electrochemical, optical, and acoustic) at the microscale level and in microfluidic platforms.

12.4.1 Electrochemical detection

Electrochemical detection is based on a cell comprising a working electrode, where the sensing takes place and a counter reference electrode should maintain a stable potential (Rackus et al., 2015; Mir et al., 2009). The implementation of electrochemical detection systems in microdevices typically requires specific markers to promote a selective binding and detection. This biomolecular recognition takes place close to the functionalized surface of an electrode. For this reason, the electrode shape, dimension, material, and surface properties play a crucial role in the performance of these biosensors (Mir et al., 2009; Ben-Yoav et al., 2015).

For the majority of electrochemical applications, the analyte participates in a reduction–oxidation (or redox) reaction as consequence of an electric potential, measured between the electrodes.

Electrochemical sensors can be classified as amperometric, voltametric, potentiometric, impedimetric, or electrochemical impedance spectroscopy, depending on the detection working principle (Mir et al., 2009; Rackus et al., 2015). Amperometric and voltametric sensors are often used in catalytic mode. For example, in amperometric glucose sensors, the working electrode is coated with a layer of glucose oxidase. When glucose in the sample binds to the enzyme, hydrogen peroxide is formed, oxidizing at the working electrode, which generates a current, proportional to the glucose quantity.

Electrochemical impedance spectroscopy, on the other hand, is typically used for affinity biosensing, in which antibodies or nucleic acids bioreceptors are attached to the working electrode surface. The charge transfer resistance experienced by those electroactive reporters diffused through the film of bioreceptors is a measure of the amount of bound analyte. However, this technique is highly sensitive to nonspecific adsorption (Rackus et al., 2015).

Most electrochemical detection techniques require secondary antibodies with labels (such as gold nanoparticles, fluorescent dye, and chemiluminescent dye), with subsequent multiple rinsing steps. However, there are alternatives of lab-on-a-chip devices with label-free electrochemical detection that do not involve labels, for example, label-free immunoassay lab-on-a-chip. Impedimetric immunoassay lab-on-a-chip is the most popular example of these devices (Yoon and Kim, 2012; Tsekenis et al., 2008). In impedance immunoassays, antibodies are immobilized on a surface where two electrodes are patterned in a configuration called interdigitated microelectrode (Tsekenis et al., 2008). When a big target binds to the surface-bound antibodies, some of the target may be able to bridge the two electrodes, thus lowering the resistance (Yoon and Kim, 2012). Finally, impedance immunosensors have been reported for successfully detection of different substances (Tokarskyy and Marshall, 2008; Guo et al., 2012; Lin et al., 2015; Elshafey et al., 2013).

12.4.2 Optical detection

Integrated optics-based biosensors have become the most promising technology for lab-on-chip integration due to their extreme sensitivity, multiplexing, low-cost mass production, and robustness. Moreover, it is known that using optical detection in a chip results in a better coupling of the light from emitter to source, due to the decrease of the interfaces number, reducing optical losses (Duval and Lechuga, 2013).

Optical detection devices have as a major requirement the high transparency in the optical path. Different optical methods can be applied, depending on the devices' characteristics and requirements of the sensor: absorbance, SPR and nanoplasmonics devices, integrated interferometers, microring resonators, grating-coupled waveguide sensors, photonic crystal- or silicon-wire-based sensors, among others (Duval and Lechuga, 2013; Estevez et al., 2012).

Optical sensors can be divided in two types, depending on whether or not labels are used. Most of the labeled biosensors are based on fluorescence detection and generally imply sample or reagents preparation. Label-free biosensors, most of them using evanescent field detection, have advantages, such as rapid and real-time detection and are the most suitable for lab-on-chip integration (Fan and White, 2011; Duval and Lechuga, 2013; Estevez et al., 2012). In order to integrate the optical sensors in a complete and autonomous lab-on-a-chip device, the optical transducers in a multiplexed configuration must be integrated with all the required units (light sources, photodetectors, microfluidics, and control electronics), as well as with robust biofunctionalization protocols for the biological receptors (Duval and Lechuga, 2013).

The simplest optical sensing technique is based on optical absorption (also known as colorimetry when it is used with visible wavelengths) or fluorescence spectrophotometry for quantitative analysis of biomolecules (Minas et al., 2005; Cardoso et al., 2010). In absorbance, the relative intensity of light before and after passing through a sample correlates with the concentration of absorbing species (also known as chromophores) in the sample. In fluorescence (or fluorimetry), the light that is detected is emitted from fluorescent species (also known as fluorophores) after the initial absorption (or excitation). The wavelengths of light that are absorbed and emitted match differences between electronic energy levels of the chromophores and fluorophores (Rackus et al., 2015).

Absorbance and fluorescence require optical transducers, such as photodiodes or photomultiplier tubes, and they often require lenses, reflectors, and other optical components. Further information about optical absorption and fluorescence spectrophotometry can be found in Upstone (2000) and So and Dong (2001).

SPR is a label-free sensor technique that takes advantage of being implemented in lab-on-a-chip devices (Yoon and Kim, 2012; Abdulhalim et al., 2008). SPR is based on total internal reflection, due to the difference of refractive indices of the interface media when light from an external source hits a metal–fluid interface (Abdulhalim et al., 2008). When molecules adsorb to the functionalized surface, the overall refractive index of the liquid and the resonance angle change (Rackus et al., 2015). Several lab-on-a-chip applications of SPR sensors can be found in literature (Novak et al., 2015; Zhang et al., 2015b; Taylor et al., 2006; Estevez et al., 2012).

Rasooly et al. described a charged-coupled device based detector that can be integrated with a portable lab-on-a-chip assay for various optical detection modalities including fluorescence, chemiluminescence, densitometry, and colorimetric assays (Rasooly et al., 2013).

12.4.3 Acoustic detection

Acoustic signals have been widely considered for detection of biological samples. These detection methods are based on the acoustic coupling between the fluids and the device, and can be based on different sensor principles: SAW, flexural plate wave, quartz crystal microbalance (QCM), film bulk acoustic resonator (FBAR), microcantilever, or Doppler flow sensors. For these detection techniques, the selection of the materials for the substrate and for the microfluidic device needs to take into account the acoustic reflection and absorption in the materials. Many acoustic sensors integrated in lab-on-a-chip devices have been reported. Examples of acoustic sensors in microfluidic applications will be described below.

SAW piezoelectric sensor has been widely reported to detect different analytes. The principle of operation of the SAW sensor is that mass loading on the guiding layer, results in a surface acoustic velocity change, which is detected as a frequency or phase shift of a SAW (Lee et al., 2009a, 2013).

In particular, the guided shear horizontal SAW, which is a specific type of SAW—SH-SAW (also called Love wave sensor) assures high sensitivity and stability in biosensor applications. It consists in a substrate with an overlayer having a lower shear wave velocity. The overlay traps the acoustic energy near the sensing surface, improving the detection response to any physical perturbation on the surface. Several dielectric materials such as silicon dioxide, zinc oxide, and polymers can be used as waveguide material in SAW sensors (Lee et al., 2013). Other SAW applications are described in the literature (Kim et al., 2012b, 2016; Länge et al., 2008; Krishnamoorthy and Iliadis, 2008).

The QCM resonator has also been reported as a piezoelectric mass-sensitive sensor (Henne et al., 2006; Lee et al., 2008a). The binding of the analyte results in an altered mass load of the resonant sensor, resulting in a shift of the resonance frequency that can be measured (Rackus et al., 2015). Lederer et al. reported a biofunctionalized QCM sensor integrated in a digital microfluidic lab-on-a-chip system (Lederer et al., 2011).

Microcantilever, which owes its existence to atomic force microscopy, is based on the principle that binding the analyte to a biological recognition layer on the microcantilever induces surface stress, resulting in nanomechanical motion that can be measured optically or by a piezoresistive readout system (Rackus et al., 2015).

The FBARs sensor consists of a piezoelectric film sandwiched between two metal electrodes, and a micromachined air cavity in silicon substrate underneath the metal/piezo/metal structure. Since its resonance frequency is sensitive to the added mass, FBARs have been widely investigated for use as chemical and biological sensors in gaseous and aqueous environments (Zhang et al., 2015a; Qiu et al., 2011; Nirschl et al., 2009).

12.5 Diagnosis applications

The lab-on-a-chip field is an area in quick development, and many studies have been developed for different applications. The common goal is reflected in overcoming the limitations presented by such devices, preserving their advantages, which consequently enables the development of new microdevices with improved functionality, autonomy, point of care, and performance (Cardoso and Minas, 2011). Particularly, for diagnosis applications, three examples of different applications will be referred to below.

12.5.1 Analytical chemistry

The quantification of proteins, nucleic acids, and metabolites can work as a biomarker for several diseases. Metabolites (glucose, urea nitrogen, creatinine, lactate, etc.) and ionic blood chemicals (sodium, potassium, chloride, etc.) have been used as biomarkers in revealing various body conditions such as diabetes, liver disease, and acid–base homeostasis (Jung et al., 2015). Particularly, glucose has been the most frequent biomarker for diagnosis and management of diabetes and, consequently, more than 80% of the commercial biosensors detect and quantify this metabolite (Freckmann et al., 2010; Wang, 2008). Several lab-on-a-chip devices for analytical chemistry applications, for clinical diagnosis on human physiological fluids, including urine, saliva, and blood serum, have been widely reported in literature (Minas et al., 2005; Srinivasan et al., 2004; Sato et al., 2008; Myers and Lee, 2008; Ahn et al., 2004). A scheme of a lab-on-a-chip device for spectrophotometric analysis of biological fluids is presented in Fig. 12.5 (Ribeiro et al., 2005; Minas et al., 2010).

Different clinical diagnosis studies addressed the detection of biomarkers for malaria (Gascoyne et al., 2002, 2004), infectious diseases (Lee, 2005; Liao et al., 2005; Gulliksen et al., 2005), or cancer (Tsukagoshi et al., 2005; Weigum et al., 2007; Ortiz et al., 2008). Besides the lab-on-a-chip devices that have been developed for quantifying biomolecules and biomarkers in the fluids, other lab-on-a-chip devices have been developed for DNA (Gamby et al., 2007; Nestorova et al., 2016; Lafleur et al., 2016), proteins (Gubic et al., 2015; Rodríguez-Ruiz et al., 2015; Oedit et al., 2015), or cell studies (Alrifaiy et al., 2015; He et al., 2015).

12.5.2 RBCs deformability evaluation

Lab-on-a-chip technology has improved the conditions for studying the blood and its components, mainly the RBCs. From the development of microsystems for measuring the blood flow (Anandan et al., 2015; Raub et al., 2015), blood rheology properties (Calejo et al., 2015; Pinho et al., 2015; Kang and Yang, 2013) and hematocrit (Browne et al., 2011), to microsystems for measuring the deformability of RBCs (Rodrigues et al., 2015; Faustino et al., 2014; Lee et al., 2009b; Rosenbluth et al., 2008; Kim et al., 2012a), several relevant research has been achieved during the last decade. This section will focus on microfluidic devices developed to measure the deformability of the RBCs. Further reading on the measurements of blood flow phenomena happening in microfluidic devices can be found elsewhere (Lima et al., 2012; Geislinger and Franke, 2014; Karimi et al., 2013).

The deformability of the RBCs is closely related to microcirculation and diagnosis of specific diseases such as malaria, arterial sclerosis, sepsis, certain types of cancer, among others (Faustino et al., 2014; Lee et al., 2009b; Hur et al., 2011; Bow et al., 2011; Zheng et al., 2013b). The major determinants of the cells deformability include geometry and size of the microvessels, flow rate, mechanical properties of the cell membrane and its cytoskeleton, and intracellular viscosity (Abkarian et al., 2008). RBCs deformability in microfluidic devices can be evaluated through passive or active methods. Passive methods include microchannel geometrical effects, like

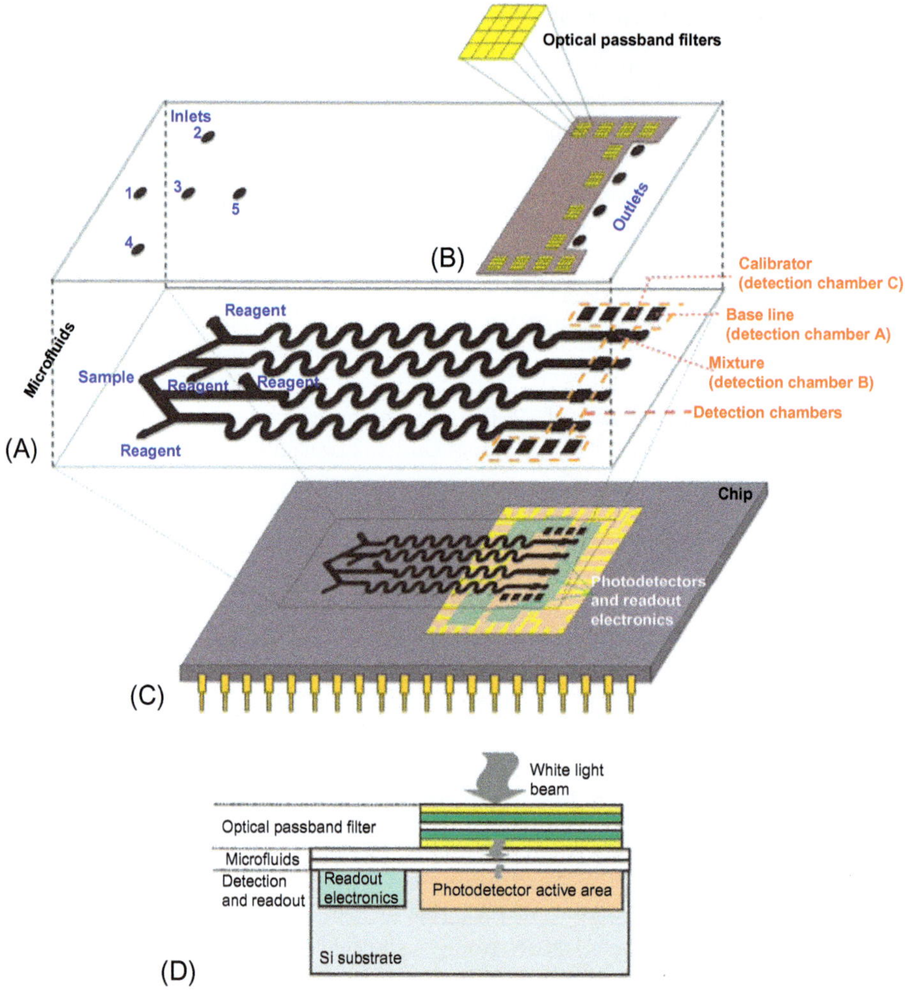

Fig. 12.5 Artist impression of the lab-on-a-chip structure for spectrophotometric analysis of biological fluids. (A) Microfluidic channels; (B) Optical filters; (C) Detection and readout chip; (D) General scheme of the lab-on-a-chip structure.
Reproduced from Minas, G., Wolffenbuttel, R.F. Correia, J.H., 2010. MCM-based microlaboratory for simultaneous measurement of several biochemical parameters by spectrophotometry. Biomed. Microdevices 12 (4), 727–736. Available at: http://link.springer.com/10.1007/s10544-010-9426-1 with permission from Springer.

hyperbolic designs, that allow the continuous monitoring of cells' deformation in an extensional flow region, reducing the experimental time (Faustino et al., 2014; Lee et al., 2009b). Different authors performed studies using soft lithography techniques to fabricate optically transparent microchannels to determine the dynamical deformation of cells (Yaginuma et al., 2013; Pinho et al., 2013; Lima et al., 2008;

Fujiwara et al., 2009; Zhao et al., 2006; Rodrigues et al., 2015). Fig. 12.6 shows RBC deformability measurements at two different constriction regions of a microfluidic device (Pinho et al., 2013).

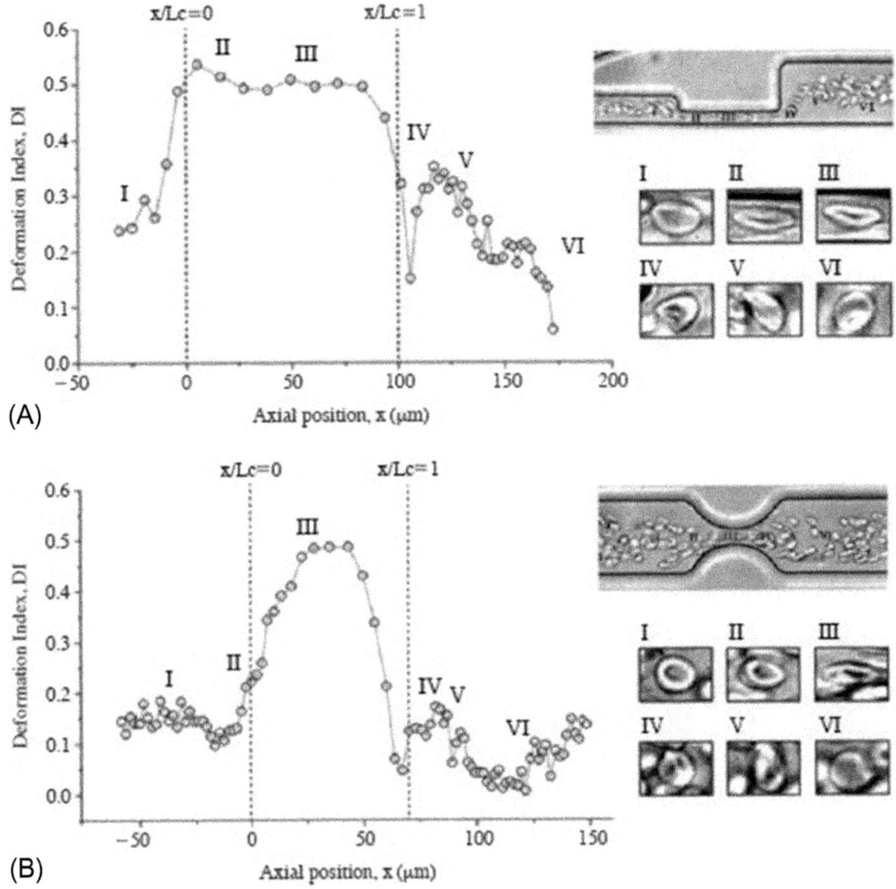

Fig. 12.6 Deformability measurements of an individual RBC flowing through (A) a sudden contraction and (B) a smooth contraction microchannel.
Reproduced from Pinho, D., Yaginuma, T., Lima, R., 2013. A microfluidic device for partial cell separation and deformability assessment. BioChip J. 7 (4), 367–374 with permission from Springer.

The assessment of RBCs deformability can also be performed by active methods, through the application of external force fields, such as acoustic, optical, electrical, and magnetic ones. Acoustic radiation force has been reported for fast and direct measurement of the mechanical properties of cells in a microfluidic chip. This method is based on the formation of an acoustic standing wave within a straight microchannel that moves the cells to the acoustic pressure nodes, with a movement speed dependent on the compressibility (Hartono et al., 2011).

Optical tweezers have been reported for studying the deformation and shape recovery of deformed RBCs, by measuring the relaxation time for each RBC (Bronkhorst et al., 1995). The deformability of RBCs can be electrically measured within a microfluidic channel, by applying a low frequency voltage signal across the microfluidic channel, and considering an electrical current signal continuously sampled when RBCs pass through the measurement areas (Zheng et al., 2013a).

A high-throughput microsystem was reported, based on the biophysical flow cytometry technique to quantify differences in blood cell deformability and prevent hematologic complications, such as microvascular occlusion, sepsis, and leukostasis (Rosenbluth et al., 2008). The deformability of cells was also studied using a microfluidic-based electroporative flow cytometry, combining electroporation with flow cytometry, for clinical applications of diagnosis and staging of cancer (Bao et al., 2008). Other studies for assessing RBCs' deformability include RBCs' filtration (Guéguen et al., 1984; Ogura et al., 1991), rheoscopy (Dobbe et al., 2002), micropipette aspiration (Mokken et al., 1992), and laser diffraction ellipsometry (Shin et al., 2005).

12.5.3 HIV diagnostics

Lab-on-a-chip devices using differential counting of lymphocytes have been developed for HIV diagnostics (Watkins et al., 2013; Holmes et al., 2009; Weaver et al., 2014). Watkins et al. reported a combination of microfluidic handling and impedance based electrical readouts to create a simple, low cost, and robust device for fast counting of both CD4+ and CD8+ T-lymphocytes, using small volumes of whole blood (10 μL), without the need for off-chip sample preparation. The device is based on differential electrical counting and relies on five on-chip modules as follows: erythrocytes are chemically lysed, lysis is quenched to preserve leukocytes, cells are electrically enumerated, the target cells (CD4 or CD8) are depleted with antibodies, and finally the remaining cells are electrically enumerated (Watkins et al., 2013). Emaminejad et al. developed a portable cytometry microdevice for counting cells and microsized particles, able to CD4 cell count for HIV diagnosis, as presented in Fig. 12.7 (Emaminejad et al., 2016).

Holmes et al. also reported a microfluidic single-cell impedance cytometer that performs a white blood cell differential count. The device consists of a microfluidic chip with microelectrodes that measure the impedance of single cells at two different frequencies (Holmes et al., 2009).

Other lab-on-a-chip devices for HIV diagnosis include a microfluidic device for monitoring the progression of the HIV infection by counting and sorting CD4 cells, using electroosmosis as a driving mechanism and a laser diode as a light source (Sun et al., 2005b). An automatic lab-on-a-chip for the clinical diagnosis of HIV, based on laser-induced fluorescence measurements for real-time monitoring of the signal after the sample preparation, reaction, and signal amplification, was also reported (Guo et al., 2005). Additionally, a fully disposable and point-of-care RT-PCR microfluidic device was developed with embedded micropinch valves on the basis of chemiluminescence assays for the rapid detection of HIV (Lee et al., 2008b).

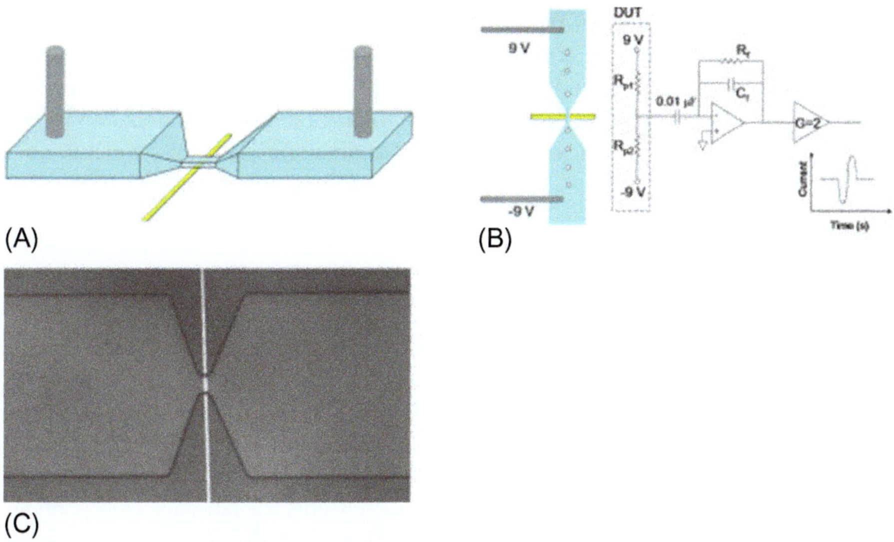

Fig. 12.7 (A) Schematic of microfluidic device integrated with open circuit electrode at the bottom surface of the micropore. Microchannels 300 μm wide taper down to smaller pore so that majority of voltage drop is across the pore. Positive and negative voltage applied at outer channel edges. (B) Circuit diagram of device under test integrated with readout electronics. Transient change in the current across the pore is amplified using integrator circuit configuration. (Inset) Bead passing through the pore results in drop in current and then rise. (C) Optical micrograph of fabricated microdevice. Electrode is fabricated on a glass substrate. Microchannel on top is embedded in PDMS.
Reproduced from Emaminejad, S. et al., 2016. Portable cytometry using microscale electronic sensing. Sens. Actuators B 224, 275–281. Available at: http://linkinghub.elsevier.com/retrieve/pii/S0925400515302951 with permission from Elsevier.

12.6 Conclusions and perspectives

In this chapter, the main microfabrication technologies for lab-on-a-chip devices were described, as well as the main advances and challenges regarding new biomaterials. We also discussed the manipulation, control, actuation of the fluids within the microchannels, and the main detection techniques. Different examples of diagnosis applications using lab-on-a-chip devices were presented.

The lab-on-a-chip research opens new possibilities for the miniaturization of (bio) chemical analysis systems. However, this research requires interdisciplinary work to integrate in a single chip the microfluidic, actuation, detection, and readout systems at such a small scale. Currently, the lab-on-a-chip technology has already gained credibility, maturity, and robustness, reflected by the exponential growth in the number of publications in this research field, the large diversity of lab-on-a-chip devices and their use in various research fields, as well as by the increasing number of commercially available products. Therefore this technology is preparing to advance to the next steps, namely the design of more challenging platforms offering novel experimentation opportunities and performance, such as the use of biomaterials as the substrate for the microfluidic platforms and lab-in-a-cell devices, using single cells as experimentation platforms.

All the developed efforts and challenges regarding the lab-on-a-chip technology rely on a main objective that consists in the development of multifunctional and commercial microdevices that are low cost, portable, autonomous, and able to achieve the same or better sensitivity as the commercially available equipment.

12.7 Future research directions

Despite all the advances in the lab-on-a-chip field, a great amount of research still needs to be performed to achieve even higher maturity and robustness, and to be more than an active academic research field. Several research directions are expected to tackle the current challenges in the bioinspired materials for the lab-on-a-chip research field.

The fabrication of complex three-dimensional systems for lab-on-a-chip applications is still a big challenge since most of the existing lab-on-a-chip devices are based on macroscopic instrumentation around microfluidic structures and polymer technologies are still difficult to integrate with some electronic components.

Several lab-on-a-chip applications are challenging to implement as traditional microdevices, since they require a high number of off-chip components. Therefore the integration of many functionalities on-chip, allowing the devices to be highly customizable for individualized applications, is still a challenge. Major challenges also remain relatively to the miniaturization of systems at the nanoscale for single-cell analysis, with the fully integration of control and readout electronics, as well as the development of new synthetic antibodies or adhesion layers for surfaces coating. Further progress is also expected in the development of new low-cost techniques for manipulating and controlling fluids at the micro- and nanoscale levels.

The use of biomaterials as substrates in lab-on-a-chip devices, overcoming the current limitations regarding the integration of microelectronics in these devices, and achieving the same performance of the silicon, glass, and polymeric systems, is also a major research area. The combination of the emerging understanding of biopolymer physics and the ability to integrate microfluidics is offering opportunities for new research directions. Combined with the study of biomaterials, paper substrates to control the fluid flow and electronic readouts have also been addressed as major challenges in lab-on-a-chip research. Paper microfluidics are being investigated as they have significant potential for low-cost point-of-care devices, in terms of fabrication methods, capable functionalities and readouts.

New trends in lab-on-a-chip research will focus the use of off-the-shelf consumer electronics for telemedicine purposes, such as smart phones, tablets, or scanners for simplified readouts and effective follow-up.

Many efforts have been addressed to the analysis of samples from heterogeneous physiological fluids (such as blood, urine, or pleural fluid), which have a low number of cells/molecules of interest. Thus, to obtain statistically meaningful data and achieve clinical relevance, techniques with high throughput are required.

Finally, as the lab-on-a-chip devices acquire innovative features and become more precise, more robust, and automated, their ability to detect and/or quantify micro- and nanofluidic samples with high sensitivity will grow, opening the possibility to develop more efficient miniaturized systems and perform new research for (bio)medical, pharmaceutical, and diagnosis applications.

Acknowledgments

This work is supported by FCT with the reference project UID/EEA/04436/2013, by FEDER funds through the COMPETE 2020—Programa Operacional Competitividade e Internacionalização (POCI) with the reference project POCI-01-0145-FEDER-006941. S.O. Catarino thanks the FCT for the SFRH/BPD/108889/2015 grant.

References

Abdelgawad, M., et al., 2008. Soft lithography: masters on demand. Lab Chip 8, 1379–1385.

Abdulhalim, I., Zourob, M., Lakhtakia, A., 2008. Surface plasmon resonance for biosensing: a mini-review. Electromagnetics 28 (3), 214–242. Available at: http://www.tandfonline.com/doi/abs/10.1080/02726340801921650.

Abgrall, P., Gué, A.-M., 2007. Lab-on-chip technologies: making a microfluidic network and coupling it into a complete microsystem—a review. J. Micromech. Microeng. 17 (5), R15–R49. Available at: http://stacks.iop.org/0960-1317/17/i=5/a=R01?key=crossref.c24504191bbdbbc35f746483f719698a.

Abkarian, M., et al., 2008. Cellular-scale hydrodynamics. Biomed. Mater. 3 (3), 034011. Available at: http://www.ncbi.nlm.nih.gov/pubmed/18765900.

Afshar, R., et al., 2011. Magnetic particle dosing and size separation in a microfluidic channel. Sens. Actuators B 154 (1), 73–80. Available at: http://linkinghub.elsevier.com/retrieve/pii/S0925400509006777.

Ahn, C.H., et al., 2004. Disposable smart lab on a chip for point-of-care clinical diagnostics. Proc. IEEE 92 (1), 154–173. Available at: http://ieeexplore.ieee.org/lpdocs/epic03/wrapper.htm?arnumber=1258178.

Alrifaiy, A., et al., 2015. A lab-on-a-chip for hypoxic patch clamp measurements combined with optical tweezers and spectroscopy—first investigations of single biological cells. Biomed. Eng. 14 (1), 36. Available at: http://www.biomedical-engineering-online.com/content/14/1/36.

Alshareef, M., et al., 2013. Separation of tumor cells with dielectrophoresis-based microfluidic chip. Biomicrofluidics 7 (1), 011803. Available at: http://scitation.aip.org/content/aip/journal/bmf/7/1/10.1063/1.4774312.

Anandan, P., et al., 2015. Red blood cells flows in rectilinear microfluidic chip. In: 2015 37th Annual International Conference of the IEEE Engineering in Medicine and Biology Society (EMBC). IEEE, pp. 3225–3228, Available at: http://ieeexplore.ieee.org/lpdocs/epic03/wrapper.htm?arnumber=7319079.

Andersson, H., Van den Berg, A., 2003. Microfluidic devices for cellomics: a review. Sens. Actuators B 92 (3), 315–325.

Antil, H., Glowinski, R., 2010. Modeling, simulation and optimization of surface acoustic wave driven microfluidic biochips. J. Comput. Math. 28, 149–169.

Auroux, P.A., et al., 2002. Micro total analysis systems. 2. Analytical standard operations and applications. Anal. Chem. 74, 2637–2652.

Aziz, N.A., et al., 2008. Characterization of HNA etchant for silicon microneedles array fabrication. In: IEEE International Conference on Semiconductor Electronics, Proceedings, ICSE, pp. 203–206.

Bai, J., et al., 2006. Regenerated spider silk as a new biomaterial for MEMS. Biomed. Microdevices 8 (4), 317–323. Available at: http://link.springer.com/10.1007/s10544-006-9820-x.

Bao, N., Zhan, Y., Lu, C., 2008. Microfluidic electroporative flow cytometry for studying single-cell biomechanics. Anal. Chem. 80 (20), 7714–7719. Available at: http://www.ncbi.nlm.nih.gov/pubmed/18798650.

Becker, H., 2002. Polymer microfluidic devices. Talanta 56 (2), 267–287. Available at: http://linkinghub.elsevier.com/retrieve/pii/S003991400100594X.

Becker, H., Gärtner, C., 2008. Polymer microfabrication technologies for microfluidic systems. Anal. Bioanal. Chem. 390 (1), 89–111. Available at: http://www.ncbi.nlm.nih.gov/pubmed/17989961.

Ben-Yoav, H., et al., 2015. A controlled microfluidic electrochemical lab-on-a-chip for label-free diffusion-restricted DNA hybridization analysis. Biosens. Bioelectron. 64, 579–585. Available at: http://linkinghub.elsevier.com/retrieve/pii/S0956566314007568.

Boozer, C., et al., 2003. Surface functionalization for self-referencing surface plasmon resonance (SPR) biosensors by multi-step self-assembly. Sens. Actuators B 90 (1–3), 22–30. Available at: http://linkinghub.elsevier.com/retrieve/pii/S0925400503000170.

Borowsky, J., Lu, Q., Collins, G.E., 2008. High pressure electroosmotic pump based on a packed bed planar microchip. Sens. Actuators B 131 (1), 333–339.

Bow, H., et al., 2011. A microfabricated deformability-based flow cytometer with application to malaria. Lab Chip 11 (6), 1065–1073.

Bradley, C.E., Bustillo, J.M., White, R.M., 1995. Flow measurements in a micromachined flow system with integrated acoustic pumping. In: 1995 IEEE Ultrasonics Symposium. Proceedings. An International Symposium. IEEE, pp. 505–510. Available at: http://ieeexplore.ieee.org/lpdocs/epic03/wrapper.htm?arnumber=495628.

Brecher, C., Baum, C., Bastuck, T., 2015. Comparison of roll-to-roll replication approaches for microfluidic and optical functions in lab-on-a-chip diagnostic devices. In: Gray, B.L., Becker, H. (Eds.), Proc. SPIE 9320, Microfluidics, BioMEMS, and Medical Microsystems XIII, 932008, Available at: http://dx.doi.org/10.1117/12.2077592.

Bridle, H., Miller, B., Desmulliez, M.P.Y., 2014. Application of microfluidics in waterborne pathogen monitoring: a review. Water Res. 55, 256–271.

Broers, A.N., Hoole Andrew, A.C.F., Ryan, J.M., 1996. Electron beam lithography—resolution limits. Microelectron. Eng. 32, 131–142.

Bronkhorst, P.J., et al., 1995. A new method to study shape recovery of red blood cells using multiple optical trapping. Biophys. J. 69 (5), 1666–1673. Available at: http://linkinghub.elsevier.com/retrieve/pii/S0006349595800846.

Brown, L.F., Mason, J.L., 1996. Disposable PVDF ultrasonic transducers for nondestructive testing applications. IEEE Trans. Ultrason. Ferroelectr. Freq. Control 43 (4), 560–568. Available at: http://ieeexplore.ieee.org/lpdocs/epic03/wrapper.htm?arnumber=503716.

Browne, A.W., et al., 2011. A lab-on-a-chip for rapid blood separation and quantification of hematocrit and serum analytes. Lab Chip 11 (14), 2440. Available at: http://xlink.rsc.org/?DOI=c1lc20144a.

Bustjllo, J.M., Howe, R.T., Muller, R.S., 1998. Surface micromachining for microelectromechanical systems. Proc. IEEE 86 (8), 1552–1573.

Cabrera, F.C., et al., 2015. A flexible lab-on-a-chip for the synthesis and magnetic separation of magnetite decorated with gold nanoparticles. Lab Chip 15 (8), 1835–1841. Available at: http://xlink.rsc.org/?DOI=C4LC01483A.

Calejo, J., et al., 2015. Particulate blood analogues reproducing the erythrocytes cell free layer in a microfluidic device containing a hyperbolic contraction. Micromachines 7 (1), 4. Available at: http://www.mdpi.com/2072-666X/7/1/4.

Cardoso, V.F., Minas, G., 2011. Micro total analysis systems. In: Microfluidics and Nanofluidics Handbook: Fabrication, Implementation and Applications. CRC Press/Taylor & Francis Group, LLC Publishers, California, pp. 319–366.

Cardoso, V.F., et al., 2010. Lab-on-a-chip with beta-poly(vinylidene fluoride) based acoustic microagitation. IEEE Trans. Bio.-Med. Eng. 57 (5), 1184–1190. Available at: http://www.ncbi.nlm.nih.gov/pubmed/19884076 (accessed 24.02.14.).

Cardoso, V.F., et al., 2011. Micro and nanofilms of poly(vinylidene fluoride) with controlled thickness, morphology and electroactive crystalline phase for sensor and actuator applications. Smart Mater. Struct. 20 (8), 087002. Available at: http://stacks.iop.org/0964-1726/20/i=8/a=087002?key=crossref.b6354c9b0f93a0cc664dc4e3e149d6e2 (accessed 14.07.14.).

Cardoso, V.F., et al., 2014. Polymer-based acoustic streaming for improving mixing and reaction times in microfluidic applications. RSC Adv. 4 (9), 4292. Available at: http://xlink.rsc.org/?DOI=c3ra46420b (accessed 24.09.14.).

Catarino, S.O., et al., 2014. Piezoelectric actuators for acoustic mixing in microfluidic devices—numerical prediction and experimental validation of heat and mass transport. Sens. Actuators B 205, 206–214. Available at: http://www.sciencedirect.com/science/article/pii/S0925400514009988 (accessed 02.09.14.).

Chen, X., Cui, D.F., 2009. Microfluidic devices for sample pretreatment and applications. Microsyst. Technol. 15, 667–676.

Cheng, J.C., Pisano, A.P., 2008. Photolithographic process for integration of the biopolymer chitosan into micro/nanostructures. J. Microelectromech. Syst. 17 (2), 402–409. Available at: http://ieeexplore.ieee.org/lpdocs/epic03/wrapper.htm?arnumber=4469666.

Cheng, J.Y., et al., 2004. Direct-write laser micromachining and universal surface modification of PMMA for device development. Sens. Actuators B 99 (1), 186–196.

Cheng, W., et al., 2006. Metabolic monitoring of the electrically stimulated single heart cell within a microfluidic platform. Lab Chip 6, 1424–1431.

Choi, Y., Kang, T., Lee, L.P., 2009. Plasmon resonance energy transfer (PRET)-based molecular imaging of cytochrome *C* in living cells. Nano Lett. 9 (1), 85–90.

Chung, Y., et al., 2004. Design of passive mixers utilizing microfluidic self-circulation in the mixing chamber. Lab Chip 4 (1), 70–77.

Chung, Y.-C., et al., 2013. Particles sorting in micro-channel system utilizing magnetic tweezers and optical tweezers. J. Magn. Magn. Mater. 333, 87–92. Available at: http://linkinghub.elsevier.com/retrieve/pii/S0304885312010153.

Clausell-Tormos, J., et al., 2008. Droplet-based microfluidic platforms for the encapsulation and screening of mammalian cells and multicellular organisms. Chem. Biol. 15 (5), 427–437.

Cowan, S.E., Liepmann, D., Keasling, J.D., 2001. Development of engineered biofilms on poly-L-lysine patterned surfaces. Biotechnol. Lett. 23 (15), 1235–1241. Available at: http://link.springer.com/10.1023/A:1010581503842.

Destgeer, G., et al., 2013. Continuous separation of particles in a PDMS microfluidic channel via travelling surface acoustic waves (TSAW). Lab Chip 13 (21), 4210. Available at: http://xlink.rsc.org/?DOI=c3lc50451d.

Dey, P.K., et al., 2010. Microstructuring of su-8 resist for MEMS and bio-applications. Int. J. Smart Sens. Intell. Syst. 3, 118–129.

Do, J., Ahn, C.H., 2008. A polymer lab-on-a-chip for magnetic immunoassay with on-chip sampling and detection capabilities. Lab Chip 8 (4), 542. Available at: http://xlink.rsc.org/?DOI=b715569g.

Dobbe, J.G.G., et al., 2002. Analyzing red blood cell-deformability distributions. Blood Cell Mol. Dis. 28 (3), 373–384. Available at: http://www.sciencedirect.com/science/article/pii/S1079979602905280.

Dragavon, J., et al., 2008. A cellular isolation system for real-time single-cell oxygen consumption monitoring. J. R. Soc. Interface/R. Soc. 5 (Suppl. 2), S151–S159. Available at: http://www.pubmedcentral.nih.gov/articlerender.fcgi?artid=2706035&tool=pmcentrez&rendertype=abstract.

Dresselhaus, M.S., Lin, Y.-M., Rabin, O., Black, M.R., Jing Kong, G.D., 2010. In: Bhushan, B. (Ed.), Handbook of Nanotechnology. Springer, Berlin, Heidelberg. Available at: http://www.springerlink.com/index/10.1007/978-3-642-02525-9 (accessed 24.07.14.).

Duffy, D.C., et al., 1998. Rapid prototyping of microfluidic systems in poly(dimethylsiloxane). Anal. Chem. 70 (23), 4974–4984. Available at: http://pubs.acs.org/doi/abs/10.1021/ac980656z.

Duval, D., Lechuga, L.M., 2013. Breakthroughs in photonics 2012: 2012 breakthroughs in lab-on-a-chip and optical biosensors. IEEE Photonics J. 5 (2), 0700906. Available at: http://ieeexplore.ieee.org/lpdocs/epic03/wrapper.htm?arnumber=6472721.

Dykstra, P., et al., 2009. An optical MEMS sensor utilizing a chitosan film for catechol detection. Sens. Actuators B 138 (1), 64–70. Available at: http://linkinghub.elsevier.com/retrieve/pii/S092540050900094X.

Edwards, T.L., et al., 2002. Rapid micromold tooling for injection molding microfluidic components. Sens. Mater. 14 (3), 167–178.

El-Ali, J., Sorger, P.K., Jensen, K.F., 2006. Cells on chips. Nature 442 (7101), 403–411. Available at: http://www.nature.com/doifinder/10.1038/nature05063.

Elshafey, R., et al., 2013. Electrochemical impedance immunosensor based on gold nanoparticles–protein G for the detection of cancer marker epidermal growth factor receptor in human plasma and brain tissue. Biosens. Bioelectron. 50, 143–149. Available at: http://linkinghub.elsevier.com/retrieve/pii/S0956566313004041.

Emaminejad, S., et al., 2016. Portable cytometry using microscale electronic sensing. Sens. Actuators B 224, 275–281. Available at: http://linkinghub.elsevier.com/retrieve/pii/S0925400515302951.

Estevez, M.C., Alvarez, M., Lechuga, L.M., 2012. Integrated optical devices for lab-on-a-chip biosensing applications. Laser Photonics Rev. 6 (4), 463–487. Available at: http://doi.wiley.com/10.1002/lpor.201100025.

Fan, X., White, I.M., 2011. Optofluidic microsystems for chemical and biological analysis. Nat. Photonics 5 (10), 591–597. Available at: http://www.nature.com/doifinder/10.1038/nphoton.2011.206.

Faustino, V., et al., 2014. Extensional flow-based microfluidic device: deformability assessment of red blood cells in contact with tumor cells. BioChip J. 8 (1), 42–47. Available at: http://link.springer.com/10.1007/s13206-014-8107-1.

Faustino, V., et al., 2015. Biomedical microfluidic devices by using low-cost fabrication techniques: a review. J. Biomech.Available at: http://www.sciencedirect.com/science/article/pii/S0021929015006739 (accessed 09.12.15.).

Ferreira, N.S., Sales, M.G.F., 2014. Disposable immunosensor using a simple method for oriented antibody immobilization for label-free real-time detection of an oxidative stress biomarker implicated in cancer diseases. Biosens. Bioelectron. 53, 193–199. Available at: http://linkinghub.elsevier.com/retrieve/pii/S095656631300674X.

Figeys, D., Pinto, D., 2000. Lab-on-a-chip: a revolution in biological and medical sciences. Anal. Chem. 72 (9), 330 A–335 A. Available at: http://pubs.acs.org/doi/abs/10.1021/ac002800y.
Fiorini, G.S., Chiu, D.T., 2005. Disposable microfluidic devices: fabrication, function, and application. Biotechniques 38, 429–446.
Foudeh, A.M., et al., 2012. Microfluidic designs and techniques using lab-on-a-chip devices for pathogen detection for point-of-care diagnostics. Lab Chip 12 (18), 3249. Available at: http://xlink.rsc.org/?DOI=c2lc40630f.
Fraden, J., 2004. Handbook of Modern Sensors—Physics, Designs and Applications, third ed. Springer-Verlag, New York. Available at: http://link.springer.com/10.1007/b97321 (accessed 13.05.15.).
Frampton, K.D., Martin, S.E., Minor, K., 2003. The scaling of acoustic streaming for application in micro-fluidic devices. Appl. Acoust. 64 (7), 681–692. Available at: http://linkinghub.elsevier.com/retrieve/pii/S0003682X03000057 (accessed 24.02.14.).
Frampton, K.D., Minor, K., Martin, S., 2004. Acoustic streaming in micro-scale cylindrical channels. Appl. Acoust. 65 (11), 1121–1129. Available at: http://linkinghub.elsevier.com/retrieve/pii/S0003682X04000696 (accessed 24.02.14.).
Freckmann, G., et al., 2010. System accuracy evaluation of 27 blood glucose monitoring systems according to DIN EN ISO 15197. Diabetes Technol. Ther. 12 (3), 221–231. Available at: http://online.liebertpub.com/doi/abs/10.1089/dia.2009.0128.
French, P.J., Sarro, P.M., 1999. Surface versus bulk micromachining: the contest for suitable applications. J. Micromech. Microeng. 8 (3), 250.
Fujii, T., 2002. PDMS-based microfluidic devices for biomedical applications. Microelectron. Eng. 61–62, 907–914.
Fujiwara, H., et al., 2009. Red blood cell motions in high-hematocrit blood flowing through a stenosed microchannel. J. Biomech. 42 (7), 838–843.
Fung, Y.C., 1997. Biomechanics—Circulation. Springer, New York, NY. Available at: http://www.springer.com/us/book/9780387943848.
Gamby, J., et al., 2007. Electroacoustic miniaturized DNA-biosensor. Lab Chip 7 (11), 1607–1609. Available at: http://www.ncbi.nlm.nih.gov/pubmed/17960294.
Gantner, A., Hoppe, R., Koster, D., Siebert, K., Wixforth, A., 2007. Numerical simulation of piezoelectrically agitated surface acoustic waves on microfluidic biochips. Comput. Visual Sci. 10, 145–161.
Gascoyne, P., et al., 2002. Microsample preparation by dielectrophoresis: isolation of malaria. Lab Chip 2 (2), 70–75. Available at: http://pubs.rsc.org/en/content/articlehtml/2002/lc/b110990c.
Gascoyne, P., Satayavivad, J., Ruchirawat, M., 2004. Microfluidic approaches to malaria detection. Acta Trop. 89 (3), 357–369. Available at: http://www.sciencedirect.com/science/article/pii/S0001706X03003164.
Geislinger, T.M., Franke, T., 2014. Hydrodynamic lift of vesicles and red blood cells in flow—from Fåhræus & Lindqvist to microfluidic cell sorting. Adv. Colloid Interface Sci. 208, 161–176. Available at: http://linkinghub.elsevier.com/retrieve/pii/S000186861400102X.
Gijs, M.A.M., 2004. Magnetic bead handling on-chip: new opportunities for analytical applications. Microfluid. Nanofluid. 1 (1), 22–40.
Gubic, J., et al., 2015. Characterization of several milk proteins in Domestic Balkan donkey breed during lactation, using lab-on-a-chip capillary electrophoresis. Chem. Ind. Chem. Eng. Q., 13. Available at: http://www.doiserbia.nb.rs/Article.aspx?ID=1451-93721500013G.
Guéguen, M., et al., 1984. Filtration pressure and red blood cell deformability: evaluation of a new device: erythrometre. Biorheology Suppl. 1, 261–265. Available at: http://www.ncbi.nlm.nih.gov/pubmed/6591984 (accessed 02.01.16.).

Guenat, O.T., et al., 2006. Development of an array of ion-selective microelectrodes aimed for the monitoring of extracellular ionic activities. Anal. Chem. 78 (21), 7453–7460.

Gulliksen, A., et al., 2005. Parallel nanoliter detection of cancer markers using polymer microchips. Lab Chip 5, 416–420.

Guo, W.-P., Ma, X.-M., Zeng, Y., 2005. Clinical laboratories on a chip for human immunodeficiency virus assay. In: Conference proceedings: … Annual International Conference of the IEEE Engineering in Medicine and Biology Society. IEEE Engineering in Medicine and Biology Society. Conference, vol. 2, pp. 1274–1277. Available at: http://www.ncbi.nlm.nih.gov/pubmed/17282427.

Guo, X., et al., 2012. Carbohydrate-based label-free detection of *Escherichia coli* ORN 178 using electrochemical impedance spectroscopy. Anal. Chem. 84 (1), 241–246. Available at: http://pubs.acs.org/doi/abs/10.1021/ac202419u.

Gupta, K., et al., 2010. Lab-on-a-chip devices as an emerging platform for stem cell biology. Lab Chip 10 (16), 2019. Available at: http://xlink.rsc.org/?DOI=c004689b.

Haeberle, S., Zengerle, R., 2007. Microfluidic platforms for lab-on-a-chip applications. Lab Chip 7 (9), 1094–1110. Available at: http://www.ncbi.nlm.nih.gov/pubmed/17713606 (accessed 24.01.14.).

Hamilton, M., Blackstock, D.T., 1998. Nonlinear Acoustics. Academic Press, San Diego, CA.

Han, M., et al., 2004. 3D microfabrication with inclined/rotated UV lithography. Sens. Actuators A 111 (1), 14–20.

Hartono, D., et al., 2011. On-chip measurements of cell compressibility via acoustic radiation. Lab Chip 11 (23), 4072. Available at: http://xlink.rsc.org/?DOI=c1lc20687g.

He, L., et al., 2015. An automated programmable platform enabling multiplex dynamic stimuli delivery and cellular response monitoring for high-throughput suspension single-cell signaling studies. Lab Chip 15 (6), 1497–1507. Available at: http://xlink.rsc.org/?DOI=C4LC01070A.

Henne, W.A., et al., 2006. Detection of folate binding protein with enhanced sensitivity using a functionalized quartz crystal microbalance sensor. Anal. Chem. 78 (14), 4880–4884. Available at: http://pubs.acs.org/doi/abs/10.1021/ac060324r.

Heuberger, A., 1988. X-ray lithography. J. Vac. Sci. Technol., B: Microelectron. Nanometer Struct. 6, 107.

Hoang, H.T., et al., 2009. Fabrication and interfacing of nanochannel devices for single-molecule studies. J. Micromech. Microeng. 19 (6), 065017.

Holmes, D., et al., 2009. Leukocyte analysis and differentiation using high speed microfluidic single cell impedance cytometry. Lab Chip 9 (20), 2881. Available at: http://xlink.rsc.org/?DOI=b910053a.

Hur, S.C., et al., 2011. Deformability-based cell classification and enrichment using inertial microfluidics. Lab Chip 11 (5), 912–920.

Jansen, H., et al., 1996. A survey on the reactive ion etching of silicon in microtechnology. J. Micromech. Microeng. 6 (1), 14–28. Available at: http://stacks.iop.org/0960-1317/6/i=1/a=002?key=crossref.7b65ee39ff4ea890d9f9927b7bbd3050.

Jung, W., et al., 2015. Point-of-care testing (POCT) diagnostic systems using microfluidic lab-on-a-chip technologies. Microelectron. Eng. 132, 46–57. Available at: http://linkinghub.elsevier.com/retrieve/pii/S0167931714004316.

Kamholz, A.E., Yager, P., 2001. Theoretical analysis of molecular diffusion in pressure-driven laminar flow in microfluidic channels. Biophys. J. 80 (1), 155–160. Available at: http://www.pubmedcentral.nih.gov/articlerender.fcgi?artid=1301222&tool=pmcentrez&rendertype=abstract.

Kane, R., 1999. Patterning proteins and cells using soft lithography. Biomaterials 20 (23–24), 2363–2376. Available at: http://linkinghub.elsevier.com/retrieve/pii/S0142961299001659.

Kang, Y.J., Yang, S., 2013. Integrated microfluidic viscometer equipped with fluid temperature controller for measurement of viscosity in complex fluids. Microfluid. Nanofluid. 14 (3–4), 657–668. Available at: http://link.springer.com/10.1007/s10404-012-1085-5.

Kang, T.G., et al., 2014. A continuous flow micro filtration device for plasma/blood separation using submicron vertical pillar gap structures. J. Micromech. Microeng. 24 (8), 087001. Available at: http://stacks.iop.org/0960-1317/24/i=8/a=087001?key=crossref.0d9dda11e85a73186e9562145967ec9a.

Karimi, A., Yazdi, S., Ardekani, A.M., 2013. Hydrodynamic mechanisms of cell and particle trapping in microfluidics. Biomicrofluidics 7 (2), 021501. Available at: http://scitation.aip.org/content/aip/journal/bmf/7/2/10.1063/1.4799787.

Kawai, T., et al., 2010. Microchip electrophoresis of oligosaccharides using large-volume sample stacking with an electroosmotic flow pump in a single channel. Anal. Chem. 82 (15), 6504–6511. Available at: http://www.ncbi.nlm.nih.gov/pubmed/20586466.

Keenan, T.M., Folch, A., 2008. Biomolecular gradients in cell culture systems. Lab Chip 8 (1), 34–57.

Khan, S.A., et al., 2015. Optical separation of heterogeneous size distributions of microparticles on silicon nitride strip waveguides. Opt. Express 23 (7), 8855. Available at: https://www.osapublishing.org/oe/abstract.cfm?uri=oe-23-7-8855.

Khine, M., et al., 2007. Single-cell electroporation arrays with real-time monitoring and feedback control. Lab Chip 7, 457–462.

Khoo, M., Liu, C., 2000. A novel micromachined magnetic membrane microfluid pump. In: Proceedings of the 22nd Annual International Conference of the IEEE Engineering in Medicine and Biology Society (Cat. No.00CH37143), vol. 3, pp. 4–7.

Khosravi Parsa, M., Hormozi, F., Jafari, D., 2014. Mixing enhancement in a passive micromixer with convergent–divergent sinusoidal microchannels and different ratio of amplitude to wave length. Comput. Fluids 105, 82–90. Available at: http://linkinghub.elsevier.com/retrieve/pii/S0045793014003612.

Kim, H.-S., et al., 2007a. Optimization of electrohydrodynamic writing technique to print collagen. Exp. Tech. 31 (4), 15–19. Available at: http://doi.wiley.com/10.1111/j.1747-1567.2007.00154.x.

Kim, J., Wang, N., Chen, Y., 2007b. Effect of chitosan and ions on actuation behavior of cellulose–chitosan laminated films as electro-active paper actuators. Cellulose 14 (5), 439–445. Available at: http://link.springer.com/10.1007/s10570-007-9134-z.

Kim, B., et al., 2008. Fabrication of cell-encapsulated alginate microfiber scaffold using microfluidic channel. J. Manuf. Sci. Eng. 130 (2), 021016. Available at: http://manufacturingscience.asmedigitalcollection.asme.org/article.aspx?articleid=1452031.

Kim, Y., Kim, K., Park, Y., 2012a. Measurement techniques for red blood cell deformability: recent advances. In: Blood Cell—An Overview of Studies in Hematology. InTech, Croatia. Available at: http://www.intechopen.com/books/blood-cell-an-overview-of-studies-in-hematology/measurement-techniques-for-red-blood-cell-deformability-recent-advances.

Kim, Y.W., et al., 2012b. An ALD aluminum oxide passivated surface acoustic wave sensor for early biofilm detection. Sens. Actuators B 163 (1), 136–145. Available at: http://linkinghub.elsevier.com/retrieve/pii/S0925400512000445.

Kim, Y.W., et al., 2016. A surface acoustic wave biofilm sensor integrated with a treatment method based on the bioelectric effect. Sens. Actuators A 238, 140–149. Available at: http://linkinghub.elsevier.com/retrieve/pii/S0924424715302491.

Koev, S.T., et al., 2007. Mechano-transduction of DNA hybridization and dopamine oxidation through electrodeposited chitosan network. Lab Chip 7 (1), 103–111. Available at: http://xlink.rsc.org/?DOI=B609149K.

Koev, S.T., et al., 2010. Chitosan: an integrative biomaterial for lab-on-a-chip devices. Lab Chip 10 (22), 3026–3042.

Kopp, M.U., Crabtree, H.J., Manz, A., 1997. Developments in technology and applications of microsystems. Curr. Opin. Chem. Biol. 1, 410–419.

Kovac, J.R., Voldman, J., 2007. Intuitive, image-based cell sorting using optofluidic cell sorting. Anal. Chem. 79 (24), 9321–9330.

Kovacs, G.T.A., Maluf, N.I., Petersen, K.E., 1998. Bulk micromachining of silicon. Proc. IEEE 86 (8), 1536–1551.

Kovarik, M.L., Jacobson, S.C., 2009. Nanofluidics in lab-on-a-chip devices. Anal. Chem. 81 (17), 7133–7140. Available at: http://pubs.acs.org/doi/abs/10.1021/ac900614k.

Krishnamoorthy, S., Iliadis, A.A., 2008. Properties of high sensitivity ZnO surface acoustic wave sensors on SiO_2/(100) Si substrates. Solid State Electron. 52 (11), 1710–1716. Available at: http://linkinghub.elsevier.com/retrieve/pii/S0038110108002293.

Lafleur, J.P., et al., 2016. Recent advances in lab-on-a-chip for biosensing applications. Biosens. Bioelectron. 76, 213–233. Available at: http://linkinghub.elsevier.com/retrieve/pii/S0956566315303298.

Laforge, F.O., et al., 2007. Electrochemical attosyringe. Proc. Natl. Acad. Sci. U. S. A. 104 (29), 11895–11900.

Länge, K., Rapp, B.E., Rapp, M., 2008. Surface acoustic wave biosensors: a review. Anal. Bioanal. Chem. 391 (5), 1509–1519. Available at: http://link.springer.com/10.1007/s00216-008-1911-5.

Lauks, I.R., 1998. Microfabricated biosensors and microanalytical systems for blood analysis. Acc. Chem. Res. 31 (5), 317–324. Available at: http://pubs.acs.org/doi/abs/10.1021/ar9700670.

Le Gac, S., van den Berg, A., 2010. Single cells as experimentation units in lab-on-a-chip devices. Trends Biotechnol. 28 (2), 55–62.

Lederer, T., et al., 2011. Utilizing a high fundamental frequency quartz crystal resonator as a biosensor in a digital microfluidic platform. Sens. Actuators A 172 (1), 161–168. Available at: http://linkinghub.elsevier.com/retrieve/pii/S0924424711002792.

Lee, V.G.B., 2005. Automatic Bio-MEMS platforms for fast disease diagnosis. In: 2005 IEEE International Conference on Robotics and Biomimetics—ROBIO. IEEE, pp. 34. Available at: http://ieeexplore.ieee.org/lpdocs/epic03/wrapper.htm?arnumber=1708580.

Lee, S.J., Lee, S.Y., 2004. Micro total analysis system (u-TAS) in biotechnology. Appl. Microbiol. Biotechnol. 64 (3), 289–299.

Lee, J., et al., 2008a. Real-time detection of airborne viruses on a mass-sensitive device. Appl. Phys. Lett. 93 (1), 013901. Available at: http://scitation.aip.org/content/aip/journal/apl/93/1/10.1063/1.2956679.

Lee, S.H., et al., 2008b. A polymer lab-on-a-chip for reverse transcription (RT)-PCR based point-of-care clinical diagnostics. Lab Chip 8 (12), 2121. Available at: http://xlink.rsc.org/?DOI=b811131f.

Lee, H.J., et al., 2009a. Surface acoustic wave immunosensor for real-time detection of hepatitis B surface antibodies in whole blood samples. Biosens. Bioelectron. 24 (10), 3120–3125. Available at: http://linkinghub.elsevier.com/retrieve/pii/S0956566309002103.

Lee, S.S., et al., 2009b. Extensional flow-based assessment of red blood cell deformability using hyperbolic converging microchannel. Biomed. Microdevices 11, 1021–1027.

Lee, C.Y., et al., 2011. Microfluidic mixing: a review. Int. J. Mol. Sci. 12 (5), 3263–3287.

Lee, J., et al., 2013. Sensitive and reproducible detection of cardiac troponin I in human plasma using a surface acoustic wave immunosensor. Sens. Actuators B 178, 19–25. Available at: http://linkinghub.elsevier.com/retrieve/pii/S0925400512012786.

Lee, G.-H., et al., 2016. Separation and sorting of cells in microsystems using physical principles. J. Micromech. Microeng. 26 (1), 013003. Available at: http://stacks.iop.org/0960-1317/26/i=1/a=013003?key=crossref.a3866242b5106e1e441a876a9a5c03ec.

Levinson, H.J., 2011. Principles of Lithography, third ed. SPIE Press, Washington.
Lewandowski, A.T., et al., 2008. Protein assembly onto patterned microfabricated devices through enzymatic activation of fusion pro-tag. Biotechnol. Bioeng. 99 (3), 499–507. Available at: http://doi.wiley.com/10.1002/bit.21580.
Li, P., et al., 2015. Acoustic separation of circulating tumor cells. Proc. Natl. Acad. Sci. 112 (16), 4970–4975. Available at: http://www.pnas.org/lookup/doi/10.1073/pnas.1504484112.
Liao, C.S., et al., 2005. Miniature RT-PCR system for diagnosis of RNA-based viruses. Nucleic Acids Res. 33 (18), 1–7.
Lidke, D.S., et al., 2004. Quantum dot ligands provide new insights into erbB/HER receptor-mediated signal transduction. Nat. Biotechnol. 22 (2), 198–203.
Lifson, M.A., Carter, J.A., Miller, B.L., 2015. A novel antibody immobilization strategy for optical biosensors. In: Miller, B.L., Fauchet, P.M., Cunningham, B.T. (Eds.), Proc. SPIE 9310, Frontiers in Biological Detection: From Nanosensors to Systems VII, 931007, Available at: http://dx.doi.org/10.1117/12.2083877.
Lim, Y.C., et al., 2015. A protocol for improving fabrication yield of thin SU-8 microcantilevers for use in an aptasensor. Microsyst. Technol. 21 (2), 371–380, Available at: http://link.springer.com/article/10.1007/s00542-013-2019-1.
Lima, R., et al., 2008. In vitro blood flow in a rectangular PDMS microchannel: experimental observations using a confocal micro-PIV system. Biomed. Microdevices 10 (2), 153–167.
Lima, R., et al., 2012. Blood flow behavior in microchannels: past, current and future trends. In Single and Two-Phase Flows on Chemical and Biomedical Engineering. Bentham Science, Dubai, UAE, pp. 513–547.
Lin, C.-H., et al., 2002. A new fabrication process for ultra-thick microfluidic microstructures utilizing SU-8 photoresist. J. Micromech. Microeng. 12, 590–597.
Lin, D., et al., 2015. A regenerating ultrasensitive electrochemical impedance immunosensor for the detection of adenovirus. Biosens. Bioelectron. 68, 129–134. Available at: http://linkinghub.elsevier.com/retrieve/pii/S0956566314009749.
Linder, C., et al., 1992. Surface micromachining. J. Micromech. Microeng. 2 (3), 122–132. Available at: http://iopscience.iop.org/0960-1317/2/3/003.
Liou, A.C., Chen, R.H., 2006. Injection molding of polymer micro- and sub-micron structures with high-aspect ratios. Int. J. Adv. Manuf. Technol. 28 (11–12), 1097–1103. Available at: http://link.springer.com/10.1007/s00170-004-2455-2.
Manz, A., Graber, N., Widmer, H.M., 1990. Miniaturized total chemical analysis systems: a novel concept for chemical sensing. Sens. Actuators B 1, 244–248.
McDonald, J.C., Whitesides, G.M., 2002. Poly(dimethylsiloxane) as a material for fabricating microfluidic devices. Acc. Chem. Res. 35 (July), 491–499.
Mehta, A., et al., 2006. A micromachined electrochemical sensor for free chlorine monitoring in drinking water. Water Sci. Technol. 53, 403–410.
Mijatovic, D., Eijkel, J.C.T., van den Berg, A., 2005. Technologies for nanofluidic systems: top-down vs. bottom-up—a review. Lab Chip 5 (5), 492–500. Available at: http://www.ncbi.nlm.nih.gov/pubmed/15856084.
Minas, G., Wolffenbuttel, R.F., Correia, J.H., 2005. A lab-on-a-chip for spectrophotometric analysis of biological fluids. Lab Chip 5 (11), 1303–1309. Available at: http://www.ncbi.nlm.nih.gov/pubmed/16234956 (accessed 24.02.14.).
Minas, G., Wolffenbuttel, R.F., Correia, J.H., 2010. MCM-based microlaboratory for simultaneous measurement of several biochemical parameters by spectrophotometry. Biomed. Microdevices 12 (4), 727–736. Available at: http://link.springer.com/10.1007/s10544-010-9426-1.

Mir, M., Homs, A., Samitier, J., 2009. Integrated electrochemical DNA biosensors for lab-on-a-chip devices. Electrophoresis 30 (19), 3386–3397. Available at: http://doi.wiley.com/10.1002/elps.200900319.

Mokken, F.C., et al., 1992. The clinical importance of erythrocyte deformability, a hemorrheological parameter. Ann. Hematol. 64 (3), 113–122.

Myers, F.B., Lee, L.P., 2008. Innovations in optical microfluidic technologies for point-of-care diagnostics. Lab Chip 8 (12), 2015–2031.

Narasimhan, J., Papautsky, I., 2003. Polymer embossing tools for rapid prototyping of plastic microfluidic devices. J. Micromech. Microeng. 14 (1), 96–103.

Nestorova, G.G., et al., 2016. Lab-on-a-chip thermoelectric DNA biosensor for label-free detection of nucleic acid sequences. Sens. Actuators B 225, 174–180. Available at: http://linkinghub.elsevier.com/retrieve/pii/S0925400515306146.

Nguyen, N., Truong, T., 2003. A fully polymeric micropump with piezoelectric actuator. Sens. Actuators B 97, 137–143.

Nguyen, N., White, R., 1999. Design and optimization of an ultrasonic flexural plate wave micropump using numerical simulation. Sens. Actuators 77, 229–236 .

Nirschl, M., et al., 2009. Film bulk acoustic resonators for DNA and protein detection and investigation of in vitro bacterial S-layer formation. Sens. Actuators A 156 (1), 180–184. Available at: http://linkinghub.elsevier.com/retrieve/pii/S0924424709000570.

Novak, R., et al., 2015. Microfluidic platform for multiplexed cell sampling and time-resolved SPR-based cytokine sensing. In: 6th European Conference of the International Federation for Medical and Biological Engineering, pp. 785–788. Available at: http://link.springer.com/10.1007/978-3-319-11128-5_195.

Nyborg, W.L., 1953. Acoustic streaming due to attenuated plane waves. J. Acoust. Soc. Am. 25 (1), 68. Available at: http://link.aip.org/link/JASMAN/v25/i1/p68/s1&Agg=doi (accessed 01.03.14.).

Nyborg, W.L., 1958. Acoustic streaming near a boundary. J. Acoust. Soc. Am. 30 (4), 329. Available at: http://link.aip.org/link/JASMAN/v30/i4/p329/s1&Agg=doi (accessed 01.03.14.).

Oedit, A., et al., 2015. Lab-on-a-chip hyphenation with mass spectrometry: strategies for bioanalytical applications. Curr. Opin. Biotechnol. 31, 79–85. Available at: http://linkinghub.elsevier.com/retrieve/pii/S0958166914001517.

Ogura, E., Abatti, P.J., Moriizumi, T., 1991. Measurement of human red blood cell deformability using a single micropore on a thin Si_3N_4 film. IEEE Trans. Biomed. Eng. 38 (8), 721–726. Available at: http://ieeexplore.ieee.org/lpdocs/epic03/wrapper.htm?arnumber=83583.

Olofsson, J., et al., 2009. Direct access and control of the intracellular solution environment in single cells. Anal. Chem. 81 (5), 1810–1818.

Ortiz, P., et al., 2008. A hybrid microfluidic system for cancer diagnosis based on MEMS biosensors. In: 2008 IEEE Biomedical Circuits and Systems Conference, pp. 337–340. Available at: http://ieeexplore.ieee.org/lpdocs/epic03/wrapper.htm?arnumber=4696943.

Ozkan, M., et al., 2003. Electro-optical platform for the manipulation of live cells. Langmuir 19 (5), 1532–1538 Available at: papers://76717a26-9e5d-4e3a-a6a9-df9fa5fe3ffe/Paper/p5479.

Pamme, N., Manz, A., 2004. On-chip free-flow magnetophoresis: continuous flow separation of magnetic particles and agglomerates. Anal. Chem. 76 (24), 7250–7256.

Park, J.J., et al., 2006. Chitosan-mediated in situ biomolecule assembly in completely packaged microfluidic devices. Lab Chip 6 (10), 1315. Available at: http://xlink.rsc.org/?DOI=b603101c.

Park, I., et al., 2007. Low temperature, low pressure nanoimprinting of chitosan as a biomaterial for bionanotechnology applications. Appl. Phys. Lett. 90 (9), 093902. Available at: http://scitation.aip.org/content/aip/journal/apl/90/9/10.1063/1.2709914.

Patel, J.N., et al., 2008. PDMS as a sacrificial substrate for SU-8-based biomedical and microfluidic applications. J. Micromech. Microeng. 18, 095028.
Piggee, C., 2009. Optical tweezers: not just for physicists anymore. Anal. Chem. 81, 16–19.
Pinho, D., Yaginuma, T., Lima, R., 2013. A microfluidic device for partial cell separation and deformability assessment. BioChip J. 7 (4), 367–374.
Pinho, D., et al., 2015. Red blood cells radial dispersion in blood flowing through microchannels: the role of temperature. J. Biomech. Available at: http://linkinghub.elsevier.com/retrieve/pii/S002192901500679X.
Pinto, E., et al., 2014a. A rapid and low-cost nonlithographic method to fabricate biomedical microdevices for blood flow analysis. Micromachines 6 (1), 121–135. Available at: http://www.mdpi.com/2072-666X/6/1/121/.
Pinto, V., et al., 2014b. Optimized SU-8 processing for low-cost microstructures fabrication without cleanroom facilities. Micromachines 5, 738–755. Available at: http://www.mdpi.com/2072-666X/5/3/738/.
Pinto, V.C., Minas, G., Correia-Neves, M., 2015. PDMS biofunctionalization study for the development of a microfluidic device: application to salivary cortisol. In: 2015 IEEE 4th Portuguese Meeting on Bioengineering (ENBENG). IEEE, pp. 1–5. Available at: http://ieeexplore.ieee.org/lpdocs/epic03/wrapper.htm?arnumber=7088852.
Postier, B., et al., 2008. Benefits of in-situ synthesized microarrays for analysis of gene expression in understudied microorganisms. J. Microbiol. Methods 74, 26–32.
Pushkarsky, I., et al., 2014. Research highlights: microfluidics and magnets. Lab Chip 14 (16), 2882–2886. Available at: http://xlink.rsc.org/?DOI=C4LC90060J.
Qin, D., Xia, Y., Whitesides, G.M., 2010. Soft lithography for micro- and nanoscale patterning. Nat. Protoc. 5 (3), 491–502. Available at: http://www.ncbi.nlm.nih.gov/pubmed/20203666 (accessed 09.07.14.).
Qiu, X., et al., 2011. The effects of temperature, relative humidity and reducing gases on the ultraviolet response of ZnO based film bulk acoustic-wave resonator. Sens. Actuators B 151 (2), 360–364. Available at: http://linkinghub.elsevier.com/retrieve/pii/S0925400510006544.
Quinto-Su, P.A., et al., 2008. Examination of laser microbeam cell lysis in a PDMS microfluidic channel using time-resolved imaging. Lab Chip 8 (3), 408–414. Available at: http://www.pubmedcentral.nih.gov/articlerender.fcgi?artid=2525503&tool=pmcentrez&rendertype=abstract.
Rackus, D.G., Shamsi, M.H., Wheeler, A.R., 2015. Electrochemistry, biosensors and microfluidics: a convergence of fields. Chem. Soc. Rev. 44 (15), 5320–5340. Available at: http://xlink.rsc.org/?DOI=C4CS00369A.
Rammohan, A., et al., 2011. One-step maskless grayscale lithography for the fabrication of 3-dimensional structures in SU-8. Sens. Actuators B 153, 125–134.
Rasooly, A., Kostov, Y., Bruck, H.A., 2013. Charged-coupled device (CCD) detectors for lab-on-a chip (LOC) optical analysis. In: Microfluidic Diagnostics: Methods and Protocols. Humana Press, New York, pp. 365–385. Available at: http://link.springer.com/10.1007/978-1-62703-134-9_23.
Raub, C.B., Lee, C., Kartalov, E., 2015. Sequestration of bacteria from whole blood by optimized microfluidic cross-flow filtration for rapid antimicrobial susceptibility testing. Sens. Actuators B 210, 120–123. Available at: http://linkinghub.elsevier.com/retrieve/pii/S0925400514012726.
Revzin, A., et al., 2001. Fabrication of poly(ethylene glycol) hydrogel microstructures using photolithography. Langmuir 17 (18), 5440–5447. Available at: http://pubs.acs.org/doi/abs/10.1021/la010075w.
Ribeiro, J.C., et al., 2005. A SU-8 fluidic microsystem for biological fluids analysis. Sens. Actuators A 123–124, 77–81.

Rife, J.C., et al., 2000. Miniature valveless ultrasonic pumps and mixers. Sens. Actuators A 86 (1–2), 135–140. Available at: http://linkinghub.elsevier.com/retrieve/pii/S0924424700004337 (accessed 17.03.14.).
Riley, N., 1998. Acoustic streaming. Theor. Comput. Fluid Dyn. 10 (1–4), 349–356. Available at: http://link.springer.com/10.1007/s001620050068 (accessed 24.02.14.).
Rodrigues, R.O., et al., 2015. A simple microfluidic device for the deformability assessment of blood cells in a continuous flow. Biomed. Microdevices 17 (6), 108. Available at: http://link.springer.com/10.1007/s10544-015-0014-2.
Rodríguez-Ruiz, I., et al., 2015. A multiple path photonic lab on a chip for parallel protein concentration measurements. Lab Chip 15 (4), 1133–1139. Available at: http://xlink.rsc.org/?DOI=C4LC01332H.
Roselli, R.J., Diller, K.R., 2011. Biotransport: Principles and Applications. Springer, New York, NY. Available at: https://books.google.com/books?id=l40-3Zgp0JUC&pgis=1 (accessed 11.12.15.).
Rosenbluth, M.J., Lam, W.A., Fletcher, D.A., 2008. Analyzing cell mechanics in hematologic diseases with microfluidic biophysical flow cytometry. Lab Chip 8 (7), 1062–1070.
Ruan, Y., et al., 2007. Methods to protect silicon microstructures from the damages in deep reactive ion etching. In: 2007 International Workshop on Electron Devices and Semiconductor Technology (EDST). IEEE, pp. 101–105. Available at: http://ieeexplore.ieee.org/ielx5/4289754/4289755/04289788.pdf?tp=&arnumber=4289788&isnumber=4289755.
Ruffien-Ciszak, A., et al., 2008. Electrochemical microsensors for cutaneous surface analysis: application to the determination of pH and the antioxidant properties of stratum corneum. ITBM-RBM 29, 162–170.
Sackmann, E.K., Fulton, A.L., Beebe, D.J., 2014. The present and future role of microfluidics in biomedical research. Nature 507, 181–189.
Sakudo, A., et al., 2015. Integration of antibody by surface functionalization of graphite-encapsulated magnetic beads using ammonia gas plasma technology for capturing influenza A virus. Bioorg. Med. Chem. Lett. 25 (9), 1876–1879. Available at: http://linkinghub.elsevier.com/retrieve/pii/S0960894X15002425.
Saliba, A.-E., et al., 2010. Microfluidic sorting and multimodal typing of cancer cells in self-assembled magnetic arrays. Proc. Natl. Acad. Sci. U. S. A. 107 (33), 14524–14529.
Sato, K., Mawatari, K., Kitamori, T., 2008. Microchip-based cell analysis and clinical diagnosis system. Lab Chip 8 (12), 1992–1998. Available at: http://www.ncbi.nlm.nih.gov/pubmed/19023462.
Schena, M., et al., 1995. Quantitative monitoring of gene expression patterns with a complementary DNA microarray. Science 270, 467–470.
Schift, H., et al., 2000. Nanoreplication in polymers using hot embossing and injection molding. Microelectron. Eng. 53, 171–174.
Sencadas, V., Gregorio Filho, R., Lanceros-Mendez, S., 2006. Processing and characterization of a novel nonporous poly(vinilidene fluoride) films in the β phase. J. Non-Cryst. Solids 352 (21–22), 2226–2229. Available at: http://linkinghub.elsevier.com/retrieve/pii/S0022309306003899 (accessed 24.02.14.).
Shim, M., et al., 2002. Functionalization of carbon nanotubes for biocompatibility and biomolecular recognition. Nano Lett. 2 (4), 285–288. Available at: http://pubs.acs.org/doi/abs/10.1021/nl015692j.
Shin, S., et al., 2005. Slit-flow ektacytometry: laser diffraction in a slit rheometer. Cytometry B Clin. Cytom. 65 (1), 6–13. Available at: http://www.ncbi.nlm.nih.gov/pubmed/15786510.
Skelley, A.M., et al., 2009. Microfluidic control of cell pairing and fusion. Nat. Methods 6 (2), 147–152.

So, P., Dong, C., 2001. Fluorescence Spectrophotometry. Encyclopedia of Life Sciences. John Wiley & Sons Ltd, Chichester. Available at: http://onlinelibrary.wiley.com/doi/10.1038/npg.els.0002978/abstract?userIsAuthenticated=false&deniedAccessCustomisedMessage=.

Song, Y., et al., 2012. DC dielectrophoresis separation of marine algae and particles in a microfluidic chip. Sci. China: Chem. 55 (4), 524–530. Available at: http://link.springer.com/10.1007/s11426-012-4533-x.

Spinks, G., et al., 2007. A novel "dual mode" actuation in chitosan/polyaniline/carbon nanotube fibers. Sens. Actuators B 121 (2), 616–621. Available at: http://linkinghub.elsevier.com/retrieve/pii/S0925400506003662.

Squires, T., Quake, S., 2005. Microfluidics: fluid physics at the nanoliter scale. Rev. Mod. Phys. 77 (3), 977–1026. Available at: http://link.aps.org/doi/10.1103/RevModPhys.77.977 (accessed 21.02.14.).

Srinivasan, V., Pamula, V.K., Fair, R.B., 2004. An integrated digital microfluidic lab-on-a-chip for clinical diagnostics on human physiological fluids. Lab Chip 4 (4), 310–315. Available at: http://www.ncbi.nlm.nih.gov/pubmed/15269796.

Suh, Y.K., Kang, S., 2010. A review on mixing in microfluidics. Micromachines 1 (3), 82–111.

Sun, C., et al., 2005a. Projection micro-stereolithography using digital micro-mirror dynamic mask. Sens. Actuators A 121 (1), 113–120.

Sun, Y., et al., 2005b. A self-contained microfluidic cell sorting system for HIV diagnosis. In: The 13th International Conference on Solid-State Sensors, Actuators and Microsystems, 2005. Digest of Technical Papers. TRANSDUCERS'05. IEEE, pp. 1708–1711. Available at: http://ieeexplore.ieee.org/lpdocs/epic03/wrapper.htm?arnumber=1497420.

Suresha, K.M., et al., 2008. Actuator, sensor and MEMS devices based on regenerated cellulose. Compos. Interfaces 15 (7–9), 679–685. Available at: http://www.tandfonline.com/doi/abs/10.1163/156855408786778393.

Takayama, S., et al., 2001. Subcellular positioning of small molecules. Nature 411 (6841), 1016.

Tamaki, E., et al., 2002. Single-cell analysis by a scanning thermal lens microscope with a microchip: direct monitoring of cytochrome *c* distribution during apoptosis process. Anal. Chem. 74 (7), 1560–1564. Available at: http://pubs.acs.org/doi/abs/10.1021/ac011092t.

Tas, N.R., et al., 2002. Nanofluidic bubble pump using surface tension directed gas injection. Anal. Chem. 74 (9), 2224–2227.

Taylor, A.D., et al., 2006. Quantitative and simultaneous detection of four foodborne bacterial pathogens with a multi-channel SPR sensor. Biosens. Bioelectron. 22 (5), 752–758. Available at: http://linkinghub.elsevier.com/retrieve/pii/S095656630600090X.

Terry, S.C., Jerman, J.H., Angell, J.B., 1979. A gas chromatographic air analyzer fabricated on a silicon wafer. IEEE Trans. Electron Dev. 26, 1880–1886.

Théry, M., Bornens, M., 2006. Cell shape and cell division. Curr. Opin. Cell Biol. 18 (6), 648–657.

Tng, D.J.H., et al., 2015. Standalone lab-on-a-chip systems toward the evaluation of therapeutic biomaterials in individualized disease treatment. ACS Biomater. Sci. Eng. 1 (11), 1055–1066. Available at: http://pubs.acs.org/doi/10.1021/acsbiomaterials.5b00369.

Tokarskyy, O., Marshall, D.L., 2008. Immunosensors for rapid detection of *Escherichia coli* O157:H7—perspectives for use in the meat processing industry. Food Microbiol. 25 (1), 1–12. Available at: http://linkinghub.elsevier.com/retrieve/pii/S0740002007000895.

Tong, H.D., et al., 2009. Novel top-down wafer-scale fabrication of single crystal silicon nanowires. Nano Lett. 9 (3), 1015–1022.

Tsekenis, G., et al., 2008. Label-less immunosensor assay for myelin basic protein based upon an AC impedance protocol. Anal. Chem. 80 (6), 2058–2062. Available at: http://pubs.acs.org/doi/abs/10.1021/ac702070e.

Tsukagoshi, K., Jinno, N., Nakajima, R., 2005. Development of a micro total analysis system incorporating chemiluminescence detection and application to detection of cancer markers. Anal. Chem. 77 (6), 1684–1688. Available at: http://www.ncbi.nlm.nih.gov/pubmed/15762572.

Upstone, S.L., 2000. In: Meyers, R.A. (Ed.), Ultraviolet/Visible Light Absorption Spectrophotometry in Clinical Chemistry. Encyclopedia of Analytical Chemistry. John Wiley & Sons Ltd, Chichester, pp. 1699–1714.

Urban, G.A., 2009. Micro- and nanobiosensors—state of the art and trends. Meas. Sci. Technol. 20 (1), 012001. Available at: http://stacks.iop.org/0957-0233/20/i=1/a=012001?key=crossref.74ada4421967e337230127f877c98fdb (accessed 22.01.14.).

Wacogne, B., et al., 2008. Measuring the mechanical behaviour of human oocytes with a very simple SU-8 micro-tool. Biomed. Microdevices 10 (3), 411–419.

Wang, J., 2008. Electrochemical glucose biosensors. Chem. Rev. 108 (2), 814–825. Available at: http://pubs.acs.org/doi/abs/10.1021/cr068123a.

Wang, Z., Zhe, J., 2011. Recent advances in particle and droplet manipulation for lab-on-a-chip devices based on surface acoustic waves. Lab Chip 11 (7), 1280. Available at: http://xlink.rsc.org/?DOI=c0lc00527d.

Wang, J., et al., 2000. Microfabricated electrophoresis chips for simultaneous bioassays of glucose, uric acid, ascorbic acid, and acetaminophen. Anal. Chem. 72 (11), 2514–2518.

Wang, M., et al., 2010. Single-cell electroporation. Anal. Bioanal. Chem. 397 (8), 3235–3248. Available at: http://www.ncbi.nlm.nih.gov/pubmed/20496058.

Watkins, N.N., et al., 2013. Microfluidic CD4+ and CD8+ T lymphocyte counters for point-of-care HIV diagnostics using whole blood. Sci. Transl. Med. 5 (214), 214ra170. Available at: http://stm.sciencemag.org/cgi/doi/10.1126/scitranslmed.3006870.

Weaver, W., et al., 2014. Research highlights: microfluidic point-of-care diagnostics. Lab Chip 14 (12), 1962. Available at: http://xlink.rsc.org/?DOI=c4lc90033b.

Weigum, S.E., et al., 2007. Cell-based sensor for analysis of EGFR biomarker expression in oral cancer. Lab Chip 7 (8), 995–1003. Available at: http://pubs.rsc.org/en/content/articlehtml/2007/lc/b703918b.

Westin, L., et al., 2000. Anchored multiplex amplification on a microelectronic chip array. Nat. Biotechnol. 18, 199–204.

Whitesides, G.M., 2006. The origins and the future of microfluidics. Nature 442 (7101), 368–373. Available at: http://www.ncbi.nlm.nih.gov/pubmed/16871203 (accessed 21.01.14.).

Whitesides, G.M., et al., 2001. Soft lithography in biology and biochemistry. Annu. Rev. Biomed. Eng. 3, 335–373.

Wilding, P., Shoffner, M.A., Kricka, L.J., 1994. PCR in a silicon microstructure. Clin. Chem. 40 (9), 1815–1818.

Williams, J.D., Wang, W., 2004. Study on the postbaking process and the effects on UV lithography of high aspect ratio SU-8 microstructures. J. Microlith. Microfab. Microsyst. 3 (4), 563.

Wong, I., Ho, C.-M., 2009. Surface molecular property modifications for poly(dimethylsiloxane) (PDMS) based microfluidic devices. Microfluid. Nanofluid. 7 (3), 291–306. Available at: http://link.springer.com/10.1007/s10404-009-0443-4.

Wu, L.-Q., et al., 2003. Spatially selective deposition of a reactive polysaccharide layer onto a patterned template. Langmuir 19 (3), 519–524. Available at: http://pubs.acs.org/doi/abs/10.1021/la026518t.

Xia, Y., Whitesides, G.M., 1998. Soft lithography. Annu. Rev. Mater. Sci. 28 (1), 153–184. Available at: http://www.annualreviews.org/doi/abs/10.1146/annurev.matsci.28.1.153.

Xia, Y., et al., 1997. Replica molding using polymeric materials : a practical step toward nanomanufacturing. Adv. Mater. 9, 147–149.

Xu, Y., Takai, M., Ishihara, K., 2010. Phospholipid polymer biointerfaces for lab-on-a-chip devices. Ann. Biomed. Eng. 38 (6), 1938–1953. Available at: http://link.springer.com/10.1007/s10439-010-0025-3.

Yaginuma, T., et al., 2013. Human red blood cell behavior under homogeneous extensional flow in a hyperbolic-shaped microchannel. Biomicrofluidics 7, 054110.

Yang, L.-J., Ou, Y.-C., 2005. The micro patterning of glutaraldehyde (GA)-crosslinked gelatin and its application to cell-culture. Lab Chip 5 (9), 979. Available at: http://xlink.rsc.org/?DOI=b505193b.

Yaralioglu, G., Wygant, I., Marentis, T., Khuri-Yakub, B., 2004. Ultrasonic mixing in microfluidic channels using integrated transducers. Anal. Chem. 76, 3694–3698.

Yi, H., et al., 2005. Biofabrication with chitosan. Biomacromolecules 6 (6), 2881–2894. Available at: http://pubs.acs.org/doi/abs/10.1021/bm050410l.

Yoon, J.-Y., Kim, B., 2012. Lab-on-a-chip pathogen sensors for food safety. Sensors 12 (12), 10713–10741. Available at: http://www.mdpi.com/1424-8220/12/8/10713/.

Yuan, D., Das, S., 2007. Experimental and theoretical analysis of direct-write laser micromachining of polymethyl methacrylate by CO_2 laser ablation. J. Appl. Phys. 101, 024901. Available at: http://link.aip.org/link/JAPIAU/v101/i2/p024901/s1&Agg=doi.

Zangmeister, R.A., et al., 2006. Electrochemical study of chitosan films deposited from solution at reducing potentials. Electrochim. Acta 51 (25), 5324–5333. Available at: http://linkinghub.elsevier.com/retrieve/pii/S0013468606001253.

Zare, R.N., Kim, S., 2010. Microfluidic platforms for single-cell analysis. Annu. Rev. Biomed. Eng. 12, 187–201.

Zhang, M., et al., 2015a. Monolithic integrated system with an electrowetting-on-dielectric actuator and a film-bulk-acoustic-resonator sensor. J. Micromech. Microeng. 25 (2), 025002. Available at: http://stacks.iop.org/0960-1317/25/i=2/a=025002?key=crossref.98f635e91ff5ad9da80f30b3f46019cb.

Zhang, Y., et al., 2015b. A SPR sensor based on twin-core fiber, In: Proc. SPIE 9634, 24th International Conference on Optical Fibre Sensors, 96347P, Available at: http://dx.doi.org/10.1117/12.2193871.

Zhao, R., et al., 2006. Microscopic investigation of erythrocyte deformation dynamics. Biorheology 43, 747–765.

Zheng, Y., Nguyen, J., Wang, C., et al., 2013a. Electrical measurement of red blood cell deformability on a microfluidic device. Lab Chip (16), 3275. Available at: http://xlink.rsc.org/?DOI=c3lc50427a.

Zheng, Y., Nguyen, J., Wei, Y., et al., 2013b. Recent advances in microfluidic techniques for single-cell biophysical characterization. Lab Chip 13 (13), 2464. Available at: http://xlink.rsc.org/?DOI=c3lc50355k.

Ziaie, B., 2004. Hard and soft micromachining for BioMEMS: review of techniques and examples of applications in microfluidics and drug delivery. Adv. Drug Deliv. Rev. 56 (2), 145–172. Available at: http://linkinghub.elsevier.com/retrieve/pii/S0169409X03001911.

Zou, Y., et al., 2008. Glucose biosensor based on electrodeposition of platinum nanoparticles onto carbon nanotubes and immobilizing enzyme with chitosan–SiO_2 sol–gel. Biosens. Bioelectron. 23 (7), 1010–1016. Available at: http://linkinghub.elsevier.com/retrieve/pii/S0956566307004356.

Electronic tongues and aptasensors

13

L.G. Dias*,†, S. G. Meirinho‡, A.C.A. Veloso‡,§, L.R. Rodrigues‡, A.M. Peres*,#
*Polytechnic Institute of Bragança, ESA, Bragança, Portugal, †University of Trás-os-Montes e Alto Douro, CQ-VR, Vila Real, Portugal, ‡University of Minho, Centre of Biological Engineering, Braga, Portugal, §Instituto Politécnico de Coimbra, ISEC, DEQB, Coimbra, Portugal, #University of Porto, LSRE-LCM, Porto, Portugal

13.1 Introduction

Multidisciplinary research within life and material sciences provide novel insights for designing bioinspired materials and devices for medical applications (Choy et al., 2010; Gentile et al., 2011). Bioinspired technologies artificially mimic the physiology sensing capabilities using several types of sensors coupled with chemometric tools (Gutiérrez et al., 2012). These sensor approaches may be used per se or as an integrated part of a chemical or biomedical sensing element, applied in stationary or flow mode and may be categorized according to their electrochemical principles, as potentiometric, amperometric, or voltammetric sensors (Liu, 2000). Sensor-based devices are alternative techniques to retrieve valuable chemical information from a specific matrix, by using appropriate multivariate statistical qualitative/quantitative data processing-modeling techniques, aiming to overcome drawbacks like the presence of nonidealities, interference effects, collinearity between measured variables and noise issues (Gutiérrez et al., 2012). These analytical electrochemistry-based sensors range from chemical applications to biomedical monitoring, from invasive to noninvasive approaches, from off-line to real-time in situ analysis, from in vitro to in vivo use, from single cell to animal and human measurement including clinical screening, diagnosis, and treatment (Mc Caffrey et al., 2015; Wang et al., 2008; Zhang et al., 2008). However, unlike wearable physical sensors for monitoring vital signs, the availability of noninvasive chemical sensors is still scarce (Bandodkar and Wang, 2014). Among them, the use of chemical sensor arrays, a simple and straightforward electrochemical sensing strategy that includes ion selective electrodes (ISE) and low-selective electrodes, such as in electronic tongues (E-tongues) and the development of more elaborate and complex aptasensors, such as RNA- and DNA-sensor based strategies, will be the focus of this chapter.

Despite the great advances of the (bio)electrochemical technologies, eg, sensor arrays/E-tongue and aptasensor devices that are recognized as promising tools for medical and pharmaceutical applications, there are still relevant challenges in the design and applications of electrochemical sensors in order to meet the demands of modern health care. Indeed, there is an urgent need to take advantage of the unique capabilities of these sensors, such as low-cost, miniaturization, portability, short response times,

Bioinspired Materials for Medical Applications. http://dx.doi.org/10.1016/B978-0-08-100741-9.00013-9

minimum, or no sample pretreatment, and wide applicability, already demonstrated at research level, in real-world applications. This chapter will review the state-of-the-art and recent developments of electrochemical sensor approaches, as well as some novel trends on this exciting on-going research field.

13.2 Electrochemical devices: Chemical sensors and aptasensors

13.2.1 General principles and apparatus

Multisensor chemical arrays and aptasensors are generally electrochemical-based sensor devices (eg, potentiometry, amperometry, voltammetry, and impedance spectroscopy).

13.2.1.1 Potentiometry

In potentiometry the potential signal is measured at zero current intensity (Scholz, 2010). The typical potentiometric analytical cell has two electrodes immersed in a solution containing the analyte, whose concentration is to be measured (Fig. 13.1). The reference electrode (RE) has a constant contribution to the signal, independently of the solution matrix. Usually it contains a metal electrode in contact with an insoluble salt of the same metal (second type of electrode) and its potential depends only on the solubility of the salt. The most used RE is the silver/silver chloride (Ag/AgCl). The second electrode is the indicator electrode (IE) that contains a membrane sensitive to the

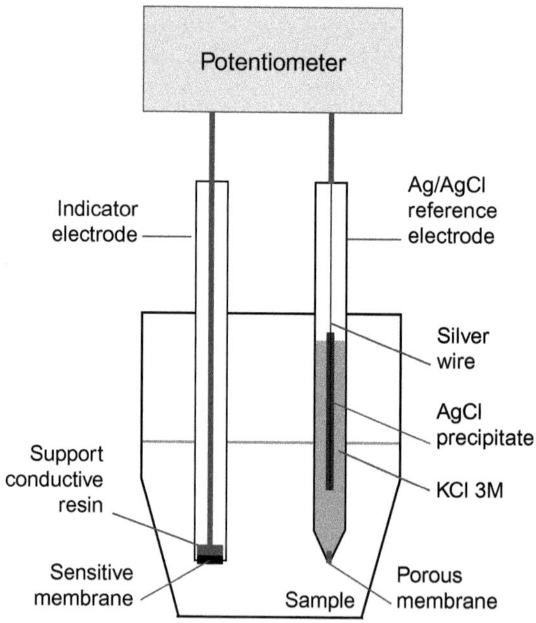

Fig. 13.1 Typical potentiometric analytical system.

compound to be analyzed, thus its potential depends on the compound's concentration. The analyte of the sample solution enters the electrode membrane causing a change in membrane potential due to the modification of the electrochemical properties. A high impedance potentiometer is used to measure the potential between the two electrodes (see Fig. 13.1).

These two electrodes (half-cells) are used separately or are combined into a single body. The most common IEs are sensitive to ion activity and not to ion concentration. The Nernst equation shows that the logarithm of the measured ion activity (a_i) is linearly related with the potential signal (Eq. 13.1), in the ideal case where the electrode only responds to a single analyte (electrodes with high selectivity towards an analyte) (Scholz, 2010):

$$E = E_0 + \frac{2.303 \times R \times T}{z_i \times F} \times \log(a_i) \tag{13.1}$$

where E is the measured potential between the indicator and reference electrode; E_0 is the temperature-dependent standard potential of the electrode; R is the general gas constant; T is the temperature in Kelvin; z is the ionic charge including the sign; and F is the Faraday constant.

Due to the temperature dependence, the potentiometric measurements must be carried out at a constant temperature. If interferences are relevant, an extended expression of the Nernst equation, the Nikolsky–Eisenman equation, should be used (Scholz, 2010):

$$E = E_0 + \frac{2.303 \times R \times T}{z_i \times F} \times \log\left(a_i + \sum_j K_{ij} \times (a_j)^{\frac{z_i}{z_j}} \right) \tag{13.2}$$

where K_{ij} is the selectivity coefficient of the indicator electrode for the interfering ion j, a factor giving the influence of the interfering ion in relationship to the analyte; z_i and z_j are the ion charge of the primary and interfering ions, respectively.

This equation predicts the linear dependency between the sensor response and the logarithm of a function of the ions activity in solution measured in the electrode membrane. The substance activity is directly related with the analytical concentration (C) via the activity coefficient (γ). The γ is a function of the solution's ionic force (I), which represents the total electrolyte content. Therefore in quantitative work, solutions should have approximately the same ionic strength, achieved by using a solution containing a high concentration of an inert salt (total ionic strength adjustment buffer solution, TISAB).

Two types of potentiometric electrodes are usually described, the ISE, which was developed to selectively recognize ions and used to analyze ions (anions or cations) in a solution; and the cross-sensitivity electrodes (CSE), used in sensor arrays for solution analysis, which due to their low selectivity gives, as output, a matrix "fingerprint." E-tongue systems (multisensor systems with several low-selective sensors) are an example of this application.

Different ISE systems have been described in the literature, including (1) glass-membrane, with a framework of silicate glass interstitial sites for H^+ and Na^+, being the pH electrode the best example; (2) crystal-membrane, defined by a crystal lattice containing defined gaps for the ion to be measured, eg, the fluoride electrode that uses a crystal of lanthanum fluoride (LaF_3) doped with europium fluoride (EuF_2) to create lattice gaps; and (3) polymer-membrane—polymeric membrane containing an additive molecule (an ionophore, ie, a high-selective molecule) that binds with high selectivity to the ion to be measured, for instance, the potassium electrode with a membrane of polyvinyl chloride (PVC) impregnated with the macrocyclic antibiotic valinomycin (Mikhelson, 2013; Wang, 2006).

In low-selective electrodes, assembled as sensor arrays, several membranes can be used for potentiometric sensors, namely chalcogenide glasses and lipid polymeric-membranes (Vlasov et al., 2005). These arrays constitute analytical tools whose performance capabilities depend on the selected electrodes but also on the practical purpose. Qualitative, semiquantitative and quantitative analysis are possible by using advanced chemometric techniques.

13.2.1.2 Amperometry and voltammetry

The most common techniques that apply a constant and/or varying potential at an electrode surface, within a three-electrode system, measuring the resulting current intensity in an electrolytic solution are amperometry, cyclic voltammetry (CV), square wave voltammetry (SWV), and differential pulse voltammetry (DPV). These electroanalytical techniques evaluate the redox properties of a single compound or a mixture of compounds. The three-electrode system (Fig. 13.2) comprises an RE, a counter electrode (CE or auxiliary electrode) and a working electrode (WE). The RE contributes with a stable and known potential.

The analyte is measured (quantification or evaluation of the redox properties) in the WE surface, where the potential varies linearly with time in relation to the constant contribution of the RE. The charge is transferred to and from the analyte at the WE surface, resulting in a current flow to or from the cell, through the auxiliary electrode. The measurements must occur in an electrolytic solution to provide ions to the electrodes during oxidation and reduction. The equipment, a so-called potentiostat, is a device that simultaneously produces an accurate potential and measures the current involved in the system comprised of the WE surface plus the analyte. The WEs are electrodes of metals or metals with its surface chemically modified, allowing high sensitive electrochemical determination of organic molecules, as well as ions (Scholz, 2010; Thomas and Henze, 2001; Zoski, 2007). When a dropping mercury electrode or a static mercury drop electrode is used as the WE, the analytical technique is usually referred to as polarography (Scholz, 2010; Thomas and Henze, 2001; Zoski, 2007).

Amperometry. In this technique, the current is continuously measured as a function of a constant potential applied to the WE. The current intensity signal from the oxidation or reduction of the substance analyzed is proportional to its concentration.

CV. A cyclic voltammogram is obtained by applying a linear sweep potential (the potential increases or decreases linearly with time) at the WE. When a potential change occurs, the current flows through the WE, oxidizing or reducing the compound under analysis. The intensity of this current is proportional to the concentration of the compound in the solution, thus enabling the use of this technique in analytical

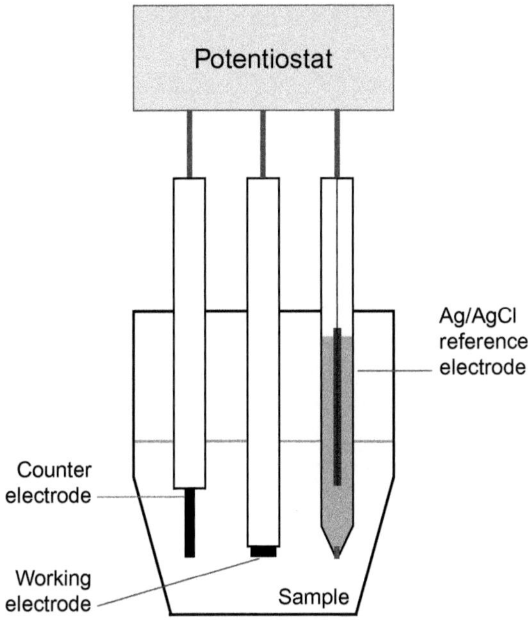

Fig. 13.2 Typical three-electrode voltammetric analytical system.

quantification. Fig. 13.3 shows the information that it is possible to obtain from a cyclic voltammogram during the course of a reversible redox reaction.

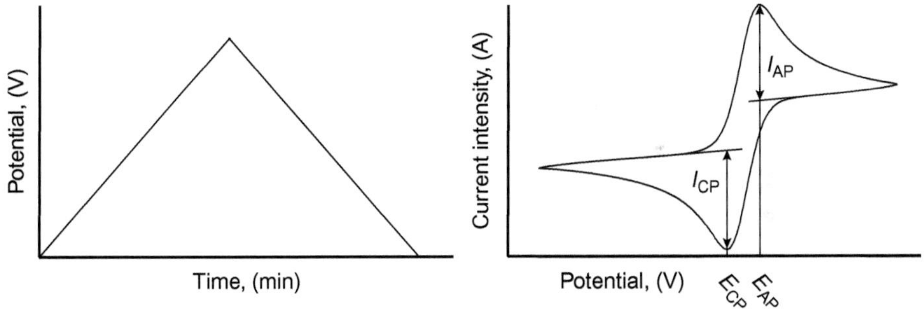

Fig. 13.3 Cyclic potential sweep and typical voltammogram of a reversible reaction using a three-electrode system (I_{AP} and I_{CP}, anode and cathode peak current intensities; E_{AP} and E_{CP}, anode and cathode potentials).

The quantitative information regarding the concentration of electroactive(s) compound(s) can be obtained from the voltammogram using the Randles–Sevcik equation, for the case of a reversible reaction. This equation expresses the relationship between the peak current intensity I_P (either anode or cathode) and the analyte concentration (C) at a given absolute temperature (T, in Kelvin or Rankine) and is given by

$$I_P = kn^{\frac{3}{2}} v^{\frac{1}{2}} D^{\frac{1}{2}} AC \qquad 13.3$$

where k contains all constants at T, n is the number of electrons that are involved in the reaction for the redox pair, v is scan rate, ie, the speed at which the potential is swept (V/s), A is the area of the electrode (cm^2), and D is the diffusion coefficient of the compound to be analyzed (cm^2/s) (Scholz, 2010; Thomas and Henze, 2001; Zoski, 2007).

This method allows the reduction potential of an analyte and its electrochemical reactivity to be assessed, and is considered nondestructive since only a very small amount of the analyte is consumed at the surface of the WE.

DPV. DPV is a pulse technique that is more sensitive towards oxidation or reduction currents (faradaic currents) than conventional voltammetry since it permits discriminating charging (capacitance) current. In this technique, the currents before the end of the pulse (I_1) and just before pulse application (I_2) are measured, using pulses superimposed on a ramp of potential changing linearly with time (applied with amplitudes between 10 and 100 mV, for several milliseconds). The difference between the two currents ($\Delta I = I_2 - I_1$) is plotted against the staircase potential and leads to a voltammogram with a peak-shaped waveform. Fig. 13.4 shows a typical voltammogram of the DPV analysis.

The peak's position (E_p) and the shape on the potential axis are dependent of the type of analyte under study and, on the other hand, its height (I_p, faradaic response current peak) is directly proportional to the concentrations of the electroactive compounds (Scholz, 2010; Thomas and Henze, 2001; Zoski, 2007). DPV allows a faster analysis and lower consumption of electroactive compounds at the electrode surface (lower adsorption).

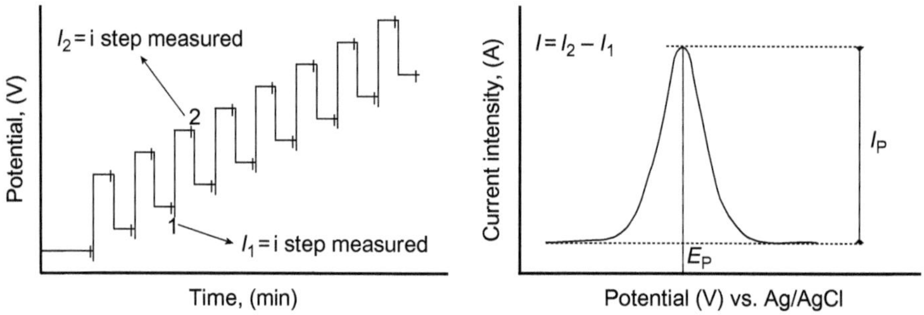

Fig. 13.4 Potential sweep and typical voltammogram of the DPV analysis for a reversible reaction (I_p, maximum peak current intensity; E_p, potential at which I_p was recorded).

SWV. The SWV is also a pulse voltammetry technique and exhibits a greater capacity to discriminate the influence of capacitive current. An SWP analysis is carried out by measuring the current in the WE, while the potential is swept in time over a range of set values by using a voltage ramp with a staircase-shaped between the WE and RE. In the square-wave cycle (potential waveform sweep), the current is measured at the end of the positive direction towards oxidation (forward pulse, I_{fwd}) and negative direction towards reduction (reverse pulse, I_{rev}) generating a peak for each of the processes, which gives information concerning the oxidation or reduction of the electroactive species at the electrode surface.

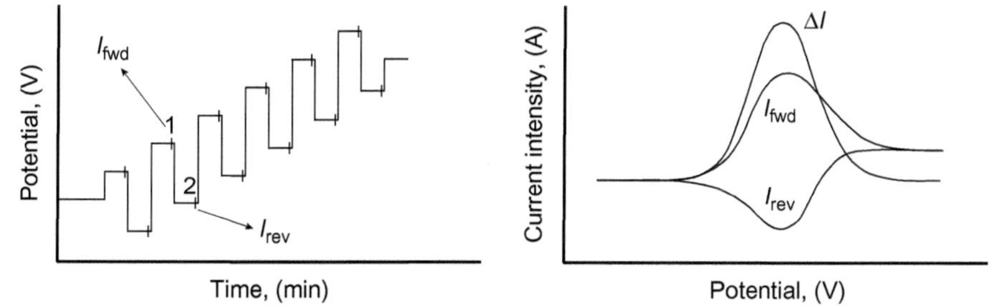

Fig. 13.5 Potential sweep and typical voltammogram of the SWV analysis for a reversible reaction (I_{fwd} and I_{rev}: forward and reverse mode peak current intensities; $\Delta I = I_{fwd} - I_{rev}$).

This double measurement minimizes the capacitive current contribution on the total current reading. The difference between these two currents (response waveform, $\Delta I = I_{fwd} - I_{rev}$) is plotted versus the sweep potential obtaining a peak-shaped voltammogram display (Fig. 13.5), where the peak height in this plot is proportional to the concentrations of the various redox active species (Scholz, 2010; Thomas and Henze, 2001; Zoski, 2007).

Since the SWV technique removes the capacitive current from the measurements, it allows a fast analysis with a wide dynamic range of electroactive species, thus resulting in higher sensitivity compared to CV technique. Moreover, this electrochemical technique does not require the exclusion of oxygen from the solution, except when it interferes with the electrode reaction in the analysis, as it has no time to diffuse to the electrode surface.

13.2.1.3 Electrochemical impedance spectroscopy

The electrochemical impedance spectroscopy (EIS) consists of varying the excitation frequency f of the applied potential E, over a range of frequencies, while the impedance (both resistance and reactance) is measured. The electrical impedance (Z) is defined as the ratio of the change of the voltage-time function $E(t)$ and the resulting change of the current-time function $I(t)$ and can be calculated by

$$Z = \frac{E(t)}{I(t)} = \frac{1}{Y} = \frac{E_0 \sin(2\pi ft)}{I_0 \sin(2\pi ft + \varphi)} \tag{13.4}$$

where E_0 and I_0 are the maximum voltage and current signals, f is the frequency, t is time, φ is the phase shift between the voltage-time and current-time functions, and Y is the complex conductance (Wang et al., 2012).

This technique enables the study of any material property or specific process, such as the resistive characterization, recombination, and corrosion. It is a useful tool in the development and analysis of new materials for biosensors, since it allows monitoring changes at the surfaces of the modified electrodes (Grieshaber et al., 2008; Wang et al., 2012).

13.2.2 E-tongues and sensor-arrays: design, development, and applications

Multisensor systems for liquid analysis based on chemical sensor arrays that attempt to mimic the human chemical senses coupled with pattern recognition methods are widely known as E-tongues (Legin et al., 2002). These devices (Fig. 13.6) allow correlating electrochemical signals with the human's ability to measure and compare taste intensities (Gutiérrez et al., 2012; Ramamoorthy et al., 2014). The human tongue contains sensors, in the form of 2000–10,000 taste buds of 50–100 taste cells each (Roper, 1995), for sweet, acid, bitter, salty and umami. So the task of designing an artificial sensing device is very complicated, since the mechanisms underlying natural or chemical perception are not fully known (Ciosek and Wróblewski, 2007).

The E-tongue uses an array of several nonspecific, low-selective chemical sensors with partial specificity (cross-sensitivity) to different compounds in solution, such as salts, acids, sugars, bitter and astringent compounds, among others (Wardencki et al., 2013). These sensors are mainly developed for the classification of foodstuffs, although the results are not necessarily comparable to those of a trained sensory panel (Ciosek and Wróblewski, 2007). The E-tongue's sensing capability is derived from its ability to detect multiple organic and inorganic compounds, from a signal spectrum-profile recorded, which contains complementary information from each sensor, generating a unique fingerprint of each matrix under evaluation, rather than information about the nature of the studied compounds (Gutiérrez et al., 2012; Ramamoorthy et al., 2014).

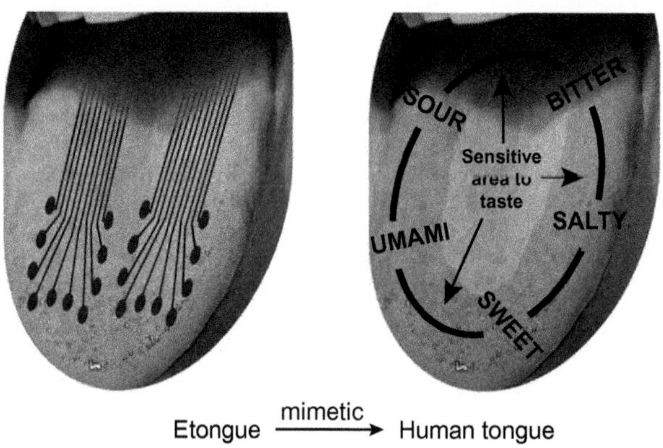

Fig. 13.6 E-tongue: mimicking the human chemical senses aiming to evaluate basic taste intensities.

E-tongue systems (Fig. 13.7) are available in different versions, from desktop to portable devices, static or flow analysis operation modes, consisting of (Baldwin et al., 2011; Wardencki et al., 2013):

- A sensor array including a RE.
- A multichannel electronic interface device (eg, data-logger) that reads the sensor output, converts it to a digital signal and sends it to a computer.
- A computer for data acquisition, storage and processing.

A variety of sensors, from optical to mass spectrometry-based, have been employed in the design of E-tongues, but the electrochemical devices are still the most common (Bagnasco et al., 2014), in particular potentiometric- and voltammetric-based devices.

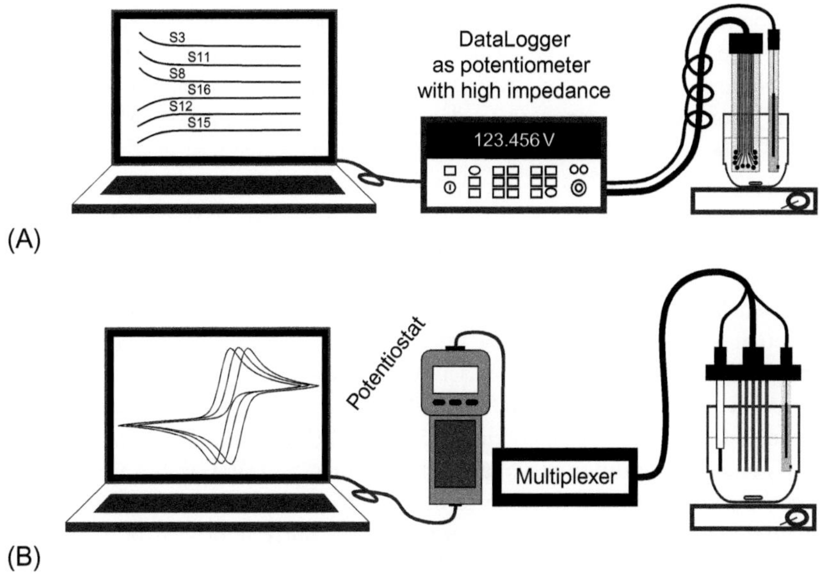

Fig. 13.7 Basic principles of potentiometric (A) and voltammetric (B) sensor arrays analytical systems.

In potentiometric electrochemical devices (Fig. 13.7A), the sensors may be ion selective membranes or polymeric membranes (eg, lipid membranes or others), comprising a mixture of sensor additive chemical compounds, plasticizers and a suitable polymeric matrix, applied using appropriate techniques (eg, drop-by-drop) to a solid support (eg, acrylic body; screen-printed) (Fig. 13.8). The type of sensors and relative

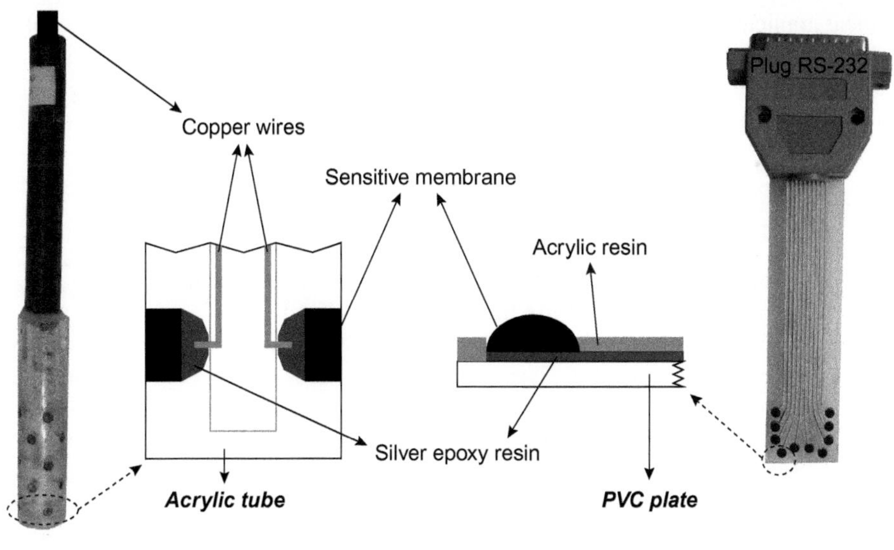

Fig. 13.8 Examples of potentiometric E-tongue devices with different geometries and built with different types of solid supports.

composition included in the E-tongue are established according to their capability to distinguish the different basic tastes and their levels (Baldwin et al., 2011). Also, a RE must be included in the setup (eg, Ag/AgCl). For signal acquisition, a conducting resin (eg, silver epoxy resin) connected to electric wires (eg, copper, silver) may be used (Dias et al., 2008, 2011, 2014).

Voltammetric or even hybrid based E-tongues, which combine sensors from different types to improve the system recognition performance, have also been reported, although with the disadvantage of requiring data processing tools with a high level of complexity (del Valle, 2011). Voltammetric E-tongues (Fig. 13.7B) show high selectivity, sensitivity and low signal-to-noise ratio compared to potentiometric systems (Bagnasco et al., 2014). Usually they are an array of noble metal WEs (eg, gold, palladium, platinum, and silver) and/or electrodes with several coating membranes (eg, polymers and epoxy-graphite). The CE and RE are coupled to the system array and are usually included in screen-printed electrodes (SPE) (Wang et al., 2015), as the signal profile recorded using different voltammetric techniques (eg, CV, SWV). In general, the experimental setup includes one or several WEs, a CE and an RE. In some situations, the potential advantages of merging molecularly imprinted polymers (MIP) with traditional voltammetric E-tongues, leading to novel synergetic hybrid MIP-based E-tongue devices, have also been evaluated (Huynh and Kutner, 2015).

E-tongues have been largely applied in several research fields, as their main applications are still focused on foodstuffs analysis and in particular in beverages evaluation (eg, Apetrei and Apetrei, 2013; de Sá et al., 2016; Phat et al., 2016; Veloso et al., 2016). Nevertheless electrochemical sensor arrays have also been studied for other purposes, such as environmental monitoring (eg, Mimendia et al., 2010; Zadorozhnaya et al., 2015), biomedical research (eg Bandodkar et al., 2013, 2014; Brett et al., 1999; Mc Caffrey et al., 2015; Guinovart et al., 2013; Tahirbegi et al., 2013, 2014) and pharmaceutical applications (eg, Guhmann et al., 2015; Pein et al., 2015; Sidel'nikov et al., 2015; Yoshida et al., 2015). Within the healthcare field, several potentiometric, voltammetric, and/or impedimetric sensor-arrays have been reported, thus highlighting their versatility for medical applications.

13.2.2.1 Potentiometric based-sensor arrays for biomedical and pharmaceutical applications

Potentiometric devices have been used to analyze several biological fluids including blood, urine, and sweat. One of the first references regarding the biomedical applications of such devices dates back to 1999 and describes the use of a chemical sensor array for multicomponent analysis of biological fluids (Legin et al., 1999). The authors developed an ISE system for the simultaneous determination of ions (Ca^{2+}, Mg^{2+}, Na^{+}, HCO_3^{-}, Cl^{-}, H^{+}, and HPO_4^{2-}) in solution modeling human blood plasma. The multisensors array, based on nonspecific original PVC materials, had cross-sensitivity towards cations and anions. The results showed that the electrochemical device coupled with pattern recognition tools (eg, partial least squares (PLS) and artificial neural networks (ANNs)) presented a satisfactory quantification precision

(1–4%) within the typical ion ranges found in human blood plasma. The ANNs simulate the biological neural network. The mathematical model uses "... a large number of parallel connected simple arithmetic units (neurons) that can be defined as nonlinear, parameterized, bounded function, so that the variables this function depends on are called the inputs of the neuron and its value is called the output" (Dreyfus, 2005; Marini et al., 2008).

Di Natale et al. (2000) showed that an E-tongue containing metalloporphyrins as sensitive substances and a mixture of PVC and a plasticizer (dibuthylphtalate) could be used for clinical analysis of urine samples. Linear correlations could be established between the sensors signal profiles and several clinical markers determined routinely (eg, pH, specific weight and blood cell concentration). Phillips et al. (2007) used a flow-through multisensor array, assembled in insulated screen-printed chips that comprised cation-selective polymeric membrane electrodes to successfully evaluate Na^+ concentration in undiluted urine after removing interfering compounds (eg, electrically neutral lipids).

Assessing sodium concentration is of clinical relevance as low urine sodium concentration may indicate dehydration, while a relatively high urine sodium concentration suggests acute renal failure. Lvova and coworkers (2009) proposed an E-tongue composed of chemical sensors to detect urinary system dysfunctions and creatinine levels. The electrochemical system was composed of miniaturized metallic sensors and ISEs with PVC solvent polymeric membranes. The device enabled the correct classification of urine samples from healthy volunteers, according to creatinine levels and to predict the creatinine content of urine.

Also, the E-tongue could be used as a noninvasive and low-cost technique for early monitoring of urinary tumors, since it allowed the distinction between urine samples of healthy patients and patients with malignant and nonmalignant tumor diagnosis of bladder. Recently, Yaroshenko et al. (2015) developed a multisensor system with ISE and CSE as an analytical tool to determine the urine ionic composition of healthy people and patients suffering with urolithiasis. The potentiometric data recorded from diluted urine samples enabled the differentiation of samples from healthy and unhealthy people and the quantitative analysis of the sodium, potassium, ammonium, calcium, magnesium, chloride, sulfate, phosphate, urate, and creatinine.

Gonzalo-Ruiz et al. (2009) developed novel and fast disposable screen-printed sensor devices capable of quantifying chloride in sweat, thus being a suitable tool for the early detection of cystic fibrosis (CF). The method relies on the direct measurement of chloride on the skin by a four-electrode configuration (ie, anode and cathode electrodes for sweat generation; WE and RE for potentiometric measurements).

The device performance was assessed using synthetic and real samples of volunteers and deviations lower than 8% were obtained as compared to values determined using conventional clinical techniques. Schazmann et al. (2010) proposed a novel real-time in situ potentiometric quantitative analysis of sodium in human sweat, using wearable ISEs platform, in-house fabricated with PVC tubing used as barrels, which could be used during exercise. The device showed good intra- and interday repeatability and was used to monitor the sweat of CF patients.

Bandodkar et al. (2013, 2014) built a novel tattoo-based solid-contact ISE for non-invasive monitoring of epidermal pH levels. The proposed device exhibited a rapid and sensitive response to a wide range of pH changes. The device was applied to several areas of the human body (eg, lower back, neck, and wrist) and was successfully used for real-time monitoring of pH levels of human perspiration during exercise. Guinovart et al. (2013) showed the potential use of a novel ion-selective all-solid state potentiometric cell containing ammonium-selective polymeric nonactin-based membrane for monitoring ammonium levels in sweat using a temporary-transfer tattoo platform. The results showed that the new wearable tattoo-sensor could be, in the near future, a promising tool for monitoring sports performance or for detecting metabolic disorders.

Tahirbegi and coworkers (2013, 2014) demonstrated the applicability of an all-solid-state differential potentiometric, miniaturized and mass producible pH and potassium ISE sensor integrated in an array, together with an RE, for detecting ischemia at low pH on stomach tissue. The sensor device was designed for enabling its insertion inside the stomach by means of an endoscopic device. The signals' profiles showed good reproducibility for sensors included in the same or in different arrays. The results indicated that ischemic and reperfusion states could be sensed in vivo and that information on tissue damage could also be assessed by the sensor arrays.

Recently, our research group studied the potential use of an E-tongue, operating in a static mode, comprising 40 lipid polymeric membranes with cross-sensitivity, for the analysis of caffeine, analgesic and antipyretic compounds (paracetamol and aspirin, also known as acetylsalicylic acid) (*unpublished data*). The lipid membranes contained PVC (~32%) mixed with different combinations of six plasticizers (~65%; bis(2-ethylhexyl)phthalate, bis(1-butylpentyl) adipate, tris(2-ethylhexyl)phosphate, dibutyl sebacate, 2-nitrophenyl-octylether, or dioctyl phenylphosphonate) and six sensor/additive compounds (~3%; octadecylamine, bis(2-ethylhexyl)phosphate, oleyl alcohol, methyltrioctylammonium chloride, tridodecylmethylammonium chloride, or oleic acid). The final lipid membranes contained lipids with alkyl chains and phosphoric groups negatively charged, and amine lipids with alkyl chains allowing hydrophobic interactions, besides exhibiting a positive charge. The E-tongue system was formed by two cylindrical sensor arrays (Fig. 13.8) built on acrylic bodies, previously described by Dias et al. (2009). Each array had 20 holes filled with conducting silver-epoxy resin connected to copper electric wires. Membranes were formed by deposition of the membrane solution on the silver conducting surface using a drop-by-drop technique. Linear discriminant analysis (LDA), based on the potentiometric profiles of the individual standard solutions of each compound, was used to assess the capability of the device to correctly classify the samples.

The results showed that the E-tongue could correctly classify all the solutions (sensitivity of 100%) for the original grouped data (Fig. 13.9), and for the leave-one-out cross-validation procedure.

The LDA model had two discriminant functions (explaining 100% of data variability) and included the information of the 12 sensors represented in Fig. 13.9, chosen by a simulated annealing (SA) metaheuristic variable selection algorithm (Bertsimas and Tsitsiklis, 1993; Cadima et al., 2004; Kirkpatrick et al., 1983). In general, the sensitivity

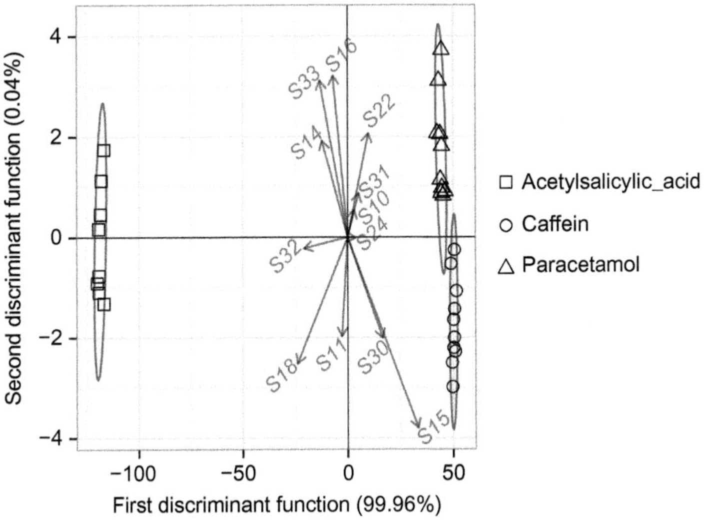

Fig. 13.9 Discrimination of standard solutions containing caffeine, paracetamol, or acetylsalicylic acid using a LDA model based on a subset of E-tongue sensors, selected by the SA variable selection algorithm.

of the lipid polymeric sensors used in the E-tongue decreased in the following order: caffeine > paracetamol > acetylsalicylic acid. The satisfactory qualitative and quantitative results obtained could be tentatively explained considering that

(i) Caffeine can interact with different functional groups present in the plasticizer/sensor additive mixtures that formed the potentiometric multisensor array, namely with the alkane-like regions, amine, and phosphoric groups (Evanics and Prosser, 2005; Shen et al., 2008).
(ii) Acetylsalicylic acid may interact with the quaternary ammonium ions present in the lipid membranes since substituted aromatic carboxylates like salicylates and aspirin are able to interact with lipophilic carriers (He et al., 1992).

Hence, the proposed potentiometric E-tongue seems adequate to quantify caffeine, paracetamol or acetylsalicylic acid in pharmaceutical formulations, although validation of this device using real samples is still required.

Regarding pharmaceutical applications, most reports focus on the use of potentiometric devices as taste-sensing tools for the development of pharmaceutical formulations. E-tongue systems have been used for taste measurement of bitter drug substances towards the development of palatable oral formulations.

Several works published in recent years strengthen the interest in using potentiometric E-tongue in the development of new pharmaceutical formulations. Choi et al. (2014) used an E-tongue to assess the taste masking effect of conventional pharmaceutical sweeteners, including neohesperidin dihydrochalcone, sucrose, sucralose and aspartame. The multichannel taste sensor system, which comprised seven sensors, was used to measure the bitterness degree of typical bitter-tasting model drugs, namely acetaminophen, ibuprofen, tramadol hydrochloride, and sildenafil citrate.

In general, the sensors exhibited a concentration-dependent pattern of the taste-masking-agents showing that the E-tongue could detect small concentration changes of a chemical in solution enabling the evaluation of taste masking using potentiometric data, thus increasing the efficiency of the formulation development process.

Guhmann et al. (2015) described the application of an E-tongue as a taste sensor for the in vitro evaluation of diclofenac taste-masked orodispersible tablet formulations. The potentiometric E-tongue contained an RE and seven lipid membrane sensors for different taste qualities like bitterness (three sensors), sourness, saltiness, umami, and astringency. The results showed that the E-tongue could discriminate the formulations prepared with the same taste-masking agent. Pein et al. (2015) compared different E-tongues for pharmaceutical analysis. Among them, the performances of three laboratory prototypes of potentiometric E-tongues, working in flow or static modes, and comprising different sensors (in number and composition) were evaluated. The potentiometric E-tongues could differentiate samples containing caffeine citrate from API (active pharmaceutical ingredient)-free samples, showing potential for use in the evaluation of taste-masking effects and drug-release kinetics. Yoshida et al. (2015) also studied the use of a potentiometric E-tongue to evaluate palatability of the original and nine generic versions of famotidine orally disintegrating tablets and the bitterness intensities predicted by the E-tongue were in accordance with those assessed by a sensory panel.

13.2.2.2 Voltammetric based-sensor arrays for biomedical and pharmaceutical applications

Voltammetric based-approaches have also been reported for healthcare applications. In 1999, Brett et al. (1999) used poly(methylene blue) (MB) modified electrodes for successfully quantifying hemoglobin in the blood samples of healthy and ill people. The analysis was based on the electro-oxidation of hemoglobin at a fixed potential, which was monitored by CV, using a typical three-electrode cell (a glassy carbon electrode (GCE) as the WE; a Pt gauze as CE and a saturated calomel electrode as the RE). The methodology identified a blood sample as belonging to a patient if the voltammetric signal showed a deviation from the linear correlation established for healthy people (electrochemical method versus conventional clinical spectrophotometric technique).

It was hypothesized that such deviations could be linked to structural changes occurring in hemoglobin variants and so, the E-tongue could be used as a diagnostic tool for anemia, leukemia or excessive loss of blood. Fan et al. (2000) used a modified iodide-silver electrode to determine by CV and DPV the hemoglobin contents in standard solutions and in solutions mimicking real biological fluids. The results showed that a linear relationship could be established between the anodic peak current of the DPV and the protein concentration (detection limit of 3×10^{-7} M).

Mitsubayashi et al. (2003) developed a wearable and flexible oxygen sensor with membrane structure, constructed using microfabrication techniques, and containing a nonpermeable sheet and a gas-permeable membrane with platinum- and Ag/AgCl-electrodes. The sensor device, applied to the skin surface of healthy male volunteers with no history of skin diseases, allowed the safe monitoring, by CV, of the transcutaneous oxygen pressure without any problems, such as skin inflammation. Iguchi et al. (2005) developed a novel wearable oxygen sensor device with gold and Ag/AgCl electrodes fabricated with gas-permeable membranes using photolithography and sputtering methods and that also contained a membrane filter and a nonpermeable membrane.

The CV and chronoamperometric data recorded showed that the wearable sensor could be used as a new transcutaneous oxygen sensor, enabling evaluating the oxygen level in the conjunctiva of a rabbit without any thermoregulation. An automatic sequential injection voltammetric E-tongue was described by Gutés et al. (2007) to determine oxidizable compounds of clinical and pharmaceutical interest, such as ascorbic acid, uric acid, and paracetamol.

The array comprised three WEs (platinum, gold, and epoxy-graphite discs with 1 mm of diameter) and one integrated RE (Ag/AgCl) for minimizing noise effects. All electrodes were built from metal wires and encased in epoxy resin in PVC tube (6 mm inner diameter) used as the system body. ANN models based on voltammograms data showed a good prediction capability, allowing quantifying ascorbic acid, uric acid, and paracetamol with average errors of 8%, 10%, and 12%, respectively.

Twomey et al. (2011) showed that a four electrodes (Au, Pt, Ir, and Rh) voltammetric E-tongue probe could be used to evaluate different biological fluids, namely gut fluids. CV was used to obtain chemical information (in vivo) from gut model fluids and the different signal profile shapes highlighted the discrimination capability and the potential of such device as a tool for gastrointestinal fluid investigation.

Recently, Mc Caffrey et al. (2015) presented a wireless swallowable multielectrode E-tongue device, incorporating different voltammetric sensing techniques (eg, CV, SWV, and DPV), which enables real-time nonspecific characterization of gut fluids, thus helping in the diagnosis of gastrointestinal diseases such as Crohn's and ulcerative colitis. The satisfactory results obtained, comparable with clinical routine conventional techniques, namely for the electrochemical examination of fecal waters proved the E-tongue's potential as an in vitro or in vivo gastrointestinal tract diagnostic tool.

Tattoo-based electrochemical devices have been recently described for evaluating different physiologically relevant compounds in sweat or skin. Windmiller et al. (2012) developed stamp transfer electrodes for electrochemical sensing on nonplanar and oversized surfaces. The concept was demonstrated towards the voltammetric detection of dopamine, ascorbic acid and acetaminophen, as well as to quantify increasing levels of uric acid in human skin.

Machini and coworkers (2013) developed a voltammetric sensor with hausmannite-type manganese oxide, as a sensing material, for improving sodium ion quantification. The device was satisfactorily used to determine, by CV, sodium ions in diluted urine samples, without prior treatment.

Some works have been reported concerning the use of voltammetric sensor devices for pharmaceutical applications. Sidel'nikov et al. (2015) showed the capability of a voltammetric E-tongue (containing carbon electrodes modified by polyarylene phthalides) to identify antiarrhythmic medicines from several producers. Overall, the results highlighted that the voltammograms of medicines could serve as "virtual prints" and be used for their identification and for quality control.

13.2.2.3 Impedimetric based-sensor arrays for biomedical and pharmaceutical applications

The use of impedimetric-based sensing strategies for biomedical applications is scarce compared to potentiometric or voltammetric bioinspired devices. Even so, some successful applications have been reported. Ivorra et al. (2003) and Genescà et al. (2005) developed miniaturized platinum four-electrode probes for in vivo electrical bio-impedance measurements. The results obtained in vivo using rat kidneys subjected to ischemia showed that this type of probe could be used as a helpful marker of tissue condition. Indeed, since impedance modulus and phase were measured at low frequency it was possible to evaluate extracellular pH and potassium levels. Moreover, the device was also partially successful in identifying kidneys that have suffered previous warm ischemia.

Gonzalez-Guillaumin et al. (2007) proposed a multisensor impedance-pH wireless capsule capable of discriminating between acidic and nonacidic gastro-esophageal reflux. The results suggested that the device could offer a minimally invasive and reliable testing of all aspects of gastro-esophageal reflux disease. Beging et al. (2010) built miniaturized field-effect capacitive Ca^{2+}-sensitive electrolyte-membrane–insulator–semiconductor sensors to determine free Ca^{2+}-ion concentration in native urine of high-risk patients (stone formation) by potentiometry/impedance. The sensor showed almost Nernstian calcium sensitivity and exhibited a detection limit around 0.01 mM, which was below the lowest concentration of Ca^{2+} in native urine.

13.2.3 Aptasensors: Design, development and application

The detection and quantification of protein biomarkers is crucial for clinic diagnostics, as well as for monitoring the treatment of certain diseases. As previously mentioned, electrochemical biosensors exhibit high sensitivity and selectivity for the monitoring of the low levels of protein biomarkers (Saberian et al., 2011; Xu et al., 2009). The use of aptamers to develop biosensors (so-called aptasensors) presents many advantages, including high selectivity and affinity, chemical stability under a wide range of buffer conditions, resistance to harsh treatments without loss of bioactivity, reversible thermal denaturation, adaptability to several targets, ease of storage, and versatility in labeling, immobilization in several surfaces (eg, gold, carbon), signaling and regeneration (Feng et al., 2008; Hianik and Wang, 2009; Li et al., 2010; Radi, 2011; Strehlitz et al., 2008). Additionally, the use of aptamers opens the possibility of performing several analyses with mild alteration of specificity and selectivity of the binding. Aptamers can be isolated by an in vitro selection technique named SELEX (systematic evolution of ligands by exponential enrichment) from random-sequences nucleic acids libraries.

DNA aptamers are suitable for designing reusable aptasensors, whereas RNA aptamers allow single shot measurements since they are more susceptible to nucleases action (Sassolas et al., 2009; Strehlitz et al., 2008). Some chemical modifications can enhance nuclease resistance (ie, biostability in serum) and increase the half-life of RNA aptamers. These chemical modifications can be introduced in the oligonucleotides libraries and either during or after the SELEX cycle (Kuwahara and Sugimoto, 2010; Stoltenburg et al., 2007).

An electrochemical aptasensor is a compact device using aptamers as the bioreceptor element immobilized onto the electrode surface. It comprises the transducer responsible for monitoring the formation of the aptamer-target complex and for the translation of this formation into a measurable signal that can be easily processed, recorded and displayed (Hong et al., 2012; Monošík et al., 2012; Sadik et al., 2009; Thévenot et al., 1999). The electrochemical transduction can be divided into voltammetric, amperometric, potentiometric, and impedimetric (Arshak et al., 2009; Velusamy et al., 2010). In the fabrication of electrochemical aptasensors, different electrode/transducer surface, immobilization methods of aptamers and design strategies can be used depending on the envisaged use (Fig. 13.10).

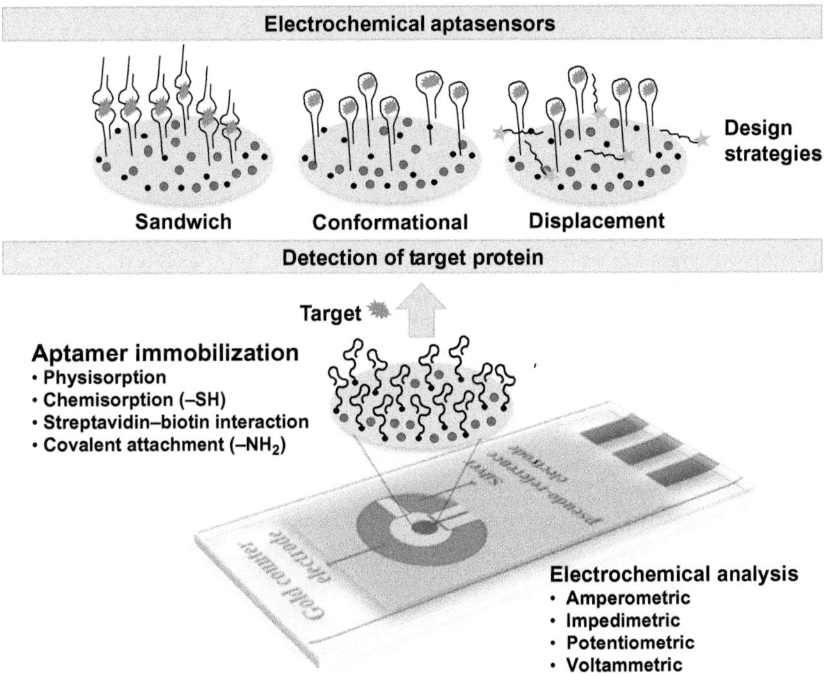

Fig. 13.10 Basic principles of electrochemical aptasensors.

The design of these aptasensors can be divided into three or four types based on the differences in the design of the DNA/RNA-modified electrodes. Cheng et al. (2009) classified electrochemical aptasensors into three categories in which the analyte/target molecule detection relies: configuration, conformation or conductivity changes. For the first, the target binding induces either an assembly or dissociation of the aptamer. In the second configuration type, the target binding induces a modification in the conformation of the aptamer immobilized onto the surface. Finally, for the latter case, the target binding "switches on" the conductivity of the surface-bound aptamer-DNA.

On the other hand, Han et al. (2010) suggested four possible design strategies, viz. target-induced structure switching mode; sandwich or sandwich-like mode;

target-induced dissociation or displacement mode; and competitive replacement mode. These strategies can be used in the development of label and label-free, as well as in "signal-on" and "signal-off" electrochemical aptasensors.

13.2.3.1 Electrochemical aptasensors based on sandwich design

The sandwich design presents an increased sensitivity and selectivity concerning the detection of the target molecule. However, two conditions are required for this sensor arrangement, namely (1) the target must have two independent binding sites (epitopes) to which two different ligands (aptamers) may bind the target molecule without affecting the binding of other targets; and (2) two or more aptamers are selected against the target (Han et al., 2010; Palchetti and Mascini, 2012).

Very few target molecules (platelet-derived growth factor (PDGF) and thrombin (THR)) have two binding sites and two or more isolated aptamers, which limits the use of this type of sensor format. This limitation can be circumvented through the use of the aptamer–protein–aptamer (using the same aptamer) and aptamer–protein–antibody (Han et al., 2010; Palchetti and Mascini, 2012) designs.

Some works have reported the use of aptasensors based on sandwich design for the detection of different proteins, namely THR, C-reactive protein (CRP), vascular endothelial growth factor (VEGF) (Ravalli et al., 2015), mucin 1 (MUC1) (Chen et al., 2015), and PDGF (Wang et al., 2009) (Table 13.1).

Centi et al. (2007) developed a labeled "signal-on" electrochemical aptasensor to detect THR in human plasma samples using the sandwich design with magnetic particles as solid supports. A biotinylated aptamer was captured onto streptavidin-coated magnetic beads through streptavidin–biotin interaction in a carbon electrode surface. The resulting aptamer-modified magnetic beads were incubated with THR. Upon binding, a biotinylated secondary aptamer was added, ready to bind in a further step to a streptavidin–alkaline phosphatase (AP) conjugate. The changes in the electrode surface were detected by DPV and a low detection limit (0.50 nM) was achieved in serum and plasma.

These authors used the same strategy for detecting the CRP. However, in this example a biotinylated RNA aptamer with affinity for CRP was immobilized on the magnetic beads (capture probe) and a biotinylated monoclonal antibody antiCRP conjugated with alkaline phosphatase (AP) (detection probe) was used. The electrochemical detection through DPV allowed a detection limit of 2 nM in serum samples (Centi et al., 2009).

In recent years nanomaterials have been explored for the signal amplification thereby promoting the sensitivity of electrochemical aptasensors. Wang et al. (2011) reported an electrochemical aptasensor for the detection of THR in which nanoparticles were used to increase the surface area (capture probe) and for signal amplification (detection probe). The authors described a sandwich design using a GCE modified with chitosan-hollow CoPt alloy nanoparticle (Cs–HcoPt) film activated with glutaraldehyde (GA) for the immobilization of aptamer-1 modified with amino group. For the signal amplification, aptamer-2 was conjugated with high-quality hollow CoPt bimetal alloy nanoparticles (HcoPt) onto reduced graphene oxide sheet (rGS) with a redox probe

Table 13.1 Examples of electrochemical aptasensors based on sandwich design

Target/aptamer	Aptasensor	Detection limit	Samples	References
THR (DNA)	Label (AP), "signal-on", voltammetric	0.50 nM	Serum and plasma samples	Centi et al. (2007)
THR (DNA)	Label (CdS-QDs), "signal-on", voltammetric	0.55 fM	Standard solutions	Ding et al. (2010)
THR (DNA)	Label (AuNPs–HRP), "signal-on", voltammetric	30 fM	Standard solutions	Zhaoet al. (2011a)
THR (DNA)	Label (NPs–rGS–Thi–HRP), "signal-on", voltammetric	0.34 pM	Standard solutions	Wang et al. (2011)
CRP (RNA)	Label (AP), "signal-on", voltammetric	2 nM	Serum samples	Centi et al. (2009)
VEGF (DNA)	Label (AuNPs–AP), "signal-on", voltammetric	30 nM	Standard solutions	Ravalli et al. (2015)
MUC1 (DNA)	Label (PoPD–AuNPs), "signal-on", voltammetric	1 pM	Serum samples	Chen et al. (2015)
PDGF (DNA)	Label (AuNPs–$[Ru(NH_3)_5Cl]^{2+}$), "signal-on", voltammetric	1 pM	Blood serum	Wang et al. (2009)
THR (DNA)	Label (Cds-QDs), "signal-on", potentiometric	0.14 nM	Standard solutions	Numnuam et al. (2008)
THR (DNA)	Label (AuNPs), impedimetric	0.3 pM	Standard solutions	Ocaña and del Valle (2014)

AP, alkaline phosphatase; *AuNPs*, gold nanoparticles; *CdS-QDs*, cadmium sulfide quantum dot; *CRP*, C-reactive protein; *HRP*, horseradish peroxidase; *MUC1*, mucin 1; *NPs*, nanoparticles; *PDGF*, platelet-derived growth factor; *PoPD*, poly(*o*-phenylenediamine); *rGS*, reduced graphene oxide sheet; *THR*, thrombin; *VEGF*, vascular endothelial growth factor.

thionine (Thi) and enzyme horseradish peroxidase (HRP). This aptasensor presented a low detection limit (0.34 pM) and a good specificity for THR in Tris–HCl buffer.

A simple and ultrasensitive aptasensor for the detection of THR was reported by Zhao et al. (2011a). The aptamer-1 (Apt1) was immobilized onto core/shell Fe_3O_4/gold magnetic nanoparticles (AuMNPs) and by chemisorption onto a gold electrode, and the aptamer-2 (Apt2) was coupled with gold nanoparticles (AuNPs) and HRP for signal amplification. This electrochemical aptasensor using DPV and containing two different aptamers (AuMNPs–Apt1/THR/Apt2–AuNPs–HRP) allowed a detection limit of 30 fM for THR in PBS buffer (phosphate buffered saline). In addition, it showed good reproducibility and selectivity for THR.

Recently Ravalli et al. (2015) described a single-use electrochemical aptasensor for the detection of VEGF based on a sandwich design with two different aptamers, AuNPs and an enzyme-amplified detection. The graphite SPEs were modified by electrodeposition of AuNPs for thiolated aptamer-1 immobilization by chemisorption. After Apt1-VEGF recognition, the biotinylated Apt2 was added and the resulting complex was coupled with streptavidin–AP for amplified detection. The electroactive product of the enzymatic reaction was detected by DPV. The "signal-on" aptasensor response was found to be linearly related to the target concentration between 0 and 250 nM in Tris buffer; the detection limit was 30 nM.

Using a similar strategy, Chen et al. (2015) reported a "signal-on" electrochemical aptasensor for the detection of MUC1. The poly(*o*-phenylenediamine)–AuNPs (PoPD–AuNPs) film was used as a capture probe for the immobilization of aptamer-1. On the other hand, the AuNPs functionalized silica/multiwalled carbon nanotubes core-shell nanocomposites (AuNPs/SiO2@MWCNTs) were used to enhance the immobilization of the secondary aptamer, as well as to load large amounts of Thi electrochemical probe. The presence of MUC1 induced the formation of one complex between the PoPD–AuNPs–Apt1 and the Thi–AuNPs/SiO2@MWCNTs–Apt2. The current changes resulting from the formation of such complex were registered by DPV and a detection limit of 1 pM was obtained in serum.

Numnuam et al. (2008) reported the first potentiometric aptasensor using ion-selective microelectrodes for THR detection. In the sandwich design, the THR was captured by a thiolated aptamer attached to the surface of the gold electrode and the measurements were based on cadmium sulfide quantum dot (CdS-QDs) label of the secondary aptamer. The potentiometric aptasensor presented good sensitivity allowing the detection of up to 28 fmol of THR in PBS buffer solutions (detection limit of 0.14 nM).

A THR impedimetric aptasensor using sandwich design was developed by Ocaña and del Valle (2014). The aptasensor used gold–streptavidin nanoparticles (strep–AuNPs), silver enhancement treatment for signal amplification and two different biotinylated THR aptamers (AptTHRBio1 and AptTHRBio2). The fabrication of the aptasensor involved several steps, namely: (1) immobilization of AptTHRBio1 onto an avidin-graphite epoxy composite electrode surface by biotin–avidin interaction; (2) sandwich formation between the AptTHRBio1–THR–AptTHRBio2; (3) binding strep–AuNPs with AptTHRBio2; and (4) silver enhancement treatment. The EIS aptasensor showed high selectivity and sensitivity for THR with a detection limit of 0.3 pM and a good linear range (0.1–100 pM) in PBS buffer.

13.2.3.2 Electrochemical aptasensors based on target binding-induced aptamer conformational changes

This strategy has been widely used in the development of electrochemical aptasensors for the detection of different proteins, such as THR (Düzgün et al., 2010; Ocaña et al., 2012; Xiao et al., 2005a), interferon gamma (IFN-γ) (Liu et al., 2010), MUC1 (Hu et al., 2014; Liu et al., 2015; Ma et al., 2013), VEGF (Zhao et al., 2011b), osteopontin (OPN) (Meirinho et al., 2015), and PDGF (Degefa and Kwak, 2008; Lai et al., 2007) (Table 13.2). It exploits the ability of aptamers to form several secondary and/or tertiary structures after binding to their target protein.

Table 13.2 Examples of electrochemical aptasensors based on target binding-induced aptamer conformational change

Target/aptamer	Aptasensor	Detection limit	Samples	References
THR (DNA)	Label (MB), "signal-off", voltammetric	6.4 nM	Blood serum	Xiao et al. (2005a)
THR (DNA)	Label-free, potentiometric	80 nM	Standard solutions	Düzgün et al. (2010)
THR (DNA)	Label-free, impedimetric	4.5 pM	Standard solutions	Ocaña et al. (2012)
IFN-γ (DNA)	Label (MB), "signal-off", voltammetric	0.06 nM	Standard solutions	Liu et al. (2010)
MUC1 (DNA)	Label (MB), "signal-off", voltammetric	50 nM	Standard solutions	Ma et al. (2013)
MUC1 (DNA)	Label (AuNPs–HRP), "signal-on", voltammetric	2.2 nM	Standard solutions	Hu et al. (2014)
MUC1 (DNA)	Label-free, "signal-off", impedimetric	0.1 nM	Standard solutions	Liu et al. (2015)
VEGF (DNA)	Label (MB), "signal-on", voltammetric	5 pM	Human whole blood	Zhao et al. (2011b)
OPN (RNA)	Label-free, "signal-off", voltammetric	3.7 nM	Standard solutions	Meirinho et al. (2015)
PDGF (DNA)	Label (MB), "signal-on", voltammetric	50 pM	Blood serum	Lai et al. (2007)
PDGF (DNA)	Label-free, "signal-off", voltammetric	1–40 nM	Standard solutions	Degefa and Kwak (2008)

HRP, horseradish peroxidase; *IFN-γ*, interferon gamma; *MB*, methylene blue; *MUC1*, mucin 1; *OPN*, osteopontin; *PDGF*, platelet-derived growth factor; *THR*, thrombin; *VEGF*, vascular endothelial growth factor.

Xiao et al. (2005a) developed a label "signal-off" aptasensor for the detection of THR in blood serum. The aptamer against THR was immobilized onto a gold electrode by chemisorption. Before binding to the protein, the 3′-end MB-label aptamer is close to the electrode surface, thus allowing the transfer of electrons with the electrode surface due to the flexible structure of the aptamer.

After THR binding, the aptamer forms a stable and rigid structure (G-quadruplex structure) and the MB-label is kept away from the electrode surface, the electron transfer is inhibited, thus resulting in a current decrease. The electrochemical measurements were performed by alternating current voltammetry (ACV) and a detection limit of 6.4 nM was reported. The same strategy was used by Liu et al. (2010) for the detection of IFN-γ. The aptamer against IFN-γ was 5′-end thiolated, conjugated with 3′-MB-label and immobilized onto a gold electrode by chemisorption. The IFN-γ binding induced an aptamer conformation change, increased the distance of MB-label from the electrode surface, led to a decrease of the electron transfer and consequently of the current. SWV was used to quantify the current decrease and a detection limit of 0.06 nM was obtained. This reusable, label "signal-off" electrochemical aptasensor proved to be sensitive and specific to IFN-γ in the presence of overabundant serum protein.

The same strategy was reported by Ma et al. (2013) for the development of a label "signal-off" aptasensor to detect MUC1. For that purpose, a specific DNA aptamer MB-label was immobilized onto a gold electrode surface by chemisorption. In the absence of MUC1, one hairpin structure was formed and the electrode transfer between MB-label and the gold electrode was facilitated. Upon MUC1 binding, a conformational change of the aptamer was induced, the MB-label was removed from the electrode surface and a decrease in the current was observed. The electrochemical measurements were performed by SWV, a detection limit of 50 nM and a large dynamic response range (up to 1.5 μM) were reported. This electrochemical aptasensor showed good specificity in the presence of other proteins and could be seen as a promising tool in clinical applications.

On the other hand, Lai et al. (2007) reported a labeled "signal-on" electrochemical aptasensor for the detection of PDGF in clinical samples. The aptasensor was constructed by immobilizing a MB-label aptamer onto a gold electrode through a thiol group. In the absence of PDG, the MB-label is far away from the electrode surface. Upon PDGF binding, the aptamer forms a stable structure holding the MB-label close to the electrode surface, improving the electron transfer. ACV was used to monitor the changes at the electrode surface and detection limits of 1 nM in blood serum and of 50 pM in serum twofold diluted with buffer were obtained. This aptasensor showed excellent stability in real samples and could be regenerated by disrupting the aptamer–PDGF complex.

Zhao et al. (2011b) reported a labeled "signal-on" aptasensor for the detection VEGF in human whole blood. The aptasensor was fabricated through self-assembly monolayer at the electrode surface, using a polycrystalline gold disk electrode as WE and thiol- and MB-modified DNA aptamer. Upon VEGF binding the partially unfolded aptamer formed a conformational stem-loop structure. This conformational change forces the MB-label to be in close proximity to the electrode, thus resulting in a significant increase in the electron transfer and current signal. A detection limit of 5 pM was achieved in 50% of blood serum.

Using AuNPs–HRP for signal amplification, Hu et al. (2014) developed an ultrasensitive electrochemical aptasensor for the detection of MUC1. AuNPs were used to manufacture this aptasensor, as well as the enzyme HRP and a GCE modified with multiwalled carbon nanotubes and streptavidin.

The aptamer was modified with thiol at the 5′-end and biotin at the 3′-end, and both aptamer and HRP were immobilized on the AuNPs (GCE–Apt–AuNPs–HRP). After the aptamer–MUC1 interaction, the aptamer was disrupted and the biotin exposed was captured by the streptavidin-modified electrode. This "signal-on" aptasensor exhibited good linear dynamic ranges (8.8–353.3 nM) and a low detection limit (2.2 nM) for MUC1 in PBS buffer.

Applying the target binding induced aptamer conformational change strategy, a label-free approach was reported by Degefa and Kwak (2008) for detecting the PDGF cancer-related protein using $[Fe(CN)_6]^{3-/4-}$ as a redox probe. The DNA aptamer against PDGF self-assembled in a monolayer onto the gold surface by chemisorption, which, in the absence of the PDGF showed a dynamic state and efficient electron transfer between the redox probe and the electrode surface. Following the PDGF binding-induced aptamer conformation change, the electron transfer was significantly affected and a linear decrease of the peak current with the protein concentration (1–40 nM) was observed. Using the same approach and the CV, our research team (Meirinho et al., 2015) developed an aptasensor for OPN detection. An RNA aptamer was immobilized on a streptavidin-modified gold surface through the streptavidin–biotin interaction. After binding the OPN, the current decreased due to the alteration of the aptamer structure. The label-free "signal-off" electrochemical aptasensor showed sensitivity and selectivity towards OPN (detection limit of 3.7 nM) and was able to detect OPN in the presence of other interfering proteins, with the exception of THR.

A potentiometric aptasensor for THR detection using single-walled carbon nanotubes (SWCNT) as a transducing element was reported by Düzgün et al. (2010)). The THR binding aptamer was covalently linked to the carboxylic groups of the SWCNT and the aptamer–THR interaction led to a direct potentiometric signal. The aptasensor showed a good response in the THR concentration range of 10^{-7}–10^{-6} M and a limit of detection of 80 nM. The aptasensor presented also good selectivity against elastase and bovine serum albumin and was easily regenerated.

On the other hand, Ocaña et al. (2012) reported a simple, label-free impedimetric aptasensor for the detection of THR in PBS buffer solutions. In the design of the aptasensor, a graphite epoxy composite was used and the aptamers were immobilized onto the electrode surface by physical adsorption. A detection limit of 4.5 pM was achieved using EIS in the presence of the $[Fe(CN)_6]^{3-/4-}$ redox probe. The aptasensor was regenerated for several cycles. Recently, Liu et al. (2015) developed an impedimetric aptasensor, using AuNPs for signal amplification and the redox probe $[Fe(CN)_6]^{3-/4-}$, for detection and quantification of MUC1 in PBS buffer solutions.

For the fabrication of the aptasensor, a complementary DNA (cDNA) sequence was designed and immobilized on the gold electrode via chemisorption. For signal amplification and to capture the MUC1 protein, the aptamer was functionalized with AuNPs (Apt–AuNPs). After MUC1 binding, a well-defined 3D structure was formed, which led to the Apt–AuNPs/MUC1 complex formation. The proposed label-free aptasensor showed a low detection limit (0.1 nM) exhibiting high sensitivity and good selectivity against carcinoembryonic antigen (CEA) and tumor necrosis factor-α (TNF-α).

13.2.3.3 Electrochemical aptasensors based on target-induced aptamer displacement

This strategy is grounded mainly in the strong affinity of the label-free aptamer to its specific target with a labeled aptamer-complementary sequence (Han et al., 2010). Upon binding of the target-aptamer, the dissociation/displacement of the complementary sequences of the aptamer occurs, resulting in detectable signals.

Xiao et al. (2005b) developed a "signal-on" aptasensor using an aptamer immobilized onto a gold electrode by chemisorption and then hybridized it with a partially cDNA sequence labeled with MB. Upon THR binding, the aptamer adopted a G-quadruplex conformation and labeled aptamer-cDNA sequence pushed MB closer to the gold electrode surface, thus leading to a detectable current that could be measured by ACV. This aptasensor allowed the detection of THR in a linear concentration range up to 80 nM with a detection limit of 3 nM in Tris–HCl buffer.

In turn, Lu et al. (2008) developed a "signal-off" aptasensor for the same protein, using a ferrocene (Fc) labeled short aptamer-cDNA sequence to form a double-strain DNA (dsDNA) with the aptamer immobilized on a gold electrode. The target binding led to the dissociation of the label-sequence that was followed by a decrease in the DPV current signal due to the distance between the Fc-label and the gold electrode. The aptasensor was found to be reusable and highly specific with a detection limit of 2 nM in Tris buffer.

This strategy has been reported by Li et al. (2010) and it used AuNPs to increase the signal of an electrochemical aptasensor designed for lysozyme (LYS) detection. The fabrication of the aptasensor included three steps, namely pretreatment of the gold electrode, self-assembly of AuNPs and immobilization of duplex DNA onto the AuNPs-modified gold electrode (aptamer hybridization with an aptamer cDNA sequence label with Fc). In the absence of LYS, the duplex DNA presumably lies down and places the Fc-label in the close proximity of the electrode to give a significantly strong faradaic current. In the presence of LYS, whenever the aptamer binds the protein, the duplex denatures and releases the aptamer complementary DNA sequence into the solution, thus producing a detectable signal decrease. The "signal-off" aptasensor showed a detection limit of 0.1 pM in PBS buffer solutions and high specificity for LYS.

13.2.3.4 Electrochemical aptasensors for multiple protein detection

For the diagnosis and monitoring of diseases, often the detection of a single target analyte is not sufficient and the simultaneous detection of multiple targets is envisaged. Therefore new designs of electrochemical aptasensors for the simultaneous detection of multiple targets are required (Xiang et al., 2011).

Some strategies with this aim have been reported using, for example, a dual-functional aptamer (Min et al., 2010; Xie and Walton, 2010), an aptamer-cDNA that hybridizes with two aptamers (Zhao et al., 2012), or nanomaterials (Bai et al., 2012; Qian et al., 2010).

Zhao et al. (2012) reported a simple label-free "signal-on" electrochemical aptasensor for simultaneous determination of two tumor markers, MUC1 and VEGF in standard solutions. In this aptasensor, the Fc-labeled aptamer-cDNA sequence was immobilized onto a gold disk electrode that hybridizes with both MUC1 and VEGF aptamers to form a long double-strand blocking the electrochemical signal. In the presence of the proteins, the hybridization reaction between the cDNA and the aptamers was inhibited and, Fc-cDNA was close to the electrode surface leading to an increase in the current that could be detected by SWV.

Based in a dual signal amplification strategy, Bai et al. (2012) reported a sandwich design for simultaneous detection of PDGF and THR in PBS buffer. The aptasensor was fabricated using AuNPs–SWCNTs as a biosensor platform to capture a large amount of primary aptamers and amplify the detection response. The redox probes toluidine blue (Tb) and Fc were attached onto the rGS coated with platinum nanoparticles (PtNPs–redox probes–rGS nanocomposites). The synthesized PtNPs–Tb/Fc–rGS nanocomposites were then used as carriers for glucose oxidase (GOD) and HRP and the aptamer-2 (PDGF- and THR-binding), respectively. Using DPV it was found that the linear range of PDGF was 0.01–35 nM with a detection limit of 8 pM, while the linear range was 0.02–45 nM with a detection limit of 11 pM for THR.

Recently, Cheng et al. (2015) reported a simple electrochemical aptasensor for multiple detection of THR and LYS proteins in Tris–HCl buffer. In this study, dabycyl-labeled aptamer modified metal nanoparticles (DLAPs) were immobilized on the β-cyclodextrins (β-CDs) modified gold electrode by means of host–guest recognition technique. During the detection, the aptamers' structure changes due to the specific binding with corresponding proteins that force DLAPs far away from the electrode (previously modified with β-CDs).

The DPV responses of the proposed aptasensor after incubation with different concentrations of both proteins showed a detection limit of 64 and 17 pM for THR and LYS, respectively. The reusable aptasensor showed good response, high specificity and practical applicability in complex biological samples.

13.3 Conclusions and future perspectives

This chapter discussed the versatility and broad range of applicability of electrochemical based-sensors, namely sensor arrays/E-tongues and aptasensors, for biomedical and pharmaceutical applications. The potential use of these low-cost, fast, and green bioinspired analytical techniques for medical purposes has been demonstrated in standard solutions, complex biological matrices, and in real samples.

Several design strategies for the development of electrochemical (bio)sensors have been presented, as well as their potential uses. The results reported in the literature offer a first clue about the feasibility of using electrochemical devices as tools for disease diagnosis and monitoring. However, nowadays, sensor arrays/E-tongue and/or aptasensors are not yet fully exploited as routine diagnosis techniques despite their promising suitability for biological applications. Transposing sensor devices from laboratory to real-world applications is one of the major challenges that must be addressed in the near future.

The success of such tasks may reside in the incorporation of new bioinspired sensor materials, which can increase selectivity and lifetime, together with the adaptation and development of new signal processing techniques that could minimize the need of chemical interpretation of sensor signals. For this purpose an interdisciplinary approach must be undertaken, by means of a collaborative effort of biologists, chemists, physicists, material scientists, and computer scientists. Although there is still a long way to go, the overall quality of the available reports and the consolidated current status of electrochemical sensors undercovers a strong driving force that might provide guidelines for the next years of research and for the application of E-tongues and aptasensors to biomedical purposes, as reliable measurement systems.

Acknowledgments

The authors acknowledge the financial support from the Strategic funding of UID/BIO/04469/2013 unit, from FCT and FEDER through COMPETE 2020 (Project UID/EQU/50020/2013—POCI-01-0145-FEDER-006984) and project ref. RECI/BBB-EBI/0179/2012 (project number FCOMP-01-0124-FEDER-027462) and S. Meirinhos's doctoral grant (ref. SFRH/BD/65021/2009) funded by Fundação para a Ciência e a Tecnologia.

References

Apetrei, I.M., Apetrei, C., 2013. Voltammetric e-tongue for the quantification of total polyphenol content in olive oils. Food Res. Int. 54, 2075–2082.

Arshak, K., Velusamy, V., Korostynska, O., Oliwa-Stasiak, K., Adley, C., 2009. Conducting polymers and their applications to biosensors: emphasizing on foodborne pathogen detection. IEEE Sensors J. 9, 1942–1951.

Bagnasco, L., Cosulich, M.E., Speranza, G., Medini, L., Oliveri, P., Lanteri, S., 2014. Application of a voltammetric electronic tongue and near infrared spectroscopy for a rapid umami taste assessment. Food Chem. 157, 421–428.

Bai, L., Yuan, R., Chai, Y., Zhuo, Y., Yuan, Y., Wang, Y., 2012. Simultaneous electrochemical detection of multiple analytes based on dual signal amplification of single-walled carbon nanotubes and multi-labeled graphene sheets. Biomaterials 33, 1090–1096.

Baldwin, E.A., Bai, J., Plotto, A., Dea, S., 2011. Electronic noses and tongues: applications for the food and pharmaceutical industries. Sensors 11, 4744–4766.

Bandodkar, A.J., Wang, J., 2014. Non-invasive wearable electrochemical sensors: a review. Trends Biotechnol. 32, 363–371.

Bandodkar, A.J., Hung, V.W.S., Jia, W., Valdés-Ramírez, G., Windmiller, J.R., Martinez, A.G., Ramírez, J., Chan, G., Kerman, K., Wang, J., 2013. Tattoo-based potentiometric ion-selective sensors for epidermal pH monitoring. Analyst 138, 123–128.

Bandodkar, A.J., Molinnus, D., Mirza, O., Guinovart, T., Windmiller, J.R., Valdés-Ramírez, G., Andrade, F.J., Schöning, M.J., Wan, J., 2014. Epidermal tattoo potentiometric sodium sensors with wireless signal transduction for continuous non-invasive sweat monitoring. Biosens. Bioelectron. 54, 603–609.

Beging, S., Mlynek, D., Hataihimakul, S., Poghossian, A., Baldsiefen, G., Busch, H., Laube, N., Kleinen, L., Schöning, M.J., 2010. Field-effect calcium sensor for the determination of the risk of urinary stone formation. Sensors Actuators B 144, 374–379.
Bertsimas, D., Tsitsiklis, J., 1993. Simulated annealing. Stat. Sci. 8, 10–15.
Brett, C.M.A., Inzeltb, G., Kertesz, V., 1999. Poly(methylene blue) modified electrode sensor for haemoglobin. Anal. Chim. Acta 385, 119–123.
Cadima, J., Cerdeira, J.O., Minhoto, M., 2004. Computational aspects of algorithms for variables election in the context of principal components. Comput. Stat. Data Anal. 47, 225–236.
Centi, S., Tombelli, S., Minunni, M., Mascini, M., 2007. Aptamer-based detection of plasma proteins by an electrochemical assay coupled to magnetic beads. Anal. Chem. 79, 1466–1473.
Centi, S., Sanmartin, B., Tombelli, S., Palchetti, I., 2009. Detection of C reactive protein (CRP) in serum by an electrochemical aptamer-based sandwich assay. Electroanalysis 21, 1309–1315.
Chen, X., Zhang, Q., Qian, C., Hao, N., Xu, L., Yao, C., 2015. Electrochemical aptasensor for mucin 1 based on dual signal amplification of poly(o-phenylenediamine) carrier and functionalized carbon nanotubes tracing tag. Biosens. Bioelectron. 64, 485–492.
Cheng, A.K.H., Sen, D., Yu, H., 2009. Design and testing of aptamer-based electrochemical biosensors for proteins and small molecules. Bioelectrochemistry 77, 1–12.
Cheng, L., Zhang, J., Lin, Y., Wang, Q., Zhang, X., Ding, Y., Cui, H., Fan, H., 2015. An electrochemical molecular recognition-based aptasensor for multiple protein detection. Anal. Biochem. 491, 31–36.
Choi, D.H., Kim, N.A., Nam, T.S., Lee, S., Jeong, S.H., 2014. Evaluation of taste-masking effects of pharmaceutical sweeteners with an electronic tongue system. Drug Dev. Ind. Pharm. 40, 308–317.
Choy, J.-H., Oh, J.-M., Choi, S.-J., Jung, H., 2010. Bioinspired layered nanomaterials in medical therapy. In: Kumar, C.S.S.R. (Ed.), Nanomaterials for Life Sciences Vol.7: Biomimetic and Bioinspired Nanomaterials, Wiley-VCH Verlag GmbH & Co KGaA, Weinheim (Chapter 6).
Ciosek, P., Wróblewski, W., 2007. Sensor arrays for liquid sensing—electronic tongue systems. Analyst 132, 963–978.
de Sá, A.C., Cipri, A., González-Calabuig, A., Stradiotto, N.R., del Valle, M., 2016. Resolution of galactose, glucose, xylose and mannose in sugarcane bagasse employing a voltammetric electronic tongue formed by metals oxy-hydroxide/MWCNT modified electrodes. Sensors Actuators B 222, 645–653.
Degefa, T.H., Kwak, J., 2008. Label-free aptasensor for platelet-derived growth factor (PDGF) protein. Anal. Chim. Acta 613, 163–168.
del Valle, M., 2011. Bioinspired sensor systems. Sensors 11, 10180–10186.
Di Natale, C., Paolesse, R., Macagnano, A., Mantini, A., D'Amico, A., Legin, A., Lvova, L., Rudnitskaya, A., Vlasov, Y., 2000. Electronic nose and electronic tongue integration for improved classification of clinical and food samples. Sensors Actuators B 64, 15–21.
Dias, L.G., Peres, A.M., Vilas-Boas, M., Rocha, A., Estevinho, L., Machado, A.A.S.C., 2008. An electronic tongue for honey classification. Microchim. Acta 163, 97–102.
Dias, L.G., Peres, A.M., Veloso, A.C.A., Reis, F.S., Vilas Boas, M., Machado, A.A.S.C., 2009. An electronic tongue taste evaluation: identification goat milk adulterations with bovine milk. Sensors Actuators B 136, 209–217.
Dias, L.G., Peres, A.M., Barcelos, T.P., Sá Morais, J., Machado, A.A.S.C., 2011. Semi-quantitative and quantitative analysis of soft drinks using an electronic tongue. Sensors Actuators B 154, 111–118.

Dias, L.G., Sequeira, C., Veloso, A.C.A., Sousa, M.E.B.C., Peres, A.M., 2014. Evaluation of healthy and sensory indexes of sweetened beverages using an electronic tongue. Anal. Chim. Acta 848, 32–42.

Ding, C., Ge, Y., Lin, J.-M., 2010. Aptamer based electrochemical assay for the determination of thrombin by using the amplification of the nanoparticles. Biosens. Bioelectron. 25, 1290–1294.

Dreyfus, G., 2005. Neural networks: an overview. In: Dreyfus, G. (Ed.), Neural Networks—Methodology and Applications. Springer, Heidelberg.

Düzgün, A., Maroto, A., Mairal, T., O'Sullivan, C., Rius, F.X., 2010. Solid-contact potentiometric aptasensor based on aptamer functionalized carbon nanotubes for the direct determination of proteins. Analyst 135, 1037–1041.

Evanics, F., Prosser, R.S., 2005. Discriminating binding and positioning of amphiphiles to lipid bilayers by ^{1}H NMR. Anal. Chim. Acta 534, 21–29.

Fan, C., Li, G., Zhuang, Y., Zhu, J., Zhu, D., 2000. Iodide modified silver electrode and its application to the electroanalysis of hemoglobin. Electroanalysis 12, 205–208.

Feng, K., Sun, C., Kang, Y., Chen, J., Jiang, J.-H., Shen, G.-L., Yu, R.-Q., 2008. Label-free electrochemical detection of nanomolar adenosine based on target-induced aptamer displacement. Electrochem. Commun. 10, 531–535.

Genescà, M., Ivorra, A., Sola, A., Palacios, L., Goujon, J.-M., Hauet, T., Villa, R., Aguiló, J., Hotter, G., 2005. Electrical bioimpedance measurement during hypothermic rat kidney preservation for assessing ischemic injury. Biosens. Bioelectron. 20, 1866–1871.

Gentile, P., Chiono, V., Tonda-Turo, C., Sartori, S., Ciardelli, G., 2011. Biomimetic materials for medical application through enzymatic modification. Adv. Biochem. Eng. Biotechnol. 125, 181–205.

Gonzalez-Guillaumin, J., Sadowski, D., Kaler, K., Mintchev, M., 2007. Ingestible capsule for impedance and pH monitoring in the esophagus. IEEE Trans. Biomed. Eng. 54, 2231–2236.

Gonzalo-Ruiz, J., Mas, R., de Haro, C., Cabruja, E., Camero, R., Alonso-Lomillo, M.A., Muñoza, F.J., 2009. Early determination of cystic fibrosis by electrochemical chloride quantification in sweat. Biosens. Bioelectron. 24, 1788–1791.

Grieshaber, D., MacKenzie, R., Vörös, J., Reimhult, E., 2008. Electrochemical biosensors—sensor principles and architectures. Sensors 8, 1400–1458.

Guhmann, M., Preis, M., Gerber, F., Pöllinger, N., Breitkreutz, J., Weitschies, W., 2015. Design, development and in-vitro evaluation of diclofenac taste-masked orodispersible tablet formulations. Drug Dev. Ind. Pharm. 41, 540–551.

Guinovart, T., Bandodkar, A.J., Windmiller, J.R., Andrade, F.J., Wang, J., 2013. A potentiometric tattoo sensor for monitoring ammonium in sweat. Analyst 138, 7031–7038.

Gutés, A., Calvo, D., Cespedes, F., del Valle, M., 2007. Automatic sequential injection analysis electronic tongue with integrated reference electrode for the determination of ascorbic acid, uric acid and paracetamol. Microchim. Acta 157, 1–6.

Gutiérrez, J.M., Leija, L., Muñoz, R., 2012. Bio-inspired systems patents: electronic tongues. Recent Pat. Signal Process. 2, 108–114.

Han, K., Liang, Z., Zhou, N., 2010. Design strategies for aptamer-based biosensors. Sensors 10, 4541–4557.

He, H., Uray, G., Wolfbeis, O., 1992. Optical sensor for salicylic acid and aspirin based on a new lipophilic carrier for aromatic carboxylic acids. Fresenius J. Anal. Chem. 343, 313–318.

Hianik, T., Wang, J., 2009. Electrochemical aptasensors—recent achievements and perspectives. Electroanalysis 21, 1223–1235.

Hong, P., Li, W., Li, J., 2012. Applications of aptasensors in clinical diagnostics. Sensors 12, 1181–1193.

Hu, R., Wen, W., Wang, Q., Xiong, H., Zhang, X., Gu, H., Wang, S., 2014. Novel electrochemical aptamer biosensor based on an enzyme-gold nanoparticle dual label for the ultrasensitive detection of epithelial tumour marker MUC1. Biosens. Bioelectron. 53, 384–389.

Huynh, T.P., Kutner, W., 2015. Molecularly imprinted polymers as recognition materials for electronic tongues. Biosens. Bioelectron. 74, 856–864.

Iguchi, S., Mitsubayashi, K., Uehara, T., Ogawa, M., 2005. A wearable oxygen sensor for transcutaneous blood gas monitoring at the conjunctiva. Sensors Actuators B 108, 733–737.

Ivorra, A., Gómez, R., Noguera, N., Villa, R., Sola, A., Palacios, L., Hotter, G., Aguilo, J., 2003. Minimally invasive silicon probe for electrical impedance measurements in small animals. Biosens. Bioelectron. 391, 393–399.

Kirkpatrick, S., Gelatt, C.D., Vecchi, M.P., 1983. Optimization by simulated annealing. Science 220, 671–680.

Kuwahara, M., Sugimoto, N., 2010. Molecular evolution of functional nucleic acids with chemical modifications. Molecules 15, 5423–5444.

Lai, R.Y., Plaxco, K.W., Heeger, A.J., 2007. Aptamer-based electrochemical detection of picomolar platelet-derived growth factor directly in blood serum. Anal. Chem. 79, 229–233.

Legin, A., Smirnova, A., Rudnitskaya, A., Lvova, L., Suglobova, E., Vlasov, Y., 1999. Chemical sensor array for multicomponent analysis of biological liquids. Anal. Chim. Acta 385, 131–135.

Legin, A., Rudnitskaya, A., Vlasov, Y., 2002. Electronic tongues: sensors, systems, applications. Sensors Update 10, 143–188.

Li, L.-D., Chen, Z.-B., Zhao, H.-T., Guo, L., Mu, X., 2010. An aptamer-based biosensor for the detection of lysozyme with gold nanoparticles amplification. Sensors Actuators B 149, 110–115.

Liu, C.-C., 2000. Electrochemical sensors. In: Bronzino, J.D. (Ed.), The Biomedical Engineering Handbook. CRC Press LLC, Boca Raton, FL (Chapter 49).

Liu, Y., Tuleouva, N., Ramanculov, E., Revzin, A., 2010. Aptamer-based electrochemical biosensor for interferon gamma detection. Anal. Chem. 82, 8131–8136.

Liu, X., Qin, Y., Deng, C., Xiang, J., Li, Y., 2015. A simple and sensitive impedimetric aptasensor for the detection of tumor markers based on gold nanoparticles signal amplification. Talanta 132, 150–154.

Lu, Y., Zhu, N., Yu, P., Mao, L., 2008. Aptamer-based electrochemical sensors that are not based on the target binding-induced conformational change of aptamers. Analyst 133, 1256–1260.

Lvova, L., Martinelli, E., Dini, F., Bergamini, A., Paolesse, R., Di Natale, C., D'Amico, A., 2009. Clinical analysis of human urine by means of potentiometric electronic tongue. Talanta 77, 1097–1104.

Ma, F., Ho, C., Cheng, A.K.H., Yu, H.Z., 2013. Immobilization of redox-labeled hairpin DNA aptamers on gold: electrochemical quantitation of epithelial tumor marker mucin 1. Electrochim. Acta 110, 139–145.

Machini, W.B.S., Martin, C.S., Martinez, M.T., Teixeira, S.R., Gomes, H.M., Teixeira, M.F.S., 2013. Development of an electrochemical sensor based on nanostructured hausmannite-type manganese oxide for detection of sodium ions. Sensors Actuators B 181, 674–680.

Marini, F., Bucci, R., Magrì, A.L., Magrì, A.D., 2008. Artificial neural networks in chemometrics: history, examples and perspectives. Microchem. J. 88, 178–185.

Mc Caffrey, C., Twomey, K., Ogurtsov, V.I., 2015. Development of a wireless swallowable capsule with potentiostatic electrochemical sensor for gastrointestinal track investigation. Sensors Actuators B 218, 8–15.

Meirinho, S.G., Dias, L.G., Peres, A.M., Rodrigues, L.R., 2015. Development of an electrochemical RNA-aptasensor to detect human osteopontin. Biosens. Bioelectron. 71, 332–341.

Mikhelson, K.N., 2013. In: Ion-Selective Electrodes. Series: Lecture Notes in Chemistry, vol. 81. Springer Science & Business Media, Berlin, Heidelberg.
Mimendia, A., Gutiérrez, J.M., Leija, L., Hernández, P.R., Favari, L., Muñoz, R., del Valle, M., 2010. A review of the use of the potentiometric electronic tongue in the monitoring of environmental systems. Environ. Model Softw. 25, 1023–1030.
Min, K., Song, K.-M., Cho, M., Chun, Y.-S., Shim, Y.-B., Ku, J.K., Ban, C., 2010. Simultaneous electrochemical detection of both PSMA (+) and PSMA (−) prostate cancer cells using an RNA/peptide dual-aptamer probe. Chem. Commun. 46, 5566–5568.
Mitsubayashi, K., Wakabayashi, Y., Murotomi, D., Yamada, T., Kawase, T., Iwagaki, S., Karube, I., 2003. Wearable and flexible oxygen sensor for transcutaneous oxygen monitoring. Sensors Actuators B 95, 373–377.
Monošík, R., Streďanský, M., Šturdík, E., 2012. Biosensors—classification, characterization and new trends. Acta Chim. Slov. 5, 109–120.
Numnuam, A., Chumbimuni-Torres, K.Y., Xiang, Y., Bash, R., Thavarungkul, P., Kanatharana, P., Pretsch, E., Wang, J., Bakker, E., 2008. Aptamer-based potentiometric measurements of proteins using ion-selective microelectrodes. Anal. Chem. 80, 707–712.
Ocaña, C., del Valle, M., 2014. Signal amplification for thrombin impedimetric aptasensor: sandwich protocol and use of gold-streptavidin nanoparticles. Biosens. Bioelectron. 54, 408–414.
Ocaña, C., Pacios, M., del Valle, M., 2012. A reusable impedimetric aptasensor for detection of thrombin employing a graphite-epoxy composite electrode. Sensors 12, 3037–3048.
Palchetti, I., Mascini, M., 2012. Electrochemical nanomaterial-based nucleic acid aptasensors. Anal. Bioanal. Chem. 402, 3103–3114.
Pein, M., Kirsanov, D., Ciosek, P., del Valle, M., Yaroshenko, I., Wesoły, M., Zabadaj, M., Gonzalez-Calabuig, A., Wróblewski, W., Legin, A., 2015. Independent comparison study of six different electronic tongues applied for pharmaceutical analysis. J. Pharm. Biomed. Anal. 114, 321–329.
Phat, C., Moon, B., Lee, C., 2016. Evaluation of umami taste in mushroom extracts by chemical analysis, sensory evaluation, and an electronic tongue system. Food Chem. 192, 1068–1077.
Phillips, F., Kaczor, K., Gandhi, N., Pendley, B.D., Danish, R.K., Neuman, M.R., Tóth, B., Horváth, V., Lindner, E., 2007. Measurement of sodium ion concentration in undiluted urine with cation-selective polymeric membrane electrodes after the removal of interfering compounds. Talanta 74, 255–264.
Qian, X., Xiang, Y., Zhang, H., Chen, Y., Chai, Y., Yuan, R., 2010. Aptamer/nanoparticle-based sensitive, multiplexed electronic coding of proteins and small biomolecules through a backfilling strategy. Chem. Eur. J. 16, 14261–14265.
Radi, A.-E., 2011. Electrochemical aptamer-based biosensors: recent advances and perspectives. Int. J. Electrochem. 2011, 1–17.
Ramamoorthy, H.V., Mohamed, S.N., Devi, D.S., 2014. E-nose and E-tongue: applications and advances in sensor technology. J. Nanosci. Nanotechnol. 2, 370–376.
Ravalli, A., Rivas, L., De La Escosura-Muñiz, A., Pons, J., Merkoçi, A., Marrazza, G., 2015. A DNA aptasensor for electrochemical detection of vascular endothelial growth factor. J. Nanosci. Nanotechnol. 15, 3411–3416.
Roper, S., 1995. Ofactory/taste receptor transduction. In: Speralakis, N. (Ed.), Cell Physiology Source Book. Academic Press, San Diego, CA, pp. 514–522 (Chapter 38).
Saberian, M., Hamzeiy, H., Aghanejad, A., Asgari, D., 2011. Aptamer-based nanosensors: juglone as an attached-redox molecule for detection of small molecules. Bioimpacts 1, 31–36.
Sadik, O.A., Aluoch, A.O., Zhou, A., 2009. Status of biomolecular recognition using electrochemical techniques. Biosens. Bioelectron. 24, 2749–2765.

Sassolas, A., Blum, L.J., Leca-Bouvier, B.D., 2009. Electrochemical aptasensors. Electroanalysis 21, 1237–1250.
Schazmann, B., Morris, D., Slater, C., Beirne, S., Fay, C., Reuveny, R., Moyna, N., Diamond, D., 2010. A wearable electrochemical sensor for the real-time measurement of sweat sodium concentration. Anal. Methods 2, 342–348.
Scholz, F., 2010. Electroanalytical Methods: Guide to Experiments and Applications. Springer, Heidelberg.
Shen, H., Habara, M., Toko, K., 2008. Development of caffeine detection using taste sensor with lipid/polymer membranes. Sensor. Mater. 20, 171–178.
Sidel'nikov, A.V., Zil'berg, R.A., Yarkaeva, Y.A., Maistrenko, V.N., Kraikin, V.A., 2015. Voltammetric identification of antiarrhythmic medicines using principal component analysis. J. Anal. Chem. 70, 1261–1266.
Stoltenburg, R., Reinemann, C., Strehlitz, B., 2007. SELEX—a (r)evolutionary method to generate high-affinity nucleic acid ligands. Biomol. Eng. 24, 381–403.
Strehlitz, B., Nikolaus, N., Stoltenburg, R., 2008. Protein detection with aptamer biosensors. Sensors 8, 4296–4307.
Tahirbegi, I.B., Mir, M., Samitier, J., 2013. Real-time monitoring of ischemia inside stomach. Biosens. Bioelectron. 40, 323–328.
Tahirbegi, I.B., Mir, M., Schostek, S., Schurr, M., Samitier, J., 2014. In vivo ischemia monitoring array for endoscopic surgery. Biosens. Bioelectron. 61, 124–130.
Thévenot, D.R., Toth, K., Durst, R.A., Wilson, G.S., 1999. Electrochemical biosensors: recommended definitions and classification (technical report). Pure Appl. Chem. 71, 2333–2348.
Thomas, F.G., Henze, G., 2001. Introduction to Voltammetric Analysis: Theory and Practice. CSIRO Publishing, Collingwood.
Twomey, K., Alvarez de Eulate, E., Marchesi, J.R., Kolida, S., Gibson, G., Arrigan, D.W.M., Ogurtsov, V.I., 2011. Characterization of the electrochemical behavior of gastrointestinal fluids using a multielectrode sensor probe, biomedical engineering. IEEE Trans. Biomed. Eng. 58, 2521–2527.
Veloso, A.C.A., Dias, L.G., Rodrigues, N., Pereira, J.A., Peres, A.M., 2016. Sensory intensity assessment of olive oils using an electronic tongue. Talanta 146, 585–593.
Velusamy, V., Arshak, K., Korostynska, O., Oliwa, K., Adley, C., 2010. An overview of foodborne pathogen detection: in the perspective of biosensors. Biotechnol. Adv. 28, 232–254.
Vlasov, Y., Legin, A., Rudnitskaya, A., Di Natale, C., D'Amico, A., 2005. Nonspecific sensor arrays ("electronic tongue") for chemical analysis of liquids (IUPAC technical report). Pure Appl. Chem. 77, 1965–1983.
Wang, J., 2006. Potentiometry. In: Wang, J. (Ed.), Analytical Electrochemistry. third ed.. John Wiley & Sons, Inc, Hoboken, NJ, pp. 165–200 (Chapter 5).
Wang, Y., Xu, H., Zhang, J., Li, G., 2008. Electrochemical sensors for clinical analysis. Sensors 8, 2043–2081.
Wang, J., Meng, W., Zheng, X., Liu, S., Li, G., 2009. Combination of aptamer with gold nanoparticles for electrochemical signal amplification: application to sensitive detection of platelet-derived growth factor. Biosens. Bioelectron. 24, 1598–1602.
Wang, Y., Yuan, R., Chai, Y., Yuan, Y., 2011. A multi-amplification aptasensor for highly sensitive detection of thrombin based on high-quality hollow CoPt nanoparticles decorated graphene. Biosens. Bioelectron. 30, 61–66.
Wang, Y., Ye, Z., Ying, Y., 2012. New trends in impedimetric biosensors for the detection of foodborne pathogenic bacteria. Sensors 12, 3449–3471.
Wang, L., Niu, Q., Hui, Y., Jin, H., 2015. Discrimination of rice with different pretreatment methods by using a voltammetric electronic tongue. Sensors 15, 17767–17785.

Wardencki, W., Chmiel, T., Dymerski, T., 2013. Gas chromatography-olfactometry (GC-O), electronic noses (e-noses) and electronic tongues (e-tongues) for in vivo food flavor measurement. In: Kilcast, D. (Ed.), Instrumental Assessment of Food Sensory Quality. A Practical Guide. Woodhead Publishing Limited, Cambridge (Chapter 7).

Windmiller, J.R., Bandodkar, A.J., Parkhomovsky, S., Wang, J., 2012. Stamp transfer electrodes for electrochemical sensing on non-planar and oversized surfaces. Analyst 137, 1570–1575.

Xiang, Y., Qian, X., Jiang, B., Chai, Y., Yuan, R., 2011. An aptamer-based signal-on and multiplexed sensing platform for one-spot simultaneous electronic detection of proteins and small molecules. Chem. Commun. 47, 4733.

Xiao, Y., Lubin, A.A., Heeger, A.J., Plaxco, K.W., 2005a. Label-free electronic detection of thrombin in blood serum by using an aptamer-based sensor. Angew. Chem. Int. Ed. 44, 5456–5459.

Xiao, Y., Piorek, B.D., Plaxco, K.W., Heeger, A.J., 2005b. A reagentless signal-on architecture for electronic, aptamer-based sensors via target-induced strand displacement. J. Am. Chem. Soc. 127, 17990–17991.

Xie, S., Walton, S.P., 2010. Development of a dual-aptamer-based multiplex protein biosensor. Biosens. Bioelectron. 25, 2663–2668.

Xu, Y., Cheng, G., He, P., Fang, Y., 2009. A review: electrochemical aptasensors with various detection strategies. Electroanalysis 21, 1251–1259.

Yaroshenko, I., Kirsanov, D., Kartsova, L., Sidorova, A., Borisova, I., Legin, A., 2015. Determination of urine ionic composition with potentiometric multi-sensor system. Talanta 131, 556–561.

Yoshida, M., Hazekawa, M., Haraguchi, T., Uchida, T., 2015. Evaluation of the palatabilities in 10 different famotidine orally disintegrating tablets by combination of disintegration device and taste sensor. Drug Dev. Ind. Pharm. 41, 1387–1392.

Zadorozhnaya, O., Kirsanov, D., Buzhinsky, I., Tsarev, F., Abramova, N., Bratov, A., Muñoz, F.J., Ribó, J., Bori, J., Riva, M.C., Legin, A., 2015. Water pollution monitoring by an artificial sensory system performing in terms of *Vibrio fischeri* bacteria. Sensors Actuators B 207, 1069–1075.

Zhang, X., Ju, H., Wang, J., 2008. Electrochemical Sensors, Biosensors and Their Biomedical Applications. Academic Press/Elsevier, New York.

Zhao, J., Zhang, Y., Li, H., Wen, Y., Fan, X., 2011a. Ultrasensitive electrochemical aptasensor for thrombin based on the amplification of aptamer–AuNPs–HRP conjugates. Biosens. Bioelectron. 26, 2297–2303.

Zhao, S., Yang, W., Lai, R.Y., 2011b. A folding-based electrochemical aptasensor for detection of vascular endothelial growth factor in human whole blood. Biosens. Bioelectron. 26, 2442–2447.

Zhao, J., He, X., Bo, B., Liu, X., Yin, Y., Li, G., 2012. A "signal-on" electrochemical aptasensor for simultaneous detection of two tumor markers. Biosens. Bioelectron. 34, 249–252.

Zoski, C.G., 2007. Handbook of Electrochemistry. Elsevier, Amsterdam.

Advances on nucleic acid delivery with nonviral vectors

14

R.M. Lopes*, N.A. Fonseca*,†, A.F. Cruz*, A.C. Gregório*, Â. Valério-Fernandes*, V. Moura*,†, S. Simões*, J.N. Moreira*
*University of Coimbra, Coimbra, Portugal, †TREAT U, Coimbra, Portugal

14.1 From the genome to gene-based therapy

The discovery of the DNA molecule and its fundamental role in the codification of life as we perceive it, has revolutionized the way the biology underlying a given biological process or phenotype is interpreted. It has enabled the interpretation of pathological conditions from a different perspective, associating diseases with mutations in the genetic code and, subsequently, the "correction" of those mutations as a therapeutic strategy.

One of the first strategies attempted to correct a genetic mutation underlying a pathological condition, such as cancer, relied on the reexpression of a wild-type copy of the affected gene (Ibraheem et al., 2014). In this respect, mutations of the tumor suppressor p53 protein have been associated with cancers of different histological origin, and therefore they became an important target for genetic intervention (Bieging et al., 2014). Different authors have proposed the reexpression of the wild-type p53 protein as a means to reestablish its function as the "genome guardian" and a tumor suppressor. Using adenovirus-mediated p53 delivery, a decrease was shown in the growth of different cancer cell lines expressing various p53-mutant proteins as well as a prolonged mice survival relative to controls (Harris et al., 1996). A similar observation was later reported by Xu et al. (2001) using a nonviral vector for the systemic delivery of *TP53* gene.

Nevertheless, full length gene delivery has some significant technological limitations, including the complexity of producing recombinant plasmids to encode the wild-type gene. Gene size may also be restrictive to plasmid cloning hindering viral packing or encapsulation in nonviral systems (Ibraheem et al., 2014).

14.1.1 RNA interference: Reachable protein modulation

The introduction of the RNA interference (RNAi) mechanism, including micro-RNA (miRNA) and small-interference RNA (siRNA)-mediated gene silencing, had an extensive impact on the manipulation of a cell phenotype by enabling the use of shorter oligonucleotide sequences for the specific modulation of a particular gene or set of genes at the posttranscriptional level (Fire et al., 1998; Ipsaro and Joshua-Tor, 2015; Gomes-Da-Silva et al., 2012a).

At the start of the chain of events, long hairpinned primary miRNAs (pri-miRNAs, encoded in the genome as noncoding small RNAs) are cropped at the nucleus by a

Bioinspired Materials for Medical Applications. http://dx.doi.org/10.1016/B978-0-08-100741-9.00014-0

heterodimeric complex, which includes Drosha, into the 70 nucleotides (nt) precursor miRNA (pre-miRNA). The pre-miRNAs are exported from the nucleus and processed by Dicer endonuclease into a 21–25 nt mature miRNA (dsRNA), which is then loaded into RISC (RNA-induced silencing complex; Ipsaro and Joshua-Tor, 2015). Despite not being exclusive, the guide strand-loaded Argonaute 2 (Ago2) in the RISC (which includes also Dicer), finally mediates gene silencing through imperfect target messenger RNA (mRNA) recognition at the 3′UTR (untranslated region), thus impairing translation (Ipsaro and Joshua-Tor, 2015).

The processing of exogenous dsRNA (imported directly into the cytoplasm) is similar to that of pre-miRNAs. The exogenous dsRNA is processed by Dicer into interfering dsRNAs–siRNAs–(as mature miRNA), which are subsequently loaded into the RISC. In the case of exogenous dsRNA-mediated generation of siRNAs, there is a perfect complementarity of the guide strand, normally at the open reading frame (ORF) region, leading to target mRNA degradation (Ipsaro and Joshua-Tor, 2015; Gomes-Da-Silva et al., 2012a; Elbashir et al., 2001). Accordingly, siRNAs generated endogenously may regulate several targets (owing to absence of full complementarity), whereas siRNAs generated from exogenous dsRNA can only regulate one target protein (Zhang et al., 2013).

From the above-described mechanism, two different strategies have emerged to perform gene silencing. The first relies in the delivery of short hairpin RNA (shRNA), consisting of two complementary 19–22 bp RNA sequences linked by a short loop of 4–11 nt, similar to the hairpin found in naturally occurring miRNA. These will be processed in the nucleus, in a similar manner to the pri-miRNAs (Moore et al., 2010; Svoboda and Di Cara, 2006). Delivery of shRNA into mammalian cells is normally achieved through infection with viral vectors encoding the corresponding nucleotide sequence. This enables the stable integration of shRNA in the cell genome, therefore sustaining the long-term knockdown of the target gene (Moore et al., 2010). As an alternative, direct cytosolic delivery of siRNA represents an accessible manner to achieve gene silencing without the compromise of long-term knockdown, as well as enabling the use of delivery systems with higher translational potential (Fig. 14.1; Gomes-Da-Silva et al., 2012a).

14.1.2 DNA/RNA in vivo delivery: Challenges and limitations

Different attempts have been made to explore the therapeutic potential of full gene delivery and shRNA or siRNA gene silencing in different pathological settings (Zuckerman and Davis, 2015; Haussecker, 2014; Boudreau and Davidson, 2012). Despite their potential, when studied in clinical trials, many of those technologies suffered some drawbacks, often unanticipated. The delivery of a full length gene, a shRNA or even a siRNA, often implied the use of viral vectors, the best known vehicle for the efficient transduction of DNA-based oligonucleotide sequences into mammalian cells (Boudreau and Davidson, 2012; Brummelkamp et al., 2002a,b). Although being highly efficient delivery agents, viral vectors present several drawbacks, including the high complexity in their preparation and handling; being potentially oncogenic; and being able to trigger immunogenic responses (Zhang et al., 2013). These issues have limited their use to some specific situations, such as talimogene laherparepvec (T-VEC), a

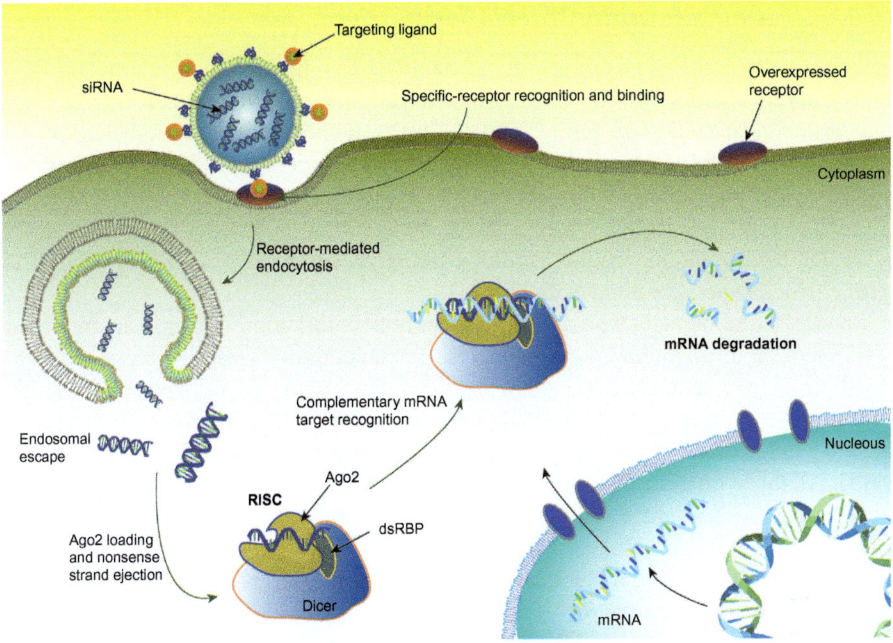

Fig. 14.1 Receptor-mediated endocytosis of small interfering RNA (siRNA)-containing ligand-mediated targeted nanoparticles. Following binding of ligand-mediated targeted nanoparticles containing siRNA to membrane overexpressed receptors, siRNA escape from the endocytic pathway into the cytoplasm takes place. siRNA available in the cytosol is incorporated into RNA-induced silencing complex (RISC) where the passenger strand is cleaved by Ago2. The activated RISC incorporating the antisense strand recognizes complementary mRNA, mediating cleavage of the latter, thus preventing protein translation.

herpes simplex virus-based vector for delivery of GM-CSF (granulocyte-macrophage colony-stimulating factor), recently approved by FDA (Food and Drug Administration) for melanoma treatment (Ledford, 2015; Andtbacka et al., 2015).

Synthetic oligonucleotides, including siRNAs, are an alternative approach to viral vectors-based strategies. However, upon systemic administration, the therapeutic activity of free oligonucleotides can be limited by a number of different extracellular and intracellular barriers.

14.1.2.1 Extracellular barriers

Once in the blood stream, oligonucleotides face a highly unfavorable pharmacokinetics (PKs) that limits their accumulation in a given target tissue, other than the liver. Underlying this poor PK is their negative charge, causing a strong renal clearance (Gomes-Da-Silva et al., 2012a) and facilitating their capture and accumulation by the mononuclear phagocytic system (MPS), mainly at the liver. Furthermore, oligonucleotides bind to serum proteins and are easily degraded by blood endonucleases (Ozpolat et al., 2014; Gomes-Da-Silva et al., 2012a).

14.1.2.2 Cellular and intracellular barriers

The negatively charged nature of oligonucleotides also impairs their interaction with the negatively charged cell membrane, thus limiting the diffusion into the intracellular compartment, and they are further affected by their molecular size. As such, oligonucleotides may be internalized by energy-consuming processes, such as endocytosis. However, since their action occurs at the cytoplasm, especially for siRNAs, once internalized oligonucleotides need to further escape the endosomal compartment to avoid degradation, a feature that is highly limited for free oligonucleotides (Ozpolat et al., 2014; Gomes-Da-Silva et al., 2012a).

In order to counteract some of the aforementioned limitations, chemically modified siRNAs, often through incorporation of 2′OMe nucleotides (2′OMe-guanine, 2′OMe-uracil, or 2′OMe-adenosine residues), and devoid of immunostimulatory CpG motifs, were used in an attempt to improve the biocompatibility of free siRNA, with limited success (Judge et al., 2009; Tagami et al., 2009, 2010; Wan et al., 2014; Zhang et al., 2013). All those hindrances severely limit the systemic administration of free oligonucleotides, as siRNAs, funneling their use towards topical administration (Whitehead et al., 2009; Sarett et al., 2015).

Encapsulation of oligonucleotides in delivery systems has been one the most promising strategies to overcome the described hindrances associated with their use in the free form. From the different delivery systems described to date, lipid-based nonviral vectors are among the best characterized delivery systems that may enable systemic delivery of oligonucleotides.

14.2 Lipid- and polymer-based nonviral vectors for systemic siRNA and DNA delivery

14.2.1 Lipoplexes and liposomes

The first formulations of nucleic acid–lipid complexes (a.k.a. *lipoplex*) were described by Felgner et al. (1987) for the development of novel DNA transfection vectors. The electrostatic attraction between the anionic nucleic acids and cationic lipid (DOTMA, *N*-[1-(2,3-dioleyloxy)propyl]-*N*,*N*,*N*-trime-thylammonium chloride) enabled a positively charged lipid–DNA complex, responsible for the interaction with the negatively charged cell membranes and subsequent DNA uptake and protein expression in the transfected cell (Felgner et al., 1987). The high therapeutic potential associated with the intracellular delivery of nucleic acids led to a fast transposition of this strategy to in vivo application (both in mice and humans; Brigham et al., 1989; Nabel et al., 1993). However, unlike DNA, siRNAs are smaller and present lower charge density and stiffer backbone structure. This leads to a lower binding affinity to cationic lipids, which results in low siRNA loading efficiency and less compact and stable lipoplexes (Kwok and Hart, 2011; Shu et al., 2011). Attempts to improve their structural stability in vivo relied on the use of higher amounts of cationic lipids which, however, have been associated with severe toxicity (such as activation of a complement system and immune or inflammatory responses) and off-target effects (Dokka et al., 2000; Lv et al., 2006; Yew and Scheule, 2005).

The excessive amount of cationic lipid required to stabilize the nucleic acids led to extensive research into increasing the diversity of cationic lipids. Bouxsein et al. observed that siRNA complexes containing a pentavalent lipid MVL5 and DOPE exhibited superior silencing efficiency in vitro when compared to a similar formulation containing the monovalent DOTAP (Bouxsein et al., 2007). The pentavalent lipid allowed the formation of siRNA complexes with five times fewer lipid molecules than DOTAP and resulted in reduced toxicity (Bouxsein et al., 2007). Although the use of multivalent lipids (with higher charge per area) could improve the lipoplex–cell interaction and the endosomal escape, the strong siRNA–MLV (multilamelar vesicles) interaction may compromise the dissociation of the nucleic acid in the cytoplasm after endosomal escape (Ahmad et al., 2005). Other examples of multivalent cationic lipids used for nucleic acid stabilization included di-octadecyl-amido-glycyl-spermine (DOGS; Behr et al., 1989) or β-L-arginyl-2,3-L-diaminopropionic acid-*N*-palmityl-*N*-oleyl-amide trihydrochloride (AtuFECT; Aleku et al., 2008). In addition to the high toxicity, the highly positive surface charge of the complex induced strong interactions with negatively charged serum proteins leading to changes in the complex surface charge and size, accelerating blood clearance by the MPS (Levchenko et al., 2002). Surface coating with hydrophilic molecules, such as poly(ethylene glycol), PEG, may be one of the strategies to overcome this sort of limitation.

The hydrophilic nature of PEG provides an aqueous surface shield that reduces plasma protein binding onto the liposome surface (opsonization) and the subsequent uptake by macrophages from the MPS, resulting in enhanced blood circulation half-life (Suk et al., 2016). Santel et al. developed a siRNA-lipoplex (AtuPLEX) composed of a multivalent cationic lipid (AtuFECT), a neutral phospholipid and a PEGylated lipid (*N*-(carbonyl-methoxypolyethyleneglycol-2000)-1,2-distearoyl-sn-glycero-3-phospho-ethanolamine sodium salt (DSPE-PEG); Santel et al., 2006a). Using siRNAs targeting endothelia-specifically expressed genes, *CD31* (platelet endothelial cell adhesion molecule-1) or *TIE-2*, AtuPLEX enabled the downregulation of the corresponding mRNAs and proteins in mice (Santel et al., 2006a,b), inhibiting tumor growth and reducing the volume of lymph node metastases in two different xenograft mouse models (Santel et al., 2006a).

This led to the development of siRNA-lipoplex formulation (Atu027) targeting the expression of protein kinase N3 (known to control metastases formation; Aleku et al., 2008). In vivo efficacy of Atu027 was demonstrated in orthotopic mouse models of prostate and pancreatic cancers, with significant inhibition of tumor growth and metastization to the lymph nodes (Aleku et al., 2008). Moreover, inhibition of pulmonary metastasis was shown in experimental and spontaneous mouse metastases models (Santel et al., 2010). Silence Therapeutics GmbH presented promising results with its Atu027 formulation in a phase I clinical trial, with 41% of the patients with advanced solid tumors demonstrating stable disease at the end of treatment. Atu027 was well tolerated at a dose level of 336 μg/kg, with residual toxicity (Schultheis et al., 2014). A combination study with Gemcitabine has been initiated in a phase I/II trial for advanced pancreatic cancer (NCT01808638; Table 14.1).

Table 14.1 **Current clinical trials using lipid- and polymer-based nonviral vectors containing siRNA (identification numbers of the clinical trial from https://clinicaltrials.gov/)**

Candidate	Target	Vehicle/ formulation	Route	Condition	Phase	Status	Clinical trial ID	Sponsor
Atu027	*PKN3*	AtuPLEX and AtuRNAi	i.v.	Advanced solid tumors Advanced or metastatic pancreatic adenocarcinoma	I Ib/IIa	Completed Ongoing	NCT00938574 NCT01808638	Silence Therapeutics GmbH
siRNA-EphA2-DOPC	*EphA2*	Neutral liposomes	i.v.	Advanced cancers	I	Recruiting	NCT01591356	M.D. Anderson Cancer Center
TKM 080301	*PLK1*	SNALP	HAI	Colorectal cancer with liver metastases Pancreatic cancer with liver metastases Gastric cancer with liver metastases Breast cancer with liver metastases Ovarian cancer with liver metastases	I	Completed	NCT01437007	National Cancer Institute (NCI)/Arbutus Biopharma Corporation
ND-L02-s0201	*HSP47*	Vitamin A-coupled lipid nanoparticle	i.v.	METAVIR F3-4	I Ib/II	Completed Recruiting	NCT01858935 NCT02227459	Nitto Denko Corporation
DCR-MYC	*MYC*	EnCore lipid nanoparticle	i.v.	Hepatocellular carcinoma Solid tumors Multiple myeloma Nonhodgkins lymphoma	Ib/II I	Recruiting Recruiting	NCT02314052 NCT02110563	Dicerna Pharmaceuticals, Inc.

ALN-TTR01	*TTR*	SNALP	i.v.	ATTR	I	Completed	NCT01148953	Alnylam Pharmaceuticals Inc.
Patisiran (ALN-TTR02)	*TTR*	SNALP	i.v.	ATTR	I II II III III	Completed Completed Ongoing Recruiting Recruiting by invitation	NCT02053454 NCT01617967 NCT01961921 NCT01960348 NCT02510261	Alnylam Pharmaceuticals Inc.
ALN-PCS02	*PCSK9*	SNALP	i.v.	Elevated LDL-C	I	Completed	NCT01437059	Alnylam Pharmaceuticals Inc.
ALN-VSP02	*KSP* and *VEGF*	SNALP	i.v.	Advanced solid tumors with liver involvement	I	Completed	NCT01158079 NCT00882180	Alnylam Pharmaceuticals Inc.
TKM-100201	Multiple	SNALP	i.v.	Ebola virus infection	I	Terminated	NCT01518881	Arbutus Biopharma Corporation
TKM-100802	L polymerase, viral protein 24, viral protein 35	SNALP	i.v.	Ebola virus infection	I	Terminated	NCT02041715	Arbutus Biopharma Corporation
TKM-HBV	Multiple	SNALP	i.v.	HBV	II	Recruiting	NCT02631096	Arbutus Biopharma Corporation

Continued

Table 14.1 Continued

Candidate	Target	Vehicle/ formulation	Route	Condition	Phase	Status	Clinical trial ID	Sponsor
TKM 080301 (TKM-PLK1)	*PLK1*	SNALP	i.v.	Colorectal cancer with liver metastases Gastric cancer with liver metastases Breast cancer with liver metastases Ovarian cancer with liver metastases	I	Completed	NCT01437007	Arbutus Biopharma Corporation
				Neuroendocrine tumors adrenocortical carcinoma	I/II	Completed	NCT01262235	
				Advanced hepatocellular carcinoma	I/II	Recruiting	NCT02191878	
siG12D LODER	*KRAS*^{G12D}	LODER polymer	Implant	Pancreatic ductal adenocarcinoma	I	Completed	NCT01188785	Silenseed Ltd.
				Pancreatic cancer	II	Not yet recruiting	NCT01676259	
SNS01-T	*eIF5A*	PEI-based nanoparticle	i.v.	Multiple myeloma B-cell lymphoma Plasma cell leukemia	I/II	Ongoing	NCT01435720	Senesco Technologies Inc.

ATTR, transthyretin mediated amyloidosis; *HAI*, hepatic arterial infusion; *LDL-C*, LDL-cholesterol; *METAVIR F3-4*, moderate to extensive hepatic fibrosis; *TTR*, transthyretin.

Further efforts in reducing toxicity and reduced blood circulation half-life arising from the positive charge of cationic lipids at physiological pH, primed the development of several ionizable cationic lipids, in particular with a pK_a lower than 7 (Semple et al., 2001). At low pH values (pH ~4), these ionizable lipids display a positive charge that can interact with the negative charged siRNA, enabling efficient encapsulation into liposomes. Moreover, at physiological pH, liposomes exhibit a low positive surface charge that reduces toxicity and increases blood circulation times.

Once in the acidic environment of the endosomes, the positively charged ionizable lipid promotes the destabilization of the endosomal membranes and siRNA release into the cytoplasm. The first ionizable cationic lipid used for the encapsulation of nucleic acids was 1,2-dioleoyl-3-dimethylammonium propane (DODAP; Semple et al., 2001). Since then, several other new ionizable lipids have been synthesized, such as YSK05 (Sato et al., 2012) and 1,2-dilinoleyloxy-3-dimethylaminopropane (DLin-DMA; Morrissey et al., 2005), leading to significant improvements in the in vivo delivery and efficacy of nucleic acid nanoparticles.

These advances led to a hallmark in liposome technology with the development of stabilized nucleic acid lipid particles (SNALP). SNALP are formed by a mixture of ionizable lipid, cholesterol, a high-transition temperature lipid (as 1,2-distearoyl-sn-glycero-3-phosphocholine—DSPC) and a PEG-derivatized lipid that provides a neutral, hydrophilic exterior that shields the lipid bilayer in vivo, preventing rapid blood clearance (Gomes-Da-Silva et al., 2012a). Morrissey et al. successfully demonstrated the persistent in vivo gene silencing activity against a model of hepatitis B upon systemic administration of SNALP, incorporating the ionizable lipid DLin-DMA and containing a siRNA targeting the hepatitis B virus (Morrissey et al., 2005).

The versatility of SNALPs as a delivery platform for siRNA has been extended to the downregulation of polo-like kinase 1 (*PLK1*) and kinesin spindle protein (*KSP*), which are involved in the deregulated proliferation of cancer cells of tumors of diverse histological origins (Judge et al., 2009). The systemic administration of SNALP containing a mixture of anti*PLK1* and anti*KSP* siRNAs displayed potent antitumor efficacy in animal models bearing hepatic orthotopic (tumor growth in the same organ as in the human disease) or subcutaneous tumors, without measurable immune responses (Judge et al., 2009). The potential of this strategy led Tekmira Pharmaceuticals Corporation (now Arbutus Biopharma Corporation) and Alnylam Pharmaceuticals Inc. to apply SNALP to the development of siRNA therapeutics. Tekmira Pharmaceuticals Corporation completed a phase I clinical trial of SNALP-encapsulating siRNA targeting *PLK1* (TKM 080301) in patients with advanced hepatocellular carcinoma (Table 14.1), and SNALP-encapsulating siRNA targeting apolipoprotein B (TKM-ApoB) in patients suffering from hypercholesterolemia. Although TKM-ApoB was well-tolerated and effective in lowering LDL (low density lipoprotein) cholesterol, the trial was terminated owing to the potential for immune stimulation and transient reductions in cholesterol levels (Ozcan et al., 2015).

Alnylam Pharmaceuticals Inc. (in a partnership with Tekmira Pharmaceuticals Corporation) completed a phase I clinical trial with a SNALP formulation (ALN-VSP02), containing two siRNAs targeting *KSP* and vascular endothelial growth factor

(*VEGF*) in patients with advanced solid tumors with liver involvement (Tabernero et al., 2013). Using the DLin-DMA, Alnylam Pharmaceuticals Inc. developed another SNALP encapsulating a siRNA targeting transthyretin (ALN-TTR01) for the treatment of transthyretin mediated amyloidosis (ATTR) that in 2012 completed a phase I clinical trial (Table 14.1).

DLin-DMA, as a starting point for a structure–activity relationship study, primed the identification of other ionizable cationic lipid even more potent for hepatic gene silencing in vivo, such as 1,2-dilinoleyloxy-keto-*N*,*N*-dimethyl-3-aminopropane (DLin-K-DMA), 1,2-dilinoleyl-4-(2-dimethylaminoethyl)-[1,3]-dioxolane (DLin-KC2-DMA; Semple et al., 2010) and heptatriaconta-6,9,28,31-tetraen-19-yl 4-(dimethylamino) butanoate (DLin-MC3-DMA; Jayaraman et al., 2012). This later promising cationic lipid was used for the preparation of second-generation SNALP-siRNA formulations by Alnylam Pharmaceuticals Inc.

In 2012, Alnylam Pharmaceuticals Inc. initiated phase I clinical trials for second generation formulation of antitransthyretin (*TTR*) siRNAs (ALN-TTR02, a.k.a. Patisiran) for the treatment of TTR-mediated amyloidosis, as well as for the ALN-PCS02 formulation, targeting protein convertase subtilisin/kexin type 9 (*PCSK9*) in subjects with elevated LDL cholesterol (Table 14.1). Despite encouraging results in clinical trials with SNALP formulations, Alnylam Pharmaceuticals Inc. has started to apply a novel and promising siRNA-conjugate technology to the ALN-PCS and ALN-TTR development programs. The only exception is the formulation ALN-TTR02 that recently entered a phase III clinical trial (NCT01960348).

After very promising preclinical studies in nonhuman primates (Geisbert et al., 2010), Tekmira Pharmaceuticals Corporation initiated a phase I clinical trial with a formulation (TKM-100201) targeting various Ebola virus components. However, in the same year, the trial was terminated by corporate decision to reformulate the product. In 2014, in collaboration with the United States Department of Defense, a new phase I trial was initiated for the second siRNA-based therapeutic targeting Ebola (TKM-100802, a.k.a. TKM-Ebola-Guine) in healthy volunteers, using the lipid 3-(dilinoleylmethoxy)-*N*,*N*-dimethylpropan-1-amine (DLin-MP-DMA; Table 14.1).

14.2.2 Neutral liposomes

As an alternative strategy to overcome the limitations associated with the systemic administration of positively charged nanoparticles, there has been an increased interest in the use of neutral liposomes. In contrast to charged liposomes, neutral ones present reduced interaction with serum proteins, thereby achieving longer circulation times and presenting lower toxicity (Ozpolat et al., 2014). In 2005, a neutral liposomal formulation composed of 1,2-dioleoyl-sn-glycero-3-phosphatidylcholine (DOPC) for the systemic delivery of siRNA against the oncoprotein *EphA2* was described (Landen et al., 2005). This was translated by a significant in vivo reduction of *EphA2* expression 48 h after a single dose, as well as a tumor growth inhibition (relative to a nonsilencing siRNA), in an orthotropic mouse model of ovarian cancer (Landen et al., 2005).

This formulation has also been shown to be active in other animal models of cancer, including colorectal carcinoma (targeting *Id2*), pancreatic (targeting *TG2*;

Shao et al., 2012), lung and colon (targeting *KRAS*; Pecot et al., 2014), prostatic (targeting TMPRSS2/ERG fusion junctions; Shao et al., 2012), melanoma (targeting *PAR-1*; Villares et al., 2008), and estrogen receptor (−) and (+) breast cancer (targeting *Bcl-2*; Tekedereli et al., 2013), with limited toxicity or immune responses observed after single and repeated administration over 4 weeks (Landen et al., 2005; Ozcan et al., 2015; Shao et al., 2012). Currently, the anti*EphA2* siRNA-encapsulating DOPC liposomes is in a phase I clinical trial for ovarian cancer, sponsored by the M.D. Anderson Cancer Center (NCT01591356; Table 14.1).

14.2.3 Polymeric nonviral vectors

Alternatively to the use of lipids for the development of delivery systems, polymeric materials can be also used as building blocks. As with lipid-based delivery systems for nucleic acids, polymers were first used in gene delivery as a part of the development of new DNA transfection vectors (Wu and Wu, 1987). Polymers can be synthesized in different lengths, with different geometry (linear versus branched), and with substitution or addition of functional groups. As such, there is a wide variety of natural and synthetic polymers currently used for siRNA and DNA delivery, such as chitosan (Yao et al., 2015), polylactic-co-glycolic acid (Lee et al., 2011), or polyethylenimine (PEI; Francis et al., 2014).

Despite the recent advances in the development of polymer-based nonviral vectors for siRNA or DNA delivery, the number of formulations that entered clinical trials has been substantially lower than lipid-based nonviral vectors. In this respect, the first-in-human trial for siRNA delivery was a transferrin-targeted cyclodextrin, CALAA-01 (Fonseca et al., 2014). In 2008, Calando Pharmaceuticals (now part of Arrowhead Research Corporation) started a phase I clinical trial with CALAA-01 for the treatment of melanoma (Zuckerman et al., 2014). The rationale relied on the downregulation of ribonuclease reductase (*RRM2*) upon transferrin-mediated endocytosis of the siRNA-containing nanoparticle (Zuckerman et al., 2014). However, this nanoparticle was further withdrawn (Fonseca et al., 2014).

In 2011, Senesco Technologies Inc. (now Sevion Therapeutics Inc.) initiated a phase I clinical trial (still ongoing, NCT01435720) for safety and tolerability evaluation of SNS01-T in relapsed or refractory B cell malignancies (multiple myeloma, B-cell lymphoma and plasma cell leukemia; Table 14.1). SNS01-T is a nonviral PEI-based nanoparticle designed to target the eukaryotic translational initiation factor 5A (*eIF5A*), which is involved in many cellular functions, including cell proliferation and apoptosis (Francis et al., 2014). The polymeric nanoparticle comprises an anti-*eIF5A* siRNA and a plasmid expressing a pro-apoptotic mutant of *elF5A* to induce apoptosis in B-cell cancers. In preclinical studies, SNS01-T was preferentially taken up by malignant B cells and inhibited tumor growth in multiple xenograft models of B-cell lymphoma (Francis et al., 2014). SNS01-T presented only residual toxicity against normal B-cells and was well-tolerated in all xenograft models evaluated, without significant changes in body weight and behavior (Francis et al., 2014).

In addition, Silenseed Ltd. has developed a miniaturized biodegradable polymeric matrix designed to release regionally, within a pancreatic tumor (SiG12D-LODER), the anti$KRAS^{G12D}$ siRNA (Zorde Khvalevsky et al., 2013). This approach provided a controlled and prolonged local siRNA release within the tumor over several months, while protecting the nucleic acid from degradation. The siRNA remained stable and intact for at least 97 days in saline and 60 days in mouse liver tissue (Zorde Khvalevsky et al., 2013). Preclinical studies demonstrated that when implanted in subcutaneous and orthotopic pancreatic tumors, it significantly reduced tumor volume and prolonged mouse survival. Implantation of siG12D-LODER into the pancreas did not affect either body or liver weight, or animal behavior (Zorde Khvalevsky et al., 2013).

In 2013, Silenseed Ltd. has completed an open label, multicenter, phase I/IIa study (NCT01188785) in patients with nonoperable, locally advanced pancreatic cancer (LAPC) in combination with chemotherapy (Gemcitabine and FOLFIRINOX; Golan et al., 2015). From 15 patients enrolled in the trial, 12 did not demonstrate evidence of tumor progression, with the majority (10 of 12) presenting stable disease and two demonstrating partial response as evaluated by computerized tomography (Golan et al., 2015). Decrease in the level of pancreatic tumor biomarker CA19-9 was observed in 70% of patients, with a median overall survival of 15.12 months (Golan et al., 2015). This was in contrast with the median overall survival of 9–13 months for patients receiving only Gemcitabine (Golan et al., 2015; Loehrer et al., 2011; Chauffert et al., 2008). The combination of siG12D-LODER and chemotherapy was well-tolerated and no dose-limiting toxicity events were observed during the study (Golan et al., 2015). siG12D-LODER is currently entering phase II trial for LAPC (NCT01676259; Table 14.1).

Despite the overall success with lipid and polymeric-based nucleic acid delivery, it has been conceptualized that simpler systems may achieve similar results in terms of delivery and knockdown efficacy. As such, siRNA-conjugates are being explored as therapeutic platforms.

14.3 siRNA-conjugate delivery systems: Down to the essential

The use of conjugation techniques enabling the covalent link of an active molecule to another molecule with the objective of modulating and improving their physicochemical and PK properties, as well as the biological activity, is well-established. Successful examples of this strategy that have been clinically approved include (PEG)-interferon alpha-2b (PegIntron) for the treatment of hepatitis B; or anti-CD30 antibody conjugated to a microtubule inhibitor, monomethyl auristatin for the treatment of Hodgkin lymphoma (Adcetris). Most importantly, several other conjugates are currently in preclinical phase or in clinical trials, including oligonucleotide-conjugates, such as those containing siRNAs. In recent years, there have been promising advances in siRNA-conjugates aimed at improving their ability to overcome extracellular and intracellular barriers in vivo. Cholesterol and alpha-tocopherol (Nishina et al., 2008), peptides (Moschos et al., 2007), carbohydrates (Nair et al., 2014), and polymers (Kim et al., 2006) are currently being investigated in preclinical studies for conjugation with siRNA. Among these, two siRNA-conjugates are currently in clinical trials and have produced some promising results: dynamic polyconjugates (DPCs) developed by Arrowhead Research Corporation and GalNAc-conjugated siRNA developed by Alnylam Pharmaceuticals Inc. (Table 14.2).

14.3.1 Dynamic polyconjugates

DPCs are small nanoparticles, 5–20 nm in size, that combine an amphipathic polymer to which an siRNA is linked by a disulfide bond, while a shielding agent and a targeting ligand towards hepatocytes are reversibly attached by an acid-labile maleamate linkage that masks the membrane active moieties of the polymer (Rozema et al., 2007). Upon cell internalization, the acidic pH in the endosome triggers the release of the shielding agent and targeting ligand, exposing the endosomolytic activity of the polymer that enables the destabilization of the endosome membrane and escape of the siRNA from the endocytic pathway into the cytoplasm. The siRNA is further released from the polymer via cleavage of disulfide bond in the reductive environment of the cytoplasm, becoming bioavailable to exert its action (Rozema et al., 2007).

This multifunctional platform was initially described by Rozema et al., using an amphipathic polybutylamino vinyl ether polymer (PBAVE; Wakefield et al., 2005), PEG as the shielding agent and the hepatocyte targeting ligand *N*-acetylgalactosamine (NAG; Rozema et al., 2007). Anti-apoB and antiperoxisome proliferator-activated receptor alpha siRNAs DPCs demonstrated an effective knockdown of the two endogenous genes in mouse liver, following intravenous administration, with 64% and 76% mRNA and protein downregulation, respectively. Furthermore, this effect was achieved without major toxicity as assessed by serum levels of hepatic enzymes and cytokines (Rozema et al., 2007). In a later report, Wong et al., demonstrated that the cholesterol-siRNA silencing effect in mouse hepatocytes could be significantly improved by co-administration with the NAG–PEG–PBAVE complex, without the need of siRNA chemical bonding. This observation allowed a simplification in the formulation procedure and enabled the use of other endosomolytic agents for siRNA delivery to liver hepatocytes (Wong et al., 2012).

This was the basis for the development of a *second generation* DPC, named ARC-520, which is currently in phase II clinical trial for the treatment of hepatitis B (Table 14.2). In ARC-520, the previous endosomolytic PBAVE polymer was replaced with a melittin-like peptide (MLP) with a well-defined structure. In addition, there is no chemical link between the siRNA and the polymer. Thus, ARC-520 consists of two individual components: cholesterol–siRNA conjugates and hepatocyte-targeting membrane-active peptides linked to the MLP polymer.

In preclinical studies, single administration of 6 mg ARC-520/kg into transient and transgenic mouse models of HBV infection demonstrated a significant and long-term decrease (over 3 weeks) of viral RNA, proteins and viral DNA. In nonhuman primates chronically infected with hepatitis B virus, a low dose of ARC-520 induced a 95% reduction in circulating viral DNA and, approximately, 90% reduction in hepatitis e-antigen and s-antigen (Wooddell et al., 2013). Besides Arrowhead, other companies like Alnylam, Benitec Biopharma and Tekmira are also developing siRNA delivery strategies for the treatment of hepatitis B.

In addition to ARC-520, Arrowhead is further exploring the DPC delivery platform for the treatment of the liver disease associated with alpha-1 antitrypsin (*AAT*) deficiency (ARC-AAT). In a transgenic mouse model, it induced 95% reduction in circulating AAT after a single dose. This effect was confirmed in a nonhuman primate, where knockdown of serum AAT persisted for over 10 weeks, with a greater than 80% knockdown observed at the 6-week time point. ARC-AAT is now in phase I clinical trial (NCT02363946; Table 14.2). Despite the focus on liver targeting, the versatility of the DPC to incorporate different targeting peptides or siRNAs led Arrowhead to expand their preclinical development programs for the treatment of several types of tumors (in particular hepatocellular carcinoma), thrombosis and angioedema and cardiovascular diseases.

14.3.2 GalNAc-conjugated siRNA

Despite the success on intravenous siRNA delivery using SNALP for the treatment of transthyretin-mediated amyloidosis (ALN-TTR02, Patisiran) or the regulation of blood cholesterol (ALN-PCS02; Akinc et al., 2010), Alnylam Pharmaceuticals Inc. is currently taking an alternate delivery approach. This approach involves the covalent linkage of engineered siRNA with trivalent *N*-acetylgalactosamine (*triantennary* GalNAc), a ligand targeting for the asialoglycoprotein receptor expressed in hepatocytes.

More recently, in 2014, Alnylam Pharmaceuticals Inc. announced their Enhanced Stabilization Chemistry (ESC)-GalNAc-conjugate delivery platform, involving siRNA chemical modifications (with 2′-F, 2′-O-Me sugar modification and phosphorothioate linkage). The ability to enhance the in vitro stability against nuclease degradation was demonstrated, enabling increased in vivo liver exposure and potency, as well as durability of effect as compared with early GalNAc-conjugates.

A subcutaneous administration in mice of a single dose of 25 mg of siRNA/kg, resulted in a downregulation of hepatic TTR mRNA higher than 80%, 24 h post dose (ED50 at 1 mg/kg), representing a fivefold improvement in efficacy over the parent design control (Nair et al., 2014). Furthermore, these data demonstrated the potential for subcutaneous administration at therapeutically relevant doses and, most importantly, at dose volumes lower than 1 mL, a significant advantage over the large volumes needed intravenous infusion of lipid or polymeric-based siRNA delivery (Nair et al., 2014).

Using the GalNAc platform, Alnylam Pharmaceuticals Inc. is currently focused in three strategic areas (Genetic medicines, Cardio-metabolic diseases and hepatic infectious diseases) with more than 15 siRNA therapies under development, including five currently in clinical trials for the treatment of transthyretin amyloidosis (ALN-TTRsc, revusiran), hemophilia (ALN-AT3), complement-mediated diseases (ALN-AS1), hepatic porphyrias (ALN-CC5) and hypercholesterolemia (ALN-PCSsc). Currently on phase II open-label extension studies, Alnylam Pharmaceuticals Inc. reported that ALN-TTRsc (revusiran, RNAi targeting transthyretin, TTR) demonstrated robust and sustained knockdown of serum TTR. It appeared to be generally well-tolerated in the majority of patients with TTR cardiac amyloidosis, up to 10 months of treatment, the longest human dosing experience for a GalNAc-siRNA conjugate reported to date.

Table 14.2 **Current clinical trials using siRNA-conjugates (identification numbers of the clinical trial from https://clinicaltrials.gov/)**

Candidate	Target	Vehicle/formulation	Route	Condition	Phase	Status	Clinical trial ID	Sponsor
ALN-AT3SC	*AT*	GalNAc-siRNA conjugate	s.c.	Hemophilia A	I	Recruiting	NCT02035605	Alnylam Pharmaceuticals Inc.
				Hemophilia B	I/II	Recruiting	NCT02554773	
ALN-CC5	*C5*	GalNAc-siRNA conjugate	s.c.	PNH	I/II	Recruiting	NCT02352493	
ALN-AAT	*AAT*	GalNAc-siRNA conjugate	s.c.	ZZ type alpha-1 antitrypsin deficiency liver disease	I/II	Recruiting	NCT02503683	
ALN-PCSSC	*PCSK9*	GalNAc-siRNA conjugate	s.c.	Hypercholesterolemia	I	Ongoing	NCT02314442	
ALN-AS1	*ALAS1*	GalNAc-siRNA conjugate	s.c.	AIP	I	Recruiting	NCT02452372	
Revusiran (ALN-TTRSC)	*TTR*	GalNAc-siRNA conjugate	s.c.	TTR-mediated amyloidosis	I	Ongoing	NCT01814839	
					II	Completed	NCT01981837	
					II	Ongoing	NCT02292186	
				TTR-mediated familial amyloidotic cardiomyopathy	III	Recruiting	NCT02319005	
ARC-520	Conserved HBV sequences	DPC	i.v.	Hepatitis B	II	Recruiting	NCT02604199	Arrowhead Research Corporation
				Hepatitis B	II	Recruiting	NCT02604212	
				Chronic hepatitis B	II	Recruiting	NCT02452528	
				Healthy	I	Completed	NCT01872065	
				Hepatitis B	II	Recruiting	NCT02577029	
				Chronic hepatitis B	II	Recruiting	NCT02065336	
				Healthy	I	Recruiting	NCT02535416	
ARC-AAT	*AAT*	DPC	i.v.	AATD	I	Recruiting	NCT02363946	

AIP, acute intermittent porphyria; *PNH*, paroxysmal nocturnal hemoglobinuria.

More recently, the ALN-AT3 (RNAi targeting antithrombin; Sehgal et al., 2015) entered a phase I clinical trial with healthy volunteers (NCT02035605) and then patients with moderate or severe hemophilia A and B (NCT02554773).

ALN-CC5 (RNAi targeting complement component C5) is currently on a phase I/II clinical trials to evaluate the safety, tolerability, PKs and pharmacodynamics in healthy adult volunteers and subjects with paroxysmal nocturnal hemoglobinuria (NCT02352493). Recently, Alnylam reported that ALN-CC5 achieved up to 99% knockdown of serum C5 complement component. Most importantly, ALN-CC5 was shown to be generally well-tolerated, with no clinically significant drug-related adverse events. Additionally, ALN-AS1 an RNAi therapeutic agent targeting aminolevulinic acid synthase 1, demonstrated in a phase I clinical trial, following a single subcutaneous administration, a downregulation up to 82% of delta-aminolevulinic acid and 93% downregulation of porphobilinogen (the toxic heme entity that mediates porphyria; NCT02452372).

In 2015, Alnylam Pharmaceuticals Inc. presented initial data from a phase I trial of ALN-PCSsc (NCT02314442) in subjects with elevated LDL cholesterol (LDL-C). Subcutaneous administration of ALN-PCSsc resulted in 83% lowering of LDL-C, at dose of 300 mg. The effects were highly durable, with clinically significant reductions in LDL-C maintained for over 140 days, thus supporting a once-quarterly and possibly bi-annual subcutaneous dose regimen.

14.4 Future perspectives and challenges

Many of the principles discussed throughout this chapter may be applied to other molecules mediating RNAi, such as miRNAs. In contrast with siRNA technology, miRNAs enable the simultaneous silencing of multiple targets (Wang et al., 2015). As an example, a liposomal formulation of miR-34 (MRX34) is entering phase I clinical trial (NCT01829971). miR-34 is a potent antitumor miRNA known to modulate different target proteins involved in the cell cycle, differentiation and apoptosis (Misso et al., 2014). Yet, either siRNA- or miRNA-based therapeutics rely solely on RNAi to achieve its effect.

The advent of novel genomic-editing tools is a potential game changer on gene therapy-based strategies. Gene editing has been used for quite some time, but has remained mainly limited to basic science. Nevertheless, the introduction of programmable nucleases, like TALEN (transcription activator-like effector nucleases) and more recently the CRISPR/Cas9 (clustered regularly interspaced short palindromic repeat-associated nuclease Cas9) opened the door to the development of genomic-editing therapeutics for different diseases (Cox et al., 2015). These technologies have been adapted to introduce double strand breaks in a sequence-specific manner, to trigger the action of various DNA repair pathways, such as homology-directed repair or nonhomologous end joining, enabling the excision of a defective gene or the insertion of wild-type or enhanced genes (Seah et al., 2015).

Despite effective, the TALENs recognize the DNA by specific protein–DNA interaction, whereas CRISPR/Cas9 system is targeted to specific DNA sequences by a short RNA guide molecule that base-pairs directly with the target DNA and by protein–DNA interactions, unleashing unprecedented specificity for editing (Cox et al., 2015). Upon engineering the guide RNA, Cas endonucleases (most commonly Cas9 from *Streptococcus pyogenes*) can be programmed to trigger a double-strand break at any desired genomic locus, followed by a DNA repair that can result in precise changes in the gene of interest (Jinek et al., 2012). In contrast to other nuclease systems, CRISPR/Cas9 system is cheap, quick and easy to construct and does not need protein engineering for redirecting the system to new target sites, thus supporting the relevance that this technology is gaining (Seah et al., 2015).

The programmable nucleases have enabled gene editing in several models of diseases (Cox et al., 2015), and despite it being simple to achieve, the delivery of such nucleases is currently limited to the use of viral vectors, which has limited its use to ex vivo applications, such as correction of T cell function (Perez et al., 2008). Nevertheless, systemic delivery of nuclease systems with nonviral vectors may be developed encompassing all the currently available knowledge associated with oligonucleotide delivery, exploring the potential of lipid-based nonviral vectors, cell penetrating peptides, as well as the novel and more efficient nucleases (Hsu et al., 2014; Zetsche et al., 2015).

In addition, the described technologies may benefit from active targeting, promoting the accumulation and internalization of the therapeutic agent in cells of tissues other than the liver (Gomes-Da-Silva et al., 2012a; Fonseca et al., 2014). Several new technologies are undergoing preclinical study, presenting the potential to change landscape of targeted therapeutic strategies (Lorenzer et al., 2015) and exploiting different targeting moieties, including peptides, aptamers, or monoclonal antibodies (Meissner et al., 2015; Sato et al., 2012; Hada et al., 2015; Gomes-Da-Silva et al., 2012b, 2013a,b).

The different paths and technologies herein explored are examples of how the knowledge of genome and gene manipulation may reflect the future of therapeutic intervention on a vast range of diseases. From RNAi to gene editing, the different strategies have advantages and disadvantages, which will have to be considered and likely may be a part of a truly personalized therapeutic intervention.

Acknowledgments

R. Lopes was a recipient of a post-doc fellowship from "Incentivo 2014—Estímulo à contratação e retenção de recursos humanos" from the Portuguese Foundation for Science and Technology (FCT). A.F. Cruz was a recipient of the fellowship SFRH/BD/85554/2012 from FCT. Ana C. Gregório and Ângela Valério-Fernandes were students of PhD Program in Experimental Biology and Biomedicine (PDBEB), Center for Neuroscience and Cell Biology, University of Coimbra, and recipients of the FCT fellowships SFRH/BD/51190/2010 and SFRH/BD/51191/2010, respectively. The work was supported by the grant PEst-C/SAU/LA0001/2013-2014.

References

Ahmad, A., Evans, H.M., Ewert, K., George, C.X., Samuel, C.E., Safinya, C.R., 2005. New multivalent cationic lipids reveal bell curve for transfection efficiency versus membrane charge density: lipid-DNA complexes for gene delivery. J. Gene Med. 7, 739–748.

Akinc, A., Querbes, W., De, S., Qin, J., Frank-Kamenetsky, M., Jayaprakash, K.N., Jayaraman, M., Rajeev, K.G., Cantley, W.L., Dorkin, J.R., Butler, J.S., Qin, L., Racie, T., Sprague, A., Fava, E., Zeigerer, A., Hope, M.J., Zerial, M., Sah, D.W., Fitzgerald, K., Tracy, M.A., Manoharan, M., Koteliansky, V., Fougerolles, A., Maier, M.A., 2010. Targeted delivery of RNAi therapeutics with endogenous and exogenous ligand-based mechanisms. Mol. Ther. 18, 1357–1364.

Aleku, M., Schulz, P., Keil, O., Santel, A., Schaeper, U., Dieckhoff, B., Janke, O., Endruschat, J., Durieux, B., Roder, N., Loffler, K., Lange, C., Fechtner, M., Mopert, K., Fisch, G., Dames, S., Arnold, W., Jochims, K., Giese, K., Wiedenmann, B., Scholz, A., Kaufmann, J., 2008. Atu027, a liposomal small interfering RNA formulation targeting protein kinase N3, inhibits cancer progression. Cancer Res. 68, 9788–9798.

Andtbacka, R.H., Kaufman, H.L., Collichio, F., Amatruda, T., Senzer, N., Chesney, J., Delman, K.A., Spitler, L.E., Puzanov, I., Agarwala, S.S., Milhem, M., Cranmer, L., Curti, B., Lewis, K., Ross, M., Guthrie, T., Linette, G.P., Daniels, G.A., Harrington, K., Middleton, M.R., Miller Jr., W.H., Zager, J.S., Ye, Y., Yao, B., Li, A., Doleman, S., Vanderwalde, A., Gansert, J., Coffin, R.S., 2015. Talimogene laherparepvec improves durable response rate in patients with advanced melanoma. J. Clin. Oncol. 33, 2780–2788.

Behr, J.P., Demeneix, B., Loeffler, J.P., Perez-Mutul, J., 1989. Efficient gene transfer into mammalian primary endocrine cells with lipopolyamine-coated DNA. Proc. Natl. Acad. Sci. USA 86, 6982–6986.

Bieging, K.T., Mello, S.S., Attardi, L.D., 2014. Unravelling mechanisms of p53-mediated tumour suppression. Nat. Rev. Cancer 14, 359–370.

Boudreau, R.L., Davidson, B.L., 2012. Generation of hairpin-based RNAi vectors for biological and therapeutic application. Methods Enzymol. 507, 275–296.

Bouxsein, N.F., McAllister, C.S., Ewert, K.K., Samuel, C.E., Safinya, C.R., 2007. Structure and gene silencing activities of monovalent and pentavalent cationic lipid vectors complexed with siRNA. Biochemistry 46, 4785–4792.

Brigham, K.L., Meyrick, B., Christman, B., Magnuson, M., King, G., Berry Jr., L.C., 1989. In vivo transfection of murine lungs with a functioning prokaryotic gene using a liposome vehicle. Am. J. Med. Sci. 298, 278–281.

Brummelkamp, T.R., Bernards, R., Agami, R., 2002a. Stable suppression of tumorigenicity by virus-mediated RNA interference. Cancer Cell 2, 243–247.

Brummelkamp, T.R., Bernards, R., Agami, R., 2002b. A system for stable expression of short interfering RNAs in mammalian cells. Science 296, 550–553.

Chauffert, B., Mornex, F., Bonnetain, F., Rougier, P., Mariette, C., Bouche, O., Bosset, J.F., Aparicio, T., Mineur, L., Azzedine, A., Hammel, P., Butel, J., Stremsdoerfer, N., Maingon, P., Bedenne, L., 2008. Phase III trial comparing intensive induction chemoradiotherapy (60 Gy, infusional 5-FU and intermittent cisplatin) followed by maintenance gemcitabine with gemcitabine alone for locally advanced unresectable pancreatic cancer. Definitive results of the 2000-01 FFCD/SFRO study. Ann. Oncol. 19, 1592–1599.

Cox, D.B., Platt, R.J., Zhang, F., 2015. Therapeutic genome editing: prospects and challenges. Nat. Med. 21, 121–131.

Dokka, S., Toledo, D., Shi, X.G., Castranova, V., Rojanasakul, Y., 2000. Oxygen radical-mediated pulmonary toxicity induced by some cationic liposomes. Pharm. Res. 17, 521–525.

Elbashir, S.M., Harborth, J., Lendeckel, W., Yalcin, A., Weber, K., Tuschl, T., 2001. Duplexes of 21-nucleotide RNAs mediate RNA interference in cultured mammalian cells. Nature 411, 494–498.

Felgner, P.L., Gadek, T.R., Holm, M., Roman, R., Chan, H.W., Wenz, M., Northrop, J.P., Ringold, G.M., Danielsen, M., 1987. Lipofection: a highly efficient, lipid-mediated DNA-transfection procedure. Proc. Natl. Acad. Sci. USA 84, 7413–7417.

Fire, A., Xu, S., Montgomery, M.K., Kostas, S.A., Driver, S.E., Mello, C.C., 1998. Potent and specific genetic interference by double-stranded RNA in Caenorhabditis elegans. Nature 391, 806–811.

Fonseca, N.A., Gregorio, A.C., Valerio-Fernandes, A., Simoes, S., Moreira, J.N., 2014. Bridging cancer biology and the patients' needs with nanotechnology-based approaches. Cancer Treat. Rev. 40, 626–635.

Francis, S.M., Taylor, C.A., Tang, T., Liu, Z., Zheng, Q., Dondero, R., Thompson, J.E., 2014. SNS01-T modulation of eIF5A inhibits B-cell cancer progression and synergizes with bortezomib and lenalidomide. Mol. Ther. 22, 1643–1652.

Geisbert, T.W., Lee, A.C., Robbins, M., Geisbert, J.B., Honko, A.N., Sood, V., Johnson, J.C., De Jong, S., Tavakoli, I., Judge, A., Hensley, L.E., Maclachlan, I., 2010. Postexposure protection of non-human primates against a lethal Ebola virus challenge with RNA interference: a proof-of-concept study. Lancet 375, 1896–1905.

Golan, T., Khvalevsky, E.Z., Hubert, A., Gabai, R.M., Hen, N., Segal, A., Domb, A., Harari, G., David, E.B., Raskin, S., Goldes, Y., Goldin, E., Eliakim, R., Lahav, M., Kopleman, Y., Dancour, A., Shemi, A., Galun, E., 2015. RNAi therapy targeting KRAS in combination with chemotherapy for locally advanced pancreatic cancer patients. Oncotarget 6, 24560–24570.

Gomes-Da-Silva,L.C.,Fonseca,N.A.,Moura,V.,PedrosoDeLima,M.C.,Simoes,S.,Moreira,J.N., 2012a. Lipid-based nanoparticles for siRNA delivery in cancer therapy: paradigms and challenges. Acc. Chem. Res. 45, 1163–1171.

Gomes-Da-Silva, L.C., Santos, A.O., Bimbo, L.M., Moura, V., Ramalho, J.S., Lima, M.C., Simoes, S., Moreira, J.N., 2012b. Towards a siRNA-containing nanoparticle targeted to breast cancer cells and the tumor microenvironment. Int. J. Pharm. 434, 9–19.

Gomes-Da-Silva, L.C., Fernandez, Y., Abasolo, I., Schwartz Jr., S., Ramalho, J.S., Pedroso De Lima, M.C., Simoes, S., Moreira, J.N., 2013a. Efficient intracellular delivery of siRNA with a safe multitargeted lipid-based nanoplatform. Nanomedicine (Lond.) 8, 1397–1413.

Gomes-Da-Silva, L.C., Ramalho, J.S., Pedroso De Lima, M.C., Simoes, S., Moreira, J.N., 2013b. Impact of anti-PLK1 siRNA-containing F3-targeted liposomes on the viability of both cancer and endothelial cells. Eur. J. Pharm. Biopharm. 85, 356–364.

Hada, T., Sakurai, Y., Harashima, H., 2015. Optimization of a siRNA carrier modified with a pH-sensitive cationic lipid and a cyclic RGD peptide for efficiently targeting tumor endothelial cells. Pharmaceutics 7, 320–333.

Harris, M.P., Sutjipto, S., Wills, K.N., Hancock, W., Cornell, D., Johnson, D.E., Gregory, R.J., Shepard, H.M., Maneval, D.C., 1996. Adenovirus-mediated p53 gene transfer inhibits growth of human tumor cells expressing mutant p53 protein. Cancer Gene Ther. 3, 121–130.

Haussecker, D., 2014. Current issues of RNAi therapeutics delivery and development. J. Control. Release 195, 49–54.

Hsu, P.D., Lander, E.S., Zhang, F., 2014. Development and applications of CRISPR-Cas9 for genome engineering. Cell 157, 1262–1278.

Ibraheem, D., Elaissari, A., Fessi, H., 2014. Gene therapy and DNA delivery systems. Int. J. Pharm. 459, 70–83.

Ipsaro, J.J., Joshua-Tor, L., 2015. From guide to target: molecular insights into eukaryotic RNA-interference machinery. Nat. Struct. Mol. Biol. 22, 20–28.
Jayaraman, M., Ansell, S.M., Mui, B.L., Tam, Y.K., Chen, J., Du, X., Butler, D., Eltepu, L., Matsuda, S., Narayanannair, J.K., Rajeev, K.G., Hafez, I.M., Akinc, A., Maier, M.A., Tracy, M.A., Cullis, P.R., Madden, T.D., Manoharan, M., Hope, M.J., 2012. Maximizing the potency of siRNA lipid nanoparticles for hepatic gene silencing in vivo. Angew. Chem. Int. Ed. Engl. 51, 8529–8533.
Jinek, M., Chylinski, K., Fonfara, I., Hauer, M., Doudna, J.A., Charpentier, E., 2012. A programmable dual-RNA-guided DNA endonuclease in adaptive bacterial immunity. Science 337, 816–821.
Judge, A.D., Robbins, M., Tavakoli, I., Levi, J., Hu, L., Fronda, A., Ambegia, E., Mcclintock, K., Maclachlan, I., 2009. Confirming the RNAi-mediated mechanism of action of siRNA-based cancer therapeutics in mice. J. Clin. Invest. 119, 661–673.
Kim, S.H., Jeong, J.H., Lee, S.H., Kim, S.W., Park, T.G., 2006. PEG conjugated VEGF siRNA for anti-angiogenic gene therapy. J. Control. Release 116, 123–129.
Kwok, A., Hart, S.L., 2011. Comparative structural and functional studies of nanoparticle formulations for DNA and siRNA delivery. Nanomedicine 7, 210–219.
Landen, C.N., Chavez-Reyes, A., Bucana, C., Schmandt, R., Deavers, M.T., Lopez-Berestein, G., Sood, A.K., 2005. Therapeutic EphA2 gene targeting in vivo using neutral liposomal small interfering RNA delivery. Cancer Res. 65, 6910–6918.
Ledford, H., 2015. Cancer-fighting viruses win approval. Nature 526, 622–623.
Lee, S.H., Mok, H., Lee, Y., Park, T.G., 2011. Self-assembled siRNA–PLGA conjugate micelles for gene silencing. J. Control. Release 152, 152–158.
Levchenko, T.S., Rammohan, R., Lukyanov, A.N., Whiteman, K.R., Torchilin, V.P., 2002. Liposome clearance in mice: the effect of a separate and combined presence of surface charge and polymer coating. Int. J. Pharm. 240, 95–102.
Loehrer Sr., P.J., Feng, Y., Cardenes, H., Wagner, L., Brell, J.M., Cella, D., Flynn, P., Ramanathan, R.K., Crane, C.H., Alberts, S.R., Benson 3rd., A.B., 2011. Gemcitabine alone versus gemcitabine plus radiotherapy in patients with locally advanced pancreatic cancer: an Eastern Cooperative Oncology Group trial. J. Clin. Oncol. 29, 4105–4112.
Lorenzer, C., Dirin, M., Winkler, A.M., Baumann, V., Winkler, J., 2015. Going beyond the liver: progress and challenges of targeted delivery of siRNA therapeutics. J. Control. Release 203, 1–15.
Lv, H., Zhang, S., Wang, B., Cui, S., Yan, J., 2006. Toxicity of cationic lipids and cationic polymers in gene delivery. J. Control. Release 114, 100–109.
Meissner, J.M., Toporkiewicz, M., Czogalla, A., Matusewicz, L., Kuliczkowski, K., Sikorski, A.F., 2015. Novel antisense therapeutics delivery systems: in vitro and in vivo studies of liposomes targeted with anti-CD20 antibody. J. Control. Release 220, 515–528.
Misso, G., Di Martino, M.T., De Rosa, G., Farooqi, A.A., Lombardi, A., Campani, V., Zarone, M.R., Gulla, A., Tagliaferri, P., Tassone, P., Caraglia, M., 2014. Mir-34: a new weapon against cancer? Mol. Ther. Nucleic Acids 3, e194.
Moore, C.B., Guthrie, E.H., Huang, M.T., Taxman, D.J., 2010. Short hairpin RNA (shRNA): design, delivery, and assessment of gene knockdown. Methods Mol. Biol. 629, 141–158.
Morrissey, D.V., Lockridge, J.A., Shaw, L., Blanchard, K., Jensen, K., Breen, W., Hartsough, K., Machemer, L., Radka, S., Jadhav, V., Vaish, N., Zinnen, S., Vargeese, C., Bowman, K., Shaffer, C.S., Jeffs, L.B., Judge, A., Maclachlan, I., Polisky, B., 2005. Potent and persistent in vivo anti-HBV activity of chemically modified siRNAs. Nat. Biotechnol. 23, 1002–1007.

Moschos, S.A., Jones, S.W., Perry, M.M., Williams, A.E., Erjefalt, J.S., Turner, J.J., Barnes, P.J., Sproat, B.S., Gait, M.J., Lindsay, M.A., 2007. Lung delivery studies using siRNA conjugated to TAT(48-60) and penetratin reveal peptide induced reduction in gene expression and induction of innate immunity. Bioconjug. Chem. 18, 1450–1459.

Nabel, G.J., Nabel, E.G., Yang, Z.Y., Fox, B.A., Plautz, G.E., Gao, X., Huang, L., Shu, S., Gordon, D., Chang, A.E., 1993. Direct gene transfer with DNA-liposome complexes in melanoma: expression, biologic activity, and lack of toxicity in humans. Proc. Natl. Acad. Sci. USA 90, 11307–11311.

Nair, J.K., Willoughby, J.L., Chan, A., Charisse, K., Alam, M.R., Wang, Q., Hoekstra, M., Kandasamy, P., Kel'in, A.V., Milstein, S., Taneja, N., O'Shea, J., Shaikh, S., Zhang, L., Van Der Sluis, R.J., Jung, M.E., Akinc, A., Hutabarat, R., Kuchimanchi, S., Fitzgerald, K., Zimmermann, T., Van Berkel, T.J., Maier, M.A., Rajeev, K.G., Manoharan, M., 2014. Multivalent N-acetylgalactosamine-conjugated siRNA localizes in hepatocytes and elicits robust RNAi-mediated gene silencing. J. Am. Chem. Soc. 136, 16958–16961.

Nishina, K., Unno, T., Uno, Y., Kubodera, T., Kanouchi, T., Mizusawa, H., Yokota, T., 2008. Efficient in vivo delivery of siRNA to the liver by conjugation of alpha-tocopherol. Mol. Ther. 16, 734–740.

Ozcan, G., Ozpolat, B., Coleman, R.L., Sood, A.K., Lopez-Berestein, G., 2015. Preclinical and clinical development of siRNA-based therapeutics. Adv. Drug Deliv. Rev. 87, 108–119.

Ozpolat, B., Sood, A.K., Lopez-Berestein, G., 2014. Liposomal siRNA nanocarriers for cancer therapy. Adv. Drug Deliv. Rev. 66, 110–116.

Pecot, C.V., Wu, S.Y., Bellister, S., Filant, J., Rupaimoole, R., Hisamatsu, T., Bhattacharya, R., Maharaj, A., Azam, S., Rodriguez-Aguayo, C., Nagaraja, A.S., Morelli, M.P., Gharpure, K.M., Waugh, T.A., Gonzalez-Villasana, V., Zand, B., Dalton, H.J., Kopetz, S., Lopez-Berestein, G., Ellis, L.M., Sood, A.K., 2014. Therapeutic silencing of KRAS using systemically delivered siRNAs. Mol. Cancer Ther. 13, 2876–2885.

Perez, E.E., Wang, J., Miller, J.C., Jouvenot, Y., Kim, K.A., Liu, O., Wang, N., Lee, G., Bartsevich, V.V., Lee, Y.L., Guschin, D.Y., Rupniewski, I., Waite, A.J., Carpenito, C., Carroll, R.G., Orange, J.S., Urnov, F.D., Rebar, E.J., Ando, D., Gregory, P.D., Riley, J.L., Holmes, M.C., June, C.H., 2008. Establishment of HIV-1 resistance in CD4+ T cells by genome editing using zinc-finger nucleases. Nat. Biotechnol. 26, 808–816.

Rozema, D.B., Lewis, D.L., Wakefield, D.H., Wong, S.C., Klein, J.J., Roesch, P.L., Bertin, S.L., Reppen, T.W., Chu, Q., Blokhin, A.V., Hagstrom, J.E., Wolff, J.A., 2007. Dynamic polyconjugates for targeted in vivo delivery of siRNA to hepatocytes. Proc. Natl. Acad. Sci. USA 104, 12982–12987.

Santel, A., Aleku, M., Keil, O., Endruschat, J., Esche, V., Fisch, G., Dames, S., Loffler, K., Fechtner, M., Arnold, W., Giese, K., Klippel, A., Kaufmann, J., 2006a. A novel siRNA-lipoplex technology for RNA interference in the mouse vascular endothelium. Gene Ther. 13, 1222–1234.

Santel, A., Aleku, M., Keil, O., Endruschat, J., Esche, V., Durieux, B., Loffler, K., Fechtner, M., Rohl, T., Fisch, G., Dames, S., Arnold, W., Giese, K., Klippel, A., Kaufmann, J., 2006b. RNA interference in the mouse vascular endothelium by systemic administration of siRNA-lipoplexes for cancer therapy. Gene Ther. 13, 1360–1370.

Santel, A., Aleku, M., Roder, N., Mopert, K., Durieux, B., Janke, O., Keil, O., Endruschat, J., Dames, S., Lange, C., Eisermann, M., Loffler, K., Fechtner, M., Fisch, G., Vank, C., Schaeper, U., Giese, K., Kaufmann, J., 2010. Atu027 prevents pulmonary metastasis in experimental and spontaneous mouse metastasis models. Clin. Cancer Res. 16, 5469–5480.

Sarett, S.M., Nelson, C.E., Duvall, C.L., 2015. Technologies for controlled, local delivery of siRNA. J. Control. Release 218, 94–113.

Sato, Y., Hatakeyama, H., Sakurai, Y., Hyodo, M., Akita, H., Harashima, H., 2012. A pH-sensitive cationic lipid facilitates the delivery of liposomal siRNA and gene silencing activity in vitro and in vivo. J. Control. Release 163, 267–276.

Schultheis, B., Strumberg, D., Santel, A., Vank, C., Gebhardt, F., Keil, O., Lange, C., Giese, K., Kaufmann, J., Khan, M., Drevs, J., 2014. First-in-human phase I study of the liposomal RNA interference therapeutic Atu027 in patients with advanced solid tumors. J. Clin. Oncol. 32, 4141–4148.

Seah, Y.F., El Farran, C.A., Warrier, T., Xu, J., Loh, Y.H., 2015. Induced pluripotency and gene editing in disease modelling: perspectives and challenges. Int. J. Mol. Sci. 16, 28614–28634.

Sehgal, A., Barros, S., Ivanciu, L., Cooley, B., Qin, J., Racie, T., Hettinger, J., Carioto, M., Jiang, Y., Brodsky, J., Prabhala, H., Zhang, X., Attarwala, H., Hutabarat, R., Foster, D., Milstein, S., Charisse, K., Kuchimanchi, S., Maier, M.A., Nechev, L., Kandasamy, P., Kel'in, A.V., Nair, J.K., Rajeev, K.G., Manoharan, M., Meyers, R., Sorensen, B., Simon, A.R., Dargaud, Y., Negrier, C., Camire, R.M., Akinc, A., 2015. An RNAi therapeutic targeting antithrombin to rebalance the coagulation system and promote hemostasis in hemophilia. Nat. Med. 21, 492–497.

Semple, S.C., Klimuk, S.K., Harasym, T.O., Dos Santos, N., Ansell, S.M., Wong, K.F., Maurer, N., Stark, H., Cullis, P.R., Hope, M.J., Scherrer, P., 2001. Efficient encapsulation of antisense oligonucleotides in lipid vesicles using ionizable aminolipids: formation of novel small multilamellar vesicle structures. Biochim. Biophys. Acta Biomembr. 1510, 152–166.

Semple, S.C., Akinc, A., Chen, J., Sandhu, A.P., Mui, B.L., Cho, C.K., Sah, D.W., Stebbing, D., Crosley, E.J., Yaworski, E., Hafez, I.M., Dorkin, J.R., Qin, J., Lam, K., Rajeev, K.G., Wong, K.F., Jeffs, L.B., Nechev, L., Eisenhardt, M.L., Jayaraman, M., Kazem, M., Maier, M.A., Srinivasulu, M., Weinstein, M.J., Chen, Q., Alvarez, R., Barros, S.A., De, S., Klimuk, S.K., Borland, T., Kosovrasti, V., Cantley, W.L., Tam, Y.K., 2010. Rational design of cationic lipids for siRNA delivery. Nat. Biotechnol. 28, 172–176.

Shao, L., Tekedereli, I., Wang, J., Yuca, E., Tsang, S., Sood, A., Lopez-Berestein, G., Ozpolat, B., Ittmann, M., 2012. Highly specific targeting of the TMPRSS2/ERG fusion gene using liposomal nanovectors. Clin. Cancer Res. 18, 6648–6657.

Shu, D., Shu, Y., Haque, F., Abdelmawla, S., Guo, P., 2011. Thermodynamically stable RNA three-way junction for constructing multifunctional nanoparticles for delivery of therapeutics. Nat. Nanotechnol. 6, 658–667.

Suk, J.S., Xu, Q., Kim, N., Hanes, J., Ensign, L.M., 2016. PEGylation as a strategy for improving nanoparticle-based drug and gene delivery. Adv. Drug Deliv. Rev. 99, 28–51.

Svoboda, P., Di Cara, A., 2006. Hairpin RNA: a secondary structure of primary importance. Cell. Mol. Life Sci. 63, 901–908.

Tabernero, J., Shapiro, G.I., Lorusso, P.M., Cervantes, A., Schwartz, G.K., Weiss, G.J., Paz-Ares, L., Cho, D.C., Infante, J.R., Alsina, M., Gounder, M.M., Falzone, R., Harrop, J., White, A.C., Toudjarska, I., Bumcrot, D., Meyers, R.E., Hinkle, G., Svrzikapa, N., Hutabarat, R.M., Clausen, V.A., Cehelsky, J., Nochur, S.V., Gamba-Vitalo, C., Vaishnaw, A.K., Sah, D.W., Gollob, J.A., Burris 3rd., H.A., 2013. First-in-humans trial of an RNA interference therapeutic targeting VEGF and KSP in cancer patients with liver involvement. Cancer Discov. 3, 406–417.

Tagami, T., Nakamura, K., Shimizu, T., Ishida, T., Kiwada, H., 2009. Effect of siRNA in PEG-coated siRNA-lipoplex on anti-PEG IgM production. J. Control. Release 137, 234–240.

Tagami, T., Nakamura, K., Shimizu, T., Yamazaki, N., Ishida, T., Kiwada, H., 2010. CpG motifs in pDNA-sequences increase anti-PEG IgM production induced by PEG-coated pDNA-lipoplexes. J. Control. Release 142, 160–166.

Tekedereli, I., Alpay, S.N., Akar, U., Yuca, E., Ayugo-Rodriguez, C., Han, H.D., Sood, A.K., Lopez-Berestein, G., Ozpolat, B., 2013. Therapeutic silencing of Bcl-2 by systemically administered siRNA nanotherapeutics inhibits tumor growth by autophagy and apoptosis and enhances the efficacy of chemotherapy in orthotopic xenograft models of ER (-) and ER (+) Breast cancer. Mol. Ther. Nucleic Acids 2.

Villares, G.J., Zigler, M., Wang, H., Melnikova, V.O., Wu, H., Friedman, R., Leslie, M.C., Vivas-Mejia, P.E., Lopez-Berestein, G., Sood, A.K., Bar-Eli, M., 2008. Targeting melanoma growth and metastasis with systemic delivery of liposome-incorporated protease-activated receptor-1 small interfering RNA. Cancer Res. 68, 9078–9086.

Wakefield, D.H., Klein, J.J., Wolff, J.A., Rozema, D.B., 2005. Membrane activity and transfection ability of amphipathic polycations as a function of alkyl group size. Bioconjug. Chem. 16, 1204–1208.

Wan, C., Allen, T.M., Cullis, P.R., 2014. Lipid nanoparticle delivery systems for siRNA-based therapeutics. Drug Deliv. Transl. Res. 4, 74–83.

Wang, H., Jiang, Y., Peng, H., Chen, Y., Zhu, P., Huang, Y., 2015. Recent progress in microRNA delivery for cancer therapy by non-viral synthetic vectors. Adv. Drug Deliv. Rev. 81, 142–160.

Whitehead, K.A., Langer, R., Anderson, D.G., 2009. Knocking down barriers: advances in siRNA delivery. Nat. Rev. Drug Discov. 8, 129–138.

Wong, S.C., Klein, J.J., Hamilton, H.L., Chu, Q., Frey, C.L., Trubetskoy, V.S., Hegge, J., Wakefield, D., Rozema, D.B., Lewis, D.L., 2012. Co-injection of a targeted, reversibly masked endosomolytic polymer dramatically improves the efficacy of cholesterol-conjugated small interfering RNAs in vivo. Nucleic Acid Ther. 22, 380–390.

Wooddell, C.I., Rozema, D.B., Hossbach, M., John, M., Hamilton, H.L., Chu, Q., Hegge, J.O., Klein, J.J., Wakefield, D.H., Oropeza, C.E., Deckert, J., Roehl, I., Jahn-Hofmann, K., Hadwiger, P., Vornlocher, H.P., Mclachlan, A., Lewis, D.L., 2013. Hepatocyte-targeted RNAi therapeutics for the treatment of chronic hepatitis B virus infection. Mol. Ther. 21, 973–985.

Wu, G.Y., Wu, C.H., 1987. Receptor-mediated in vitro gene transformation by a soluble DNA carrier system. J. Biol. Chem. 262, 4429–4432.

Xu, L., Tang, W.H., Huang, C.C., Alexander, W., Xiang, L.M., Pirollo, K.F., Rait, A., Chang, E.H., 2001. Systemic p53 gene therapy of cancer with immunolipoplexes targeted by anti-transferrin receptor scFv. Mol. Med. 7, 723–734.

Yao, Y., Su, Z., Liang, Y., Zhang, N., 2015. pH-Sensitive carboxymethyl chitosan-modified cationic liposomes for sorafenib and siRNA co-delivery. Int. J. Nanomedicine 10, 6185–6198.

Yew, N.S., Scheule, R.K., 2005. Toxicity of cationic lipid-DNA complexes. Adv. Genet. 53, 189–214.

Zetsche, B., Gootenberg, J.S., Abudayyeh, O.O., Slaymaker, I.M., Makarova, K.S., Essletzbichler, P., Volz, S.E., Joung, J., Van Der Oost, J., Regev, A., Koonin, E.V., Zhang, F., 2015. Cpf1 Is a single RNA-guided endonuclease of a class 2 CRISPR-Cas system. Cell 163, 759–771.

Zhang, Y., Wang, Z., Gemeinhart, R.A., 2013. Progress in microRNA delivery. J. Control. Release 172, 962–974.

Zorde Khvalevsky, E., Gabai, R., Rachmut, I.H., Horwitz, E., Brunschwig, Z., Orbach, A., Shemi, A., Golan, T., Domb, A.J., Yavin, E., Giladi, H., Rivkin, L., Simerzin, A., Eliakim, R., Khalaileh, A., Hubert, A., Lahav, M., Kopelman, Y., Goldin, E., Dancour, A., Hants, Y., Arbel-Alon, S., Abramovitch, R., Shemi, A., Galun, E., 2013. Mutant KRAS is a druggable target for pancreatic cancer. Proc. Natl. Acad. Sci. USA 110, 20723–20728.

Zuckerman, J.E., Davis, M.E., 2015. Clinical experiences with systemically administered siRNA-based therapeutics in cancer. Nat. Rev. Drug Discov. 14, 843–856.

Zuckerman, J.E., Gritli, I., Tolcher, A., Heidel, J.D., Lim, D., Morgan, R., Chmielowski, B., Ribas, A., Davis, M.E., Yen, Y., 2014. Correlating animal and human phase Ia/Ib clinical data with CALAA-01, a targeted, polymer-based nanoparticle containing siRNA. Proc. Natl. Acad. Sci. USA 111, 11449–11454.

Artificial virus particles

15

D. Ferreira, I.M. Martins
University of Minho, Centre of Biological Engineering, Braga, Portugal

15.1 Introduction

Viruses' existence goes back for as long as life forms existed on earth. They are unique organisms known to infect all types of cells including plants, animals, protozoa, fungi, and bacteria. Although they may seem like living organisms because of their reproductive abilities, they do not contain the genetic machinery to produce their own proteins. For this reason viruses are not considered living organisms and are obligate intracellular parasites of the living kingdom. A *virion* is a complete viral particle consisting of ribonucleic or deoxyribonucleic acid (RNA or DNA), surrounded by a protein shell, constituting the infective form of a virus. It depends entirely on a host cell for its multiplication and functioning taking over the host cell functions for their own benefit and forcing the infected cell to generate viral particles instead of its normal products.

Viruses vary greatly in size and complexity with only the two main component parts needed to enter the host cell being common among all species: the nucleic acid and the protein coat (capsid). During the life cycle of a virus, the capsid proteins assemble in a very accurate 3D structure around the nucleic acid molecules to form new viruses.

Through the years virology has allowed researchers to find several uses for these unique organisms, primarily known as pathogens, for humans benefit in biological studies and biomedical applications. Viruses, as the simple systems that they are, have been extensively used in molecular and cellular biology to manipulate and investigate cell functions, as well as in omic research from genes to proteins.

Traditional pharmaceuticals consisting of relatively small molecules, easily end up at the desired location, which is more difficult to achieve for newer types of drugs that are being developed, as they consist of large biomolecules such as proteins and genetic material (ie, RNA or DNA). Because viruses can efficiently penetrate cells, natural viruses that have been made harmless could be used as vectors to deliver these new types of medicines to diseased cells. Nevertheless, the process of making natural viruses harmless has not yet been accomplished and, for that reason, scientists are searching for new alternatives and research is also being conducted on alternative "virus-like" particles (VLPs) or artificial virus (meant to mimic the virus of interest in everything except the genetic material), based on synthetic molecules. Artificial viruses are able to "package" new generations of medicines and deliver them into diseased cells by a natural process.

They are being used as targeted drug and gene delivery vectors or carriers for specific treatment of a given disease. Gene therapy and cancer are the two main areas where artificial viruses are being applied (Ledford, 2015) for the introduction of genetically modified sequences of genomes to the host cells. Molecular imaging of virus-based tools is also widely used for early and specific disease detection and diagnosis.

Bioinspired Materials for Medical Applications. http://dx.doi.org/10.1016/B978-0-08-100741-9.00015-2

For prevention purposes, virus-based vaccines have been in use since the time of Edward Jenner, an English physician and scientist who in 1798 reported the discovery of the world's first vaccine, the smallpox vaccine (Riedel, 2005). Vaccines, when inoculated into a healthy individual, help the immune system to recognize and deploy an immune defense against a virus. In the event of a later infection, the body will remember the organism and attack it, allowing the organism to combat the disease. Nevertheless, despite the efficient use of vaccines, bacterial infections are very common and virus-based therapy has become an important tool against this type of illness.

In this chapter, we review and outline some of the basic characteristics of virus particles used in medicine. Additionally, we discuss important strategies for virus particles modification, towards new materials for biomedical applications including strategies for disease prevention, detection, monitoring, and treatment.

15.2 Virus particles—Basic functionalities and properties

Viruses vary greatly in size and complexity containing only the parts needed to enter the host. Most viruses can range from a few tens to a few hundreds of nanometers (nm, one-billionth of a meter), being 100 times smaller than a single bacteria cell, that is itself more than 10 times smaller than a human cell, which is 10 times smaller than the diameter of a single human hair. For that reason the majority of viruses can only be visualized under a scanning electron microscope.

All virus particles are composed of two main components, the nucleic acid genome and the protein coat (or capsid) covering the genome, together this is called the nucleocapsid (Knight, 1954). In addition, in a large number of viruses, the nucleocapsid is surrounded by a lipid bilayer membrane (or envelope), enabling the virus to survive outside the cell sufficiently long to spread elsewhere via the blood. This envelope is usually acquired from the membrane of the host cell during the viral budding process through cellular membranes and it is composed of two lipid layers interspersed with protein molecules of viral and host membrane origin. Many viruses also develop spikes made of glycoprotein on their envelopes that help them to attach to specific receptors on the host cell surface at the first stage of infection. Each virus has its specific receptor, usually a vital component of the cell surface, and it is the distribution of these receptor molecules on host cells that determines the virus's cell-preference (Lucas, 2010).

15.2.1 Viral nucleic acid

As in other cells, the nucleic acid is the core of the virus, encoding the genetic information for the synthesis of all proteins. Although double-strand (ds) DNA comprises the genomes in prokaryotic and eukaryotic cells, the genomes of viruses can comprise single strand (ss) or dsDNA or RNA. Nevertheless, only a few groups of viruses use DNA, most are RNA viruses. The replication process varies among different types of virus and it is their genomes that determine the way viruses replicate themselves to make viral proteins, more copies of the viral coat, and RNA/DNA.

15.2.2 Protein coat

The protein coat (commonly referred as capsid), is a protein shell that encloses the nucleic acid protecting it from the surrounding environment (eg, digestion by enzymes), and it is also responsible for the recognition and attachment of the viral particle to the host cell (Kaesberg, 1956; Klug and Caspar, 1960; Kushner, 1969). The capsid contains special sites on its surface that allow the viral particle to attach to a host cell enabling it to penetrate the host cell membrane or, in some cases, to inject the infectious nucleic acid into the cell's cytoplasm. It has a symmetrical structure and is composed of one or more proteins organized in subunits packed like a rod-shaped helix or polyhedral spherical-shape. During the life cycle of a virus, the capsid proteins assemble in a very accurate 3D structure around the nucleic acid molecules to form new viruses (Kushner, 1969; Perlmutter and Hagan, 2015).

This virus helical structure is commonly seen in ssRNA virus. It has a capsid with a central cavity or hollow tube that is made by proteins self-assembled in a circular fashion, creating a disc-like shape. The disc shapes are attached helically creating a tube comprising the nucleic acid in the middle. An example of a virus with a helical symmetry is the tobacco mosaic virus (TMV) (Fig. 15.1A).

The icosahedral structured virus appears near-spherical because the coat proteins assemble into a closed shell. The icosahedron is made up of equilateral triangles fused together in a spherical-shape and the genetic material is fully enclosed inside the capsid. Viruses with icosahedral structures are released into the environment lysing the cell. An example of a virus with an icosahedral structure is the adenovirus (Ad) (Fig. 15.1B).

There are also more complex virus assemblies where the capsid is neither purely helical, nor purely icosahedral, presenting a combination of icosahedral and helical shape. Extra features may be present, like a complex outer wall or a head–tail morphology. Examples of viruses with a complex structure are (i) the variola virus (which causes smallpox) presenting a unique outer wall and capsid (Fig. 15.1C) and (ii) bacteriophages, which (most of them) present a head–tail morphology structure—this is unique to viruses that only infect bacteria (Fig. 15.1D).

15.2.3 Bacteriophage

The bacteriophage era began in 1915 with the British investigator Frederick Twort and in 1917 with the French Canadian scientist Félix d'Hérelle. In their independent studies, growth inhibition and cell lysis were discovered in cultures of bacteria and attributed to an agent called bacteriophage, commonly referred to as phage (from the Greek word *phagein* which means "to devour"), now known to be a virus that specifically infects bacterial cells.

The head of the virus has an icosahedral shape with a helical-shaped tail to attach to the bacterium, creating a hole in the cell wall; it then inserts its DNA into the cell using the tail as a channel. Some phages immediately reproduce and lyse the host cell (lytic phages, eg, T4, T7, λ), while others (temperate phages) may enter into a quiescent state in which the phage genome is either integrated into the host genome or exists

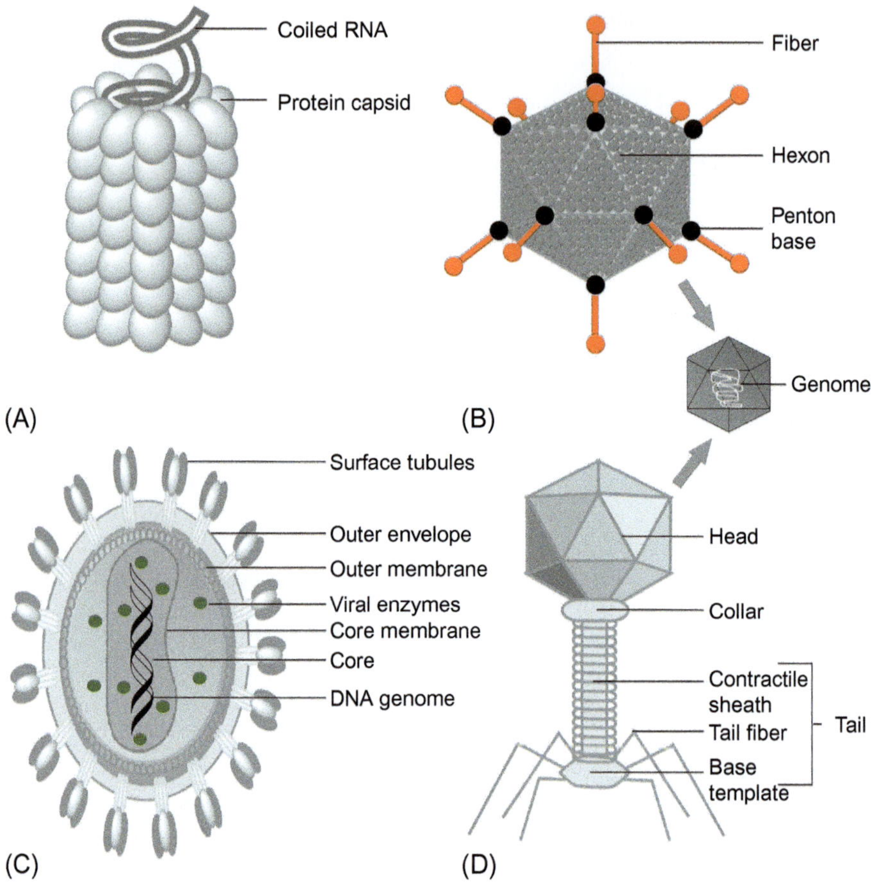

Fig. 15.1 Schematic representation of the helical, icosahedral, and complex viral structures. TMV, representative of the helical structure (A), adenovirus of the icosahedral structure (B) and smallpox virus (C), and head–tail bacteriophage (D), representing the complex structure.

as a plasmid and is maintained throughout the growth and replication of the host cell with minimal phage gene expression in a process called lysogeny (Weinbauer, 2004).

Since the early 1920s these phages have been used in clinical practice (Abedon et al., 2011); however, interest in them decreased with the discovery of antibiotics. Nevertheless, the emergence of multidrug-resistant bacteria has opened a second window of opportunity for phage therapy in bacterial infections (Kutter et al., 2010; Torres-Barcelo and Hochberg, 2016).

15.2.3.1 Filamentous phage

A group of the most commonly used phages are the collectively called Ff phages (M13, fd, f1), because of their filamentous structure and almost total dependence on the F-pilus to infect their *Escherichia coli* host (Russel et al., 1988). Unlike the lytic phage that causes cell lysis when released from the host, Ff phage does not lyse the host cell but instead converts the cell into a phage-producing factory, coupling new virus assemblage and exporting with inhibited bacterial growth (Campbell, 2003; Russel et al., 2004; Rakonjac et al., 2011). Filamentous phage consists of an ssDNA core surrounded by a tube-like capsid composed of 2700 copies of tightly packed major coat protein pVIII, capped by five copies of pIII and pVI on one end and five copies of pVII and pIX on the opposite end (Marvin et al., 2014) (Fig. 15.2A).

Ff phages have been the most widely used since the 1970s as "genetic warehouses" for DNA fragment cloning and sequencing. In 1985, George Smith introduced for the first time the phage display technology using filamentous phage as an expression vector (Smith, 1985). The usefulness of this technology derives from phage biology. Ff phage is in fact a nanofiber whose surface can be specifically modified by genetic engineering to display polypeptides on their surface while the gene encoding the polypeptide, found inside the viral particle, can be analyzed (Barbas et al., 2001; Marvin et al., 2014). Among the molecules that can be displayed on the surface of the phage we can find random peptides, antibody fragments, complementary DNA libraries and protein fragments or variants.

The M13 phage is the Ff phage most widely used in phage display experiments where, by DNA engineering, a peptide or protein can be site-specifically displayed at the tip and/or along the side wall of the phage through fusion, leading to the display of a peptide or protein on the surface of a virus particle. The foreign gene sequence is spliced between genes encoding a phage signal peptide and a portion of the coat protein, which ensures that the foreign protein is produced as a fusion with the coat protein (Molek and Bratkovic, 2015) (Fig. 15.2B).

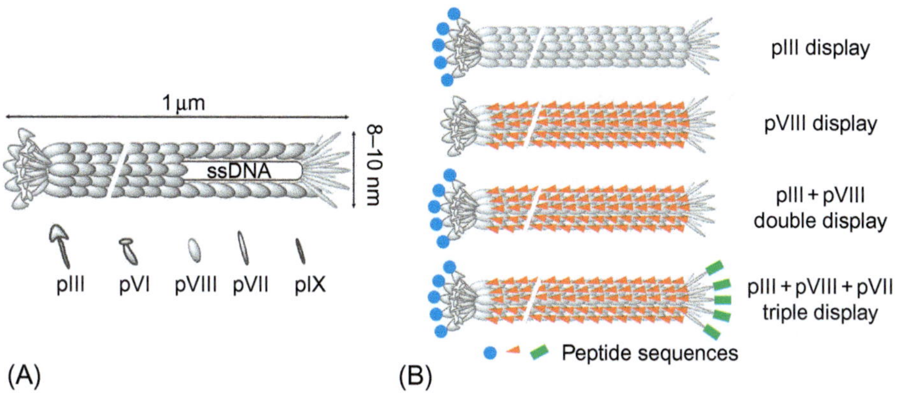

Fig. 15.2 Schematic diagram showing the structure of the filamentous phage and its different modes of display. (A) Filamentous phages are rod-like viruses with a circular ssDNA genome of about 6.4 kb. The tube-like capsid is composed of several thousand copies (up to 2700) of tightly packed major coat protein pVIII, capped by five copies of pIII and pVI on one end and five copies of pVII and pIX on the opposite end. (B) Phage display libraries can be displayed on the surface of the Ff phage by fusion to the different capsid proteins.

Despite being successfully employed to identify peptide ligands for a wide variety of targets, which can often be accessed free of charge in online databases (Huang et al., 2011, 2012), phage display has recently broadened its application, by taking advantage of the surface display and self-assembly abilities of the phage particles, for the development of (i) biologically active molecules, (ii) probes for sensing and imaging, and (iii) target drug and gene delivery vehicles (Petrenko, 2008; Farr et al., 2014). Further details are described in the following sections.

15.3 Viral particles engineering

The artificial virus formation process is in many ways similar to that of natural viruses, such as the TMV, which served as a model for artificial virus development.

Viral nanotechnology is a highly interdisciplinary field in which artificial viruses are applied in various areas, such as chemistry, virology, physics, medicine, pharmacology, and materials science (Douglas and Young, 2006). Methodologies have been established for the efficient production and modification of virus nanoparticles (VNPs) consisting of virus-based nanoparticles, which can be used as building blocks for novel materials, as well as VLPs, which mimic the structure of infectious particles expressed in heterologous systems but lack genomic nucleic acid making them noninfectious.

Viruses have emerged as platforms for synthetic manipulation. A wide range of genetic modifications, conjugation chemistries, and self-assembly/encapsulation techniques can be performed to endow VNPs with different functions. Several ligands ranging from oligonucleotides, peptides, proteins, carbohydrates, fluorescent reagents, drugs, and even additional nanoparticles, have been used to functionalize VNPs. Recent advances in the use of a myriad of different VNPs for biomedical applications will be further discussed.

15.3.1 Genetic engineering

VNPs and VLPs are assembled from protein subunits whose structure can be changed by genetic modifications (Fig. 15.3).

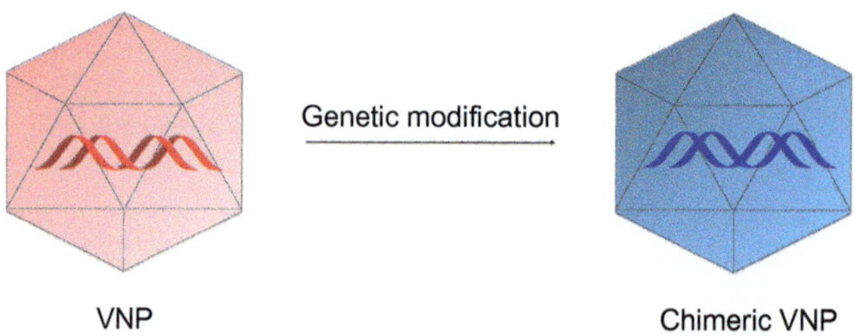

Fig. 15.3 Genetic engineering of VNPs. VNPs can be designed and modified using genetic protocols imparting new functions to protein cage architectures.

Because chemical engineering is not 100% efficient, this strategy can be advantageous over any synthetic material (Yildiz et al., 2011). The use of genetic engineering has enabled the incorporation of amino acids for bioconjugation as will be further referred to in Section 15.3.2 (Strable et al., 2008), insertion of peptide-based affinity tags (Park et al., 2009) and introduction of peptides as targeting ligands (Grifman et al., 2001) or as epitopes to stimulate the immune response.

One of the first approaches of virus engineering for direct applications was the development of phage display (Smith, 1985), as previously described. The application of phage display technologies over the past few years has proved its potential by contributing to different areas of medicine and technology, such as medical diagnostics and monitoring, molecular imaging, targeted drug and gene delivery, as well as vaccine development, as reviewed by several authors (Smith and Petrenko, 1997; Kehoe and Kay, 2005; Paschke, 2006; Bratkovic, 2010; Pande et al., 2010; Hamzeh-Mivehroud et al., 2013).

Additionally, several studies exploited the genetic manipulation of phages to allow their use as functional nanobiomaterials for tissue engineering and regenerative medicine (Chung et al., 2010; Yoo et al., 2012). In cancer research, phages have also been used to overcome detection and therapy issues (Ghosh et al., 2012a,b; Pranjol and Hajitou, 2015). Further details are described in Section 15.4.1.

15.3.2 Chemical modifications

Several chemical reactions have been developed to chemically modify the surfaces of viral nanocarriers including the capsid interior, capsid interface, and exterior (Fig. 15.4).

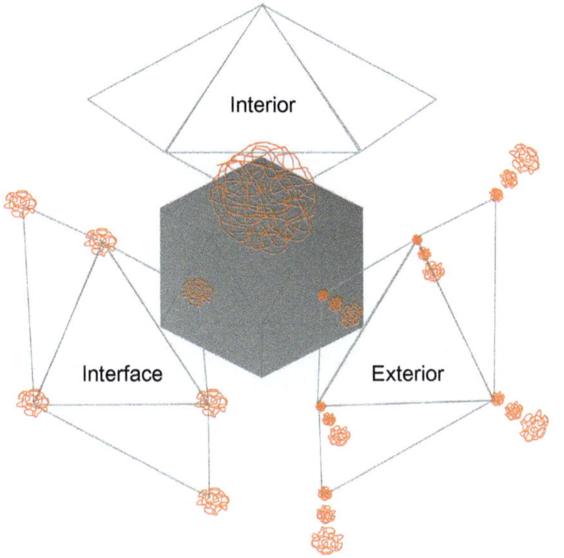

Fig. 15.4 Chemical manipulation of virus nanoparticles (VNPs). A broad range of chemical engineering protocols have been established that allow new VNP formulations.

Noncovalent VNP modification strategies include electrostatic, protein–protein, protein–nucleotide, and protein–metal interactions. This type of VNP modification is often reversible, which can be disadvantageous when permanent functionalization and ligation stability are required (Smith et al., 2013).

For the covalent approach, standard protocols include bioconjugation techniques that have been routinely used in protein derivatization (Ma et al., 2012). The most widely used reactions include the reactive side chains of lysine (Lys), cysteine (Cys), aspartic acid (Asp), glutamic acid (Glu), and tyrosine (Tyr) residues, which are available to form biocompatible covalent bonds (Fig. 15.5A). Lysine residues and N-termini provide reactive moieties in primary amines form ($R\text{-}NH_2$) that have been mainly targeted with *N*-hydroxysuccinimidyl-esters (NHS-esters) or NHS-ester sulfate derivatives (Smith et al., 2013).

Cysteine residues have been reacted with success via maleimide–thiol reactions. Although the natural amino acids lysine and cysteine are the main targets for VNP functionalization, aspartic and glutamic acids also provide carboxylic acids that can react with primary amines via carbodiimide activation (Pokorski and Steinmetz, 2011; Smith et al., 2013). Furthermore, the coupling of a tyrosine side chain and an activated aniline also provides an exclusive linkage opportunity in the form of phenol groups—diazonium method—already described as a coupling strategy for MS2 bacteriophage (Kovacs et al., 2007) and TMV (Schlick et al., 2005; Pokorski and Steinmetz, 2011) (Fig. 15.5B). Although it is a more specialized and labor-intensive coupling process, researchers found this a versatile method, when standard bioconjugation protocols are inappropriate for the introduction of new functional groups onto VNPs.

Recent advances for VNPs modification rely on the incorporation of unnatural amino acids (uAAs) into viral proteins. There are over 70 uAAs available (Liu and Schultz, 2010) and 2 predominant techniques have been used to integrate uAAs into VNPs proteins, namely global-replacement that is residue specific or the site-specific incorporation (SSI). Global-replacement residue specific (GRRS) relies on the substitution of a natural amino acid with an analogous unnatural variety during translation, and SSI uses nonsense stop codons such as tRNA (transcriptomic RNA) encoding sites to incorporate uAAs into a single or multiple location in viral proteins (Smith et al., 2013). The GRRS methodology was used to genetically incorporate azide or alkyne side chains into the capsids of Qβ bacteriophage and hepatitis B virus (HBV) (Strable et al., 2008). In this approach, the methionine residues were replaced with either homopropargyl glycine or azidohomoalanine with an efficiency superior to 95%, which proved to be accessible to click chemistry conjugation protocols. More recently Francis and coworkers (Tong et al., 2009; Stephanopoulos et al., 2010) developed a reaction using SSI methodology to incorporate the uAA *p*-aminophenylalanine into MS2 for site-selective bioconjugation of oligonucleotides (Fig. 15.5C).

Bioorthogonal chemistry is gaining increased attention. Condensation reactions between aldehyde and hydrazide groups, or aldehyde and alkoxyamine groups respectively, are also a successful VNP functionalization strategy and have been adapted for MS2 and TMV (Fig. 15.5D) (Schlick et al., 2005; Hooker et al., 2007). One powerful approach for protein conjugation, extensively used in virus manipulation, is so-called

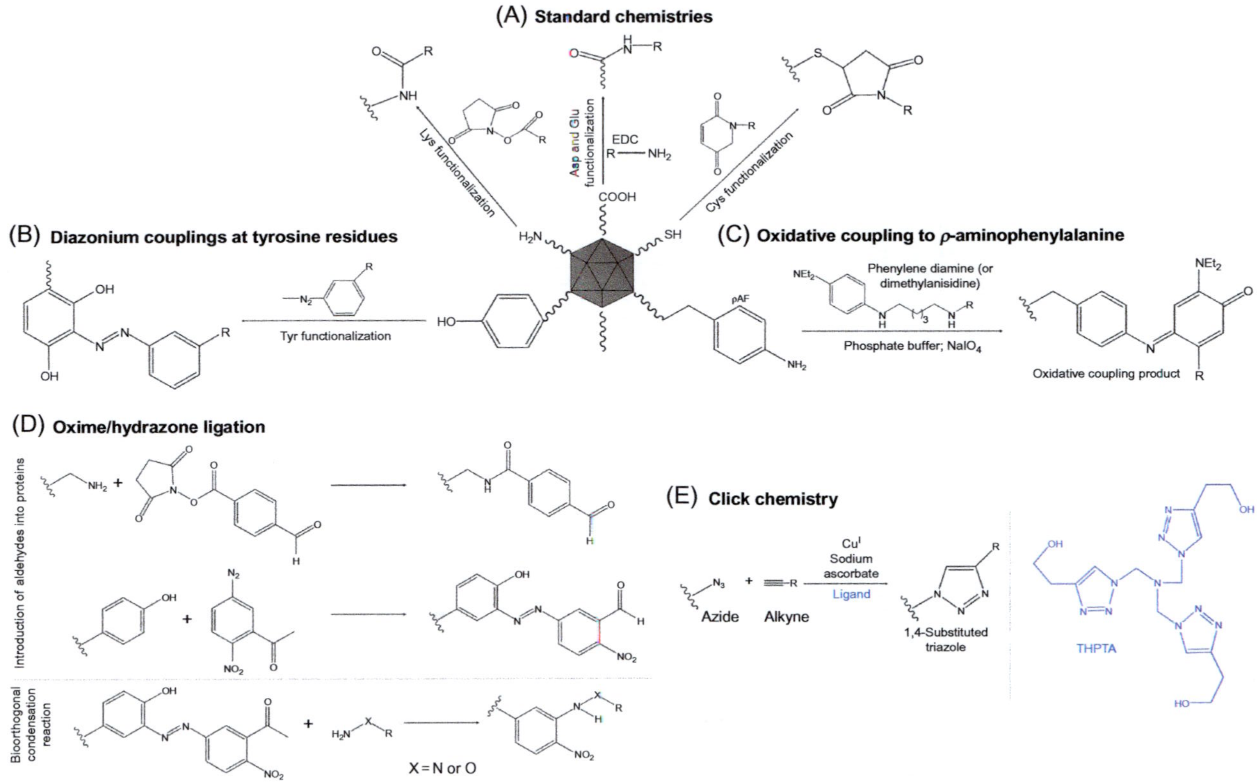

Fig. 15.5 Bioconjugation methods for VNPs. (A) An overview of the three most common bioconjugation chemistries, Lys-NHS, Cys-maleimide, and carbodiimide. (B) Diazonium coupling chemistry. (C) Oxidative coupling to the unnatural amino acid *p*-aminophenylalanine. (D) Condensation reactions to form oximes and hydrazones, two strategies for the introduction of aldehydes into proteins and bioorthogonal condensation reaction. (E) The CuAAC reaction (click chemistry).

click chemistry, or the copper-catalyzed azide–alkyne cycloaddition (CuAAC), which includes functional groups inert to most biological molecules and proceeds more quickly and with much higher fidelity than NHS or maleimide reactions (Fig. 15.5E) (Koudelka and Manchester, 2010; Pokorski and Steinmetz, 2011). The pioneering research on this reaction was performed by Finn and coworkers who used it to chemically modify cowpea mosaic virus (CPMV), HBV, and bacteriophage Qβ (Prasuhn et al., 2007; Strable et al., 2008; Steinmetz et al., 2009).

These bioconjugation chemistries have been combined with VNPs to enable their functionalization with nucleic acids, drugs, peptides, polymers, and fluorophores to the internal and external surfaces and have been extensively reviewed elsewhere (Young et al., 2008; Steinmetz, 2010).

The future of complex VNP development lies in the conjunction of molecular biology approaches and bioconjugation chemistry, particularly in terms of the ability to access both natural amino acids and uAAs side chains for modification in the same VNP. This will allow the incorporation of multiple moieties such as targeting ligands, therapeutic and imaging molecules.

15.3.3 Self-assembly/encapsulation strategies

Self-assembly strategies allowed mimicking of natural processes for the development of virus-based nanomaterials (Liu et al., 2012). VNPs have the natural properties of virus coat proteins to maintain their ability to self-assemble into shells and tubes, but at the same time allow the entrapment of artificial cargoes. A broad range of cargoes including enzymes, polymers, drugs, imaging reagents, and synthetic nanoparticles have been successfully incorporated (Fig. 15.6) (Yildiz et al., 2011).

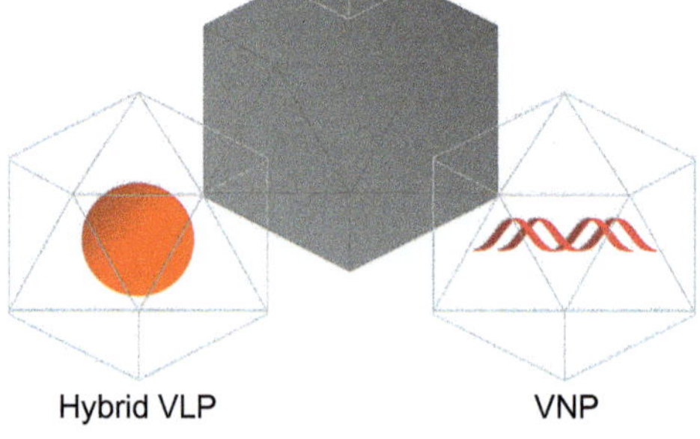

Fig. 15.6 Schematic representation of three important interfaces available for genetic and chemical engineering of virus-like particles (VLPs) and virus nanoparticles (VNPs).

Loading the interior cavity of VLPs can be performed by disassembly and reassembly, or by diffusion and entrapment within capsid by exploiting swelling mechanisms. Encapsulation of complexes of negatively charged polymers (Hu et al., 2008), enzymes (Comellas-Aragones et al., 2007), and metallic and magnetic nanoparticles (Huang et al., 2007; Loo et al., 2007) during particle self-assembly have been described. Loo and coworkers described the infusion of dye molecules into the cavity of the red clover necrotic mosaic virus. The assembled particle has a reversible gating mechanism sensitive to metal ions concentration and pH, whereby at higher pH a structural transition occurs causing swelling and pore opening. These pores allow diffusion of cargo into the interior of VNP cavity and when the reverse process occurs, the particles contract and the pores close, trapping the infused cargo inside the VNP (Loo et al., 2008).

Artificial viral coat proteins have recently been designed and produced using the natural machinery of yeast cells (Hernandez-Garcia et al., 2014). Taking into consideration recent theoretical insights on the crucial aspects of the process of packaging genetic material by natural viral coat proteins, those authors reported that when proteins were mixed with DNA, they spontaneously assembled and formed a highly protective protein coat around each DNA molecule, thus creating artificial viruses.

15.4 Virus engineering towards biomedical applications

Viruses are natural supramolecular structures, composed of multiple copies of coat proteins with the ability to assemble into different and unique shapes and sizes, and with well-defined structural features. Furthermore, their production is simple and economic and they can be easily modified either by genetic modifications, chemical modifications or both.

For the development of new materials with potential biomedical application, it is crucial to understand their overall in vivo properties. Parameters such as morphology, size, composition, surface chemistry, and associated physical properties of VNPs can greatly influence their toxicological nature, as well as accumulation and systemic clearance (Powers et al., 2006). Thus, a complete understanding of the pharmacokinetics, blood half-life, stability, biodistribution, and immunogenicity is crucial to assess the viability of virus-based nanoparticles.

Several VNP and VLP platforms are currently being developed for applications towards biomedical use and recent advances will be further highlighted.

15.4.1 Targeted delivery and therapy

Engineered virus carriers or vehicles are highly promising scaffolds that may be triggered to release their cargo, in response to changes in pH, chemical stimuli, redox status, or temperature, to the desired targets; this being the main goal of drug and gene delivery in modern medicine.

15.4.1.1 Drug carriers

Adeno-associated virus (AAV) nanoparticles have been used as platforms for the co-delivery of genes and drugs to cancer cells. Covalent conjugation of paclitaxel, a chemotherapeutic drug, onto surface-exposed lysine residues present on the virus capsid was tested for and the conjugation reaction did not adversely impact gene delivery or cytotoxicity of the VNPs (Wei et al., 2012). Another chemotherapeutic drug often used in cancer treatment is doxorubicin (DOX), whose encapsulation into hibiscus chlorotic ringspot virus targeted to cancer cells was reported (Ren et al., 2007). More recently, the use of engineered CPMV as carriers of DOX towards cancer cells has been described (Aljabali et al., 2013). CPMV externally decorated with eighty DOX molecules using two different chemical conjugation strategies, demonstrated greater cytotoxicity compared with free DOX towards HeLa cells. The use of this carrier platform for cargo delivery was also used for encapsulation of imaging and therapeutic moieties, and other molecules such as polyethylene glycol and biotin affinity tags (Wen et al., 2012; Yildiz et al., 2013). Recently, other virus-based carriers have been developed. For instance, nanoparticles formed from the potato virus X (PVX) were described as carriers of the chemotherapeutic drug Herceptin (Trastuzumab), which is currently used as a targeted therapy in ($HER2^+$) breast cancer patients (Esfandiari et al., 2015). The PVX–Herceptin conjugates enable Herceptin to specifically target breast cancer cells.

Nevertheless, phages are also being used as vectors due to their easy engineering; both genetically and chemically. A phage-based technology was developed by Rangel et al. (2012, 2013). They developed a screening internalizing phage strategy—iPhage—for phage vectors and libraries with the potential to penetrate eukaryotic cells for subcellular drug delivery. Because it enables ligand-directed discovery of signal peptides and targeting of organelles or molecular pathways within live cells, this approach is a very important tool for drug development.

For cancer treatment, the cytotoxic drugs hygromycin and DOX were covalently attached to M13 bacteriophage and targeted successfully to cancer cells in vitro (Bar et al., 2008; Ghosh et al., 2012a; Phumyen et al., 2014). However, phages have been used not only for cancer, neurosciences have also benefitted from phage applications and neuroscientists keep on exploring their use for neurological disorders treatment (Bakhshinejad and Sadeghizadeh, 2014; Bakhshinejad et al., 2015). A very important feature has been discovered when using a filamentous phage as a vector for drug delivery in the treatment of neurodegenerative diseases: it has been found that they cross the blood–brain barrier thereby being able to deliver antibodies into the brain (Frenkel and Solomon, 2002).

In regenerative medicine, phages also offer contributions. Sawada and collaborators reported the use of phage display to identify peptide sequences that interact with Integra wound-healing grafting matrices, used to promote superficial tissue regeneration (Sawada et al., 2011). These next-generation matrices for drug delivery are able to control the temporal and spatial delivery of the drug.

In a different approach, one study was published describing the use of engineered virus-based particles to deliver payloads of small interfering RNA (siRNA) to cancer cells (Galaway and Stockley, 2013). They described the use of MS2 VLP for targeted delivery of loaded siRNA against the tumor target *bcl* oncogene transcript and also showed that payload delivery by the virus-based platform is more efficient when compared with the commercial cationic lipids.

15.4.1.2 Gene carriers

Artificial viruses have been involved in several advancements in the field of gene therapy related to the process of introducing foreign genomic material into host cells in order to promote a therapeutic effect. Since many diseases have a genetic foundation, systems for nucleic acids delivery are being developed as viral vectors that incorporate virus-like functions in a single nanoparticle, to replace defective genes, correct missing genes or regulate gene expression (Mastrobattista et al., 2006).

AAV, Ad and other vectors that are derived from retroviruses, particularly lentiviruses are among the most widely used viral systems for gene delivery (Stone, 2010; Nayerossadat et al., 2012; Gaj et al., 2015), and are used in the most varied medical fields from regenerative medicine (Yungher et al., 2015; Tang et al., 2016a,b), to cancer (Hong et al., 2015; Trepel et al., 2015; Sayroo et al., 2016), cardiac and cardiovascular diseases (Merentie et al., 2015; Rincon et al., 2015), and neurological disorders (Bourdenx et al., 2014; Connor et al., 2015; Jara et al., 2016).

Viral particles are also considered appropriate options for the introduction of genome editing reagents into the target cells due to the efficient cell-entry mechanisms. Indeed, as engineered replication-deficient viruses, they are acquiring an increasingly relevant role as delivery vehicles for donor DNA templates and designer nucleases namely clustered regularly interspaced short palindromic repeats associated protein Cas9 (CRISPR–Cas9), also known as RNA-guided nucleases, zinc-finger nucleases (ZFNs), and transcription activator-like effector nucleases (TALENs) (Chen and Goncalves, 2015). Lentiviral, AAV and Ad vectors are described as holding an improved performance as genome editing devices. For instance, an integrase-defective lentivirus vectors (IDLV) was described to be used as a delivery platform of engineered ZFNs for site-specific gene correction of β-globin locus responsible by the sickle cell disease, inducing high levels of DNA cleavage in $CD34^+$ hematopoietic stem and progenitor cells (Hoban et al., 2015). The use of IDLVs as designer nuclease expression vehicles is mostly restricted to ZFNs.

Delivery of ZFNs was also achieved using AAV vectors (Li et al., 2011). A subsequent study from Anguela and coworkers extended the therapeutic potential of AAV-mediated ZFN genome editing and enabled the production of high levels of human factor IX in adult mice normalizing hemophilic clotting times (Anguela et al., 2013). Similarly to IDLVs, the use of AAV as delivery vehicles has been mostly used for ZFNs. However, the construction of a shorter Cas9 variant led to the implementation of AAV/RNA-guided nucleases tools (Senis et al., 2014). Recently, this approach was used to study the mammalian brain gene function (Swiech et al., 2015).

Ad vectors are versatile systems and have been validated as delivery platforms for TALENs and RNA-guided nucleases tools, in addition to ZFNs (Holkers et al., 2013; Maggio et al., 2014). For instance, in a recent study, Ad vectors expressing CRISPR–Cas9 led to the disruption of hyper- or hypocholesterolemia mutation associated gene *Pcsk9* in vivo with high efficiency resulting in decreased plasma PCSK9 protein and cholesterol levels (Ding et al., 2014).

15.4.2 Molecular imaging for detection, diagnosis, and monitoring

Viruses have recently proven useful for the detection of target analytes and early diagnosis of several, different diseases with high selectivity and sensitivity. Nevertheless, the samples analysis is challenging due to its heterogeneous nature, the limited volume, and the concentration of the analytes. For that reason, the development of molecular imaging tools has increased in the last two decades (Mao et al., 2009; Steinmetz, 2010).

A wide variety of design principles has been established to formulate hybrid VNP systems for imaging applications. VNPs conjugated with imaging reagents, as fluorescent labels, can be used for intravital vascular imaging. For instance, CPMV particles carrying fluorescent moieties administered intravenously allow the visualization of the vasculature and blood flow in living mouse and chick embryos to a depth of up to 500 μm and up to 72 hours (Lewis et al., 2006).

To design hybrid VNPs with fluorescent cores for application in cellular imaging, encapsulation strategies can also be used. This was demonstrated by using brome mosaic virus, whose interior is doped with the Food and Drug Administration (FDA)-approved fluorophore indocyanine green (Jung et al., 2011), and quantum-dots containing VLPs of simian virus 40 constructed by in vitro self-assembly (Li et al., 2009). Encapsulation of the imaging reagents has the advantage of enabling the incorporation of targeting ligands in the VLP external surface.

VNPs are being engineered to act as contrast agents to increase sensitivity of current in vivo imaging techniques. There is a variety of imaging strategies available for in vivo imaging, where the most commonly used are magnetic resonance imaging (MRI) and positron emission tomography (PET). Image-contrast agents in MRI include metals, such as gadolinium (Gd) or iron, and for PET isotopes, such as ^{18}F, ^{11}C, or ^{15}O (Manchester and Singh, 2006). VNPs such as CPMV, cowpea chlorotic mottle virus (CCMV), and MS2 have been developed as contrast reagents by decorating them with Gd either by chemical means or by protein engineering (Allen et al., 2005; Prasuhn et al., 2007; Datta et al., 2008). The cavity of phage P22 was also functionalized with a branched oligomer attached to Gd-based contrast agent, yielding a formulation with ionic relaxivities higher than the free contrast reagent (Qazi et al., 2013). Due to large surface area of VNPs, several hundred chelated Gd complexes can be attached to the exterior or interior surfaces, and their rigid molecular structures and large rotational correlation times can offer high relaxivity values (Yildiz et al., 2011). These indicate that VNPs are excellent candidates for MRI contrast agents.

VNPs have also been explored as potential tools for PET imaging. For instance, MS2 particles were labeled with [^{18}F]-fluorobenzaldehyde through a multistep bioconjugation strategy and its biodistribution was evaluated in rats. These experiments showed that [^{18}F]-fluorobenzaldehyde alone is rapidly cleared through the kidneys and collected in the urine, while [^{18}F]-MS2 particles exhibited prolonged circulation time in blood (Hooker et al., 2008).

In another study, superparamagnetic ferumoxide particles and ^{18}F-fluoride were encapsulated simultaneously within hemagglutinating virus of Japan envelopes.

Biodistribution in rats was analyzed using PET imaging and a higher accumulation in the liver and spleen was verified, being the results similar to the ones found for MS2 (Flexman et al., 2008).

Phages have also become an important tool in the molecular imaging field. As aforementioned, a phage capsid can be decorated with foreign molecules through phage display technology, which has become a standard technique in biotechnology. Recent studies reported the use of filamentous phages as display platforms for cancer cells imaging both in vitro and in vivo (Li et al., 2010; Ghosh et al., 2012a,b; Yi et al., 2012; Palaniappan et al., 2013; Jin et al., 2014; Soendergaard et al., 2014a,b).

A different approach developed a phage-based tool that aids in the study of phage deposition and circulation in cells and tissues (Kazmierczak et al., 2014). The authors reported a new green fluorescent protein-based methodology for T4 phage molecular imaging in living systems for the detection of inside living mammalian cells and tissues.

Recently, Chariou and coworkers used filaments formed by the plant PVX to functionalize with a 12-amino acid peptide ligand GE11 with affinity towards epidermal growth factor receptor. The fluorescently labeled PVX–GE11 enabled image and detection of different cancer cell lines (Chariou et al., 2015).

15.4.3 Vaccine applications

There is a broad range of commercially available viral vaccines against viral pathogens that can be classified into three main types: live attenuated vaccines, inactivated vaccines, and subunit vaccines (Rodrigues et al., 2015). The recent advances in molecular biology, systems biology, genomics, and engineering have contributed immensely to our understanding of human immunology (Swartz et al., 2012). Efforts have been made to design new vaccines based on VLPs that represent an advance in the development of safer and more efficient vaccines, with less side effects and improved immunogenicity compared with the live attenuated vaccines (Rodriguez-Limas et al., 2013).

VLPs are exceptional candidates as vaccines as their highly repetitive proteinaceous structure is recognized by the immune system eliciting strong humoral and cellular responses. In addition to their capability to stimulate B-cell mediated immune response generating high titers of neutralizing antibodies, VLPs have also been demonstrated to be very effective at stimulating cytotoxic T lymphocyte response without the use of adjuvant molecules (Rodriguez-Limas et al., 2013).

The first VLP-based vaccine was Recombivax HB (Merck and Co. Inc.) approved by FDA in 1986 against HBV, produced in the baker's yeast *Saccharomyces cerevisiae*. More recently, two vaccines for human papillomavirus–Gardasil (Merck and Co. Inc.) produced in *S. cerevisiae* and Cervarix (GlaxoSmithKline) produced in insect cells-baculovirus—were FDA approved in 2006 and 2009, respectively. In 2011, China's State Food and Drug Administration (SFDA) approved the vaccine Hecolin (Xiamen Innovax Biotech) produced in *E. coli* as the first vaccine against hepatitis E (Park, 2012). Other VLP-based vaccine candidates for human health in clinical trials or undergoing preclinical evaluation are the influenza virus, parvovirus, and norwalk virus (Roldao et al., 2010).

Vaccine peptide epitopes or antigens can be incorporated into a well-characterized VLP structure, either by genetic fusion into specific regions of a capsid protein gene or by chemical coupling using chemistry methodologies, thus resulting in a so-called chimeric VLP (Rodriguez-Limas et al., 2013; Rodrigues et al., 2015). Several chimeric VLP-based vaccines have entered clinical trials, including antiinfluenza A, antihuman immunodeficiency virus, two antimalaria vaccines, a vaccine for nicotine dependence and one for hypertension (Roldao et al., 2010).

15.4.4 Bacterial infections control

Bacterial biofilms are densely packed agglomerations of microbial cells and their development is one of the major reasons for hospital-based bacterial infections. The antibiotic resistance and the intrinsic resistance of microbial biofilm communities are the main hurdles of conventional antimicrobial therapy (Simoes, 2011; Venkatesan et al., 2015).

The use of virus-based particles has been reported to prevent and treat some of these bacterial infections. Suci et al. (2007) reported that target-functionalized CCMV particles were used to penetrate and kill *Staphylococcus aureus*, a common biofilm-forming pathogen. CCMV particles were genetically engineered to carry ruthenium complexes as the photosensitizer and then targeted to the *S. aureus* through conjugation with a specific antibody. Under light-emitting diodes at a wavelength of 470 nm, the exposed CCMV-targeted *S. aureus* were killed.

Recent attention has been directed to the use of bacteriophages for bacterial infection detection and treatment (Vandenheuvel et al., 2013; Yilmaz et al., 2013; Sillankorva and Azeredo, 2014). Phages have been reported as being used as targeted drug vehicles for the eradication of *S. aureus* by endowing them with a targeting moiety on their surface and the antibiotic chloramphenicol (Yacoby et al., 2006; they have also been used to inhibit *Chlamydia trachomatis* intracellular infections (Bhattarai et al., 2012).

Another approach has described that phages can be an effective topical therapy against *S. aureus* biofilm-infected wounds in vivo (Seth et al., 2013). Azeredo's group recently reported the use of phages against *Pseudomonas aeruginosa*, one of the most common causes of healthcare-associated infections. They reviewed the in vitro and in vivo results obtained by using phages to treat or prevent *P. aeruginosa* infections, as well as the major hurdles associated with this phage therapy (Pires et al., 2015).

15.5 Conclusions and future perspectives

In the medical field there is a continuous and intensive effort to seek new solutions to overcome the most varied clinical problems. In this scenario, nature over the course of evolution has provided an amazing repertoire of tailored instruments—the viruses—primarily known as pathogens, but possessing an incredible capacity for use to the benefit of humans.

Artificial viruses comprise not only virus-like particles and viral nanoparticles but also bacteriophages. These are highly versatile organisms representing a very important tool not only for use in phage display experiments, for recognition/identification purposes, but also as a prospective nanomaterial easily tailored by genetic and/or chemical manipulations. The merge of viral technologies with nanotechnology over recent years has been shown to be a valuable contribution to the biomedical field in areas such as targeted drug and gene delivery, molecular imaging for disease diagnostic and monitoring, vaccine development, and bacterial infections control. All these applications have been extended to different areas of medicine, namely cancer, tissue engineering in regenerative medicine, neurodegenerative disorders, infectious diseases, among others.

In the future, research will probably focus on understanding the in vivo behavior of artificial virus particles and, in particular, the requirements for scale-up and precise characterization. Viral nanotechnology will continue to be an inspiring and fast-moving field, holding great promise for the development of next-generation virus-based devices and bringing novel therapeutics into the clinic in years to come.

Acknowledgments

The authors acknowledge financial support from the Portuguese Foundation for Science and Technology (FCT) under the scope of the strategic funding of UID/BIO/04469/2013 unit and COMPETE 2020 (POCI-01-0145-FEDER-006684), and also under the scope of the Projects RECI/BBB-EBI/0179/2012 (FCOMP-01-0124-FEDER-027462) and Lipid NP'Phage (PTDC/SAU-BMA/121028/2010).

References

Abedon, S.T., Kuhl, S.J., Blasdel, B.G., Kutter, E.M., 2011. Phage treatment of human infections. Bacteriophage 1, 66–85.

Aljabali, A.A., Shukla, S., Lomonossoff, G.P., Steinmetz, N.F., Evans, D.J., 2013. CPMV-DOX delivers. Mol. Pharm. 10, 3–10.

Allen, M., Bulte, J.W., Liepold, L., Basu, G., Zywicke, H.A., Frank, J.A., Young, M., Douglas, T., 2005. Paramagnetic viral nanoparticles as potential high-relaxivity magnetic resonance contrast agents. Magn. Reson. Med. 54, 807–812.

Anguela, X.M., Sharma, R., Doyon, Y., Miller, J.C., Li, H., Haurigot, V., Rohde, M.E., Wong, S.Y., Davidson, R.J., Zhou, S., Gregory, P.D., Holmes, M.C., High, K.A., 2013. Robust ZFN-mediated genome editing in adult hemophilic mice. Blood 122, 3283–3287.

Bakhshinejad, B., Sadeghizadeh, M., 2014. Bacteriophages and development of nanomaterials for neural regeneration. Neural Regener. Res. 9, 1955–1958.

Bakhshinejad, B., Karimi, M., Khalaj-Kondori, M., 2015. Phage display: development of nanocarriers for targeted drug delivery to the brain. Neural Regener. Res. 10, 862–865.

Bar, H., Yacoby, I., Benhar, I., 2008. Killing cancer cells by targeted drug-carrying phage nanomedicines. BMC Biotechnol. 8, 37.

Barbas, C.F., Burton, D.R., Scott, J.K., Silverman, G.J., 2001. Phage Display: A Laboratory Manual. Cold Spring Harbor Laboratory Press, New York.

Bhattarai, S.R., Yoo, S.Y., Lee, S.W., Dean, D., 2012. Engineered phage-based therapeutic materials inhibit *Chlamydia trachomatis* intracellular infection. Biomaterials 33, 5166–5174.

Bourdenx, M., Dutheil, N., Bezard, E., Dehay, B., 2014. Systemic gene delivery to the central nervous system using Adeno-associated virus. Front. Mol. Neurosci. 7, 50.

Bratkovic, T., 2010. Progress in phage display: evolution of the technique and its application. Cell. Mol. Life Sci. 67, 749–767.

Campbell, A., 2003. The future of bacteriophage biology. Nat. Rev. Genet. 4, 471–477.

Chariou, P.L., Lee, K.L., Wen, A.M., Gulati, N.M., Stewart, P.L., Steinmetz, N.F., 2015. Detection and imaging of aggressive cancer cells using an epidermal growth factor receptor (EGFR)-targeted filamentous plant virus-based nanoparticle. Bioconjug. Chem. 26, 262–269.

Chen, X., Goncalves, M.A., 2015. Engineered viruses as genome editing devices. Mol. Ther. 24, 447–457.

Chung, W.J., Merzlyak, A., Yoo, S.Y., Lee, S.W., 2010. Genetically engineered liquid-crystalline viral films for directing neural cell growth. Langmuir 26, 9885–9890.

Comellas-Aragones, M., Engelkamp, H., Claessen, V.I., Sommerdijk, N.A., Rowan, A.E., Christianen, P.C., Maan, J.C., Verduin, B.J., Cornelissen, J.J., Nolte, R.J., 2007. A virus-based single-enzyme nanoreactor. Nat. Nanotechnol. 2, 635–639.

Connor, B., Sun, Y., Von Hieber, D., Tang, S.K., Jones, K.S., Maucksch, C., 2015. AAV-mediated BDNF gene therapy in a transgenic rat model of Huntington's disease. Gene Ther. 23, 283–295.

Datta, A., Hooker, J.M., Botta, M., Francis, M.B., Aime, S., Raymond, K.N., 2008. High relaxivity gadolinium hydroxypyridonate–viral capsid conjugates: nanosized MRI contrast agents. J. Am. Chem. Soc. 130, 2546–2552.

Ding, Q., Strong, A., Patel, K.M., Ng, S.L., Gosis, B.S., Regan, S.N., Cowan, C.A., Rader, D.J., Musunuru, K., 2014. Permanent alteration of PCSK9 with in vivo CRISPR–Cas9 genome editing. Circ. Res. 115, 488–492.

Douglas, T., Young, M., 2006. Viruses: making friends with old foes. Science 312, 873–875.

Esfandiari, N., Arzanani, M.K., Soleimani, M., Kohi-Habibi, M., Svendsen, W.E., 2015. A new application of plant virus nanoparticles as drug delivery in breast cancer. Tumour Biol. 37, 1229–1236.

Farr, R., Choi, D.S., Lee, S.W., 2014. Phage-based nanomaterials for biomedical applications. Acta Biomater. 10, 1741–1750.

Flexman, J.A., Cross, D.J., Lewellen, B.L., Miyoshi, S., Kim, Y., Minoshima, S., 2008. Magnetically targeted viral envelopes: a PET investigation of initial biodistribution. IEEE Trans. Nanobioscience 7, 223–232.

Frenkel, D., Solomon, B., 2002. Filamentous phage as vector-mediated antibody delivery to the brain. Proc. Natl. Acad. Sci. U. S. A. 99, 5675–5679.

Gaj, T., Epstein, B.E., Schaffer, D.V., 2015. Genome engineering using Adeno-associated virus: basic and clinical research applications. Mol. Ther. 24, 458–464.

Galaway, F.A., Stockley, P.G., 2013. MS2 viruslike particles: a robust, semisynthetic targeted drug delivery platform. Mol. Pharm. 10, 59–68.

Ghosh, D., Kohli, A.G., Moser, F., Endy, D., Belcher, A.M., 2012a. Refactored M13 bacteriophage as a platform for tumor cell imaging and drug delivery. ACS Synth. Biol. 1, 576–582.

Ghosh, D., Lee, Y., Thomas, S., Kohli, A.G., Yun, D.S., Belcher, A.M., Kelly, K.A., 2012b. M13-templated magnetic nanoparticles for targeted in vivo imaging of prostate cancer. Nat. Nanotechnol. 7, 677–682.

Grifman, M., Trepel, M., Speece, P., Gilbert, L.B., Arap, W., Pasqualini, R., Weitzman, M.D., 2001. Incorporation of tumor-targeting peptides into recombinant adeno-associated virus capsids. Mol. Ther. 3, 964–975.

Hamzeh-Mivehroud, M., Alizadeh, A.A., Morris, M.B., Church, W.B., Dastmalchi, S., 2013. Phage display as a technology delivering on the promise of peptide drug discovery. Drug Discov. Today 18, 1144–1157.
Hernandez-Garcia, A., Kraft, D.J., Janssen, A.F., Bomans, P.H., Sommerdijk, N.A., Thies-Weesie, D.M., Favretto, M.E., Brock, R., De Wolf, F.A., Werten, M.W., Van Der Schoot, P., Stuart, M.C., De Vries, R., 2014. Design and self-assembly of simple coat proteins for artificial viruses. Nat. Nanotechnol. 9, 698–702.
Hoban, M.D., Cost, G.J., Mendel, M.C., Romero, Z., Kaufman, M.L., Joglekar, A.V., Ho, M., Lumaquin, D., Gray, D., Lill, G.R., Cooper, A.R., Urbinati, F., Senadheera, S., Zhu, A., Liu, P.Q., Paschon, D.E., Zhang, L., Rebar, E.J., Wilber, A., Wang, X., Gregory, P.D., Holmes, M.C., Reik, A., Hollis, R.P., Kohn, D.B., 2015. Correction of the sickle cell disease mutation in human hematopoietic stem/progenitor cells. Blood 125, 2597–2604.
Holkers, M., Maggio, I., Liu, J., Janssen, J.M., Miselli, F., Mussolino, C., Recchia, A., Cathomen, T., Goncalves, M.A., 2013. Differential integrity of TALE nuclease genes following adenoviral and lentiviral vector gene transfer into human cells. Nucleic Acids Res. 41, e63.
Hong, S.H., Park, S.J., Lee, S., Cho, C.S., Cho, M.H., 2015. Aerosol gene delivery using viral vectors and cationic carriers for in vivo lung cancer therapy. Expert Opin. Drug Deliv. 12, 977–991.
Hooker, J.M., Datta, A., Botta, M., Raymond, K.N., Francis, M.B., 2007. Magnetic resonance contrast agents from viral capsid shells: a comparison of exterior and interior cargo strategies. Nano Lett. 7, 2207–2210.
Hooker, J.M., O'Neil, J.P., Romanini, D.W., Taylor, S.E., Francis, M.B., 2008. Genome-free viral capsids as carriers for positron emission tomography radiolabels. Mol. Imaging Biol. 10, 182–191.
Hu, Y., Zandi, R., Anavitarte, A., Knobler, C.M., Gelbart, W.M., 2008. Packaging of a polymer by a viral capsid: the interplay between polymer length and capsid size. Biophys. J. 94, 1428–1436.
Huang, X., Bronstein, L.M., Retrum, J., Dufort, C., Tsvetkova, I., Aniagyei, S., Stein, B., Stucky, G., McKenna, B., Remmes, N., Baxter, D., Kao, C.C., Dragnea, B., 2007. Self-assembled virus-like particles with magnetic cores. Nano Lett. 7, 2407–2416.
Huang, J., Ru, B., Dai, P., 2011. Bioinformatics resources and tools for phage display. Molecules 16, 694–709.
Huang, J., Ru, B., Zhu, P., Nie, F., Yang, J., Wang, X., Dai, P., Lin, H., Guo, F.B., Rao, N., 2012. MimoDB 2.0: a mimotope database and beyond. Nucleic Acids Res. 40, 271–277.
Jara, J.H., Stanford, M.J., Zhu, Y., Tu, M., Hauswirth, W.W., Bohn, M.C., Devries, S.H., Ozdinler, P.H., 2016. Healthy and diseased corticospinal motor neurons are selectively transduced upon direct AAV2-2 injection into the motor cortex. Gene Ther. 23, 272–282.
Jin, H.E., Farr, R., Lee, S.W., 2014. Collagen mimetic peptide engineered M13 bacteriophage for collagen targeting and imaging in cancer. Biomaterials 35, 9236–9245.
Jung, B., Rao, A.L., Anvari, B., 2011. Optical nano-constructs composed of genome-depleted brome mosaic virus doped with a near infrared chromophore for potential biomedical applications. ACS Nano 5, 1243–1252.
Kaesberg, P., 1956. Structure of small "spherical" viruses. Science 124, 626–628.
Kazmierczak, Z., Piotrowicz, A., Owczarek, B., Hodyra, K., Miernikiewicz, P., Lecion, D., Harhala, M., Gorski, A., Dabrowska, K., 2014. Molecular imaging of T4 phage in mammalian tissues and cells. Bacteriophage 4, e28364.
Kehoe, J.W., Kay, B.K., 2005. Filamentous phage display in the new millennium. Chem. Rev. 105, 4056–4072.
Klug, A., Caspar, D.L., 1960. The structure of small viruses. Adv. Virus Res. 7, 225–325.

Knight, C.A., 1954. The chemical constitution of viruses. Adv. Virus Res. 2, 153–182.

Koudelka, K.J., Manchester, M., 2010. Chemically modified viruses: principles and applications. Curr. Opin. Chem. Biol. 14, 810–817.

Kovacs, E.W., Hooker, J.M., Romanini, D.W., Holder, P.G., Berry, K.E., Francis, M.B., 2007. Dual-surface-modified bacteriophage MS2 as an ideal scaffold for a viral capsid-based drug delivery system. Bioconjug. Chem. 18, 1140–1147.

Kushner, D.J., 1969. Self-assembly of biological structures. Bacteriol. Rev. 33, 302–345.

Kutter, E., De Vos, D., Gvasalia, G., Alavidze, Z., Gogokhia, L., Kuhl, S., Abedon, S.T., 2010. Phage therapy in clinical practice: treatment of human infections. Curr. Pharm. Biotechnol. 11, 69–86.

Ledford, H., 2015. Cancer-fighting viruses win approval. Nature 526, 622–623.

Lewis, J.D., Destito, G., Zijlstra, A., Gonzalez, M.J., Quigley, J.P., Manchester, M., Stuhlmann, H., 2006. Viral nanoparticles as tools for intravital vascular imaging. Nat. Med. 12, 354–360.

Li, F., Zhang, Z.P., Peng, J., Cui, Z.Q., Pang, D.W., Li, K., Wei, H.P., Zhou, Y.F., Wen, J.K., Zhang, X.E., 2009. Imaging viral behavior in Mammalian cells with self-assembled capsid–quantum-dot hybrid particles. Small 5, 718–726.

Li, K., Chen, Y., Li, S., Nguyen, H.G., Niu, Z., You, S., Mello, C.M., Lu, X., Wang, Q., 2010. Chemical modification of M13 bacteriophage and its application in cancer cell imaging. Bioconjug. Chem. 21, 1369–1377.

Li, H., Haurigot, V., Doyon, Y., Li, T., Wong, S.Y., Bhagwat, A.S., Malani, N., Anguela, X.M., Sharma, R., Ivanciu, L., Murphy, S.L., Finn, J.D., Khazi, F.R., Zhou, S., Paschon, D.E., Rebar, E.J., Bushman, F.D., Gregory, P.D., Holmes, M.C., High, K.A., 2011. In vivo genome editing restores haemostasis in a mouse model of haemophilia. Nature 475, 217–221.

Liu, C.C., Schultz, P.G., 2010. Adding new chemistries to the genetic code. Annu. Rev. Biochem. 79, 413–444.

Liu, Z., Qiao, J., Niu, Z., Wang, Q., 2012. Natural supramolecular building blocks: from virus coat proteins to viral nanoparticles. Chem. Soc. Rev. 41, 6178–6194.

Loo, L., Guenther, R.H., Lommel, S.A., Franzen, S., 2007. Encapsidation of nanoparticles by red clover necrotic mosaic virus. J. Am. Chem. Soc. 129, 11111–11117.

Loo, L., Guenther, R.H., Lommel, S.A., Franzen, S., 2008. Infusion of dye molecules into Red clover necrotic mosaic virus. Chem. Commun. (Camb.) 88–90.

Lucas, W. 2010. Viral capsids and envelopes: structure and function. In: eLS, John Wiley & Sons Ltd, Chichester.

Ma, Y., Nolte, R.J., Cornelissen, J.J., 2012. Virus-based nanocarriers for drug delivery. Adv. Drug Deliv. Rev. 64, 811–825.

Maggio, I., Holkers, M., Liu, J., Janssen, J.M., Chen, X., Goncalves, M.A., 2014. Adenoviral vector delivery of RNA-guided CRISPR/Cas9 nuclease complexes induces targeted mutagenesis in a diverse array of human cells. Sci. Rep. 4, 5105.

Manchester, M., Singh, P., 2006. Virus-based nanoparticles (VNPs): platform technologies for diagnostic imaging. Adv. Drug Deliv. Rev. 58, 1505–1522.

Mao, C., Liu, A., Cao, B., 2009. Virus-based chemical and biological sensing. Angew. Chem. Int. Ed. Engl. 48, 6790–6810.

Marvin, D.A., Symmons, M.F., Straus, S.K., 2014. Structure and assembly of filamentous bacteriophages. Prog. Biophys. Mol. Biol. 114, 80–122.

Mastrobattista, E., Van Der Aa, M.A., Hennink, W.E., Crommelin, D.J., 2006. Artificial viruses: a nanotechnological approach to gene delivery. Nat. Rev. Drug Discov. 5, 115–121.

Merentie, M., Lottonen-Raikaslehto, L., Parviainen, V., Huusko, J., Pikkarainen, S., Mendel, M., Laham-Karam, N., Karja, V., Rissanen, R., Hedman, M., Yla-Herttuala, S., 2015. Efficacy

and safety of myocardial gene transfer of adenovirus, adeno-associated virus and lentivirus vectors in the mouse heart. Gene Ther. 23, 296–305.
Molek, P., Bratkovic, T., 2015. Bacteriophages as scaffolds for bipartite display: designing swiss army knives on a nanoscale. Bioconjug. Chem. 26, 367–378.
Nayerossadat, N., Maedeh, T., Ali, P.A., 2012. Viral and nonviral delivery systems for gene delivery. Adv. Biol. Res. 1, 27.
Palaniappan, K.K., Ramirez, R.M., Bajaj, V.S., Wemmer, D.E., Pines, A., Francis, M.B., 2013. Molecular imaging of cancer cells using a bacteriophage-based 129Xe NMR biosensor. Angew. Chem. Int. Ed. Engl. 52, 4849–4853.
Pande, J., Szewczyk, M.M., Grover, A.K., 2010. Phage display: concept, innovations, applications and future. Biotechnol. Adv. 28, 849–858.
Park, S.B., 2012. Hepatitis E vaccine debuts. Nature 491, 21–22.
Park, J.S., Cho, M.K., Lee, E.J., Ahn, K.Y., Lee, K.E., Jung, J.H., Cho, Y., Han, S.S., Kim, Y.K., Lee, J., 2009. A highly sensitive and selective diagnostic assay based on virus nanoparticles. Nat. Nanotechnol. 4, 259–264.
Paschke, M., 2006. Phage display systems and their applications. Appl. Microbiol. Biotechnol. 70, 2–11.
Perlmutter, J.D., Hagan, M.F., 2015. Mechanisms of virus assembly. Annu. Rev. Phys. Chem. 66, 217–239.
Petrenko, V., 2008. Evolution of phage display: from bioactive peptides to bioselective nanomaterials. Expert Opin. Drug Deliv. 5, 825–836.
Phumyen, A., Jantasorn, S., Jumnainsong, A., Leelayuwat, C., 2014. Doxorubicin-conjugated bacteriophages carrying anti-MHC class I chain-related A for targeted cancer therapy in vitro. OncoTargets Ther. 7, 2183–2195.
Pires, D.P., Vilas Boas, D., Sillankorva, S., Azeredo, J., 2015. Phage therapy: a step forward in the treatment of *Pseudomonas aeruginosa* infections. J. Virol. 89, 7449–7456.
Pokorski, J.K., Steinmetz, N.F., 2011. The art of engineering viral nanoparticles. Mol. Pharm. 8, 29–43.
Powers, K.W., Brown, S.C., Krishna, V.B., Wasdo, S.C., Moudgil, B.M., Roberts, S.M., 2006. Research strategies for safety evaluation of nanomaterials. Part VI. Characterization of nanoscale particles for toxicological evaluation. Toxicol. Sci. 90, 296–303.
Pranjol, M.Z., Hajitou, A., 2015. Bacteriophage-derived vectors for targeted cancer gene therapy. Viruses 7, 268–284.
Prasuhn Jr., D.E., Yeh, R.M., Obenaus, A., Manchester, M., Finn, M.G., 2007. Viral MRI contrast agents: coordination of Gd by native virions and attachment of Gd complexes by azide–alkyne cycloaddition. Chem. Commun. (Camb.), 1269–1271.
Qazi, S., Liepold, L.O., Abedin, M.J., Johnson, B., Prevelige, P., Frank, J.A., Douglas, T., 2013. P22 viral capsids as nanocomposite high-relaxivity MRI contrast agents. Mol. Pharm. 10, 11–17.
Rakonjac, J., Bennett, N.J., Spagnuolo, J., Gagic, D., Russel, M., 2011. Filamentous bacteriophage: biology, phage display and nanotechnology applications. Curr. Issues Mol. Biol. 13, 51–76.
Rangel, R., Guzman-Rojas, L., Le Roux, L.G., Staquicini, F.I., Hosoya, H., Barbu, E.M., Ozawa, M.G., Nie, J., Dunner Jr., K., Langley, R.R., Sage, E.H., Koivunen, E., Gelovani, J.G., Lobb, R.R., Sidman, R.L., Pasqualini, R., Arap, W., 2012. Combinatorial targeting and discovery of ligand–receptors in organelles of mammalian cells. Nat. Commun. 3, 788.
Rangel, R., Dobroff, A.S., Guzman-Rojas, L., Salmeron, C.C., Gelovani, J.G., Sidman, R.L., Pasqualini, R., Arap, W., 2013. Targeting mammalian organelles with internalizing phage (iPhage) libraries. Nat. Protoc. 8, 1916–1939.
Ren, Y., Wong, S.M., Lim, L.Y., 2007. Folic acid-conjugated protein cages of a plant virus: a novel delivery platform for doxorubicin. Bioconjug. Chem. 18, 836–843.

Riedel, S., 2005. Edward Jenner and the history of smallpox and vaccination. Proc. (Baylor Univ. Med. Cent.) 18, 21–25.
Rincon, M.Y., Vandendriessche, T., Chuah, M.K., 2015. Gene therapy for cardiovascular disease: advances in vector development, targeting, and delivery for clinical translation. Cardiovasc. Res. 108, 4–20.
Rodrigues, A.F., Soares, H.R., Guerreiro, M.R., Alves, P.M., Coroadinha, A.S., 2015. Viral vaccines and their manufacturing cell substrates: new trends and designs in modern vaccinology. Biotechnol. J. 10, 1329–1344.
Rodriguez-Limas, W.A., Sekar, K., Tyo, K.E., 2013. Virus-like particles: the future of microbial factories and cell-free systems as platforms for vaccine development. Curr. Opin. Biotechnol. 24, 1089–1093.
Roldao, A., Mellado, M.C., Castilho, L.R., Carrondo, M.J., Alves, P.M., 2010. Virus-like particles in vaccine development. Expert Rev. Vaccines 9, 1149–1176.
Russel, M., Whirlow, H., Sun, T.P., Webster, R.E., 1988. Low-frequency infection of F- bacteria by transducing particles of filamentous bacteriophages. J. Bacteriol. 170, 5312–5316.
Russel, M., Lowman, H.B., Clackson, T., 2004. Introduction to phage biology and phage display. In: Lowman, T.C.A.H. (Ed.), Phage Display: A Pratical Approach. Oxford University Press, Oxford.
Sawada, R., Peterson, C.Y., Gonzalez, A.M., Potenza, B.M., Mueller, B., Coimbra, R., Eliceiri, B.P., Baird, A., 2011. A phage-targeting strategy for the design of spatiotemporal drug delivery from grafted matrices. Fibrogenesis Tissue Repair 4, 7.
Sayroo, R., Nolasco, D., Yin, Z., Colon-Cortes, Y., Pandya, M., Ling, C., Aslanidi, G., 2016. Development of novel AAV serotype 6 based vectors with selective tropism for human cancer cells. Gene Ther. 23, 18–25.
Schlick, T.L., Ding, Z., Kovacs, E.W., Francis, M.B., 2005. Dual-surface modification of the tobacco mosaic virus. J. Am. Chem. Soc. 127, 3718–3723.
Senis, E., Fatouros, C., Grosse, S., Wiedtke, E., Niopek, D., Mueller, A.K., Borner, K., Grimm, D., 2014. CRISPR/Cas9-mediated genome engineering: an adeno-associated viral (AAV) vector toolbox. Biotechnol. J. 9, 1402–1412.
Seth, A.K., Geringer, M.R., Nguyen, K.T., Agnew, S.P., Dumanian, Z., Galiano, R.D., Leung, K.P., Mustoe, T.A., Hong, S.J., 2013. Bacteriophage therapy for *Staphylococcus aureus* biofilm-infected wounds: a new approach to chronic wound care. Plast. Reconstr. Surg. 131, 225–234.
Sillankorva, S., Azeredo, J., 2014. Bacteriophage attack as an anti-biofilm strategy. Methods Mol. Biol. 1147, 277–285.
Simoes, M., 2011. Antimicrobial strategies effective against infectious bacterial biofilms. Curr. Med. Chem. 18, 2129–2145.
Smith, G.P., 1985. Filamentous fusion phage: novel expression vectors that display cloned antigens on the virion surface. Science 228, 1315–1317.
Smith, G.P., Petrenko, V.A., 1997. Phage display. Chem. Rev. 97, 391–410.
Smith, M.T., Hawes, A.K., Bundy, B.C., 2013. Reengineering viruses and virus-like particles through chemical functionalization strategies. Curr. Opin. Biotechnol. 24, 620–626.
Soendergaard, M., Newton-Northup, J.R., Deutscher, S.L., 2014a. In vitro high throughput phage display selection of ovarian cancer avid phage clones for near-infrared optical imaging. Comb. Chem. High Throughput Screen. 17, 859–867.
Soendergaard, M., Newton-Northup, J.R., Deutscher, S.L., 2014b. In vivo phage display selection of an ovarian cancer targeting peptide for SPECT/CT imaging. Am. J. Nucl. Med. Mol. Imaging 4, 561–570.
Steinmetz, N.F., 2010. Viral nanoparticles as platforms for next-generation therapeutics and imaging devices. Nanomedicine 6, 634–641.

Steinmetz, N.F., Hong, V., Spoerke, E.D., Lu, P., Breitenkamp, K., Finn, M.G., Manchester, M., 2009. Buckyballs meet viral nanoparticles: candidates for biomedicine. J. Am. Chem. Soc. 131, 17093–17095.
Stephanopoulos, N., Tong, G.J., Hsiao, S.C., Francis, M.B., 2010. Dual-surface modified virus capsids for targeted delivery of photodynamic agents to cancer cells. ACS Nano 4, 6014–6020.
Stone, D., 2010. Novel viral vector systems for gene therapy. Viruses 2, 1002–1007.
Strable, E., Prasuhn Jr., D.E., Udit, A.K., Brown, S., Link, A.J., Ngo, J.T., Lander, G., Quispe, J., Potter, C.S., Carragher, B., Tirrell, D.A., Finn, M.G., 2008. Unnatural amino acid incorporation into virus-like particles. Bioconjug. Chem. 19, 866–875.
Suci, P.A., Varpness, Z., Gillitzer, E., Douglas, T., Young, M., 2007. Targeting and photodynamic killing of a microbial pathogen using protein cage architectures functionalized with a photosensitizer. Langmuir 23, 12280–12286.
Swartz, M.A., Hirosue, S., Hubbell, J.A., 2012. Engineering approaches to immunotherapy. Sci. Transl. Med. 4, 148rv9.
Swiech, L., Heidenreich, M., Banerjee, A., Habib, N., Li, Y., Trombetta, J., Sur, M., Zhang, F., 2015. In vivo interrogation of gene function in the mammalian brain using CRISPR–Cas9. Nat. Biotechnol. 33, 102–106.
Tang, J.B., Wu, Y.F., Cao, Y., Chen, C.H., Zhou, Y.L., Avanessian, B., Shimada, M., Wang, X.T., Liu, P.Y., 2016a. Basic FGF or VEGF gene therapy corrects insufficiency in the intrinsic healing capacity of tendons. Sci. Rep. 6, 1–12.
Tang, J.B., Zhou, Y.L., Wu, Y.F., Liu, P.Y., Wang, X.T., 2016b. Gene therapy strategies to improve strength and quality of flexor tendon healing. Expert Opin. Biol. Ther. 1–11.
Tong, G.J., Hsiao, S.C., Carrico, Z.M., Francis, M.B., 2009. Viral capsid DNA aptamer conjugates as multivalent cell-targeting vehicles. J. Am. Chem. Soc. 131, 11174–11178.
Torres-Barcelo, C., Hochberg, M.E., 2016. Evolutionary rationale for phages as complements of antibiotics. Trends Microbiol. 24, 249–256.
Trepel, M., Korbelin, J., Spies, E., Heckmann, M.B., Hunger, A., Fehse, B., Katus, H.A., Kleinschmidt, J.A., Muller, O.J., Michelfelder, S., 2015. Treatment of multifocal breast cancer by systemic delivery of dual-targeted adeno-associated viral vectors. Gene Ther. 22, 848.
Vandenheuvel, D., Singh, A., Vandersteegen, K., Klumpp, J., Lavigne, R., Van Den Mooter, G., 2013. Feasibility of spray drying bacteriophages into respirable powders to combat pulmonary bacterial infections. Eur. J. Pharm. Biopharm. 84, 578–582.
Venkatesan, N., Perumal, G., Doble, M., 2015. Bacterial resistance in biofilm-associated bacteria. Future Microbiol. 10, 1743–1750.
Wei, F., McConnell, K.I., Yu, T.K., Suh, J., 2012. Conjugation of paclitaxel on adeno-associated virus (AAV) nanoparticles for co-delivery of genes and drugs. Eur. J. Pharm. Sci. 46, 167–172.
Weinbauer, M.G., 2004. Ecology of prokaryotic viruses. FEMS Microbiol. Rev. 28, 127–181.
Wen, A.M., Shukla, S., Saxena, P., Aljabali, A.A., Yildiz, I., Dey, S., Mealy, J.E., Yang, A.C., Evans, D.J., Lomonossoff, G.P., Steinmetz, N.F., 2012. Interior engineering of a viral nanoparticle and its tumor homing properties. Biomacromolecules 13, 3990–4001.
Yacoby, I., Shamis, M., Bar, H., Shabat, D., Benhar, I., 2006. Targeting antibacterial agents by using drug-carrying filamentous bacteriophages. Antimicrob. Agents Chemother. 50, 2087–2097.
Yi, H., Ghosh, D., Ham, M.H., Qi, J., Barone, P.W., Strano, M.S., Belcher, A.M., 2012. M13 phage-functionalized single-walled carbon nanotubes as nanoprobes for second near-infrared window fluorescence imaging of targeted tumors. Nano Lett. 12, 1176–1183.

Yildiz, I., Shukla, S., Steinmetz, N.F., 2011. Applications of viral nanoparticles in medicine. Curr. Opin. Biotechnol. 22, 901–908.

Yildiz, I., Lee, K.L., Chen, K., Shukla, S., Steinmetz, N.F., 2013. Infusion of imaging and therapeutic molecules into the plant virus-based carrier cowpea mosaic virus: cargo-loading and delivery. J. Control. Release 172, 568–578.

Yilmaz, C., Colak, M., Yilmaz, B.C., Ersoz, G., Kutateladze, M., Gozlugol, M., 2013. Bacteriophage therapy in implant-related infections: an experimental study. J. Bone Joint Surg. Am. 95, 117–125.

Yoo, S.Y., Oh, J.W., Lee, S.W., 2012. Phage-chips for novel optically readable tissue engineering assays. Langmuir 28, 2166–2172.

Young, M., Willits, D., Uchida, M., Douglas, T., 2008. Plant viruses as biotemplates for materials and their use in nanotechnology. Annu. Rev. Phytopathol. 46, 361–384.

Yungher, B.J., Luo, X., Salgueiro, Y., Blackmore, M.G., Park, K.K., 2015. Viral vector-based improvement of optic nerve regeneration: characterization of individual axons' growth patterns and synaptogenesis in a visual target. Gene Ther. 22, 811–821.

Synthetic biology strategies towards the development of new bioinspired technologies for medical applications

16

J.L. Rodrigues, D. Ferreira, L.R. Rodrigues
University of Minho, Centre of Biological Engineering, Braga, Portugal

16.1 Introduction

Synthetic biology is an exciting scientific field that has a broad application in different sectors, such as medical, chemical, food, and agriculture, and may provide innovative solutions to several challenges (Khalil and Collins, 2010; Weber and Fussenegger, 2009; Liang et al., 2011). It can be used in the production of value-added chemicals (Moon et al., 2010), biofuels (Dong et al., 2015), biopharmaceuticals (Paddon and Keasling, 2014; Ajikumar et al., 2010), biosensors (Pardee et al., 2014) and vaccines (Nogales et al., 2014), or even as tools for in vivo health applications (Duan and March, 2010; Anderson et al., 2006; Kemmer et al., 2010) or bioremediation (Schmidt and de Lorenzo, 2012).

Many definitions have been proposed for this emergent field (Calvert, 2010; Arkin et al., 2009) as it has the potential for application in diverse areas and combines knowledge from the broad scientific backgrounds of its practitioners, which include engineering disciplines (chemical engineering, mechanical engineering, electrical engineering and computer science) and biological sciences (molecular cell biology, metabolic engineering, biomedical engineering, biochemistry, systems biology, medicine and biomaterials) (Liang et al., 2011; Kitney and Freemont, 2012; Cheng and Lu, 2012). Synthetic biology can be defined as "the design and construction of biological parts, devices and systems and/or the re-design of existing, natural biological systems for useful purposes" (Royal Academy of Engineering, 2009) or as "the effort to make biology easier to engineer", a more practical definition adopted by the Synthetic Biology Engineering Research Center (SynBERC, US).

Although some of the techniques and methods being used are quite old, synthetic biology has only become a field of its own in the last decade (Hellsten and Nerlich, 2011; Liang et al., 2011). However, impressive advances have been achieved that demonstrate its huge potential. The advances in synthetic biology are mostly driven by the progress and reduced cost of tools for DNA sequencing and synthesis, as well as by the development of computational and systems biology tools (Baker, 2011; Liang et al., 2011; Boyle and Silver, 2009).

Bioinspired Materials for Medical Applications. http://dx.doi.org/10.1016/B978-0-08-100741-9.00016-4

In this chapter we revise some of the tools and fundamentals of synthetic biology, such as the use of engineering principles, genome editing tools and metabolomics. In addition, we discuss the potential of synthetic biology for medical applications in the prevention, diagnosis and treatment of diseases.

16.2 Tools and fundamentals

The engineering of biological systems is an iterative process (Fig. 16.1) that includes the design, modeling and simulation of a biological system, its construction, evaluating its performance and optimizing the design until the desired outcome is attained (Purnick and Weiss, 2009; Cheng and Lu, 2012). Over the years several tools and methods have been developed to reduce the cost and time needed to engineer biological systems (Keasling, 2012).

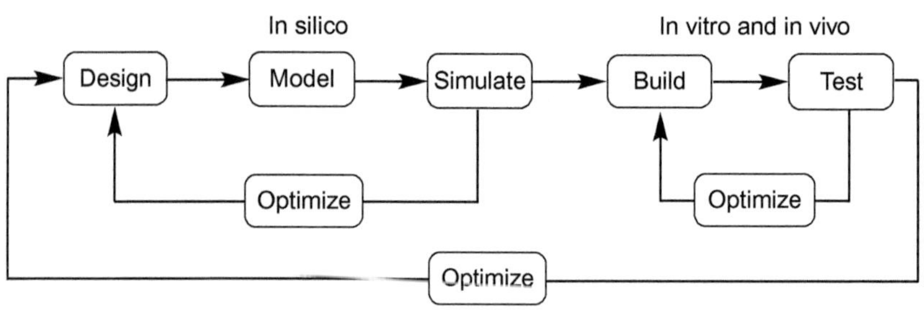

Fig. 16.1 Synthetic biology iterative cycle for engineering and optimizing biological systems.

16.2.1 Engineering principles

The use of engineering principles such as standardization/modularity, decoupling and abstraction was proposed by Endy (2005) to "make biology into an engineering discipline" (Calvert and Martin, 2009). The use of these principles allows separating synthetic biology approaches from genetic engineering ones since they reduce the complexity of biological systems (Endy, 2005; O'Malley et al., 2008). Synthetic biologists aim to program living organisms with a similar mindset of chip designers and computer programmers (Clancy and Voigt, 2010; Way et al., 2014).

The standardization/modularity principle is intended to make cloning easier and less laborious by allowing synthetic biologists to create a toolbox of well-characterized biological parts formatted according to specific rules. These standardized parts include promoter sequences, operators, ribosome-binding sites (RBS), coding DNA sequences (CDS), terminator sites, reporter proteins or antisense RNAs (Rodrigues and Kluskens, 2011; Heinemann and Panke, 2006) that can be assembled to form new biosystems in a similar way as electronic circuits are assembled in a computer motherboard (Ferber, 2004; Choffnes et al., 2011).

Decoupling is a tool that allows decomposing a complicated problem in a series of simpler ones, solving them independently and then combining the results (Endy, 2005; Andrianantoandro et al., 2006). Although all scientists need to have a sound knowledge of all the steps of the project, some scientists only need to focus on the design of useful standardized parts and others use their expertise to focus on the building of DNA circuits (Endy, 2005; Way et al., 2014; Heinemann and Panke, 2006).

The abstraction principle allows the introduction of hierarchical levels to manage the complexity of natural biological systems. There are four hierarchical levels that represent the growing levels of complexity and abstraction: "DNA" (genetic material), "Parts" (single basic biological functions), "Devices" (any arrangement of "Parts" that perform a single human-defined function) and "Systems (any combination of "Devices" with the purpose of executing a specified function) (Endy, 2005). These "Systems" are maintained in a "Chassis."

16.2.2 Parts and devices

16.2.2.1 State sensors (Promoters, RBS, riboswitches and aptamers)

Usually, gene expression is mediated by a binary state of "on" and "off" (Leonard et al., 2008). Inducible promoters are important to reduce the metabolic burden that is imposed on the organism and/or to create devices with a planned function, such as sensing the cell state. However, the number of inducible promoters available to express biosynthetic genes or pathways is very small (eg, tetracycline-inducible P_{tet}, arabinose-inducible P_{BAD} and the lactose and IPTG (isopropyl β-D-1-thiogalactopyranoside)-inducible P_{lac}) (Shiue and Prather, 2012). Bacteriophage-derived T7 promoter (P_{T7}) has also been particularly important due to its capability to drive robust gene expression (Kis et al., 2015) providing users with orthogonal control over a gene of interest. Orthogonal control is a cellular control designed to avoid undesired native host interference and regulation. In cases of complex pathways, these promoters are not enough to control specific elements (Shiue and Prather, 2012). It is also possible to use promoters that respond to specific stimuli found in the microenvironment (temperature, pH, oxygen, metabolite concentration, light, etc.). These promoters are naturally present in the cell to avoid waste of energy or inappropriate physiological responses (Garst and Batey, 2009). The use of these promoters in synthetic biology has the advantage of not requiring a chemical inducer that may not be recommended for therapeutic applications. In addition, they can be used in "state sensor" devices that can sense the microenvironment and respond accordingly, thus providing a means of control of the biological system. For example, the engineered cell can be programmed to sense toxic intermediates and to consume them. Since new orthogonal inducer promoters are needed for synthetic applications, Alper et al. (2005) used a random mutagenesis approach to modify a constitutive promoter and obtained a collection of promoters with different strengths. By using these promoter libraries it is possible to find new promoters that allow an appropriate or optimal expression level. To design stronger promoters, new promoter libraries have been created with modifications between −35 and −10 regions or in the sequence of the transcription factor binding site (Jensen and Hammer, 1998; Schlabach et al., 2010).

RBS is a RNA sequence upstream of the start codon that mediates translation initiation (Boyle and Silver, 2012) and its sequence affects the translation efficiency. Synthetic RBS sequences can be used to optimize protein expression levels. The RBS calculator, an online free software developed by Salis (2011), uses a statistical thermodynamic model that can predict the translation initiation rate (TIR) of mRNAs and also design synthetic RBS or RBS libraries with TIR from 0.1 to 100,000-fold range or more.

Riboswitches are other genetic "parts" that act as state sensors. They are RNA-based regulatory components typically found in the 5′-untranslatted regions (5′-UTR) of mRNAs that bind specific small molecules and induce conformational changes (Beisel and Smolke, 2009; Rodrigues and Kluskens, 2011; Winkler and Breaker, 2005). Riboswitches have two distinct domains, namely a metabolite receptor known as aptamer domain, and an expression platform whose secondary structure signals the regulatory response. Embedded within the aptamer domain is the switching sequence, a sequence shared between the aptamer domain and the expression platform (Garst and Batey, 2009). Aptamer domain sites form precise 3D structures composed of highly specific binding pockets in 5′-UTR. Once a ligand selectively binds an aptamer site, a conformational change leads to downstream modulation of gene expression (Isaacs et al., 2006). Aptamer domains are versatile and widely used as sensitive elements for RNA-based biosensing (Khalil and Collins, 2010).

The optimization of these regulatory genetic elements sole or combined (Fig. 16.2A) is very important for the creation of devices that require a very precise level of gene/protein expression. For a more detailed description of applications of these state sensors please refer to Section 16.4.

16.2.2.2 Spatiotemporal controllers

The timing of the expression of pathway components is very important to obtain high industrial production of a compound (Medema et al., 2011), but also in therapeutic applications for example to deliver a drug only when it reaches the diseased cell or a cell in a given condition. The "just-in-time" gene expression (Fig. 16.2B) can be very beneficial for the cell as it can help to reduce the metabolic burden imposed by the heterologous expression that requires high levels of energy and resources (Medema et al., 2011; Shiue and Prather, 2012). In *Escherichia coli* it is possible to corroborate this "just-in-time" expression, for example, in the amino acid biosynthesis. The genes encoding enzymes of the pathway are organized into operons in the sequence in which they are needed (Zaslaver et al., 2004, 2006). By using synthetic regulation (engineering of promoters, RBS and transcriptional units), the genetically modified cell can optimize the use of its limited resources by synchronizing the production of molecules with the moment when they are needed. The timing of expression can also be controlled by metabolite concentrations through allosteric control. Effector molecules can be modified or designed to be further used as switches to regulate protein activity (Medema et al., 2011).

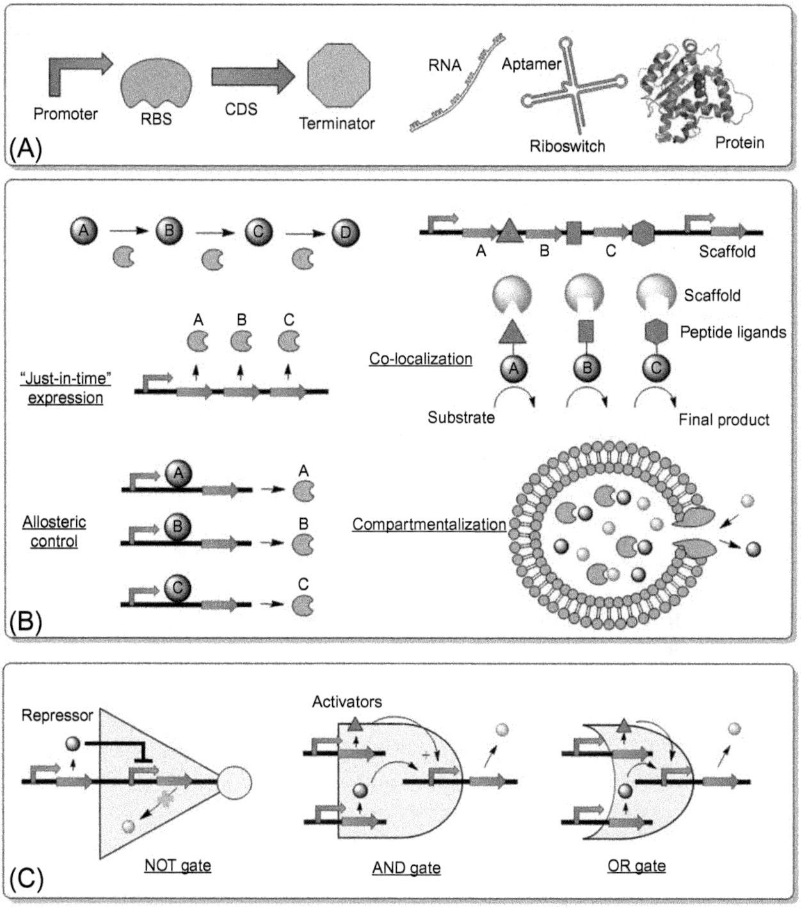

Fig. 16.2 Parts and devices. (A) Basic parts and state sensors. (B) Spatiotemporal controllers. (C) Logic gates. *CDS*, coding DNA sequence; *RBS*, ribosome binding site.

The spatial control of cellular processes can also be a powerful tool in synthetic biology since the local concentration of enzymes and metabolites can have a great influence in the rate at which the biosynthetic reactions of the pathway occur (Medema et al., 2011). Several natural systems use cellular compartmentalization as spatial controllers. The diffusion of small molecules in and out of the compartments is limited and selective, which can protect the pathway from competing reactions, increase substrate/intermediate concentrations and decrease product degradation (Shiue and Prather, 2012; Boyle and Silver, 2012; Parsons et al., 2010; Chessher et al., 2015). In addition, in eukaryotic systems this type of spatial control is frequently used to isolate sensitive metabolic processes from the rest of the cellular environmental (Shiue and Prather, 2012). For example, in plants the last biosynthetic steps of secondary metabolites are performed in vesicles to avoid selftoxicity (Sirikantaramas et al., 2008). In *Salmonella enterica*, specific-amino terminal sequences were found to direct proteins to the microcompartment where possible toxic compounds are produced (Fan et al., 2010; Parsons et al., 2010). In the future, microcompartments may be used to encapsulate, target and deliver therapeutic cargoes to specific cell types and/or tissues (Corchero and Cedano, 2011). Co-localization is also used in natural systems to improve flux through metabolic pathways. For instance, the polyketide synthases are modular enzymes organized in catalytic modules and the intermediates are channeled through them like an assembly line (Khosla et al., 2009). The use of scaffold proteins can reduce the need of highly specific enzymes, since the rates of unwanted side-reactions are lower due to co-localization (Medema et al., 2011). Synthetic protein scaffolds have already been successfully used to improve production titers of several pathways (Moon et al., 2010; Dueber et al., 2009). Cell surface display techniques using scaffolds can also be used for the efficient expression of enzymes on the cell membrane, which allows increasing productivity (Tanaka and Kondo, 2014). In recent years, efforts to construct stable co-culture (microbial consortia), where each cell type is specifically tuned to a part of the production pathway, have also been intensified (Medema et al., 2011; Boyle and Silver, 2012).

16.2.2.3 Logic gates

As mentioned before, synthetic biologists aim to program cells as computer engineers program computers. Devices comprise biochemical reactions that regulate the flow of information and manipulate physical processes, which can be equivalent to engineered digital logic gates that perform computations in a computer (Andrianantoandro et al., 2006). A logic gate implements the Boolean logic (such as AND, OR, or NOT) on one or more logic inputs to produce a logic output. Similar genetic logic gates can be constructed to integrate the sensory signals and to generate an appropriate response (Brophy and Voigt, 2014). NOT gates (or genetic inverters) can find application, for example, when a reduction of gene expression is needed (Shiue and Prather, 2012) (Fig. 16.2C). They consist of a repressor that shuts down the expression of a target gene in response to an input signal. AND gates find use in synthetic biology when multiple inputs need to be processed. For instance, in Anderson et al. (2007) an AND gate was constructed in *E. coli*. This gate integrates information from two promoters as inputs (P_{sal} and P_{BAD}) and only activates a promoter output (P_{T7}) when both input promoters are transcriptionally active. In OR gates, the output gene expression is activated even if only one of the input promoters is activated. These types of gates and other types, such as NAND and NOR, are being extensively explored in synthetic biology (Kis et al., 2015; Song et al., 2011; Kobayashi et al., 2006; Brophy and Voigt, 2014).

16.2.3 DNA sequencing and synthesis

DNA sequencing and synthesis are two essential tools in the reading and writing of DNA and as processes they are advancing exponentially and becoming cheaper and less complex as the years go by (Rothberg and Leamon, 2008; Way et al., 2014; Endy, 2005). DNA synthesis and sequencing allows precise and rapid generation of genetic parts. To rationally design new DNA sequences, restriction sites and undesirable

RNA secondary structures are eliminated and codons for gene expression optimized (Rodrigues and Kluskens, 2011; Liang et al., 2011). In addition to being used in the most synthetic biology applications, these tools are very important to design and create very large and complex circuits like biosynthetic pathways or artificial genomes (Liang et al., 2011; Stähler et al., 2006; Shao et al., 2009) or even cells to be used as data storage devices (Church et al., 2012; Grass et al., 2015; Goldman et al., 2013).

16.2.4 Chassis

The chassis or host cells supply the necessary resources for full functionality of the "Systems" previously mentioned. Depending on the application, the chassis should have different characteristics. In cases where the goal is to use microorganisms as microbial chemical factories, the chassis needs to be genetically stable for long periods of cultivations, they should be robust to industrial processing conditions and they need to be able to grow on minimal, inexpensive carbon sources to minimize production costs (Keasling, 2008, 2012). The ability to switch on the biosynthetic pathway at an exact time is also important since the pathway should be completely repressed during nonproductive phases (Keasling, 2008). *E. coli* and *Saccharomyces cerevisiae* are the two most used chassis (Paddon and Keasling, 2014; Du et al., 2011; Kitney and Freemont, 2012; Pósfai et al., 2006) since their physiology and genetics are well-characterized, they have fast growth rates on minimal inexpensive carbon sources and numerous genetic tools are available for their manipulation (Du et al., 2011). Other well-characterized chassis include *Pseudomonas putida*, *Bacillus subtilis* and *Streptomyces* species (Nikel et al., 2014; Du et al., 2011; Kitney and Freemont, 2012).

Most of the robust strains needed for synthetic biology applications are able to inactivate or eliminate foreign genes to minimize metabolic burden (Keasling, 2008). By using synthetic biology tools it is possible to create a strain that will stably maintain foreign DNA over long periods of time and reduce unexpected interactions between the added material and the host functions (Way et al., 2014). Several studies showed that precise genome reductions (removal of transposons, insertion sequence elements, integrase genes, cryptic phages, damaged genes and genes with unknown function) improve electroporation, metabolic efficiency and accurate propagation of recombinant DNA that was unstable in other strains (Kolisnychenko et al., 2002; Pósfai et al., 2006; Sharma et al., 2007a,b).

According to Piñero-Lambea et al. (2015) and Claesen and Fischbach (2014), synthetic bacteria for biomedical applications should act as "autonomous physicians" and combine the competence to diagnose, decide on the appropriate treatment, administrate the treatment and in the end to selfeliminate from the human body when they are no longer needed. To do that they should have a minimal chassis carrying different genetic modules useful for therapy: a sensory module responsible for the detection of environmental signals and respond by activating the decision making process and the transcription payload module, the delivery module and/or reporter modules; the chemotactic and adhesion modules that can control the migration of bacteria in response to environmental signals of interest and only "administrate" the treatment in a specific target cell or tissue; and finally a containment module that prevents environmental spread of the synthetic bacterium. Most of synthetic systems are tested as a proof-of-principle in an *E. coli* chassis because of the advantages described above. However, for in vivo applications, commensal bacteria already used as probiotics, such as *Lactococcus lactis* and *Streptococcus salivarius* K12, might be a more appropriate chassis since they are already capable of colonizing the human body, are harmless under normal conditions and interact positively with the host immune system (Claesen and Fischbach, 2014).

Mammalian chassis for synthetic-biology circuits would have great utility and impact in disease treatment. However, microbial synthetic biology is more advanced than the mammalian one since the current mammalian chassis technologies do not feature the same feasibility and effectiveness as the technologies available in microbial synthetic technology (Way et al., 2014). Nevertheless, some success in engineering genetic circuits in mammalian cells has been reported (Wieland and Fussenegger, 2012; Guye et al., 2013; Kemmer et al., 2010, 2011). Mammalian synthetic biology can be applied in the modification of disease-related signaling pathways in new interventions at gene level (gene therapy) or in therapies involving the insertion of modified immune cells into patients (cell therapy) (Kis et al., 2015).

16.2.5 Genome editing tools

Targeted genome editing allows modifying a predefined genome loci in a specific manner (Sun and Zhao, 2013; Perez-Pinera et al., 2012). The desired genetic modifications can be introduced by costume-designed nucleases that cause a DNA double-strand break (DSB) (Sun and Zhao, 2013; Cai and Yang, 2014). After DSB, the DNA can be repaired by homologous recombination (recombineering) or by nonhomologous end joining (NHEJ) and generate modifications that include insertions, disruptions and replacements of genomic DNA. Recombineering is more precise than NHEJ (Sun and Zhao, 2013; Cai and Yang, 2014) and is a strategy for efficient genetic manipulation of bacteria mediated by phage-related recombination proteins based on homologous recombination systems (eg, Gam, Beta and Exo recombinases from bacteriophage λ Red system) to introduce targeted modifications to loci within cells (Citorik et al., 2014; Sharan et al., 2009). It has been used to induce genomic modifications to various bacterial species such as *E. coli* (Datsenko and Wanner, 2000), *S. enterica* (Husseiny and Hensel, 2005), *Shigella flexneri* (Beloin et al., 2003), and *Vibrio cholera* (Yamamoto et al., 2009).

In recent years, several important genome editing tools have been developed including zinc-finger nucleases (ZFNs), meganucleases, transcription activator-like effector nucleases (TALENs) and the clustered regularly interspaced short palindromic repeats (CRISPR)—in combination with the Cas9 endonuclease (CRISPR/Cas9 system) (Hsu et al., 2014; Sun and Zhao, 2013; Perez-Pinera et al., 2012; Gaj et al., 2013). These tools are being increasingly used in disease modeling and gene therapy (Cai and Yang, 2014; Pan et al., 2013), for example to disrupt the human immunodeficiency virus (HIV) co-receptor C-C chemokine receptor type 5 (CCR5) gene. This disruption confers HIV-1 resistance in primary T cells and hematopoietic stem/progenitor cells (Pan et al., 2013; Holt et al., 2010). Meganuclease, ZFN and TALEN proteins recognize specific DNA sequences through DNA-protein interactions (Hsu et al., 2014).

Therefore these approaches require engineering of new enzymes for each target sequence (Jiang et al., 2013). CRISPR/Cas9 technology is originated from CRISPR-Cas systems that provide bacteria with adaptive defense mechanism to plasmids and viruses (Makarova et al., 2006). In this technology, the targeted DNA is recognized by a short guide RNA via Watson-Crick base pairing whereby it only requires the design of the short CRISPR RNA (crRNA), which is simpler to design (Hsu et al., 2014). At the 3′ side the RNA structure has a sequence that binds to Cas9, which in turn introduces a site-specific DSB in the DNA (Doudna and Charpentier, 2014). Due to its simplicity and efficiency CRISPR/Cas9 genome editing tool has been widely used in different cells and organisms to introduce different types of modification, including mutation, deletion and insertion.

For large-scale programming and evolution of cells, Wang et al. (2009) developed a method—Multiplex Automated Genome Engineering (MAGE)—that allows editing many locations on the chromosome simultaneously using short oligonucleotides. This method was used to modify 24 genetic components simultaneously in lycopene biosynthetic pathway in *E. coli* and to obtain variants that showed a fivefold increase in lycopene production. Bonde et al. (2014) developed a method called Microarray-Oligonucleotide (MO)-MAGE where the oligonucleotides needed are amplified from microarray chips for direct use in MAGE. This method allows oligonucleotides that are costly to synthesize to be obtained in a more cost-effective way.

16.2.6 Genomics, transcriptomics, proteomics and metabolomics tools

Advances in bioinformatics, genome sequencing and high-throughput genome-wide enabled the collection of large sets of data and marked the beginning of a new era of systems and synthetic biology (Tang and Zhao, 2009; Bruggeman and Westerhoff, 2007). Nowadays it is possible to analyze and optimize entire cellular networks to develop strains for biomedical applications. A variety of "omics" techniques have been developed, such as genomics (study of the genome), transcriptomics (study of the complete set of RNA transcripts that are produced by the genome), proteomics (identification, quantification and analysis of structure and function of proteins and their interactions) and metabolomics (identification and quantification of all metabolites of a biological system at a specific time point to access the complete metabolic response to a specific stimulus) (Tang and Zhao, 2009).

The most important tool of genomics is DNA sequencing and the analysis of raw sequencing data is assisted by bioinformatics that integrate computer science and mathematics to interpret biological data (Liu et al., 2013). To analyze the transcriptome, high-throughput methods such as microarray analysis have been developed. This method allows comparing transcriptomes and identifying the genes that are differentially expressed in distinct cell populations, or in response to different treatments or environments (Liang et al., 2011). Other techniques were developed to identify different DNA sequences associated to a specific protein, such as Chromatin immunoprecipitation (ChIP) combined with microarrays (ChIP-chip) or sequencing (ChIP-seq) (Collas, 2010).

Genome and its mRNA expression profile are relatively easy to characterize, however the protein expression level can be decoupled from the mRNA expression level due to translational control, posttranslational modification and localization (Liang et al., 2011), which makes proteomic tools essential. Protein purification and mass spectrometry (MS) are two of the techniques often used for proteomic analysis. For example, selected reaction monitoring (SRM) has emerged as a promising MS technique that can quantitatively detect small numbers of a specific protein in complex backgrounds (Liu et al., 2013; Picotti and Aebersold, 2012). SRM is used in a liquid chromatography—mass spectrometry (LC-MS). Other techniques for peptide/protein identification or mass fingerprinting include matrix-assisted laser desorption/ionization—time of flight—(MALDI-ToF-MS), electrospray ionization (ESI-MS), Fourier transform ion cyclotron resonance (FT-ICR) coupling with MS/MS and multidimensional protein identification technology (MudPIT), in combination with the metabolic or in vitro labeling of proteins (Duan, 2011). Metabolomics is a complementary tool to proteomics as proteomics can give information on what and how much proteins are present but metabolomics informs what those proteins are doing to a chemical molecule (Liang et al., 2011). MS and nuclear magnetic resonance (NMR) spectroscopy are two of the techniques most used in metabolomics and are essential to unambiguously identify known and novel compounds (Hill et al., 2015).

16.2.7 In silico models

Since synthetic biology cannot rely on endless trial and error methods, computational and modeling tools are a key asset to leverage the design of microorganisms towards the desired phenotype (Tyo et al., 2010; Rodrigues and Kluskens, 2011). Genome-scale metabolic modeling tools, such as flux balance analysis (FBA) and metabolic flux analysis (MFA), are formed around the basic premise that metabolites and reaction fluxes must obey the laws of conservation of mass and are based on stoichiometric calculation of metabolic reaction rates under pseudo steady-state assumptions. These models use linear programming optimization to maximize or minimize a preset objective function (frequently biomass production) (Curran and Alper, 2012; Liu et al., 2013). OptKnock is one of the first strain design algorithms developed to be used with genome-scale metabolic models to predict network behavior and select optimal engineering strategies (Burgard et al., 2003). This algorithm was developed with the goal of suggesting gene knockout strategies for biochemical overproduction and strain optimization and at the same time a maximal growth rate (Burgard et al., 2003). After the development of OptKnock, other algorithms have been proposed including OptStrain (Pharkya et al., 2004), OptReg (Pharkya and Maranas, 2006), OptCircuit (Dasika and Maranas, 2008), OptForce (Ranganathan et al., 2010), OptFlux (Rocha et al., 2010) and OptORF (Kim and Reed, 2010). All these models (except OptForce) predict mutant behaviors by finding solutions that maximize the growth rate. However, it is possible that the resulting strains need to undergo adaptive evolution to improve growth and biochemical production (Kim et al., 2011).

Other algorithms or bioinformatics tools for the design of synthetic DNA and codon optimization such as Gene Designer 2.0 (Villalobos et al., 2006), or RBS optimization, like RBS Calculator (Salis, 2011; Salis et al., 2009), RBS Designer (Na and Lee, 2010) or UTR Designer (Seo et al., 2013), are also available. SynBioSS is a software package that combines a mixture of bioinformatics tools (sequence analysis, biological design, assembly design) and also allows access to online repositories of biological parts (BioBricks) (Weeding et al., 2010). In addition, Vector NTI Express (Lu and Moriyama, 2004) is an interesting software to design vectors and for DNA/RNA sequence and protein characterization. Its other packages, including alignment tools and phylogenetic analysis tools, can likewise be very useful.

The development of user-friendly databases such as EcoCyc/BioCyc/MetaCyc, BRENDA, KEGG, ExPASy, RebiT (Retro-Biosynthesis Tool) and Parts Registry are helpful for identifying and constructing metabolic routes that allow a given molecule/drug to be produced.

16.3 Prevention

16.3.1 Vaccine development

Since the successful development of the smallpox vaccine by Edward Jenner in 1798 (Smith, 2011), several vaccines (live, killed, attenuated, subunits and nucleic acid-based vaccines) have been developed using different approaches and their development has different drawbacks. For example, attenuated vaccines may tend to revert to the virulent form. Synthetic biology provides new approaches for the development of attenuated pathogens for use as vaccines (Weber and Fussenegger, 2012). Vaccine developers instead of optimizing codon usage to improve cross-species expression can do large-scale codon de-optimization (Mueller et al., 2006; Coleman et al., 2008; Burns et al., 2006) by using *de novo* gene synthesis technology. Coleman et al. (2008) took advantage of the redundancy of the genetic code and introduced genome-scale changes to attenuate poliovirus, one of the most well characterized viruses, which for this reason is used as model system. For that purpose, they used under-represented synonymous codon pairs, which decreased the translation efficiency of poliovirus capsid protein (Fig. 16.3A). The attenuated virus proved to be suitable to provide protective immunity and since the attenuation occurs due to many hundreds of silent nucleotide changes in the viral genome, the probability of reversion of the attenuated virus to a virulent form is very low (Mueller et al., 2010). This strategy, termed SAVE (synthetic attenuated virus engineering), that uses viral genome redesign can be in the future used to attenuate many kinds of virus. In fact, this strategy has been applied to conduct the rational design of live attenuated influenza virus vaccine candidates (Mueller et al., 2010; Nogales et al., 2014).

Other types of vaccines that do not have the drawbacks of attenuated vaccines are nucleic acid-based vaccines, such as DNA vaccines that are comprised of naked plasmid DNA. These vaccines are being investigated and developed. However, they have one major limitation related with delivering the DNA to the target cells

(Jain et al., 2012). Amidi et al. (2011) used liposomes to encapsulate a bacterial transcription-and-translation network and the DNA encoding antigen β-galactosidase (Fig. 16.3B). This system expressed the antigen in vitro and in vivo and generated higher specific humoral immune responses against the produced antigen as compared to control vaccines. This system can be used in the future for other antigens by simply changing the DNA template (Ruder et al., 2011). RNA-based vaccines are also gaining increasing attention given their advantages comparing to DNA vaccines, as RNA can be directly delivered into the host cytoplasm to be translated to protein and it is not possible for the RNA to integrate and mutate the host genome (Geall et al., 2013).

Besides providing new approaches for the development of vaccines, synthetic biology can also help to develop new vaccine candidates in less time (Jain, 2013; Dormitzer et al., 2013). Synthetic and systems biology combined with the availability of complete genome sequences of different organisms have also enabled the so-called reverse vaccinology (Fig. 16.3C). This allows filtering and selecting novel protein-based vaccine candidates using bioinformatics tools and in silico methods

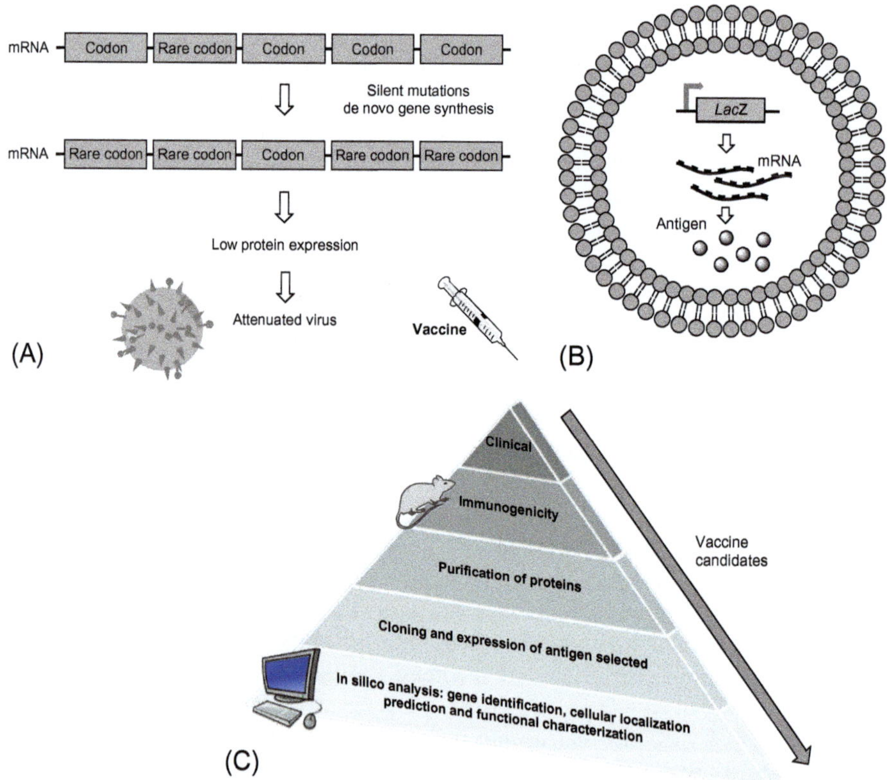

Fig. 16.3 Development of vaccines using synthetic and systems biology strategies.
(A) Synthetic attenuated virus engineering (SAVE) using codon de-optimization. (B) Antigen expression in liposomes. (C) Reverse vaccinology.

(Palumbo et al., 2012). This approach was found to be very effective in the *Neisseria meningitides* serogroup B and can be easily applied to any pathogen.

16.3.2 Engineering insect populations for vector control

The control of insect borne diseases such as malaria and dengue depends on the ability to control the mosquito populations that transmit and spread these diseases (Hemingway, 2014). By using synthetic biology strategies, insects are being engineered to spread parasite resistance, antifertility, or conditional lethal genetic components across wild-type populations (Fu et al., 2007, 2010; de Valdez et al., 2011; Labbé et al., 2012). The two most recognized synthetic biology strategies include the release of insects carrying a dominant lethal genetic system (RIDL) and the synthetic homing endonuclease-based gene (HEG) drive system. The RIDL technology has been used, for example, to control the transmission of dengue viruses caused by vector *Aedes aegypti*. This vector was engineered to express an intron-containing variant of the tetracycline (TET)-dependent transactivator (tTA) (de Valdez et al., 2011; Fu et al., 2010). In female mosquitoes (the ones that propagate the disease), the intron is spliced out by sex-specific mRNA splicing and tTA is expressed. In the absence of TET in the insect food, tTA induces the expression of a toxic gene that incapacitates female mosquitoes by removing their ability to fly. These females are unable to attract and mate with males, whereby they are effectively sterile, which eventually results in the reduction of the wild-type population (Fu et al., 2010; de Valdez et al., 2011). This technology has been successfully tested in field trials in Cayman Islands (Harris et al., 2011, 2012). Since this lethal gene is female-specific and only engineered males are released, the daughters die but heterozygous sons live and mate and only half of their offspring inherit the female-lethal transgene, allowing wild females to be obtained (Alphey, 2014).

The synthetic HEG drive system can be used to spread genetic modifications from laboratory mosquitoes to field populations such as wild-type populations of the malaria mosquitoes *Anopheles gambiae* (Windbichler et al., 2011). HEG are a class of parasitic genes that exist naturally in many microbes that encode proteins causing double-strands breaks in the genome at the precise position opposite to HEG. If the break is repaired by homologous recombination—HEG copies itself into the corresponding location of the sister chromosome in a process referred to as homing—the HEG becomes homozygous (Deredec et al., 2008). Windbichler et al. (2011) demonstrated that HEG can function on mosquitoes (*A. gambiae*) by placing the HEG *I-SceI* under the control of a male testis-specific β2-tubulin promoter. They verified that *I-SceI* rapidly invades the wild-type mosquito population. Other studies also concluded that by releasing HEGs targeting fertility genes, populations of *A. gambiae* could be suppressed (Deredec et al., 2011; Galizi et al., 2014). This principle can also be exploited in the future to knock out the gene necessary for mosquitoes to transmit malaria (Burt, 2003) or for genome engineering or gene therapy (Redondo et al., 2008; Muñoz et al., 2011).

Other approaches such as *Wolbachia* (*Wolbachia pipientis* are intracellular bacteria that occur in a majority of insect species and that manipulate their host's reproductive biology to facilitate their spread) (O'Connor et al., 2012; Hoffmann et al., 2015) and maternal-effect dominant embryonic arrest (*Medea*) (Hay et al., 2010; Chen et al., 2007) also hold a great promise (Alphey, 2014).

16.4 Biosensing and triggering

16.4.1 Quorum sensing

Quorum sensing is a chemical language that allows cell–cell communication (Hooshangi and Bentley, 2008). Chemical-signaling molecules (auto-inducers) are produced and secreted into the extracellular matrix and accumulate as the population grows (Weber and Fussenegger, 2012). These molecules are then detected and can bind to receptors that control changes in gene regulation and cell growth or manipulate the behavior of other bacterial populations (Weber and Fussenegger, 2012; Hooshangi and Bentley, 2008). Synthetic biology enables the design and implementation of cellular interactions that are not native to living cells and can be further explored for biomedical applications. Basu et al. (2004) built a synthetic multicellular pulse generator to study the spatiotemporal response of one cell population to another. The modified sender cells of *E. coli* were engineered with *Vibrio fischeri* quorum-sensing circuit (*lux*) and produced the inducer acyl-homoserine lactone (AHL) that freely diffused to the nearby pulse generating receiver cells and resulted in a transient activation of expression of green fluorescent protein (GFP) (Fig. 16.4). You et al. (2004) replaced GFP with a killer gene (*ccdB*). Anderson et al. (2006) also engineered *E. coli* with the *V. fischeri* quorum-sensing circuit that allows the expression of a gene of interest to be triggered only when the bacterial population has reached a threshold size at the desired area. Dai et al. (2013) and Swofford et al. (2015) also tested the same *lux* circuit in *Salmonella*. These quorum sensing mechanisms can be used in the future in cancer treatment or to treat some diseases associated with bacterial pathogenicity and virulence without damaging healthy tissues (see Section 16.7.1).

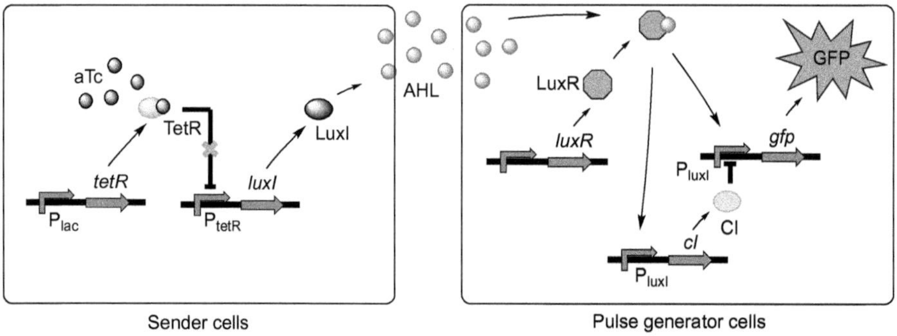

Fig. 16.4 Bacterial population control using quorum sensing. *Escherichia coli* was engineered with *luxI* and *luxR* of *Vibrio fisheri*. In the presence of anhydrotetracycline (aTc), LuxI is expressed and synthesizes the quorum-sensing molecule acyl-homoserine lactone (AHL). The transcriptional regulator LuxR is also expressed and activated by AHL. Then, the AHL-LuxR complex activates P_{luxI} and induces the expression of green fluorescent protein (GFP) and the transcriptional repressor CI. GFP expression is only activated at low concentrations of AHL; at high concentrations P_{luxI} is repressed by CI.

16.4.2 Other types of environmental induction

Controlled expression of therapeutic genes can be performed resorting to the presence of specific signaling molecules, metabolites or pathogenic toxins associated with the disease state, but also with exogenous input signals (Heng et al., 2015), such as temperature, pH, light and oxygen variation, among others. Heat shock promoters have been evaluated regarding their usefulness in synthetic biology to reprogram and trigger the expression of novel components, networks and pathways (Rodrigues et al., 2014; Valdez-Cruz et al., 2010). The increase of temperature can occur via an external trigger, such as ultrasonic waves. This type of trigger allows the drug release and location to be controlled and has proven to be very effective (Schroeder et al., 2009). Ultrasound and laser treatment are two of the techniques used to treat solid tumors. However, these techniques are not always successful, as sometimes they just heat the tumor without destroying it. If these treatments could be linked with the expression/release of a therapeutic agent, the combination could be more effective. Therefore we are currently engineering the heat shock response machinery of *E. coli* to trigger the release of a therapeutic agent *in situ* concurrent with ultrasound or laser treatment (Rodrigues, 2014). This strategy could be very useful for the administration of drugs that require *in situ* synthesis because of poor bioavailability (eg, curcuminoids) as it avoids the need for administrating repetitive oral doses to achieve enough concentration inside the cells (Rodrigues and Kluskens, 2011; Rodrigues, 2014; Rodrigues et al., 2015).

Flentie et al. (2012) identified five *Salmonella* promoters that are specifically activated by cancer cells, as well as acidic pH, a property of most tumors (Tannock, 2001). One of these promoters was used to express *Shiga toxin 2* (*Stx2*), a toxic transgene of bacterial origin in *Salmonella typhimurium* to selectively induce tumor cell death. This approach provided a potent and selective antitumor activity in vitro and in vivo (Flentie et al., 2012). Many tumors contain regions that are also hypoxic (Forbes, 2006). Several promoters (eg, *pfle* and *ansB* promoters) from *Salmonella* are known to be induced in hypoxic conditions (Arrach et al., 2008). Mengesha et al. (2006) studied fumarate and nitrate reduction regulator (FNR) in *Salmonella* that regulates the global response to the transition between aerobic and anaerobic growth. FNR is a protein that acts as a hypoxic sensor and as a hypoxia-responsive transcription factor. FNR-dependent promoters are being studied to improve the targeting of drug delivery in tumors.

Another type of exogenous input signal that can generate a biological response is light, since there are proteins from bacteria, plants and algae that are photosensitive (eg, opsins). The response mechanisms from these organisms can be used to engineer circuits that are controlled by light (Shankar and Pillai, 2011) and in the future to remotely control cells therapeutic applications (Lim, 2010; Shankar and Pillai, 2011; Ye et al., 2011). These engineered circuits are called optogenetic devices (Lim, 2010). Several devices have been developed to express a protein of interest in response to blue, red or infrared light (Ye et al., 2011; Levskaya et al., 2005, 2009; Möglich and Moffat, 2007).

16.4.3 Aptamers and biosensing

Aptamers are short single-stranded RNA and DNA oligonucleotides, or peptide molecules that can specifically recognize and tightly bind with high affinity a broad variety of targets ranging from small ions, single molecules to proteins, and even whole cells (Stoltenburg et al., 2007; Bunka and Stockley, 2006). Nucleic acid aptamers are 10–100 base-pairs long, and these folded into unique 3D conformations (Ku et al., 2015). The identification of full-length aptamers with unique properties from very large random sequence oligonucleotide libraries was first described in 1990 through a process termed SELEX (Systematic Evolution of Ligands by Exponential Enrichment) (Ellington and Szostak, 1990; Tuerk and Gold, 1990). Among SELEX technologies, cell-SELEX is a strategy that uses whole living cells as targets for aptamer selection based on differences at the molecular level between cell lines (Ye et al., 2012). Using cell-SELEX, several aptamers that specifically bind to target cell lines were described without requiring prior molecular signature information of cell surface proteins, including myeloid leukemia (Sefah et al., 2009), small lung cancer (Kunii et al., 2011; Chen et al., 2008), prostate cancer (Wang et al., 2014) and ovarian cancer cells (Van Simaeys et al., 2010).

Aptamers are able to recognize molecular moieties as biomarkers, which are recognition molecules widely defined as indicators of a biological state. As stated, aptamers generated by cell-SELEX can target and detect small differences between pathological and normal cells. Thus, it is expected that aptamers selected by this methodology open the door for identification of novel biomarkers (Ye et al., 2012). Using aptamers as sensors for biomarker discovery and the cell-SELEX screening strategy, many research groups have identified aptamers that recognize different membrane proteins such as tenascin-C from glioblastoma cells (Daniels et al., 2003), immunoglobulin μ heavy chain from Burkitt's lymphoma cells (Mallikaratchy et al., 2007) and stress-induced phosphoprotein 1 from ovarian cancer (Van Simaeys et al., 2014). Aptamers that have been raised against cell membrane biomarkers have a great potential use for early diagnosis, monitoring and efficient treatment.

16.5 Targeting

16.5.1 Targeting cancer cells using bacteria

The major problems of chemotherapy are associated with the nonselectivity and nonspecificity of the drugs being used, resulting in severe toxic side effects. Therefore, more selective and effective tumor-specific treatments are urgently needed. Many tumor regions are hypoxic and conventional cancer drugs cannot efficiently reach them (Forbes, 2006). However, in recent years many anaerobic or facultative anaerobic bacteria, including *Salmonella* (Ganai et al., 2011; Zhang and Forbes, 2015), *Escherichia* (Jiang et al., 2010; Zhou et al., 2011), *Clostridium* (Dang et al., 2001, 2004; Roberts et al., 2014) and *Bifidobacterium* (Zhu et al., 2011), have been shown to selectively accumulate in tumors. Since many of these strains are intrinsically pathogenic, their toxicity has to be eliminated before their use in bacterial therapies can be considered. In the case of *Clostridium* and *Salmonella*, nonpathogenic strains or strains with pathogenicity- and immunogenicity-related genes deleted have been used (Clairmont et al., 2000; Liu et al., 2002; Low et al., 1999; Zhang et al., 2014). Obligate anaerobes like *Clostridium* and *Bifidobacterium* germinate only in hypoxic regions of tumors and cannot target nonhypoxic tumor regions (Forbes, 2006). Therefore these bacteria are nontoxic to healthy tissue (St Jean et al., 2008). Facultative anaerobic bacteria like *S. typhimurium* and *E. coli* have the advantage of being able to colonize both small metastatic lesions and large quiescent and apoptotic tumor regions (Kasinskas and Forbes, 2006; Thamm et al., 2005). *Salmonella* has been shown to selectively accumulate in tumors in amounts 1000- to 10,000-fold higher than in any other healthy tissue in mice (Clairmont et al., 2000; Forbes et al., 2003; Ganai et al., 2009). Also, facultative anaerobes, unlike *Clostridium*, can be administered as active motile bacteria. These differences allow the tuning of the target mechanism of facultative anaerobes, while the targeting mechanism of obligate anaerobes is fixed (Forbes, 2006; Toley and Forbes, 2012).

Engineered *E. coli* was used to target and invade cancer cells in an hypoxic environment (Anderson et al., 2006). For that purpose, invasin (*inv*) adhesion protein from *Yersinia pseudotuberculosis* was expressed in *E. coli* under the control of an anaerobically induced formate hydrogenase promoter or *V. fischeri* quorum-sensing circuit (*lux*). The quorum-sensing circuit allows triggering invasin expression only when the bacterial population reaches a high level in the tumor area. The production of invasin enabled bacteria to selectively invade mammalian cells expressing β1-integrins receptors by phagocytosis. The invasion can be enhanced by co-expression of the gene *HlyA* for listeriolysin O from *Listeria monocytogenes* that triggers the breakdown of phagosome/lysosome membranes, thus releasing its content into the host-cell cytoplasm (Mathew et al., 2003; Grillot-Courvalin et al., 1998; Xiang et al., 2006; Critchley et al., 2004). This is also facilitated by the fact that the *E. coli* strain used is auxotrophic for diaminopimelic acid (DAP) due to the deletion of aspartate semialdehyde dehydrogenase, an enzyme necessary for DAP synthesis. DAP is usually present in the peptidoglycan layer of gram-negative bacteria cell wall and its deficiency impairs cell-wall synthesis inducing cell lysis. Piñero-Lambea et al. (2014) also studied the use of synthetic adhesins that allow the rational design of robust and specific adhesion properties of *E. coli*. The authors showed that lower doses of engineered *E. coli*, compared to the wild-type *E. coli*, are sufficient to colonize solid tumors expressing an antigen recognized by the synthetic adhesin.

Tumor-targeting can also be controlled by the creation of auxotrophic bacteria that are not able to survive without nutrients from specific microenvironments and apparently they only receive sufficient nutritional support from tumors (Zhao et al., 2005, 2006, 2007; Hayashi et al., 2009).

16.5.2 Targeting cancer cells using cell penetrating peptides (CPPs)

Cell penetrating peptides (CPPs) are small peptides that have the ability to enter cells on their own or together with cargoes independently of the membrane receptor (Regberg et al., 2012). A great number of CPP-conjugated therapies comprise a strong clinical promise (Bolhassani, 2011).

Each healthy or diseased tissue has specific molecular tags on its vasculature that constitute a vascular "zip code" system (Enbäck and Laakkonen, 2007). The number of cell-specific sequences, like for instance homing peptides, is increasing each day. The advantage of these peptides is their ability to recognize specific phenotypes. Furthermore, some of these peptides not only identify the targeted cells, but also have the capability to translocate across the cellular membrane. These peptides are the so-called cell-penetrating-homing-peptides (Laakkonen et al., 2008). They are suitable carriers for therapeutic and diagnostic purposes due to their selectivity. Phage display screening is frequently employed to identify these high-affinity peptides that selectively recognize molecular markers. This technique first described by Smith (1985) consists of unbiased selection for the screening of random peptide libraries. It is a powerful in vitro selection approach that takes advantage of the extensive genetic flexibility of bacteriophages to create a variety of modifications on their surface (Huang et al., 2011). The selection process consists of several iterative cycles of enrichment in phage particles that bind with high affinity to the target of interest, which are then eluted and propagated in *E. coli*. Filamentous bacteriophage M13 is mostly used for this procedure, mainly due to its ability to display peptides on its coat proteins pIII and pVIII. Kim et al. (2006) described the selection of cyclic 13-mer Pep42 peptide by phage display screening, which internalized melanoma cells Me6652/4. The cellular receptor for Pep42 was identified as the surface membrane form of glucose regulated protein 78 (GRP78), specifically overexpressed on the cancer cell surface. Higher expression of this membrane receptor has been related to a greater recurrence and poor patient survival in breast, liver, prostate, colon and gastric cancers (Lee, 2007).

Colorectal cancer is the third most common cancer in males and the second in females worldwide, with nearly 693,900 deaths occurring in 2012 (Torre et al., 2015). In order to find new diagnostic and therapeutic approaches for colon cancer, Kelly and Jones (2003) studied a new peptide (RPMrel) selected by phage display. The selected peptide was able to bind five distinct colon cancer cell lines. Moreover, when conjugated with fluorescein (fluorescein-RPMrel peptide), this peptide stained *ex vivo* sections of colon tumor tissues from four patients, but not healthy colon tissue or other tissues such as lungs, liver or stomach. The authors also described the effectiveness of this peptide in delivering a mitochondrial toxin to tumor colon cells, thereby inducing cell death. The identification of a peptide that selectively targets and penetrates colon cancer cells represents a promising tool to develop new colon cancer diagnostic and therapeutic platforms.

Identifying a cell-specific peptide with cell-penetrating characteristics is not always an easy task. The major drawback of conventional CPPs, such as TAT from HIV-TAT (Vives et al., 1997) and penetratin from the *Antennapedia* homeodomain (Derossi et al., 1994) are their lack of cell specificity, hampering their clinical development (Vivès et al., 2008).

It has also been described that combining a CPP with a cancer-related peptide yields a chimeric peptide with tumor specificity that can carry cargo molecules inside cells (Mäe et al., 2008). For instance, Myrberg et al. (2008) successfully attached the breast tumor cyclic nonapeptide named PEGA (Essler and Ruoslahti, 2002) to the well-studied CPP *p*VEC (Elmquist et al., 2001). These authors demonstrated that the peptide alone does not cross the plasma membrane. However, when conjugated with

CPP it was taken up by different breast cancer cells in vitro. Moreover, the homing ability of PEGA-*p*VEC chimeric peptide was conserved in vivo due to its accumulation in blood vessels of tumor cells. Furthermore, they also showed that the effectiveness of the anticancer drug chlorambucil against breast cancer cells was four times higher when it was conjugated to the resultant PEGA-*p*VEC peptide. Afterwards, the chimeric peptide was enhanced combining a new linear breast tumor homing peptide called CREKA, with the CPP reported in the previous referred study (Mäe et al., 2008). The tumor-related peptide was identified in breast tumors in transgenic mice by using in vivo phage display screening. This new chimeric peptide, CREKA-*p*VEC proved to be better in translocating cargo molecules inside cancer cells as compared to PEGA-*p*VEC peptide. Such peptides provide a good tool for tumor targeting and drug delivery.

16.6 Detection: Medical diagnosis

Synthetic biology already allowed obtaining diagnostic tools that can be found today in the clinics. One example is the Bayer VERSANT™ branched DNA (bDNA) assay that uses a signal amplification technique and enables the detection of hepatitis C virus (HCV) infections and monitoring HCV, hepatitis B virus (HBV) and HIV-1 viral loads during and after antiviral therapy (Elbeik et al., 2004a,b). The target RNA molecule is detected by hybridization using several capture probes. After the RNA is captured it complexes with fluorescent label probes, a preamplifier and an amplifier. To reduce the amplification background and increase the specificity of the assay they incorporated components of the artificial genetic alphabet (alternative nucleotides) in the fluorescent probe, preamplifier and amplifier. This way nontarget DNA present in the sample is not able to hybridize with the artificial DNA (Collins et al., 1997).

Other approach to detect several diseases is the use of bacteria, such as bacterial sensors in in vitro diagnostic tests (IVDs). Courbet et al. (2015) designed a whole-cell biosensor to detect clinically relevant biomarkers in human urine and blood. The authors tested glucose as the biomarker, as it has a relevant clinical interest—for instance it can be used to monitor or diagnose diabetes (high levels of glucose in blood or urine). The synthetic circuit was composed by the promoter pCpxP to drive target expression since it is activated in the presence of glucose and the reporter gene that encodes GFP or the far-red fluorescent protein (mKate2). Biomarker detection occurred at a selected threshold by using specific amplifying genetic switches and logic gates that can sense and remember the environmental stimuli.

Bacteria are also being evaluated for in vivo diagnosis (Danino et al., 2015; Kotula et al., 2014). The probiotic *E. coli* Nissle 1917 was used to develop an orally administered diagnostic agent that can noninvasively indicate the presence of liver metastasis (Danino et al., 2015). *E. coli* Nissle colonized tumor tissue in mice after oral delivery (but did not colonize healthy organs) and expressed a *lacZ* reporter that cleaves the substrate LuGal (a soluble conjugate of luciferin and galactose) to produce luciferase that can be detected in urine using luminescence assays. LuGal was only administered intravenously after tumor colonization.

Bacteriophages can also be engineered and used to transform target pathogenic bacteria into cell factories for the production of detectable molecules (Smartt et al., 2012; Schofield et al., 2012; Lu et al., 2013; Citorik et al., 2014). Engineered bacteriophage-based detectors/biosensors exhibit high sensitivity, specificity, and robustness, and are able to detect live cells (Smartt et al., 2012; Tawil et al., 2014), thus making them the ideal recognitions elements for bacterial detection. A common design strategy consists of the genetic engineering of phages to express reporter payloads upon their target bacterium infection leading to the production of detectable outputs such as luminescence, fluorescence and colorimetric signals (Schofield et al., 2012; Piuri et al., 2009). Moreover, sensor-based constructs can also include manipulated bacteriophages that express a product that causes ice nucleation (Wolber and Green, 1990) or include tags for linking to detectable moieties such as quantum dots (Edgar et al., 2006). These engineered bacteriophage-based sensors can also be used for imaging specific molecular targets, and in vivo system imaging, and are therefore ideal for medical use (Kelly et al., 2006; Newton et al., 2006).

Genetic circuits that can selectively identify if a given miRNA (micro RNA) is expressed at high or low levels can be also very useful in medical diagnosis. If the expression level matches the profiles of interest, then a cellular response is triggered. This strategy can be used in the detection of cancer, but also in the treatment if the expression of a pro-apoptosis protein is put under the conditional control of miRNAs (Xie et al., 2011). Liu et al. (2014) constructed a circuit in mammalian cells based on the CRISPR/Cas9 system by combining the bladder-specific promoter of human uroplakin II gene (hUP II) with the cancer-specific promoter of human telomerase reverse transcriptase (hTERT) gene and tested the ability of these circuits to selectively identify bladder cancer cells. The authors concluded that these systems could detect human bladder cancer by the presence of luciferase and also could treat it when functional genes were used as outputs. They tested the hBAX, p21 and E-cadherin genes that induced apoptosis, growth arrest or low cell motility, respectively, in cancer cells.

Kwong et al. (2013) used an interesting method to detect different diseases at the same time in urine samples. They used a synthetic biomarker library composed of mass-encoded tandem peptides conjugated onto nanoworm nanoparticles. These conjugated nanoworm nanoparticles were administered intravenously into living mice and accumulated in disease tissues. Due to deregulated proteases activity frequently found in disease tissues, the peptides are cleaved from nanoworms, thus allowing fragments to filter into the urine. The biomarkers are then recovered by UV irradiation and quantified by LC-MS/MS. Different methods to quantify the biomarker have been tested by the same research group (Warren et al., 2014a,b) including a method that may allow low-cost diagnosis of diseases at the point of care in resource-limited settings.

Other diagnostic tools are being developed using synthetic biology principles. For example, Ausländer et al. (2014b) designed a histamine biosensor device to diagnose allergy disorders. Pardee et al. (2014) developed a programmable in vitro paper-based synthetic platform (composed of commercially available cell-free systems and synthetic gene networks freeze dried onto paper) for different biosensors (eg, glucose sensors and strain-specific Ebola virus sensors) that generate colorimetric outputs that can be detected by naked eye. Griss et al. (2014) have also developed semisynthetic bioluminescent sensors that allow precise measurements of drug concentrations (immunosuppressant, antiepileptic, anticancer agent and antiarrhythmic) in patient samples by handling minimal volumes on paper and recording the luminescence signal using a simple digital camera. These paper-based low-cost point-of-care methods could move diagnostics from the lab to the patient, by making therapeutic drug monitoring available in regions with poor infrastructure (Griss et al., 2014; Struss et al., 2010; Pardee et al., 2014). These are only some of the examples of biomedical diagnosis tools being developed using synthetic biology. For a more extensive review please refer to Courbet (2015).

16.7 Treatment

16.7.1 Engineering commensal bacteria against pathogens and virus

Quorum sensing mechanisms can be used to reprogram the behavior of pathogens instead of killing them (Weber and Fussenegger, 2012). Duan and March (2008, 2010) used commensal bacteria to inhibit the cholera disease. *V. cholera*, during cholera infection, secretes virulence factors (cholera toxin) at low population density. To control its own density *V. cholerae* secretes and detects auto-inducer signaling molecules (cholera auto-inducer 1, CAI-1, and auto-inducer 2, AI-2) and when both levels of these molecules are high they trigger the repression of the virulence factor. An *E. coli* that naturally produces AI-2 was engineered to produce CAI-1. Next, it was fed to mice 8 hours before ingesting *V. cholerae* and it was found to increase the mice survival rate in 80% (Duan and March, 2010). By using this strategy that does not confer selection pressure as with antibiotics, the development of pathogen resistance is less likely to occur (Weber and Fussenegger, 2012). Thus, strategies like this can be very useful, for example, when dealing with human pathogens, such as *Pseudomonas aeruginosa*, that cause life-threatening infections and are resistant to many antibiotics and antimicrobials. Saeidi et al. (2011), using quorum sensing, designed and constructed an *E. coli* that was able to sense and kill *P. aeruginosa*. *E. coli* senses the production of AHL by *P. aeruginosa* and produces and releases pyocin S5 and E7 lysis protein. E7 lysis protein is produced to lyse *E. coli* cells so that the produced pyocin is released from the cells and kills the pathogen (Fig. 16.5A). This system inhibited the growth of the pathogen by 99% and the biofilm formation by 90%. In another study, *L. lactis* was engineered to detect and inhibit multiresistant *Enterococcus faecalis*. The detection system is based in the enterococcal sex pheromone cCF10. *L. lactis* detects the pheromone since it binds to the pCF10-encoded master protein regulator PrgX engineered in the lactic acid bacteria and in response it expresses genes for three bacteriocins (enterocin A, hiracin JM79 and enterocin P) that have potent antimicrobial activity against *E. faecalis* and inhibit its growth.

Chen et al. (2010) engineered probiotic *Lactobacillus casei* to express human lactoferrin to protect the host against pathogenic *E. coli* infection. The engineered probiotic bacteria orally administered to the infected mice reduced the growth of pathogenic bacteria in the duodenal fluid.

The engineering of bacteria to produce antiviral molecules has also been investigated. In women, most HIV transmission takes place through the cervicovaginal mucosa where the commensal bacterium *Lactobacillus jensenii* is present. This bacterium was genetically engineered to produce antiviral peptides (cyanovirin-N) that showed activity against HIV (Lagenaur et al., 2011). The colonization of macaques with engineered *L. jensenii* and afterwards challenged with the simian virus showed a 63% reduction of virus transmission. Similar strategies have also been studied by Pusch et al. (2006), Vangelista et al.(2010), and Liu et al. (2008). Rao et al. (2005)

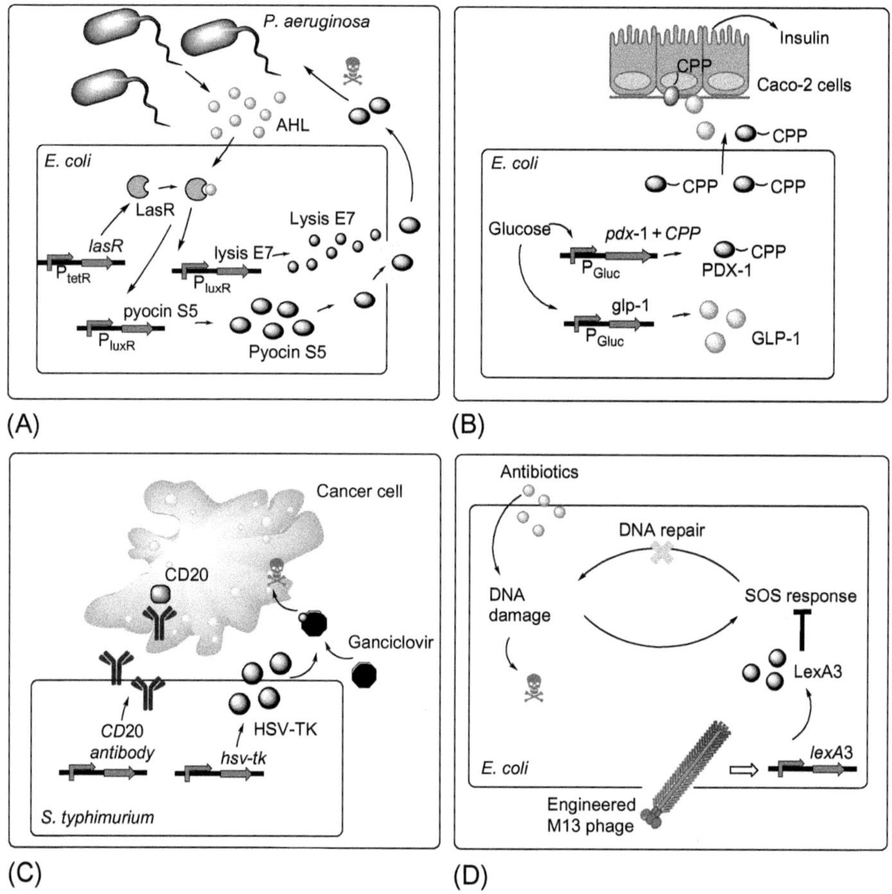

Fig. 16.5 Synthetic biology possible treatments for several diseases. (A) *Escherichia coli* was engineered to sense and kill *Pseudomonas aeruginosa*, a human pathogen. (B) *E. coli* was engineered to express proteins that will stimulate the production of insulin by mammalian cells. (C) Anticancer bacteria (*Salmonella typhimurium*) that specifically infects and kills tumor cells. (D) Combination therapy using engineered M13 bacteriophage carrying the *lexA3* gene and antibiotics. AHL: acyl-homoserine lactone; CPP: cell penetrating peptide; GLP-1: glucagon-like peptide 1; HSV-TK: herpes simplex virus thymidine kinase; PDX-1: pancreatic and duodenal homeobox gene 1.

used a different strategy for the prevention of HIV infection using other commensal bacteria. The authors engineered *E. coli* to secrete HIV-gp41-hemolysin A peptides that block HIV fusion and penetration into target cells. They further demonstrated that the bacteria were capable of colonizing the large intestine of mice where they secrete the antiHIV peptide in inhibitory concentrations. *Lactobacillus paracasei* was also modified to deliver antibodies against rotavirus infections in mice (Pant et al., 2006).

16.7.2 Engineering commensal bacteria for the treatment of metabolic diseases

Engineered commensal bacteria can also be used in the treatment of metabolic diseases. Examples of these metabolic diseases are obesity, high blood pressure, diabetes and hyperlipidemia that arises from unhealthy lifestyles and diet, and that needs to be treated using pills and injections in specified doses at particular time-points (Heng et al., 2015), thus reducing a patient's quality of life.

Type 1 diabetes is a metabolic disease featured by high blood glucose levels that are caused by the autoimmune destruction of insulin-producing β cells in the pancreas (Heng et al., 2015). So far, there is no cure for this disease and the current treatments include subcutaneous injection of insulin and monitoring blood glucose levels. This demands suitable care, preparation and discipline, and in the case of children and elderly patients this is very challenging. Duan et al. (2008) engineered *E. coli* for potential diabetes treatment. *E. coli* was modified to secrete GLP-1 (glucagon-like peptide 1) and PDX-1 (pancreatic and duodenal homeobox gene 1), two proteins that stimulate intestinal epithelial cells to synthesize insulin in response to glucose (Suzuki et al., 2003). PDX-1 was secreted as a fusion with a CPP to enable rapid entry into the epithelial cells (Caco-2 cells) after secretion (Duan et al., 2008) (Fig. 16.5B). A similar approach with *Lactobacillus gasseri* also showed that the secretion of GLP allows the reprogramming of intestinal cells as insulin-secreting cells (Duan et al., 2015). The use of these engineered commensal strains by simple oral dosing can reduce or even eliminate the need for insulin injection (Duan et al., 2008; March and Duan, 2011, 2014).

In order to control obesity, Chen et al. (2014) modified *E. coli* Nissle to express an *N*-acyltransferase that synthesizes *N*-acylphosphatidylethanolamines (NAPEs), which are precursors of the *N*-acylethanolamide (NAE) family of lipids. These compounds are synthesized in the small intestine in response to feeding and cause a reduction of food intake and obesity. The authors demonstrated that the incorporation of engineered bacteria in drinking water for 8 weeks reduced the food intake in mice and, consequently, obesity and insulin resistance. The positive effects granted by the bacteria persisted at least 4 weeks after their removal from the water.

16.7.3 Engineering bacteria to treat cancer

Bacterial therapies may be, in the future, the next generation of cancer therapeutics (Forbes, 2006, 2010; Lehouritis et al., 2013) since they possess unique features to overcome conventional therapy deficiencies. Anaerobic bacteria are already able to invade specifically tumor tissues (Section 16.5.1) and there are several studies demonstrating that they can cause tumor regression and eradication in mouse models (Arrach et al., 2008; Hayashi et al., 2009; Zhao et al., 2005, 2006, 2007) or even in dogs and humans (Roberts et al., 2014). All these bacterial therapies make use of the synthetic biology fundamentals since they include the modification of bacteria to target more specifically the tumor or to eliminate its toxicity to the human body (for example, in the cases of *Salmonella* and *Clostridium*). In addition, in some cases, they include engineering of the organism to deliver anticancer genetic material or drugs (Ganai et al., 2009; Xiang et al., 2006). Xiang et al. (2006) engineered *E. coli* to produce a short hairpin RNA (shRNA) to target and knock down a specific mammalian oncogene—CTNNB1 (encoding β-1 catenin)—that initiates many colon cancers upon its overexpression or oncogenic mutation (Ruder et al., 2011). Oral or intravenous administration of the modified *E. coli* resulted in significant gene silencing in tumor cells. The authors chose CTNNB1 since it is commonly stabilized in cancer cells and it is ideal in proof-of-concept experiments to test the potency of new RNA interference (RNAi) approaches (Xiang et al., 2006). In the future, the plasmid (that also allows the expression of invasion gene *inv* and listeriolysin O gene *HlyA*) can be modified to express RNAi against other genes of interest.

E. coli was also engineered to produce *Staphylococcus aureus* α-hemolysin (SAH) (Jean et al., 2014), a pore-forming protein/toxin that has been recently found to be naturally secreted in a fully functional form in *E. coli* and to aggressively kill mammalian cancer cells (Swofford et al., 2014). Microbial synthesized SAH was found to increase necrotic tissue and quickly reduce tumor volume (Jean et al., 2014) by creating pores that disrupt and destroy mammalian cellular membranes, as well as induce cell swelling and lysis (Swofford et al., 2014).

Other bacteria, such as attenuated *Salmonella*, were also engineered to be used in cancer therapeutics. For example, Ganai et al. (2009) engineered *S. typhimurium* to secrete murine TNF- (tumor necrosis factor) related apoptosis-inducing ligand (TRAIL). The expression was under the control of RecA promoter, induced by γ-irradiation. The results obtained showed that the engineered bacteria effectively reduced tumor growth and extended host survival. Nguyen et al. (2010) obtained similar results engineering this bacteria to express cytotoxic protein cytolysin A to kill tumor cells and the bacterial luciferase gene *lux* to generate imaging signals. Since cytolysin A is toxic to the liver and spleen, they used P_{BAD} promoter from the *E. coli* arabinose operon, which can be activated by arabinose, for tumor-specific therapy with reduced toxicity in normal organs. Massa et al. (2013) used another approach to increase *S. typhimurium* target specificity. They expressed on the bacterial cell surface a single-domain antibody directed to a human tumor-associated antigen (CD20), which decreased nonspecific cell invasion and destroyed $CD20^+$ lymphoma xenografts in mice (Fig. 16.5C). Moreover, the authors expressed the herpes simplex virus type-1 thymidine kinase (HSV-TK) that kills the cancer cells in the presence of the prodrug ganciclovir by converting it into an apoptosis- inducing derivative. *S. enterica* was also engineered with a *P. putida* circuit activated by acetyl salicylic acid (ASA) that allows the control of the expression of cytosine deaminase, which is not present in mammalian cells and is needed to convert the prodrug 5-fluorocytosine into the cytotoxic molecule 5-fluorouracil (Royo et al., 2007). The administration of ASA before 5-fluorocytosine showed a significant tumor regression.

All these results highlight that it is very important to use regulatory control circuits to selectively switch on gene expression during bacterial infection in order to increase the safety, specificity and efficiency of bacterial therapies.

16.7.4 Engineering virus to treat cancer

One of the most recent advances in the development of new treatment strategies against cancer includes the use of engineered tumor-specific oncolytic viruses (Miest and Cattaneo, 2014; Cattaneo et al., 2008). A nonlimiting list of current and recently completed oncolytic virotherapy trials includes OncoVEX, an oncolytic herpes simplex virus coding for granulocyte/macrophage colony stimulating factor (GM-CSF), which is currently in Phase III of clinical trials for metastatic malignant melanoma treatment (Senzer et al., 2009); H101, a reprogrammed E1B gene-deleted adenovirus combined with cisplatin-based chemotherapy has been administered to hundreds of patients with head and neck carcinoma in China and it is currently in Phase III of clinical trials (Xia et al., 2004); and JX-594, a modified oncolytic vaccine virus expressing GM-CSF for the treatment of hepatocellular carcinoma, which is presently in Phase IIb of clinical trials (Heo et al., 2011).

Advances in synthetic biology have also led to the development of several bacteriophage therapeutic platforms. In Bar et al. (2008), filamentous bacteriophages were genetically modified to endow them with the ability to display a host-specific conferring ligand and to be chemically loaded with a large payload of a cytotoxic drug resulting in growth inhibition of cancer cells in vitro. More recently, Ghosh et al. (2012) re-engineered the genome of M13 bacteriophage to use as a platform for tumor cell imaging and drug delivery. As stated, this type of bacteriophage is routinely used for peptide display; however, the handling of phage genome is limited by the presence of overlapping gene regions making it difficult to alter one gene without disrupting the other. In this report, the authors showed that refactoring the M13 genome enabled simultaneous prostate cancer cell imaging and targeted drug delivery. DePorter and McNaughton (2014) manipulated a M13 bacteriophage equipping it with a prostate cancer CPP on pIII coat protein and streptavidin-horseradish peroxidase (HRP) in biotin-pIX protein. HRP-dependent oxidation of indole-3-acetic acid (IAA) produces a peroxyl radical that led to toxicity in mammalian cells. Treatment of prostate cancer cells with engineered phage and IAA resulted in appreciable cell death.

16.7.5 Engineering virus to treat infections

Biofilms are structured bacteria consortia that are embedded in a selfproduced extracellular polymeric substance (EPS) matrix consisting of polysaccharides, proteins, nucleic acids and lipids. These biofilm-growing bacteria cause chronic infections characterized by persistent inflammation and tissue damage due to its increased tolerance to antibiotics, as well as resistance to the body's defense system. With this bacterial antibiotic resistance becoming a real and increasing concern, synthetic biology is turning back to an old idea of using bacteriophages to treat bacterial pathogens (Henry and Debarbieux, 2012). For instance, Lu and Collins (2007) successfully engineered an *E. coli* bacteriophage T7 to express the biofilm-degrading enzyme dispersin B (DspB) upon infection—an enzyme that hydrolyses an adhesin required for biofilm formation and integrity in *Staphylococcus* spp. and *E. coli* clinical isolates. The efficacy of biofilm dispersal by this enzymatic bacteriophage was about two orders of magnitude better than the nonenzymatic one and resulted in the removal of 99.997% of biofilm bacterial cells.

In a follow-up study, a filamentous nonlytic M13 bacteriophage was engineered to inhibit the infection of *Chlamydia trachomatis*, a sexually transmitted pathogen for which there are no effective vaccines and/or microbicides (Bhattarai et al., 2012). The bacteriophage was manipulated in order to carry two functional peptides, integrin binding peptide (RGD) and a segment of the polymorphic membrane protein (PmpD). Engineered bacteriophage enhanced cellular internalization into bacteria-containing inclusions in mammalian host cells and significant amelioration of bacterial infection in HeLa and primary endocervical cells.

Rather than encoding killing functions, bacteriophages can also be genetically engineered to reverse pathogen drug resistance, thereby restoring and enhancing their sensitivity to antibiotics. M13 was engineered to enhance the efficacy of antibiotics in a phage-drug approach (Lu and Collins, 2009). The phage was modified to express LexA3, which suppresses the SOS DNA-damage system in *E. coli* (Fig. 16.5D). The designer phage expressively enhanced killing using quinolones by several orders of magnitude in vitro and significantly increased the survival of *E. coli* infected mice in vivo. Furthermore, the engineered bacteriophage also proved that it can be used to produce other effective antibiotic adjuvants. In another study, the phage λ was used as chassis to promote antibiotic sensitization through delivery of dominant sensitive genes encoding wild-type enzymes such as *gyrA* and *rpsL* (Edgar et al., 2012).

Endolysins, which are bacteriophage-encoded peptidoglycan hydrolases, also represent a promising novel alternative class of antibacterial agents due to its modular nature making them amenable for synthetic biology applications. *S. aureus* is one of the major pathogens responsible for fatal infections. In Pastagia et al. (2011), a *Staphylococcus*-specific phage lysin was engineered and applied in a mouse model of skin infection with *S. aureus*. This antibacterial agent eradicated significantly a great number of methicillin-susceptible *S. aureus* and resistant *S. aureus* bacteria.

16.7.6 Aptamers applied to cancer treatment

Aptamers can be virtually selected against any target and their mode of action is strongly dependent of it. The aptamer-target binding inhibits its biological activity, which can be due to interference with the enzymatic catalytic site, or to the ligand-receptor recognition sites, or possibly to the induction of allosteric effects with subsequent loss of function (Missailidis and Hardy, 2009; Ulrich and Wrenger, 2009). Up to now, aptamer commercialization is limited to only one RNA aptamer-based drug (Macugen, Pfizer) for macular degeneration treatment receiving US Food and Drug Administration (FDA) approval (Ng et al., 2006). However, their uniqueness constitutes a great promise to the medical field. Of particular interest is an antitumor aptamer AS1411 against acute myeloid leukemia (from Antisoma Research) that has completed Phase II clinical trials. Likewise, aptamers raised against other diseases, such as

ARC1779 (Archemix Corporation), NOX-E36 and NOX-H94 (NOXXON Pharma AG) are at the same stage of clinical trials. Other aptamers are recruiting patients for Phase III, namely REG1 (Regado Biosciences) against coronary artery disease, and E10030 (Ophthotech Corporation) against age-related macular degeneration (Sun et al., 2014; Ni and Castanares, 2011; Sundaram et al., 2013). All these clinical studies illustrate the many possible uses that aptamers may have in several biomedical fields.

16.7.7 Prosthetic gene networks: Synthetic gene circuits in mammalian cells

Prosthetic gene networks are synthetic devices that act as molecular prosthesis (Weber and Fussenegger, 2012; Folcher and Fussenegger, 2012). These molecular prosthesis are integrated into mammalian cells and functionally coupled to their metabolism and can sense, monitor and correct metabolic disturbances by triggering therapeutic responses in a selfsufficient, timely and automatic way (Kemmer et al., 2010; Heng et al., 2015). These synthetic devices, also called theranostic devices, as they are able to diagnose a disease state and to trigger a therapy (Haellman and Fussenegger, 2016), can be particularly promising in the treatment of metabolic disorders caused by dysfunctional regulation and imbalance of specific metabolites, but also in other type of diseases such as cancer (Nissim and Bar-Ziv, 2010).

The first known example of a prosthetic network was designed and constructed by Kemmer et al. (2010) to sense metabolites in order to improve the control of urate homeostasis and treat hyperuricemia. This disease can be originated after disruption of normal uric acid homeostasis and is associated with tumor lysis syndrome and gout. The human cells containing the prosthetic network (Fig. 16.6A) were designed by combining different genetic parts, namely the uric acid sensor HucR from *Deinococcus radiodurans* fused to the transcriptional-silencing domain KRAB (Krüppel associated box), that manages oxidative stress protection (Wilkinson and Grove, 2004); the human uric acid transporter URAT1, which increases the intercellular levels of uric acid in the cell and, consequently, the sensitivity of the prosthetic circuit; and *Aspergillus flavus* urate oxidase (smUOX) that is used for the treatment of tumor lysis syndrome (Legoux et al., 1992). The presence of the transported uric acid prevents the binding of the uric acid-sensitive trans-silencer to the operator that controls the expression of smUOX ($hucO_8$). Therefore smUOX can be expressed when uric acid concentration reaches pathological levels and mediates the conversion of uric acid into the more soluble and renally secretable allantoin, thus decreasing blood uric acid concentration. Transplantation of cells containing the prosthetic gene network into hyperuricemic mice allowed restoring uric acid homeostasis and reducing uric acid crystal deposits in kidneys (Kemmer et al., 2010).

One possible strategy for the treatment of obesity would be to reduce food intake by suppressing appetite and promoting satiety (Heng et al., 2015). Rössger et al. (2013a) designed a genetic circuit that continuously monitors blood fatty acid levels and coordinates reversible and adjustable expression of the appetite-suppressing peptide hormone pramlintide (Fig. 16.6B). In the presence of fatty acids, the lipid sensor receptor that combines the phloretin-responsive repressor (TtgR) and the ligand-binding domain of human peroxisome proliferator-associated receptor alpha (PPARα) binds to

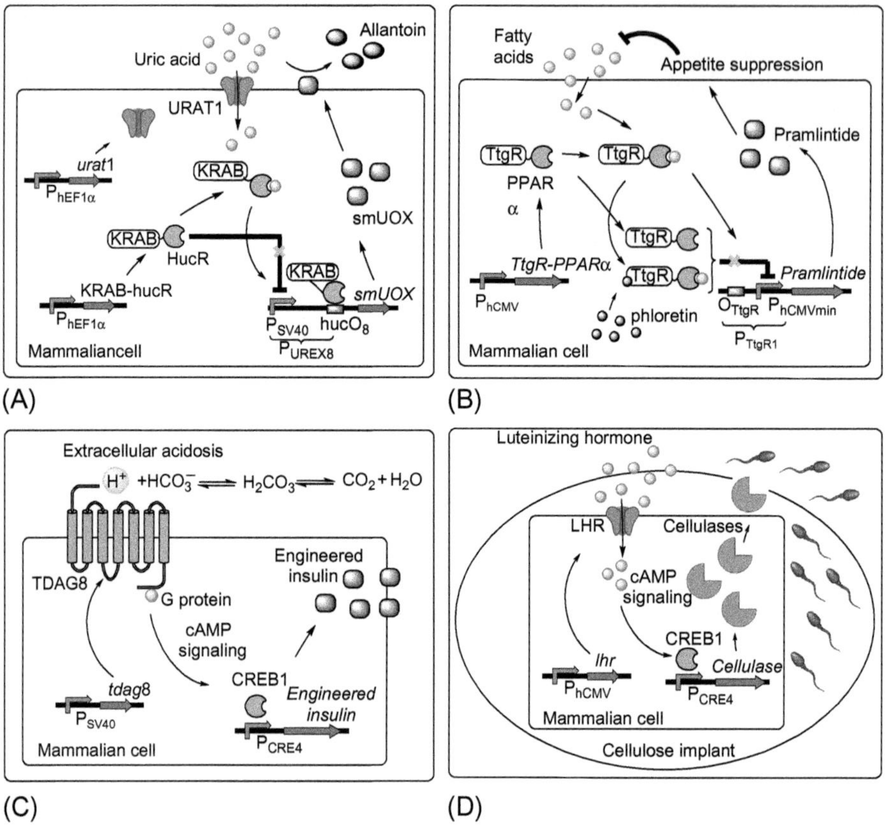

Fig. 16.6 Prosthetic gene networks. (A) Selfsufficient synthetic circuit to control blood-urate homeostasis. (B) Obesity treatment. (C) Diabetic ketoacidosis treatment. (D) Artificial insemination. *cAMP*, cyclic adenosine monophosphate; *CREB1*, cAMP-responsive element binding protein 1; *KRAB*, Krüppel associated box; *LHR*, luteinizing hormone receptor; O_{TtgR}, TtgR-specific operator; P_{CRE4}, promoter activated by CREB1; P_{hCMV}, human cytomegalovirus promoter; $P_{hEF1\alpha}$, human elongation factor 1 alpha promoter; P_{SV40}, simian virus 40 promoter; *PPARα*, human peroxisome proliferator-associated receptor alpha; *smUOX*, urate oxidase; *TDAG8*, G-protein-coupled receptor; *TtgR*, phloretin-responsive repressor; *URAT1*, uric acid transporter.

TtgR-specific operator (O_{TtgR}) and activates transcription. In the absence of fatty acids or in the presence of phloretin, the expression is inhibited. This provides a potential safety switch. The cells containing the genetic circuit were microencapsulated and implanted into mice with hyperlipidemia. Afterwards, it was observed a significant attenuation of hyperlipidemia, reduction in food consumption and body weight.

Type 1 diabetes is a disease for which the use of prosthetic networks is also being considered. The deficiency in insulin decreases the insulin-dependent glucose transporter (GLUT-4) that mediates glucose uptake in fat and muscle. Therefore the body needs to find alternative energy sources. This leads to an excessive uncontrolled lipolysis in the adipose tissues resulting in excessive production of acidic ketone bodies in the liver, which accumulate in the bloodstream, overwhelm the acid–base homeostasis maintained by the CO_2-bicarbonate buffering system and lower the pH in blood. Diabetic ketoacidosis can cause edema, coma and death (Heng et al., 2015). Ausländer et al. (2014a) created a synthetic signaling cascade that allows extracellular pH to be monitored (Fig. 16.6C). This pH-sensing device can be very useful in the treatment of type 1 diabetes when linked to the production of engineered insulin (furin-cleavable proinsulin I) via a synthetic promoter (P_{CRE}). This promoter is activated due to a cascade of events triggered by pH changes. The alginate-microencapsulated cells (human embryonic kidney cells—HEK293) containing the synthetic network, when implanted in type 1 diabetic mice, attenuated diabetic ketoacidosis and restored glucose homeostasis by coordinating insulin production (Ausländer et al., 2014a). Ye et al. (2011) used a different strategy. The authors constructed an optogenetic device that used light-controlled expression of GLP-1 to attenuate glycemic excursions in diabetic mice. A variant of GLP-1 was put under the transcriptional control of the heterologous G-protein-coupled receptor (GPCR) melanopsin and after blue light irradiation a cascade of events was triggered. GPCRs are essential for the cell to be able to sense chemical or physical inputs. Therefore GPCRs are being engineered to be used as synthetic biology tools that respond to synthetic ligands (RASSL—receptors activated solely by synthetic ligands) or designer drugs (DREADD—designer receptor exclusively activated by designer drugs) with different specificities and to be integrated into artificial gene networks (Haellman and Fussenegger, 2016).

Mammalian cells are also being reprogrammed using synthetic trigger-controlled devices to monitor pathological levels of other metabolites in the body such as bile acids (Rössger et al., 2014) and dopamine (Rössger et al., 2013b) to treat other metabolic diseases. Several anticancer strategies have also been developed using synthetic gene circuits (Ye and Fussenegger, 2014; Folcher and Fussenegger, 2012). For example, Nissim and Bar-Ziv (2010) constructed a dual-promoter integrator that consists of two expression units that receive independent input from different transcription factors (AND gate circuit). In the presence of two neoplastic markers, the activation of the two tumor specific promoters occurs and two chimeric proteins are simultaneously expressed and dimerize to form a functional trans-activator that activates P_{GAL4} promoter. This promoter triggers the expression of the HSV-TK that kills the cancer cells.

Synthetic gene circuits in mammalian cells can have other biomedical applications besides treating diseases. For example, they can be used as artificial insemination devices since, due to broad variations in estrus cycle and ovulation timing, synchronizing sperm delivery with female estrus is still a major challenge for optimizing artificial insemination in livestock farming (Weber and Fussenegger, 2012). Kemmer et al. (2011) designed an artificial insemination device that consists of cellulose-based implants containing sensor cells and bull sperm (Fig. 16.6D). The implant was positioned in the uterus of the cow. The cells (HEK293) were engineered to express luteinizing hormone receptor (LHR) constitutively. When the luteinizing hormone binds to the receptor the ovulation occurs. When expression of LHR is activated it also triggers a signaling cascade activating the target promoter P_{CRE4}. This promoter controlled the production of a secreted *B. subtilis*-derived cellulase that degrades the implanted capsule wall enabling the sperm release and leading to successful fertilization of the cow. The optimization and tailoring of this synthetic device could allow its use in humans or other species (Weber and Fussenegger, 2012; Kemmer et al., 2011).

16.7.8 CRISPR/Cas9 system and gene therapy

CRISPR/Cas9 system is revolutionizing the field of genome engineering since it allows altering the genome of organisms in a relatively rapid and easy way. This technology is recent and widely used in research laboratories and holds a very high potential, however it has yet to make an impact in the clinics. In the future, it may be used to correct genetic mutations responsible for inherited disorders (Doudna and Charpentier, 2014; Yin et al., 2014). For example, Wu et al. (2013) used CRISPR/Cas9 to correct a dominant mutation in the *Crygc* gene that causes cataracts in mouse. Cas9 mRNA and single-guide RNA targeting the mutant allele were administered by injection into the zygotes and the correction occurred by homology-directed repair. Moreover, it was found that the resulting mice were able to transmit the corrected allele to the next generation. Recent studies also suggest that the CRISPR/Cas9 system may be useful for curing HIV-1 infection by editing the viral genome and blocking its expression (Ebina et al., 2013; Zhu et al., 2015; Liao et al., 2015; Hu et al., 2014; Limsirichai et al., 2016). Cancer is another disease where the application of CRISPR/Cas9 technology has been widely explored in the pursuit of its cure (Chiou et al., 2015; Sánchez-Rivera and Jacks, 2015). One of the applications of CRISPR/Cas9 in this area consists of developing next-generation models of human cancer. These models are used to understand the evolution and progression of cancer cells (screen for tumor growth and metastasis) and identify new approaches to be tested for cancer treatment (Mou et al., 2015; Sánchez-Rivera and Jacks, 2015; Chen et al., 2015).

16.8 Conclusions and future perspectives

Despite being a relatively new research field, synthetic biology holds great promise for the development of novel therapeutic approaches and diagnosis (bio)devices. In this chapter, we discussed some of the recent developments in synthetic biology in preventing, diagnosing, targeting and treating diseases. We described bacterial and viral devices, as well as treatments developed from model organisms with well-established genome manipulation, thus presenting a toolbox with great potential for use in the design and construction of even more complex devices. We also explored some of the first mammalian synthetic circuits developed for therapeutic applications (prosthetic networks) in the last years. However, their level of development is still very far from the one achieved with bacterial and viral devices. There are several reasons for this, namely the number of functional and orthogonal parts is still limited and unpredictable, the gene circuit is more complex and genome engineering strategies for mammalian cells are not so advanced and robust. Since most of human health problems are inherently problems with mammalian systems, a more concerted effort towards advancing mammalian synthetic biology is crucial for the next-generation of therapeutic solutions. In addition, most of the reported studies on mammalian synthetic biology used immortalized cell lines (eg, HEK293, HeLa) that can be used as an indefinite source of cells as they can proliferate *ad infinitum* due to mutation. These mutations required for immortality can occur naturally (such as the ones isolated from a naturally occurring cancer) or be intentionally induced for experimental purposes. The introduction of these cells to the human body raises a number of safety concerns, including immunocompatibility and carcinogenicity. In the future, these concerns can be overcome by the use of stem cells. Indeed, stem cells could be the ideal vehicles for the delivery of prosthetic networks to the human body, since they can integrate *in situ* within the target tissue or organ. In addition, induced pluripotent stem cell (iPSC) technology also provides a way to produce and engineer autologous cells from patients of all ages.

Synthetic biology can also be used for biomaterial engineering in order to create smart materials—those that dynamically interact with surrounding tissues. The capability to manipulate genetically the sequence and structure enables the application of both evolutionary and rational approaches (Cheng and Lu, 2012). In addition, the use of synthetic biology selection techniques for the identification of material components and scaffolds may lead to the construction of new biomaterials that meet a set of desired criteria (Bryksin et al., 2014). For instance the potential use of engineered bacteriophage-based scaffolds as nanoplatforms for drug delivery to hepatocellular carcinoma has been described (Min et al., 2014). In the future, biomaterial manipulation may yield new smart materials for many biomedical applications, including tissue engineering and enhanced surgical materials.

Recently, an important breakthrough in synthetic biology was reported by Farzadfard and Lu (2014). These scientists were able to store encoded environmental data (eg, exposure to a given chemical or to light) in DNA in such a way that scientists can read it. Since the data are stored in the DNA, the information is not lost if the cell dies and it is possible to determine the magnitude and duration of the signal by sequencing the genes. This approach called "synthetic cellular recorders integrating biological events" (SCRIBE), can be considered a genome editing tool, and relies on retrons, which are DNA structures found naturally in some bacteria that use reverse transcriptase and two RNA transcripts to produce hybrid RNA-ssDNA. This DNA is expressed due to a stimulus and it is targeted into a specific place in the genome where it is recombined (using viral enzymes) and converted in permanent memory. In the future, this can be used in several biomedical applications. For instance, the probiotic bacteria could be used as sensors and record events in the gut, such as inflammation. Additionally, this design could also be adapted to eukaryotic systems and CRISPR/Cas9.

Although synthetic biology still has a long way to go before becoming a commonly used treatment, one day the use of bacteriophages or commensal bacteria against pathogenic organisms or tumor cells, as well as the use of sensor-effector devices and smart materials for personalized medicine may become a reality.

Acknowledgments

The authors acknowledge financial support from the Strategic Project UID/BIO/04469/2013 unit and COMPETE 2020 (POCI-01-0145-FEDER-006684), the project RECI/BBB-EBI/0179/2012 (FCOMP-01-0124-FEDER-027462), the project LipidNPPhage (PTDC/SAU-BMA/121028/2010) and Post-doctoral grant (UMINHO/BPD/37/2015) to J. L. Rodrigues funded by Fundação para a Ciência e a Tecnologia.

References

Ajikumar, P.K., Xiao, W.-H., Tyo, K.E., Wang, Y., Simeon, F., Leonard, E., Mucha, O., Phon, T.H., Pfeifer, B., Stephanopoulos, G., 2010. Isoprenoid pathway optimization for Taxol precursor overproduction in Escherichia coli. Science 330, 70–74.

Alper, H., Fischer, C., Nevoigt, E., Stephanopoulos, G., 2005. Tuning genetic control through promoter engineering. Proc. Natl. Acad. Sci. U. S. A. 102, 12678–12683.

Alphey, L., 2014. Genetic control of mosquitoes. Annu. Rev. Entomol. 59, 205–224.

Amidi, M., De Raad, M., Crommelin, D.J., Hennink, W.E., Mastrobattista, E., 2011. Antigen-expressing immunostimulatory liposomes as a genetically programmable synthetic vaccine. Syst. Synth. Biol. 5, 21–31.

Anderson, J.C., Clarke, E.J., Arkin, A.P., Voigt, C.A., 2006. Environmentally controlled invasion of cancer cells by engineered bacteria. J. Mol. Biol. 355, 619–627.

Anderson, J.C., Voigt, C.A., Arkin, A.P., 2007. Environmental signal integration by a modular AND gate. Mol. Syst. Biol. 3, 1–8.

Andrianantoandro, E., Basu, S., Karig, D.K., Weiss, R., 2006. Synthetic biology: new engineering rules for an emerging discipline. Mol. Syst. Biol. 2, 1–14.

Arkin, A., Berry, D., Church, G., Arnold, F., Boldt, J., Muller, O., Ellington, A.D., Endy, D., Fussenegger, M., Gold, E., 2009. What's in a name? Nat. Biotechnol. 27, 1071–1073.

Arrach, N., Zhao, M., Porwollik, S., Hoffman, R.M., McClelland, M., 2008. *Salmonella* promoters preferentially activated inside tumors. Cancer Res. 68, 4827–4832.

Ausländer, D., Ausländer, S., Charpin-El Hamri, G., Sedlmayer, F., Müller, M., Frey, O., Hierlemann, A., Stelling, J., Fussenegger, M., 2014a. A synthetic multifunctional mammalian pH Sensor and CO2 transgene-control device. Mol. Cell 55, 397–408.

Ausländer, D., Eggerschwiler, B., Kemmer, C., Geering, B., Ausländer, S., Fussenegger, M., 2014b. A designer cell-based histamine-specific human allergy profiler. Nat. Commun. 5, 1–8.

Baker, M., 2011. The next step for the synthetic genome. Nature 473, 403–408.

Bar, H., Yacoby, I., Benhar, I., 2008. Killing cancer cells by targeted drug-carrying phage nanomedicines. BMC Biotechnol. 8, 37.

Basu, S., Mehreja, R., Thiberge, S., Chen, M.-T., Weiss, R., 2004. Spatiotemporal control of gene expression with pulse-generating networks. Proc. Natl. Acad. Sci. U. S. A. 101, 6355–6360.

Beisel, C.L., Smolke, C.D., 2009. Design principles for Riboswitch function. PLoS Comput. Biol. 5, e1000363.

Beloin, C., Deighan, P., Doyle, M., Dorman, C.J., 2003. Shigella flexneri 2a strain 2457T expresses three members of the H-NS-like protein family: characterization of the Sfh protein. Mol. Genet. Genomics 270, 66–77.

Bhattarai, S.R., Yoo, S.Y., Lee, S.-W., Dean, D., 2012. Engineered phage-based therapeutic materials inhibit Chlamydia trachomatis intracellular infection. Biomaterials 33, 5166–5174.

Bolhassani, A., 2011. Potential efficacy of cell-penetrating peptides for nucleic acid and drug delivery in cancer. Biochim. Biophys. Acta 1816, 232–246.

Bonde, M.T., Kosuri, S., Genee, H.J., Sarup-Lytzen, K., Church, G.M., Sommer, M.O., Wang, H.H., 2014. Direct mutagenesis of thousands of genomic targets using microarray-derived oligonucleotides. ACS Synth. Biol. 4, 17–22.

Boyle, P.M., Silver, P.A., 2009. Harnessing nature's toolbox: regulatory elements for synthetic biology. J. R. Soc. Interface 6, S535–S546.

Boyle, P.M., Silver, P.A., 2012. Parts plus pipes: synthetic biology approaches to metabolic engineering. Metab. Eng. 14, 223–232.

Brophy, J.A., Voigt, C.A., 2014. Principles of genetic circuit design. Nat. Methods 11, 508–520.

Bruggeman, F.J., Westerhoff, H.V., 2007. The nature of systems biology. Trends Microbiol. 15, 45–50.

Bryksin, A.V., Brown, A.C., Baksh, M.M., Finn, M., Barker, T.H., 2014. Learning from nature–novel synthetic biology approaches for biomaterial design. Acta Biomater. 10, 1761–1769.

Bunka, D.H.J., Stockley, P.G., 2006. Aptamers come of age—at last. Nat. Rev. Microbiol. 4, 588–596.

Burgard, A.P., Pharkya, P., Maranas, C.D., 2003. Optknock: a bilevel programming framework for identifying gene knockout strategies for microbial strain optimization. Biotechnol. Bioeng. 84, 647–657.

Burns, C.C., Shaw, J., Campagnoli, R., Jorba, J., Vincent, A., Quay, J., Kew, O., 2006. Modulation of poliovirus replicative fitness in HeLa cells by deoptimization of synonymous codon usage in the capsid region. J. Virol. 80, 3259–3272.

Burt, A., 2003. Site-specific selfish genes as tools for the control and genetic engineering of natural populations. Proc. R. Soc. Lond. B Biol. Sci. 270, 921–928.

Cai, M., Yang, Y., 2014. Targeted genome editing tools for disease modeling and gene therapy. Curr. Gene Ther. 14, 2–9.

Calvert, J., 2010. Synthetic biology: constructing nature? Sociol. Rev. 58, 95–112.

Calvert, J., Martin, P., 2009. The role of social scientists in synthetic biology. EMBO Rep. 10, 201–204.

Cattaneo, R., Miest, T., Shashkova, E.V., Barry, M.A., 2008. Reprogrammed viruses as cancer therapeutics: targeted, armed and shielded. Nat. Rev. Microbiol. 6, 529–540.

Chen, C.-H., Huang, H., Ward, C.M., Su, J.T., Schaeffer, L.V., Guo, M., Hay, B.A., 2007. A synthetic maternal-effect selfish genetic element drives population replacement in Drosophila. Science 316, 597–600.

Chen, H.W., Medley, C.D., Sefah, K., Shangguan, D., Tang, Z., Meng, L., Smith, J.E., Tan, W., 2008. Molecular recognition of small-cell lung cancer cells using aptamers. ChemMedChem 3, 991–1001.

Chen, H.-L., Lai, Y.-W., Chen, C.-S., Chu, T.-W., Lin, W., Yen, C.-C., Lin, M.-F., Tu, M.-Y., Chen, C.-M., 2010. Probiotic Lactobacillus casei expressing human lactoferrin elevates antibacterial activity in the gastrointestinal tract. Biometals 23, 543–554.

Chen, Z., Guo, L., Zhang, Y., Walzem, R.L., Pendergast, J.S., Printz, R.L., Morris, L.C., Matafonova, E., Stien, X., Kang, L., 2014. Incorporation of therapeutically modified bacteria into gut microbiota inhibits obesity. J. Clin. Invest. 124, 3391–3406.

Chen, S., Sanjana, N.E., Zheng, K., Shalem, O., Lee, K., Shi, X., Scott, D.A., Song, J., Pan, J.Q., Weissleder, R., 2015. Genome-wide CRISPR screen in a mouse model of tumor growth and metastasis. Cell 160, 1246–1260.

Cheng, A.A., Lu, T.K., 2012. Synthetic biology: an emerging engineering discipline. Annu. Rev. Biomed. Eng. 14, 155–178.

Chessher, A., Breitling, R., Takano, E., 2015. Bacterial microcompartments: biomaterials for synthetic biology-based compartmentalization strategies. ACS Biomater. Sci. Eng. 1, 345–351.

Chiou, S.-H., Winters, I.P., Wang, J., Naranjo, S., Dudgeon, C., Tamburini, F.B., Brady, J.J., Yang, D., Grüner, B.M., Chuang, C.-H., 2015. Pancreatic cancer modeling using retrograde viral vector delivery and in vivo CRISPR/Cas9-mediated somatic genome editing. Genes Dev. 29, 1576–1585.

Choffnes, E.R., Relman, D.A., Pray, L., 2011. The Science and Applications of Synthetic and Systems Biology: Workshop Summary. National Academies Press, Washington.

Church, G.M., Gao, Y., Kosuri, S., 2012. Next-generation digital information storage in DNA. Science 337, 1628.

Citorik, R.J., Mimee, M., Lu, T.K., 2014. Bacteriophage-based synthetic biology for the study of infectious diseases. Curr. Opin. Microbiol. 19, 59–69.

Claesen, J., Fischbach, M.A., 2014. Synthetic microbes as drug delivery systems. ACS Synth. Biol. 4, 358–364.

Clairmont, C., Lee, K., Pike, J., Ittensohn, M., Low, K., Pawelek, J., Bermudes, D., Brecher, S., Margitich, D., Turnier, J., 2000. Biodistribution and genetic stability of the novel antitumor agent VNP20009, a genetically modified strain of *Salmonella typhimuvium*. J. Infect. Dis. 181, 1996–2002.

Clancy, K., Voigt, C.A., 2010. Programming cells: towards an automated 'Genetic Compiler'. Curr. Opin. Biotechnol. 21, 572–581.

Coleman, J.R., Papamichail, D., Skiena, S., Futcher, B., Wimmer, E., Mueller, S., 2008. Virus attenuation by genome-scale changes in codon pair bias. Science 320, 1784–1787.

Collas, P., 2010. The current state of chromatin immunoprecipitation. Mol. Biotechnol. 45, 87–100.

Collins, M.L., Irvine, B., Tyner, D., Fine, E., Zayati, C., Chang, C.-A., Horn, T., Ahle, D., Detmer, J., Shen, L.-P., 1997. A branched DNA signal amplification assay for quantification of nucleic acid targets below 100 molecules/ml. Nucleic Acids Res. 25, 2979–2984.

Corchero, J.L., Cedano, J., 2011. Self-assembling, protein-based intracellular bacterial organelles: emerging vehicles for encapsulating, targeting and delivering therapeutical cargoes. Microb. Cell Factories 10, 1–8.

Courbet, A., 2015. Engineering next generation diagnostics through synthetic biology. PhD thesis, University of Montpellier.

Courbet, A., Endy, D., Renard, E., Molina, F., Bonnet, J., 2015. Detection of pathological biomarkers in human clinical samples via amplifying genetic switches and logic gates. Sci. Transl. Med. 7, 1–11.

Critchley, R., Jezzard, S., Radford, K., Goussard, S., Lemoine, N., Grillot-Courvalin, C., Vassaux, G., 2004. Potential therapeutic applications of recombinant, invasive *E. coli*. Gene Ther. 11, 1224–1233.

Curran, K.A., Alper, H.S., 2012. Expanding the chemical palate of cells by combining systems biology and metabolic engineering. Metab. Eng. 14, 289–297.

Dai, Y., Toley, B.J., Swofford, C.A., Forbes, N.S., 2013. Construction of an inducible cell-communication system that amplifies *Salmonella* gene expression in tumor tissue. Biotechnol. Bioeng. 110, 1769–1781.

Dang, L.H., Bettegowda, C., Huso, D.L., Kinzler, K.W., Vogelstein, B., 2001. Combination bacteriolytic therapy for the treatment of experimental tumors. Proc. Natl. Acad. Sci. 98, 15155–15160.

Dang, L.H., Bettegowda, C., Agrawal, N., Cheong, I., Huso, D., Frost, P., Loganzo, F., Greenberger, L., Barkoczy, J., Pettit, G.R., 2004. Targeting vascular and avascular compartments of tumors with *C. novyi*-NT and anti-microtubule agents. Cancer Biol. Ther. 3, 326–337.

Daniels, D.A., Chen, H., Hicke, B.J., Swiderek, K.M., Gold, L., 2003. A tenascin-C aptamer identified by tumor cell SELEX: systematic evolution of ligands by exponential enrichment. Proc. Natl. Acad. Sci. U. S. A. 100, 15416–15421.

Danino, T., Prindle, A., Kwong, G.A., Skalak, M., Li, H., Allen, K., Hasty, J., Bhatia, S.N., 2015. Programmable probiotics for detection of cancer in urine. Sci. Transl. Med. 7, 1–12.

Dasika, M.S., Maranas, C.D., 2008. OptCircuit: an optimization based method for computational design of genetic circuits. BMC Syst. Biol. 2, 1–19.

Datsenko, K.A., Wanner, B.L., 2000. One-step inactivation of chromosomal genes in Escherichia coli K-12 using PCR products. Proc. Natl. Acad. Sci. U. S. A. 97, 6640–6645.

De Valdez, M.R.W., Nimmo, D., Betz, J., Gong, H.-F., James, A.A., Alphey, L., Black, W.C., 2011. Genetic elimination of dengue vector mosquitoes. Proc. Natl. Acad. Sci. 108, 4772–4775.

Deporter, S.M., Mcnaughton, B.R., 2014. Engineered M13 bacteriophage nanocarriers for intracellular delivery of exogenous proteins to human prostate cancer cells. Bioconjug. Chem. 25, 1620–1625.

Deredec, A., Burt, A., Godfray, H.C.J., 2008. The population genetics of using homing endonuclease genes in vector and pest management. Genetics 179, 2013–2026.

Deredec, A., Godfray, H.C.J., Burt, A., 2011. Requirements for effective malaria control with homing endonuclease genes. Proc. Natl. Acad. Sci. 108, E874–E880.

Derossi, D., Joliot, A.H., Chassaing, G., Prochiantz, A., 1994. The third helix of the Antennapedia homeodomain translocates through biological membranes. J. Biol. Chem. 269, 10444–10450.

Dong, H., Zhao, C., Zhang, T., Lin, Z., Li, Y., Zhang, Y., 2015. Engineering *Escherichia coli* Cell Factories for n-Butanol Production. Advances in Biochemical Engineering/Biotechnology, Springer, Berlin Heidelberg.

Dormitzer, P.R., Suphaphiphat, P., Gibson, D.G., Wentworth, D.E., Stockwell, T.B., Algire, M.A., Alperovich, N., Barro, M., Brown, D.M., Craig, S., 2013. Synthetic generation of influenza vaccine viruses for rapid response to pandemics. Sci. Transl. Med. 5, 1–12.

Doudna, J.A., Charpentier, E., 2014. The new frontier of genome engineering with CRISPR-Cas9. Science 346, 1–10.

Du, J., Shao, Z., Zhao, H., 2011. Engineering microbial factories for synthesis of value-added products. J. Ind. Microbiol. Biotechnol. 38, 873–890.

Duan, D.D., 2011. Proteomics and functional proteomics. In: Yuan, J.X., Garcia, J.G.N., Hales, C.A., Rich, S., Archer, S.L., West, J.B. (Eds.), Textbook of Pulmonary Vascular Disease. Springer, New York.

Duan, F., March, J.C., 2008. Interrupting Vibrio cholerae infection of human epithelial cells with engineered commensal bacterial signaling. Biotechnol. Bioeng. 101, 128–134.

Duan, F., March, J.C., 2010. Engineered bacterial communication prevents Vibrio cholerae virulence in an infant mouse model. Proc. Natl. Acad. Sci. 107, 11260–11264.

Duan, F., Curtis, K.L., March, J.C., 2008. Secretion of insulinotropic proteins by commensal bacteria: rewiring the gut to treat diabetes. Appl. Environ. Microbiol. 74, 7437–7438.

Duan, F.F., Liu, J.H., March, J.C., 2015. Engineered commensal bacteria reprogram intestinal cells into glucose-responsive insulin-secreting cells for the treatment of diabetes. Diabetes 64, 1794–1803.

Dueber, J.E., Wu, G.C., Malmirchegini, G.R., Moon, T.S., Petzold, C.J., Ullal, A.V., Prather, K.L., Keasling, J.D., 2009. Synthetic protein scaffolds provide modular control over metabolic flux. Nat. Biotechnol. 27, 753–759.

Ebina, H., Misawa, N., Kanemura, Y., Koyanagi, Y., 2013. Harnessing the CRISPR/Cas9 system to disrupt latent HIV-1 provirus. Sci. Rep. 3, 1–7.

Edgar, R., Mckinstry, M., Hwang, J., Oppenheim, A.B., Fekete, R.A., Giulian, G., Merril, C., Nagashima, K., Adhya, S., 2006. High-sensitivity bacterial detection using biotin-tagged phage and quantum-dot nanocomplexes. Proc. Natl. Acad. Sci. U. S. A. 103, 4841–4845.

Edgar, R., Friedman, N., Molshanski-Mor, S., Qimron, U., 2012. Reversing bacterial resistance to antibiotics by phage-mediated delivery of dominant sensitive genes. Appl. Environ. Microbiol. 78, 744–751.

Elbeik, T., Markowitz, N., Nassos, P., Kumar, U., Beringer, S., Haller, B., Ng, V., 2004a. Simultaneous runs of the Bayer VERSANT HIV-1 version 3.0 and HCV bDNA version 3.0 quantitative assays on the system 340 platform provide reliable quantitation and improved work flow. J. Clin. Microbiol. 42, 3120–3127.

Elbeik, T., Surtihadi, J., Destree, M., Gorlin, J., Holodniy, M., Jortani, S.A., Kuramoto, K., Ng, V., Valdes, R., Valsamakis, A., 2004b. Multicenter evaluation of the performance characteristics of the Bayer VERSANT HCV RNA 3.0 assay (bDNA). J. Clin. Microbiol. 42, 563–569.

Ellington, A.D., Szostak, J.W., 1990. In vitro selection of RNA molecules that bind specific ligands. Nature 346, 818–822.

Elmquist, A., Lindgren, M., Bartfai, T., Langel, U., 2001. VE-cadherin-derived cell-penetrating peptide, pVEC, with carrier functions. Exp. Cell Res. 269, 237–244.

Enbäck, J., Laakkonen, P., 2007. Tumour-homing peptides: tools for targeting, imaging and destruction. Biochem. Soc. Trans. 35, 780–783.

Endy, D., 2005. Foundations for engineering biology. Nature 438, 449–453.

Essler, M., Ruoslahti, E., 2002. Molecular specialization of breast vasculature: a breast-homing phage-displayed peptide binds to aminopeptidase P in breast vasculature. Proc. Natl. Acad. Sci. U. S. A. 99, 2252–2257.

Fan, C., Cheng, S., Liu, Y., Escobar, C.M., Crowley, C.S., Jefferson, R.E., Yeates, T.O., Bobik, T.A., 2010. Short N-terminal sequences package proteins into bacterial microcompartments. Proc. Natl. Acad. Sci. 107, 7509–7514.

Farzadfard, F., Lu, T.K., 2014. Genomically encoded analog memory with precise in vivo DNA writing in living cell populations. Science 346, 825–833.

Ferber, D., 2004. Synthetic biology. Microbes made to order. Science 303, 158–161.

Flentie, K., Kocher, B., Gammon, S.T., Novack, D.V., Mckinney, J.S., Piwnica-Worms, D., 2012. A bioluminescent transposon reporter-trap identifies tumor-specific microenvironment-induced promoters in Salmonella for conditional bacterial-based tumor therapy. Cancer Discov. 2, 624–637.

Folcher, M., Fussenegger, M., 2012. Synthetic biology advancing clinical applications. Curr. Opin. Chem. Biol. 16, 345–354.

Forbes, N.S., 2006. Profile of a bacterial tumor killer. Nat. Biotechnol. 24, 1484–1485.

Forbes, N.S., 2010. Engineering the perfect (bacterial) cancer therapy. Nat. Rev. Cancer 10, 785–794.

Forbes, N.S., Munn, L.L., Fukumura, D., Jain, R.K., 2003. Sparse initial entrapment of systemically injected *Salmonella typhimurium* leads to heterogeneous accumulation within tumors. Cancer Res. 63, 5188–5193.

Fu, G., Condon, K.C., Epton, M.J., Gong, P., Jin, L., Condon, G.C., Morrison, N.I., Dafa'alla, T.H., Alphey, L., 2007. Female-specific insect lethality engineered using alternative splicing. Nat. Biotechnol. 25, 353–357.

Fu, G., Lees, R.S., Nimmo, D., Aw, D., Jin, L., Gray, P., Berendonk, T.U., White-Cooper, H., Scaife, S., Phuc, H.K., 2010. Female-specific flightless phenotype for mosquito control. Proc. Natl. Acad. Sci. 107, 4550–4554.

Gaj, T., Gersbach, C.A., Barbas, C.F., 2013. ZFN, TALEN, and CRISPR/Cas-based methods for genome engineering. Trends Biotechnol. 31, 397–405.

Galizi, R., Doyle, L.A., Menichelli, M., Bernardini, F., Deredec, A., Burt, A., Stoddard, B.L., Windbichler, N., Crisanti, A., 2014. A synthetic sex ratio distortion system for the control of the human malaria mosquito. Nat. Commun. 5, 1–8.

Ganai, S., Arenas, R., Forbes, N., 2009. Tumour-targeted delivery of TRAIL using *Salmonella typhimurium* enhances breast cancer survival in mice. Br. J. Cancer 101, 1683–1691.

Ganai, S., Arenas, R.B., Sauer, J.P., Bentley, B., Forbes, N.S., 2011. In tumors *Salmonella* migrate away from vasculature toward the transition zone and induce apoptosis. Cancer Gene Ther. 18, 457–466.

Garst, A.D., Batey, R.T., 2009. A switch in time: detailing the life of a riboswitch. Biochim. Biophys. Acta 1789, 584–591.

Geall, A.J., Mandl, C.W., Ulmer, J.B., 2013. RNA: the new revolution in nucleic acid vaccines. Semin. Immunol. 25, 152–159.
Ghosh, D., Kohli, A.G., Moser, F., Endy, D., Belcher, A.M., 2012. Refactored M13 bacteriophage as a platform for tumor cell imaging and drug delivery. ACS Synth. Biol. 1, 576–582.
Goldman, N., Bertone, P., Chen, S., Dessimoz, C., Leproust, E.M., Sipos, B., Birney, E., 2013. Towards practical, high-capacity, low-maintenance information storage in synthesized DNA. Nature 494, 77–80.
Grass, R.N., Heckel, R., Puddu, M., Paunescu, D., Stark, W.J., 2015. Robust chemical preservation of digital information on DNA in silica with error-correcting codes. Angew. Chem. Int. Ed. 54, 2552–2555.
Grillot-Courvalin, C., Goussard, S., Huetz, F., Ojcius, D.M., Courvalin, P., 1998. Functional gene transfer from intracellular bacteria to mammalian cells. Nat. Biotechnol. 16, 862–866.
Griss, R., Schena, A., Reymond, L., Patiny, L., Werner, D., Tinberg, C.E., Baker, D., Johnsson, K., 2014. Bioluminescent sensor proteins for point-of-care therapeutic drug monitoring. Nat. Chem. Biol. 10, 598–604.
Guye, P., Li, Y., Wroblewska, L., Duportet, X., Weiss, R., 2013. Rapid, modular and reliable construction of complex mammalian gene circuits. Nucleic Acids Res. 41, 1–6.
Haellman, V., Fussenegger, M., 2016. Synthetic biology—toward therapeutic solutions. J. Mol. Biol. 428, 945–962.
Harris, A.F., Nimmo, D., Mckemey, A.R., Kelly, N., Scaife, S., Donnelly, C.A., Beech, C., Petrie, W.D., Alphey, L., 2011. Field performance of engineered male mosquitoes. Nat. Biotechnol. 29, 1034–1037.
Harris, A.F., Mckemey, A.R., Nimmo, D., Curtis, Z., Black, I., Morgan, S.A., Oviedo, M.N., Lacroix, R., Naish, N., Morrison, N.I., 2012. Successful suppression of a field mosquito population by sustained release of engineered male mosquitoes. Nat. Biotechnol. 30, 828–830.
Hay, B.A., Chen, C.-H., Ward, C.M., Huang, H., Su, J.T., Guo, M., 2010. Engineering the genomes of wild insect populations: challenges, and opportunities provided by synthetic Medea selfish genetic elements. J. Insect Physiol. 56, 1402–1413.
Hayashi, K., Zhao, M., Yamauchi, K., Yamamoto, N., Tsuchiya, H., Tomita, K., Hoffman, R.M., 2009. Cancer metastasis directly eradicated by targeted therapy with a modified Salmonella typhimurium. J. Cell. Biochem. 106, 992–998.
Heinemann, M., Panke, S., 2006. Synthetic biology—putting engineering into biology. Bioinformatics 22, 2790–2799.
Hellsten, I., Nerlich, B., 2011. Synthetic biology: building the language for a new science brick by metaphorical brick. New Genet. Soc. 30, 375–397.
Hemingway, J., 2014. The role of vector control in stopping the transmission of malaria: threats and opportunities. Phil. Trans. R. Soc. Lond. B Biol. Sci. 369, 1–5.
Heng, B.C., Aubel, D., Fussenegger, M., 2015. Prosthetic gene networks as an alternative to standard pharmacotherapies for metabolic disorders. Curr. Opin. Biotechnol. 35, 37–45.
Henry, M., Debarbieux, L., 2012. Tools from viruses: bacteriophage successes and beyond. Virology 434, 151–161.
Heo, J., Breitbach, C.J., Moon, A., Kim, C.W., Patt, R., Kim, M.K., Lee, Y.K., Oh, S.Y., Woo, H.Y., Parato, K., Rintoul, J., Falls, T., Hickman, T., Rhee, B.-G., Bell, J.C., Kirn, D.H., Hwang, T.-H., 2011. Sequential therapy with JX-594, a targeted oncolytic poxvirus, followed by sorafenib in hepatocellular carcinoma: preclinical and clinical demonstration of combination efficacy. Mol. Ther. 19, 1170–1179.
Hill, C.B., Czauderna, T., Klapperstück, M., Roessner, U., Schreiber, F., 2015. Metabolomics, standards and metabolic modeling for synthetic biology in plants. Front. Bioeng. Biotechnol. 3, 1–12.

Hoffmann, A.A., Ross, P.A., Rašić, G., 2015. Wolbachia strains for disease control: ecological and evolutionary considerations. Evol. Appl. 8, 751–768.

Holt, N., Wang, J., Kim, K., Friedman, G., Wang, X., Taupin, V., Crooks, G.M., Kohn, D.B., Gregory, P.D., Holmes, M.C., 2010. Human hematopoietic stem/progenitor cells modified by zinc-finger nucleases targeted to CCR5 control HIV-1 in vivo. Nat. Biotechnol. 28, 839–847.

Hooshangi, S., Bentley, W.E., 2008. From unicellular properties to multicellular behavior: bacteria quorum sensing circuitry and applications. Curr. Opin. Biotechnol. 19, 550–555.

Hsu, P.D., Lander, E.S., Zhang, F., 2014. Development and applications of CRISPR-Cas9 for genome engineering. Cell 157, 1262–1278.

Hu, W., Kaminski, R., Yang, F., Zhang, Y., Cosentino, L., Li, F., Luo, B., Alvarez-Carbonell, D., Garcia-Mesa, Y., Karn, J., 2014. RNA-directed gene editing specifically eradicates latent and prevents new HIV-1 infection. Proc. Natl. Acad. Sci. 111, 11461–11466.

Huang, R., Pershad, K., Kokoszka, M., Kay, B.K., 2011. In: Hughes, A.B. (Ed.), Phage-Displayed Combinatorial Peptides. Wiley-VCH Verlag GmbH & Co. KGaA, Weinheim, Germany.

Husseiny, M.I., Hensel, M., 2005. Rapid method for the construction of Salmonella enterica Serovar Typhimurium vaccine carrier strains. Infect. Immun. 73, 1598–1605.

Isaacs, F.J., Dwyer, D.J., Collins, J.J., 2006. RNA synthetic biology. Nat. Biotechnol. 24, 545–554.

Jain, K., 2013. Synthetic biology and personalized medicine. Med. Princ. Pract. 22, 209–219.

Jain, A., Bhatia, P., Chugh, A., 2012. Microbial synthetic biology for human therapeutics. Syst. Synth. Biol. 6, 9–22.

Jean, A.T.S., Swofford, C.A., Panteli, J.T., Brentzel, Z.J., Forbes, N.S., 2014. Bacterial delivery of *Staphylococcus aureus* α-hemolysin causes regression and necrosis in murine tumors. Mol. Ther. 22, 1266–1274.

Jensen, P.R., Hammer, K., 1998. The sequence of spacers between the consensus sequences modulates the strength of prokaryotic promoters. Appl. Environ. Microbiol. 64, 82–87.

Jiang, S.-N., Phan, T.X., Nam, T.-K., Nguyen, V.H., Kim, H.-S., Bom, H.-S., Choy, H.E., Hong, Y., Min, J.-J., 2010. Inhibition of tumor growth and metastasis by a combination of *Escherichia coli*-mediated cytolytic therapy and radiotherapy. Mol. Ther. 18, 635–642.

Jiang, W., Bikard, D., Cox, D., Zhang, F., Marraffini, L.A., 2013. RNA-guided editing of bacterial genomes using CRISPR-Cas systems. Nat. Biotechnol. 31, 233–239.

Kasinskas, R.W., Forbes, N.S., 2006. Salmonella typhimurium specifically chemotax and proliferate in heterogeneous tumor tissue in vitro. Biotechnol. Bioeng. 94, 710–721.

Keasling, J.D., 2008. Synthetic biology for synthetic chemistry. ACS Chem. Biol. 3, 64–76.

Keasling, J.D., 2012. Synthetic biology and the development of tools for metabolic engineering. Metab. Eng. 14, 189–195.

Kelly, K.A., Jones, D.A., 2003. Isolation of a colon tumor specific binding peptide using phage display selection. Neoplasia 5, 437–444.

Kelly, K.A., Waterman, P., Weissleder, R., 2006. In vivo imaging of molecularly targeted phage. Neoplasia 8, 1011–1018.

Kemmer, C., Gitzinger, M., Daoud-El Baba, M., Djonov, V., Stelling, J., Fussenegger, M., 2010. Self-sufficient control of urate homeostasis in mice by a synthetic circuit. Nat. Biotechnol. 28, 355–360.

Kemmer, C., Fluri, D.A., Witschi, U., Passeraub, A., Gutzwiller, A., Fussenegger, M., 2011. A designer network coordinating bovine artificial insemination by ovulation-triggered release of implanted sperms. J. Control. Release 150, 23–29.

Khalil, A.S., Collins, J.J., 2010. Synthetic biology: applications come of age. Nat. Rev. Genet. 11, 367–379.
Khosla, C., Kapur, S., Cane, D.E., 2009. Revisiting the modularity of modular polyketide synthases. Curr. Opin. Chem. Biol. 13, 135–143.
Kim, J., Reed, J.L., 2010. OptORF: optimal metabolic and regulatory perturbations for metabolic engineering of microbial strains. BMC Syst. Biol. 4, 1–19.
Kim, Y., Lillo, A.M., Steiniger, S.C.J., Liu, Y., Ballatore, C., Anichini, A., Mortarini, R., Kaufmann, G.F., Zhou, B., Felding-Habermann, B., Janda, K.D., 2006. Targeting heat shock proteins on cancer cells: selection, characterization, and cell-penetrating properties of a peptidic GRP78 ligand. Biochemistry 45, 9434–9444.
Kim, J., Reed, J.L., Maravelias, C.T., 2011. Large-scale bi-level strain design approaches and mixed-integer programming solution techniques. PLoS One 6, 1–13.
Kis, Z., Pereira, H.S.A., Homma, T., Pedrigi, R.M., Krams, R., 2015. Mammalian synthetic biology: emerging medical applications. J. R. Soc. Interface 12, 1–18.
Kitney, R., Freemont, P., 2012. Synthetic biology—the state of play. FEBS Lett. 586, 2029–2036.
Kobayashi, A., Hirakawa, H., Hirata, T., Nishino, K., Yamaguchi, A., 2006. Growth phase-dependent expression of drug exporters in *Escherichia coli* and its contribution to drug tolerance. J. Bacteriol. 188, 5693–5703.
Kolisnychenko, V., Plunkett, G., Herring, C.D., Fehér, T., Pósfai, J., Blattner, F.R., Pósfai, G., 2002. Engineering a reduced *Escherichia coli* genome. Genome Res. 12, 640–647.
Kotula, J.W., Kerns, S.J., Shaket, L.A., Siraj, L., Collins, J.J., Way, J.C., Silver, P.A., 2014. Programmable bacteria detect and record an environmental signal in the mammalian gut. Proc. Natl. Acad. Sci. 111, 4838–4843.
Ku, T.-H., Zhang, T., Luo, H., Yen, T., Chen, P.-W., Han, Y., Lo, Y.-H., 2015. Nucleic acid aptamers: an emerging tool for biotechnology and biomedical sensing. Sensors 15, 16281–16313.
Kunii, T., Ogura, S.-I., Mie, M., Kobatake, E., 2011. Selection of DNA aptamers recognizing small cell lung cancer using living cell-SELEX. Analyst 136, 1310–1312.
Kwong, G.A., Von Maltzahn, G., Murugappan, G., Abudayyeh, O., Mo, S., Papayannopoulos, I.A., Sverdlov, D.Y., Liu, S.B., Warren, A.D., Popov, Y., 2013. Mass-encoded synthetic biomarkers for multiplexed urinary monitoring of disease. Nat. Biotechnol. 31, 63–70.
Laakkonen, P., Zhang, L., Ruoslahti, E., 2008. Peptide targeting of tumor lymph vessels. Ann. N. Y. Acad. Sci. 1131, 37–43.
Labbé, G.M., Scaife, S., Morgan, S.A., Curtis, Z.H., Alphey, L., 2012. Female-specific flightless (fsRIDL) phenotype for control of Aedes albopictus. PLoS Negl. Trop. Dis. 6, 1–8.
Lagenaur, L.A., Sanders-Beer, B.E., Brichacek, B., Pal, R., Liu, X., Liu, Y., Yu, R., Venzon, D., Lee, P.P., Hamer, D.H., 2011. Prevention of vaginal SHIV transmission in macaques by a live recombinant Lactobacillus. Mucosal Immunol. 4, 648–657.
Lee, A.S., 2007. GRP78 induction in cancer: therapeutic and prognostic implications. Cancer Res. 67, 3496–3499.
Legoux, R., Delpech, B., Dumont, X., Guillemot, J.-C., Ramond, P., Shire, D., Caput, D., Ferrara, P., Loison, G., 1992. Cloning and expression in Escherichia coli of the gene encoding Aspergillus flavus urate oxidase. J. Biol. Chem. 267, 8565–8570.
Lehouritis, P., Springer, C., Tangney, M., 2013. Bacterial-directed enzyme prodrug therapy. J. Control. Release 170, 120–131.
Leonard, E., Nielsen, D., Solomon, K., Prather, K.J., 2008. Engineering microbes with synthetic biology frameworks. Trends Biotechnol. 26, 674–681.
Levskaya, A., Chevalier, A.A., Tabor, J.J., Simpson, Z.B., Lavery, L.A., Levy, M., Davidson, E.A., Scouras, A., Ellington, A.D., Marcotte, E.M., Voigt, C.A., 2005. Engineering *Escherichia coli* to see light. Nature 438, 441–442.

Levskaya, A., Weiner, O.D., Lim, W.A., Voigt, C.A., 2009. Spatiotemporal control of cell signalling using a light-switchable protein interaction. Nature 461, 997–1001.

Liang, J., Luo, Y., Zhao, H., 2011. Synthetic biology: putting synthesis into biology. Wiley Interdiscip. Rev. Syst. Biol. Med. 3, 7–20.

Liao, H.-K., Gu, Y., Diaz, A., Marlett, J., Takahashi, Y., Li, M., Suzuki, K., Xu, R., Hishida, T., Chang, C.-J., 2015. Use of the CRISPR/Cas9 system as an intracellular defense against HIV-1 infection in human cells. Nat. Commun. 6, 1–10.

Lim, W.A., 2010. Designing customized cell signalling circuits. Nat. Rev. Mol. Cell Biol. 11, 393–403.

Limsirichai, P., Gaj, T., Schaffer, D.V., 2016. CRISPR-mediated activation of latent HIV-1 expression. Mol. Ther. 24, 499–507.

Liu, S., Minton, N., Giaccia, A., Brown, J., 2002. Anticancer efficacy of systemically delivered anaerobic bacteria as gene therapy vectors targeting tumor hypoxia/necrosis. Gene Ther. 9, 291–296.

Liu, X., Lagenaur, L.A., Lee, P.P., Xu, Q., 2008. Engineering of a human vaginal Lactobacillus strain for surface expression of two-domain CD4 molecules. Appl. Environ. Microbiol. 74, 4626–4635.

Liu, D., Hoynes-O'Connor, A., Zhang, F., 2013. Bridging the gap between systems biology and synthetic biology. Front. Microbiol. 4, 1–8.

Liu, Y., Zeng, Y., Liu, L., Zhuang, C., Fu, X., Huang, W., Cai, Z., 2014. Synthesizing AND gate genetic circuits based on CRISPR-Cas9 for identification of bladder cancer cells. Nat. Commun. 5, 1–7.

Low, K.B., Ittensohn, M., Le, T., Platt, J., Sodi, S., Amoss, M., Ash, O., Carmichael, E., Chakraborty, A., Fischer, J., 1999. Lipid A mutant Salmonella with suppressed virulence and TNFα induction retain tumor-targeting in vivo. Nat. Biotechnol. 17, 37–41.

Lu, T.K., Collins, J.J., 2007. Dispersing biofilms with engineered enzymatic bacteriophage. Proc. Natl. Acad. Sci. 104, 11197–11202.

Lu, T.K., Collins, J.J., 2009. Engineered bacteriophage targeting gene networks as adjuvants for antibiotic therapy. Proc. Natl. Acad. Sci. U. S. A. 106, 4629–4634.

Lu, G., Moriyama, E.N., 2004. Vector NTI, a balanced all-in-one sequence analysis suite. Brief. Bioinform. 5, 378–388.

Lu, T.K., Bowers, J., Koeris, M.S., 2013. Advancing bacteriophage-based microbial diagnostics with synthetic biology. Trends Biotechnol. 31, 325–327.

Mäe, M., Myrberg, H., El-Andaloussi, S., Langel, Ü., 2008. Design of a tumor homing cell-penetrating peptide for drug delivery. Int. J. Pept. Res. Ther. 15, 11–15.

Makarova, K.S., Grishin, N.V., Shabalina, S.A., Wolf, Y.I., Koonin, E.V., 2006. A putative RNA-interference-based immune system in prokaryotes: computational analysis of the predicted enzymatic machinery, functional analogies with eukaryotic RNAi, and hypothetical mechanisms of action. Biol. Direct 1, 7.

Mallikaratchy, P., Tang, Z., Kwame, S., Meng, L., Shangguan, D., Tan, W., 2007. Aptamer directly evolved from live cells recognizes membrane bound immunoglobin heavy mu chain in Burkitt's lymphoma cells. Mol. Cell. Proteomics 6, 2230–2238.

March, J.C., Duan, F.F., 2011. Compositions and methods for treating endocrine, gastrointestinal or autoimmune disorders. US 2014/0105861.

March, J.C., Duan, F.F., 2014. Commensal bacteria as signal mediators within a mammalian host. US 2014/0234256.

Massa, P.E., Paniccia, A., Monegal, A., De Marco, A., Rescigno, M., 2013. Salmonella engineered to express CD20-targeting antibodies and a drug-converting enzyme can eradicate human lymphomas. Blood 122, 705–714.

Mathew, E., Hardee, G., Bennett, C., Lee, K., 2003. Cytosolic delivery of antisense oligonucleotides by listeriolysin O-containing liposomes. Gene Ther. 10, 1105–1115.

Medema, M.H., Breitling, R., Bovenberg, R., Takano, E., 2011. Exploiting plug-and-play synthetic biology for drug discovery and production in microorganisms. Nat. Rev. Microbiol. 9, 131–137.

Mengesha, A., Dubois, L., Lambin, P., Landuyt, W., Chiu, R.K., Wouters, B.G., Theys, J., 2006. Development of a flexible and potent hypoxia-inducible promoter for tumor-targeted gene expression in attenuated s almonella. Cancer Biol. Ther. 5, 1120–1128.

Miest, T.S., Cattaneo, R., 2014. New viruses for cancer therapy: meeting clinical needs. Nat. Rev. Microbiol. 12, 23–34.

Min, J., Moon, H., Yang, H.J., Shin, H.H., Hong, S.Y., Kang, S., 2014. Development of P22 viral capsid nanocomposites as anti-cancer drug, bortezomib (BTZ), delivery nanoplatforms. Macromol. Biosci. 14, 557–564.

Missailidis, S., Hardy, A., 2009. Aptamers as inhibitors of target proteins. Expert Opin. Ther. Pat. 19, 1073–1082.

Möglich, A., Moffat, K., 2007. Structural basis for light-dependent signaling in the dimeric LOV domain of the photosensor YtvA. J. Mol. Biol. 373, 112–126.

Moon, T.S., Dueber, J.E., Shiue, E., Prather, K.L.J., 2010. Use of modular, synthetic scaffolds for improved production of glucaric acid in engineered *E. coli*. Metab. Eng. 12, 298–305.

Mou, H., Kennedy, Z., Anderson, D.G., Yin, H., Xue, W., 2015. Precision cancer mouse models through genome editing with CRISPR-Cas9. Gen. Med. 7, 1–11.

Mueller, S., Papamichail, D., Coleman, J.R., Skiena, S., Wimmer, E., 2006. Reduction of the rate of poliovirus protein synthesis through large-scale codon deoptimization causes attenuation of viral virulence by lowering specific infectivity. J. Virol. 80, 9687–9696.

Mueller, S., Coleman, J.R., Papamichail, D., Ward, C.B., Nimnual, A., Futcher, B., Skiena, S., Wimmer, E., 2010. Live attenuated influenza virus vaccines by computer-aided rational design. Nat. Biotechnol. 28, 723–726.

Muñoz, I.G., Prieto, J., Subramanian, S., Coloma, J., Redondo, P., Villate, M., Merino, N., Marenchino, M., D'Abramo, M., Gervasio, F.L., 2011. Molecular basis of engineered meganuclease targeting of the endogenous human RAG1 locus. Nucleic Acids Res. 39, 729–743.

Myrberg, H., Zhang, L., Mäe, M., Langel, U., 2008. Design of a tumor-homing cell-penetrating peptide. Bioconjug. Chem. 19, 70–75.

Na, D., Lee, D., 2010. RBSDesigner: software for designing synthetic ribosome binding sites that yields a desired level of protein expression. Bioinformatics 26, 2633–2634.

Newton, J.R., Kelly, K.A., Mahmood, U., Weissleder, R., Deutscher, S.L., 2006. In vivo selection of phage for the optical imaging of PC-3 human prostate carcinoma in mice. Neoplasia 8, 772–780.

Ng, E.W.M., Shima, D.T., Calias, P., Cunningham, E.T., Guyer, D.R., Adamis, A.P., 2006. Pegaptanib, a targeted anti-VEGF aptamer for ocular vascular disease. Nat. Rev. Drug Discov. 5, 123–132.

Nguyen, V.H., Kim, H.-S., Ha, J.-M., Hong, Y., Choy, H.E., Min, J.-J., 2010. Genetically engineered Salmonella typhimurium as an imageable therapeutic probe for cancer. Cancer Res. 70, 18–23.

Ni, X., Castanares, M., 2011. Nucleic acid aptamers: clinical applications and promising new horizons. Curr. Med. Chem. 18, 4206–4214.

Nikel, P.I., Martínez-García, E., De Lorenzo, V., 2014. Biotechnological domestication of pseudomonads using synthetic biology. Nat. Rev. Microbiol. 12, 368–379.

Nissim, L., Bar-Ziv, R.H., 2010. A tunable dual-promoter integrator for targeting of cancer cells. Mol. Syst. Biol. 6, 1–9.

Nogales, A., Baker, S.F., Ortiz-Riaño, E., Dewhurst, S., Topham, D.J., Martínez-Sobrido, L., 2014. Influenza A virus attenuation by codon deoptimization of the NS gene for vaccine development. J. Virol. 88, 10525–10540.

O'Connor, L., Plichart, C., Sang, A.C., Brelsfoard, C.L., Bossin, H.C., Dobson, S.L., 2012. Open release of male mosquitoes infected with a Wolbachia biopesticide: field performance and infection containment. PLoS Negl. Trop. Dis. 6, 1–7.

O'Malley, M.A., Powell, A., Davies, J.F., Calvert, J., 2008. Knowledge-making distinctions in synthetic biology. BioEssays 30, 57–65.

Paddon, C.J., Keasling, J.D., 2014. Semi-synthetic artemisinin: a model for the use of synthetic biology in pharmaceutical development. Nat. Rev. Microbiol. 12, 355–367.

Palumbo, E., Fiaschi, L., Brunelli, B., Marchi, S., Savino, S., Pizza, M., 2012. Antigen identification starting from the genome: a "Reverse Vaccinology" approach applied to MenB. In: Christodoulides, M. (Ed.), Neisseria meningitidis. Springer, New York.

Pan, Y., Xiao, L., Li, A.S., Zhang, X., Sirois, P., Zhang, J., Li, K., 2013. Biological and biomedical applications of engineered nucleases. Mol. Biotechnol. 55, 54–62.

Pant, N., Hultberg, A., Zhao, Y., Svensson, L., Pan-Hammarström, Q., Johansen, K., Pouwels, P.H., Ruggeri, F.M., Hermans, P., Frenken, L., 2006. Lactobacilli expressing variable domain of llama heavy-chain antibody fragments (lactobodies) confer protection against rotavirus-induced diarrhea. J. Infect. Dis. 194, 1580–1588.

Pardee, K., Green, A.A., Ferrante, T., Cameron, D.E., Daleykeyser, A., Yin, P., Collins, J.J., 2014. Paper-based synthetic gene networks. Cell 159, 940–954.

Parsons, J.B., Frank, S., Bhella, D., Liang, M., Prentice, M.B., Mulvihill, D.P., Warren, M.J., 2010. Synthesis of empty bacterial microcompartments, directed organelle protein incorporation, and evidence of filament-associated organelle movement. Mol. Cell 38, 305–315.

Pastagia, M., Euler, C., Chahales, P., Fuentes-Duculan, J., Krueger, J.G., Fischetti, V.A., 2011. A novel chimeric lysin shows superiority to mupirocin for skin decolonization of methicillin-resistant and -sensitive Staphylococcus aureus strains. Antimicrob. Agents Chemother. 55, 738–744.

Perez-Pinera, P., Ousterout, D.G., Gersbach, C.A., 2012. Advances in targeted genome editing. Curr. Opin. Chem. Biol. 16, 268–277.

Pharkya, P., Maranas, C.D., 2006. An optimization framework for identifying reaction activation/inhibition or elimination candidates for overproduction in microbial systems. Metab. Eng. 8, 1–13.

Pharkya, P., Burgard, A.P., Maranas, C.D., 2004. OptStrain: a computational framework for redesign of microbial production systems. Genome Res. 14, 2367–2376.

Picotti, P., Aebersold, R., 2012. Selected reaction monitoring-based proteomics: workflows, potential, pitfalls and future directions. Nat. Methods 9, 555–566.

Piñero-Lambea, C., Bodelón, G., Fernández-Periáñez, R., Cuesta, A.M., Álvarez-Vallina, L., Fernández, L.A.N., 2014. Programming controlled adhesion of E. coli to target surfaces, cells, and tumors with synthetic adhesins. ACS Synth. Biol. 4, 463–473.

Piñero-Lambea, C., Ruano-Gallego, D., Fernández, L.Á., 2015. Engineered bacteria as therapeutic agents. Curr. Opin. Biotechnol. 35, 94–102.

Piuri, M., Jacobs, W.R., Hatfull, G.F., 2009. Fluoromycobacteriophages for rapid, specific, and sensitive antibiotic susceptibility testing of Mycobacterium tuberculosis. PLoS One 4, e4870.

Pósfai, G., Plunkett, G., Fehér, T., Frisch, D., Keil, G.M., Umenhoffer, K., Kolisnychenko, V., Stahl, B., Sharma, S.S., De Arruda, M., 2006. Emergent properties of reduced-genome *Escherichia coli*. Science 312, 1044–1046.

Purnick, P.E., Weiss, R., 2009. The second wave of synthetic biology: from modules to systems. Nat. Rev. Mol. Cell Biol. 10, 410–422.

Pusch, O., Kalyanaraman, R., Tucker, L.D., Wells, J.M., Ramratnam, B., Boden, D., 2006. An anti-HIV microbicide engineered in commensal bacteria: secretion of HIV-1 fusion inhibitors by lactobacilli. AIDS 20, 1917–1922.
Ranganathan, S., Suthers, P.F., Maranas, C.D., 2010. OptForce: an optimization procedure for identifying all genetic manipulations leading to targeted overproductions. PLoS Comput. Biol. 6, 1–11.
Rao, S., Hu, S., Mchugh, L., Lueders, K., Henry, K., Zhao, Q., Fekete, R.A., Kar, S., Adhya, S., Hamer, D.H., 2005. Toward a live microbial microbicide for HIV: commensal bacteria secreting an HIV fusion inhibitor peptide. Proc. Natl. Acad. Sci. U. S. A. 102, 11993–11998.
Redondo, P., Prieto, J., Muñoz, I.G., Alibés, A., Stricher, F., Serrano, L., Cabaniols, J.-P., Daboussi, F., Arnould, S., Perez, C., 2008. Molecular basis of xeroderma pigmentosum group C DNA recognition by engineered meganucleases. Nature 456, 107–111.
Regberg, J., Srimanee, A., Langel, U., 2012. Applications of cell-penetrating peptides for tumor targeting and future cancer therapies. Pharmaceuticals 5, 991–1007.
Roberts, N.J., Zhang, L., Janku, F., Collins, A., Bai, R.-Y., Staedtke, V., Rusk, A.W., Tung, D., Miller, M., Roix, J., 2014. Intratumoral injection of *Clostridium novyi*-NT spores induces antitumor responses. Sci. Transl. Med. 6, 1–11.
Rocha, I., Maia, P., Evangelista, P., Vilaça, P., Soares, S., Pinto, J.P., Nielsen, J., Patil, K.R., Ferreira, E.C., Rocha, M., 2010. OptFlux: an open-source software platform for in silico metabolic engineering. BMC Syst. Biol. 4, 1–12.
Rodrigues, J.L., 2014. Heterologous production of curcuminoids in E. coli through an artificial biosynthetic pathway. PhD thesis, University of Minho.
Rodrigues, L.R., Kluskens, L.D., 2011. Synthetic biology & bioinformatics prospects in the cancer arena. In: Lopes, H.S., Cruz, L.M. (Eds.), Computational Biology and Applied Bioinformatics. InTech, Rijeka.
Rodrigues, J.L., Sousa, M., Prather, K.L., Kluskens, L.D., Rodrigues, L.R., 2014. Selection of *Escherichia coli* heat shock promoters towards their application as stress probes. J. Biotechnol. 188, 61–71.
Rodrigues, J.L., Prather, K.L., Kluskens, L., Rodrigues, L., 2015. Heterologous production of curcuminoids. Microbiol. Mol. Biol. Rev. 79, 39–60.
Rössger, K., Charpin-El-Hamri, G., Fussenegger, M., 2013a. A closed-loop synthetic gene circuit for the treatment of diet-induced obesity in mice. Nat. Commun. 4, 1–9.
Rössger, K., Charpin-El Hamri, G., Fussenegger, M., 2013b. Reward-based hypertension control by a synthetic brain–dopamine interface. Proc. Natl. Acad. Sci. 110, 18150–18155.
Rössger, K., Charpin-El-Hamri, G., Fussenegger, M., 2014. Bile acid-controlled transgene expression in mammalian cells and mice. Metab. Eng. 21, 81–90.
Rothberg, J.M., Leamon, J.H., 2008. The development and impact of 454 sequencing. Nat. Biotechnol. 26, 1117–1124.
Royal Academy Of Engineering, 2009. Synthetic Biology: Scope, Applications and Implications. The Royal Academy of Engineering, London.
Royo, J.L., Becker, P.D., Camacho, E.M., Cebolla, A., Link, C., Santero, E., Guzmán, C.A., 2007. In vivo gene regulation in Salmonella spp. by a salicylate-dependent control circuit. Nat. Methods 4, 937–942.
Ruder, W.C., Lu, T., Collins, J.J., 2011. Synthetic biology moving into the clinic. Science 333, 1248–1252.
Saeidi, N., Wong, C.K., Lo, T.M., Nguyen, H.X., Ling, H., Leong, S.S.J., Poh, C.L., Chang, M.W., 2011. Engineering microbes to sense and eradicate Pseudomonas aeruginosa, a human pathogen. Mol. Syst. Biol. 7, 1–11.
Salis, H.M., 2011. The ribosome binding site calculator. Methods Enzymol. 498, 19–42.

Salis, H.M., Mirsky, E.A., Voigt, C.A., 2009. Automated design of synthetic ribosome binding sites to control protein expression. Nat. Biotechnol. 27, 946–950.

Sánchez-Rivera, F.J., Jacks, T., 2015. Applications of the CRISPR-Cas9 system in cancer biology. Nat. Rev. Cancer 15, 387–395.

Schlabach, M.R., Hu, J.K., Li, M., Elledge, S.J., 2010. Synthetic design of strong promoters. Proc. Natl. Acad. Sci. 107, 2538–2543.

Schmidt, M., De Lorenzo, V., 2012. Synthetic constructs in/for the environment: managing the interplay between natural and engineered biology. FEBS Lett. 586, 2199–2206.

Schofield, D., Sharp, N.J., Westwater, C., 2012. Phage-based platforms for the clinical detection of human bacterial pathogens. Bacteriophage 2, 105–121.

Schroeder, A., Kost, J., Barenholz, Y., 2009. Ultrasound, liposomes, and drug delivery: principles for using ultrasound to control the release of drugs from liposomes. Chem. Phys. Lipids 162, 1–16.

Sefah, K., Tang, Z.W., Shangguan, D.H., Chen, H., Lopez-Colon, D., Li, Y., Parekh, P., Martin, J., Meng, L., Phillips, J.A., Kim, Y.M., Tan, W.H., 2009. Molecular recognition of acute myeloid leukemia using aptamers. Leukemia 23, 235–244.

Senzer, N.N., Kaufman, H.L., Amatruda, T., Nemunaitis, M., Reid, T., Daniels, G., Gonzalez, R., Glaspy, J., Whitman, E., Harrington, K., Goldsweig, H., Marshall, T., Love, C., Coffin, R., Nemunaitis, J.J., 2009. Phase II clinical trial of a granulocyte-macrophage colony-stimulating factor-encoding, second-generation oncolytic herpesvirus in patients with unresectable metastatic melanoma. J. Clin. Oncol. 27, 5763–5771.

Seo, S.W., Yang, J.-S., Kim, I., Yang, J., Min, B.E., Kim, S., Jung, G.Y., 2013. Predictive design of mRNA translation initiation region to control prokaryotic translation efficiency. Metab. Eng. 15, 67–74.

Shankar, S., Pillai, M.R., 2011. Translating cancer research by synthetic biology. Mol. BioSyst. 7, 1802–1810.

Shao, Z., Zhao, H., Zhao, H., 2009. DNA assembler, an in vivo genetic method for rapid construction of biochemical pathways. Nucleic Acids Res. 37, 1–10.

Sharan, S.K., Thomason, L.C., Kuznetsov, S.G., Court, D.L., 2009. Recombineering: a homologous recombination-based method of genetic engineering. Nat. Protoc. 4, 206–223.

Sharma, S.S., Blattner, F.R., Harcum, S.W., 2007a. Recombinant protein production in an *Escherichia coli* reduced genome strain. Metab. Eng. 9, 133–141.

Sharma, S.S., Campbell, J.W., Frisch, D., Blattner, F.R., Harcum, S.W., 2007b. Expression of two recombinant chloramphenicol acetyltransferase variants in highly reduced genome *Escherichia coli* strains. Biotechnol. Bioeng. 98, 1056–1070.

Shiue, E., Prather, K.L., 2012. Synthetic biology devices as tools for metabolic engineering. Biochem. Eng. J. 65, 82–89.

Sirikantaramas, S., Yamazaki, M., Saito, K., 2008. Mechanisms of resistance to self-produced toxic secondary metabolites in plants. Phytochem. Rev. 7, 467–477.

Smartt, A.E., Xu, T., Jegier, P., Carswell, J.J., Blount, S.A., Sayler, G.S., Ripp, S., 2012. Pathogen detection using engineered bacteriophages. Anal. Bioanal. Chem. 402, 3127–3146.

Smith, G.P., 1985. Filamentous fusion phage: novel expression vectors that display cloned antigens on the virion surface. Science 228, 1315–1317.

Smith, K.A., 2011. Edward jenner and the small pox vaccine. Front. Immunol. 2, 1–6.

Song, H., Payne, S., Tan, C., You, L., 2011. Programming microbial population dynamics by engineered cell–cell communication. Biotechnol. J. 6, 837–849.

St Jean, A.T., Zhang, M., Forbes, N.S., 2008. Bacterial therapies: completing the cancer treatment toolbox. Curr. Opin. Biotechnol. 19, 511–517.

Stähler, P., Beier, M., Gao, X., Hoheisel, J.D., 2006. Another side of genomics: synthetic biology as a means for the exploitation of whole-genome sequence information. J. Biotechnol. 124, 206–212.
Stoltenburg, R., Reinemann, C., Strehlitz, B., 2007. SELEX—a (r)evolutionary method to generate high-affinity nucleic acid ligands. Biomol. Eng. 24, 381–403.
Struss, A., Pasini, P., Ensor, C.M., Raut, N., Daunert, S., 2010. Paper strip whole cell biosensors: a portable test for the semiquantitative detection of bacterial quorum signaling molecules. Anal. Chem. 82, 4457–4463.
Sun, N., Zhao, H., 2013. Transcription activator-like effector nucleases (TALENs): a highly efficient and versatile tool for genome editing. Biotechnol. Bioeng. 110, 1811–1821.
Sun, H., Zhu, X., Lu, P.Y., Rosato, R.R., Tan, W., Zu, Y., 2014. Oligonucleotide aptamers: new tools for targeted cancer therapy. Mol. Ther. Nucleic acids 3, e182.
Sundaram, P., Kurniawan, H., Byrne, M.E., Wower, J., 2013. Therapeutic RNA aptamers in clinical trials. Eur. J. Pharm. Sci. 48, 259–271.
Suzuki, A., Nakauchi, H., Taniguchi, H., 2003. Glucagon-like peptide 1 (1–37) converts intestinal epithelial cells into insulin-producing cells. Proc. Natl. Acad. Sci. 100, 5034–5039.
Swofford, C.A., St Jean, A.T., Panteli, J.T., Brentzel, Z.J., Forbes, N.S., 2014. Identification of Staphylococcus aureus α-hemolysin as a protein drug that is secreted by anticancer bacteria and rapidly kills cancer cells. Biotechnol. Bioeng. 111, 1233–1245.
Swofford, C.A., Van Dessel, N., Forbes, N.S., 2015. Quorum-sensing Salmonella selectively trigger protein expression within tumors. Proc. Natl. Acad. Sci. 112, 3457–3462.
Tanaka, T., Kondo, A., 2014. Cell-surface display of enzymes by the yeast Saccharomyces cerevisiae for synthetic biology. FEMS Yeast Res. 1, 1–11.
Tang, W.L., Zhao, H., 2009. Industrial biotechnology: tools and applications. Biotechnol. J. 4, 1725–1739.
Tannock, I.F., 2001. Tumor physiology and drug resistance. Cancer Metastasis Rev. 20, 123–132.
Tawil, N., Sacher, E., Mandeville, R., Meunier, M., 2014. Bacteriophages: biosensing tools for multi-drug resistant pathogens. Analyst 139, 1224–1236.
Thamm, D.H., Kurzman, I.D., King, I., Li, Z., Sznol, M., Dubielzig, R.R., Vail, D.M., MacEwen, E.G., 2005. Systemic administration of an attenuated, tumor-targeting Salmonella typhimurium to dogs with spontaneous neoplasia: phase I evaluation. Clin. Cancer Res. 11, 4827–4834.
Toley, B.J., Forbes, N.S., 2012. Motility is critical for effective distribution and accumulation of bacteria in tumor tissue. Integr. Biol. 4, 165–176.
Torre, L.A., Bray, F., Siegel, R.L., Ferlay, J., Lortet-Tieulent, J., Jemal, A., 2015. Global cancer statistics, 2012. CA Cancer J. Clin. 65, 87–108.
Tuerk, C., Gold, L., 1990. Systematic evolution of ligands by exponential enrichment: RNA ligands to bacteriophage T4 DNA polymerase. Science 249, 505–510.
Tyo, K.E., Kocharin, K., Nielsen, J., 2010. Toward design-based engineering of industrial microbes. Curr. Opin. Microbiol. 13, 255–262.
Ulrich, H., Wrenger, C., 2009. Disease-specific biomarker discovery by aptamers. Cytometry A 75, 727–733.
Valdez-Cruz, N.A., Caspeta, L., Pérez, N.O., Ramírez, O.T., Trujillo-Roldán, M.A., 2010. Production of recombinant proteins in *E. coli* by the heat inducible expression system based on the phage lambda pL and/or pR promoters. Microb. Cell Factories 9, 1–16.
Van Simaeys, D., López-Colón, D., Sefah, K., Sutphen, R., Jimenez, E., Tan, W., 2010. Study of the molecular recognition of aptamers selected through ovarian cancer cell-SELEX. PLoS One 5, 1–7.

Van Simaeys, D., Turek, D., Champanhac, C., Vaizer, J., Sefah, K., Zhen, J., Sutphen, R., Tan, W., 2014. Identification of cell membrane protein stress-induced phosphoprotein 1 as a potential ovarian cancer biomarker using aptamers selected by cell systematic evolution of ligands by exponential enrichment. Anal. Chem. 86, 4521–4527.

Vangelista, L., Secchi, M., Liu, X., Bachi, A., Jia, L., Xu, Q., Lusso, P., 2010. Engineering of Lactobacillus jensenii to secrete RANTES and a CCR5 antagonist analogue as live HIV-1 blockers. Antimicrob. Agents Chemother. 54, 2994–3001.

Villalobos, A., Ness, J.E., Gustafsson, C., Minshull, J., Govindarajan, S., 2006. Gene Designer: a synthetic biology tool for constructing artificial DNA segments. BMC Bioinformatics 7, 1–8.

Vives, E., Brodin, P., Lebleu, B., 1997. A truncated HIV-1 tat protein basic domain rapidly translocates through the plasma membrane and accumulates in the cell nucleus. J. Biol. Chem. 272, 16010–16017.

Vivès, E., Schmidt, J., Pèlegrin, A., 2008. Cell-penetrating and cell-targeting peptides in drug delivery. Biochim. Biophys. Acta 1786, 126–138.

Wang, H.H., Isaacs, F.J., Carr, P.A., Sun, Z.Z., Xu, G., Forest, C.R., Church, G.M., 2009. Programming cells by multiplex genome engineering and accelerated evolution. Nature 460, 894–898.

Wang, Y., Luo, Y., Bing, T., Chen, Z., Lu, M., Zhang, N., Shangguan, D., Gao, X., 2014. DNA aptamer evolved by cell-SELEX for recognition of prostate cancer. PLoS One 9, 1–10.

Warren, A.D., Gaylord, S.T., Ngan, K.C., Dumont Milutinovic, M., Kwong, G.A., Bhatia, S.N., Walt, D.R., 2014a. Disease detection by ultrasensitive quantification of microdosed synthetic urinary biomarkers. J. Am. Chem. Soc. 136, 13709–13714.

Warren, A.D., Kwong, G.A., Wood, D.K., Lin, K.Y., Bhatia, S.N., 2014b. Point-of-care diagnostics for noncommunicable diseases using synthetic urinary biomarkers and paper microfluidics. Proc. Natl. Acad. Sci. 111, 3671–3676.

Way, J.C., Collins, J.J., Keasling, J.D., Silver, P.A., 2014. Integrating biological redesign: where synthetic biology came from and where it needs to go. Cell 157, 151–161.

Weber, W., Fussenegger, M., 2009. The impact of synthetic biology on drug discovery. Drug Discov. Today 14, 956–963.

Weber, W., Fussenegger, M., 2012. Emerging biomedical applications of synthetic biology. Nat. Rev. Genet. 13, 21–35.

Weeding, E., Houle, J., Kaznessis, Y.N., 2010. SynBioSS designer: a web-based tool for the automated generation of kinetic models for synthetic biological constructs. Brief. Bioinform. 11, 394–402.

Wieland, M., Fussenegger, M., 2012. Engineering molecular circuits using synthetic biology in mammalian cells. Annu. Rev. Chem. Biomol. Eng. 3, 209–234.

Wilkinson, S.P., Grove, A., 2004. HucR, a novel uric acid-responsive member of the MarR family of transcriptional regulators from Deinococcus radiodurans. J. Biol. Chem. 279, 51442–51450.

Windbichler, N., Menichelli, M., Papathanos, P.A., Thyme, S.B., Li, H., Ulge, U.Y., Hovde, B.T., Baker, D., Monnat, R.J., Burt, A., 2011. A synthetic homing endonuclease-based gene drive system in the human malaria mosquito. Nature 473, 212–215.

Winkler, W.C., Breaker, R.R., 2005. Regulation of bacterial gene expression by riboswitches. Annu. Rev. Microbiol. 59, 487–517.

Wolber, P.K., Green, R.L., 1990. Detection of bacteria by transduction of ice nucleation genes. Trends Biotechnol. 8, 276–279.

Wu, Y., Liang, D., Wang, Y., Bai, M., Tang, W., Bao, S., Yan, Z., Li, D., Li, J., 2013. Correction of a genetic disease in mouse via use of CRISPR-Cas9. Cell Stem Cell 13, 659–662.

Xia, Z.-J., Chang, J.-H., Zhang, L., Jiang, W.-Q., Guan, Z.-Z., Liu, J.-W., Zhang, Y., Hu, X.-H., Wu, G.-H., Wang, H.-Q., Chen, Z.-C., Chen, J.-C., Zhou, Q.-H., Lu, J.-W., Fan, Q.-X., Huang, J.-J., Zheng, X., 2004. Phase III randomized clinical trial of intratumoral injection of E1B gene-deleted adenovirus (H101) combined with cisplatin-based chemotherapy in treating squamous cell cancer of head and neck or esophagus. Chinese J. Cancer 23, 1666–1670.

Xiang, S., Fruehauf, J., Li, C.J., 2006. Short hairpin RNA-expressing bacteria elicit RNA interference in mammals. Nat. Biotechnol. 24, 697–702.

Xie, Z., Wroblewska, L., Prochazka, L., Weiss, R., Benenson, Y., 2011. Multi-input RNAi-based logic circuit for identification of specific cancer cells. Science 333, 1307–1311.

Yamamoto, S., Izumiya, H., Morita, M., Arakawa, E., Watanabe, H., 2009. Application of lambda Red recombination system to Vibrio cholerae genetics: simple methods for inactivation and modification of chromosomal genes. Gene 438, 57–64.

Ye, H., Fussenegger, M., 2014. Synthetic therapeutic gene circuits in mammalian cells. FEBS Lett. 588, 2537–2544.

Ye, H., Daoud-El Baba, M., Peng, R.-W., Fussenegger, M., 2011. A synthetic optogenetic transcription device enhances blood-glucose homeostasis in mice. Science 332, 1565–1568.

Ye, M., Hu, J., Peng, M., Liu, J., Liu, J., Liu, H., Zhao, X., Tan, W., 2012. Generating aptamers by cell-SELEX for applications in molecular medicine. Int. J. Mol. Sci. 13, 3341–3353.

Yin, H., Xue, W., Chen, S., Bogorad, R.L., Benedetti, E., Grompe, M., Koteliansky, V., Sharp, P.A., Jacks, T., Anderson, D.G., 2014. Genome editing with Cas9 in adult mice corrects a disease mutation and phenotype. Nat. Biotechnol. 32, 551–553.

You, L., Cox, R.S., Weiss, R., Arnold, F.H., 2004. Programmed population control by cell–cell communication and regulated killing. Nature 428, 868–871.

Zaslaver, A., Mayo, A.E., Rosenberg, R., Bashkin, P., Sberro, H., Tsalyuk, M., Surette, M.G., Alon, U., 2004. Just-in-time transcription program in metabolic pathways. Nat. Genet. 36, 486–491.

Zaslaver, A., Mayo, A., Ronen, M., Alon, U., 2006. Optimal gene partition into operons correlates with gene functional order. Phys. Biol. 3, 183–189.

Zhang, M., Forbes, N.S., 2015. Trg-deficient Salmonella colonize quiescent tumor regions by exclusively penetrating or proliferating. J. Control. Release 199, 180–189.

Zhang, M., Swofford, C.A., Forbes, N.S., 2014. Lipid A controls the robustness of intratumoral accumulation of attenuated *Salmonella* in mice. Int. J. Cancer 135, 647–657.

Zhao, M., Yang, M., Li, X.-M., Jiang, P., Baranov, E., Li, S., Xu, M., Penman, S., Hoffman, R.M., 2005. Tumor-targeting bacterial therapy with amino acid auxotrophs of GFP-expressing Salmonella typhimurium. Proc. Natl. Acad. Sci. U. S. A. 102, 755–760.

Zhao, M., Yang, M., Ma, H., Li, X., Tan, X., Li, S., Yang, Z., Hoffman, R.M., 2006. Targeted therapy with a Salmonella typhimurium leucine-arginine auxotroph cures orthotopic human breast tumors in nude mice. Cancer Res. 66, 7647–7652.

Zhao, M., Geller, J., Ma, H., Yang, M., Penman, S., Hoffman, R.M., 2007. Monotherapy with a tumor-targeting mutant of Salmonella typhimurium cures orthotopic metastatic mouse models of human prostate cancer. Proc. Natl. Acad. Sci. 104, 10170–10174.

Zhou, S., Zhang, M., Wang, J., 2011. Tumor-targeted delivery of TAT-Apoptin fusion gene using *Escherichia coli* Nissle 1917 to colorectal cancer. Med. Hypotheses 76, 533–534.

Zhu, H., Li, Z., Mao, S., Ma, B., Zhou, S., Deng, L., Liu, T., Cui, D., Zhao, Y., He, J., 2011. Antitumor effect of sFlt-1 gene therapy system mediated by Bifidobacterium infantis on Lewis lung cancer in mice. Cancer Gene Ther. 18, 884–896.

Zhu, W., Lei, R., Le Duff, Y., Li, J., Guo, F., Wainberg, M.A., Liang, C., 2015. The CRISPR/Cas9 system inactivates latent HIV-1 proviral DNA. Retrovirology 12, 1–7.

Abbreviation

A	electrode area
A	alanine
AAT	alpha-1 antitrypsin
AAV	adeno-associated virus
ACV	alternating current voltammetry
Ad	adenovirus
ADSCs	adipose-derived stem cells
AFS	amniotic fluid
AGIO	amphiphilic gelatin-iron oxide
Ago2	Argonaute 2
AHL	acyl-homoserine lactone
a_i	ion activity
AI-2	auto-inducer 2
AIP	acute intermittent porphyria
ALP	alkaline phosphatase
AMP	antimicrobial peptide
ANN	artificial neural networks
AP	alkaline phosphatase
APCs	antigen presentation cells; adipose tissue-derived progenitor cells
API	active pharmaceutical ingredient
ApoB	apolipoprotein B
Apt	aptamer
APTES	(3-aminopropyl)-triethoxysilane
ASA	acetyl salicylic acid
Asp	aspartic acid
ATTR	transthyretin-related amyloidosis
AtuFECT	β-l-arginyl-2,3-L-diaminopropionic acid-*N*-palmityl-*N*-oleyl-amide trihydrochloride
AuMNPs	gold magnetic nanoparticles
AuNPs	gold nanoparticles
BA	boronic acids
BAI	biomaterial-associated infection
BBB	blood-brain barrier
BC	bacterial cellulose
Bcl-2	B-cell lymphoma 2
bDNA	branched DNA
bFGF	basic fibroblast growth factor, also known as FGF-2
Bio	biotinylated
BMPs	bone morphogenetic proteins
BMSCs	bone mesenchymal stem cells
C	analyte concentration
CAI-1	cholera auto-inducer 1

cAMP	cyclic adenosine monophosphate
CaP	calcium phosphate
CAs	contrast agents
CBD	collagen-binding domain
CCL	chemokine (C-C motif) ligand
CCMV	cowpea chlorotic mottle virus
CCR5	co-receptor C-C chemokine receptor type 5
CD	cluster of differentiation
CD31	platelet endothelial cell adhesion molecule-1
cDNA	complementary DNA
CDS	coding DNA sequence
CdS-QDs	cadmium sulfide quantum dot
CE	counter electrode
CEA	carcinoembryonic antigen
CF	cystic fibrosis
ChIP	chromatin immunoprecipitation
ChIP-chip	ChIP combined with microarrays
ChIP-seq	ChIP combined with sequencing
CMC	carboxymethyl-chitosan
CMs	cardiomyocytes
CNFs	carbon nanofibers
CNS	central nervous system
CNTs	carbon nanotubes
ConA	concanavalin A
CpG	DNA oligonucleotide sequences characterized by the presence of the dinucleotide CG
CPMV	cowpea mosaic virus
CPP	cell penetrating peptide
CREB1	cAMP-responsive element binding protein 1
CRISPR	clustered regularly interspaced short palindromic repeats
CRP	C-reactive protein
crRNA	short CRISPR RNA
CS	chitosan
CSE	cross-sensitivity electrodes
CTLA	cytotoxic T lymphocyte associated antigen receptor
CuAAC	copper-catalyzed azide-alkyne cycloaddition
CV	cyclic voltammetry
Cys	cysteine
D	diffusion coefficient
D	aspartic acid
DAP	diaminopimelic acid
DCs	dendritic cells
DDS	drug delivery system
DLAPs	dabycyl-labeled aptamer modified metal nanoparticles
DLin-DMA	1,2-dilinoleyloxy-3-dimethylaminopropane
DLin-KC2-DMA	1,2-dilinoleyl-4-(2-dimethylaminoethyl)-[1,3]-dioxolane
DLin-K-DMA	1,2-dilinoleyloxy-keto-*N*,*N*-dimethyl-3-aminopropane
DLin-MC3-DMA	heptatriaconta-6,9,28,31-tetraen-19-yl 4-(dimethylamino)butanoate
DLin-MP-DMA	3-(dilinoleylmethoxy)-*N*,*N*-dimethylpropan-1-amine

DNA	deoxyribonucleic acid
DODAP	1,2-dioleoyl-3-dimethylammonium propane
DOGS	di-octadecyl-amido-glycyl-spermine
DOPC	1,2-dioleoyl-sn-glycero-3-phosphatidylcholine
DOPE	1,2-dioleoyl-sn-glycero-3-phosphoethanolamine
DOTAP	*N*-[1-(2,3-dioleoyloxy)-propyl]-*N*,*N*,*N*-trimethyl ammonium methylsulfate
DOTMA	*N*-[1-(2,3-dioleyloxy)propyl]-*N*,*N*,*N*-trimethylammonium
DOX	doxorubicin
DPC	dynamic polyconjugates
DPV	differential pulse voltammetry
DREADD	designer receptor exclusively activated by designer drugs
ds	double strand
DSB	double-strand break
dsDNA	double-strain DNA
DSPC	1,2-distearoyl-sn-glycero-3-phosphocholine
DSPE-PEG	1,2-distearoyl-sn-glycero-3-phosphoethanolamine-*N*-amino(polyethylene glycol)
dsRNA	double-stranded RNA
DTPA	diethylenetriaminepentaacetic acid
E	electric potential difference
E_0	temperature-dependent standard potential of the electrode
E_{AP}	anode potential
ECM	extracellular matrix
E_{CP}	cathode potential
ECTs	engineer cardiac tissues
EEAPs	electronic electroactive polymers
EGF	epidermal growth factor
EGFR	EGF receptor
EIS	electrochemical impedance spectroscopy
elF5A	eukaryotic translational initiation factor 5A
EngNT	engineered neural tissue
E_P	potential value at peak's maximum intensity current
EphA2	ephrin receptor A2
EPR	enhanced permeation and retention
EPS	extracellular polymeric substances
ER	estrogen receptor
ESI-MS	electrospray ionization-MS
E-tongue	electronic tongue
F	Faraday constant
f	frequency
FA	folic acid
FBA	flux balance analysis
FBAR	film bulk acoustic resonator
FBS	fetal bovine serum
Fc	ferrocene
FDA	Food and Drug Administration
FDA	US Food and Drug Administration
FGF	fibroblast growth factor

FGFR	FGF receptor
f-MWCNTs	functionalized-MWCNTs
FNR	fumarate and nitrate reduction regulator
FT-ICR	Fourier Transform ion cyclotron resonance
G	glycine
G (G1, G2, G3,...)	dendrimer generations (one, two, three...)
GA	glutaraldehyde
GAGs	glycosaminoglycans
GalNAc	triantennary *N*-acetylgalactosamine
GBPs	glycan-binding proteins
GCE	glassy carbon electrode
Gd	gadolinium
GdIII	gadolinium(III)
GDNF	glial cell-derived neurotrophic factor
GFP	green fluorescent protein
GLP-1	glucagon-like peptide 1
Glu	glutamic acid
GM3	ganglioside-monosialic acid 3
GM-CSF	granulocyte macrophage-colony stimulating factor
GO	graphene oxide
GO_x	glucose oxidase
GPCR	G-protein-coupled receptor
GRRS	global-replacement residue specific
H	hydrophobic
HA	hyaluronic acid; hydroxyapatite
HAI	hepatic arterial infusion
HB-EGF	heparin binding EGF
HBGF-2	heparin binding growth factor 2
HBV	hepatitis B virus
HcoPt	hollow CoPt alloy nanoparticles
HCST	higher critical solution temperature
HCV	hepatitis C virus
HEG	homing endonuclease-based gene
HGF	hepatocyte growth factor
HIV	human immunodeficiency virus
HRP	horseradish peroxidase; streptavidin-horseradish peroxidase
HSA	human serum albumin
HSP47	heat shock protein 47
HSV-TK	herpes simplex virus thymidine kinase
hTERT	human telomerase reverse transcriptase
hUP II	human uroplakin II gene
HyA	hyaluronic acid
I	ionic force
I_1	current intensity before the end of the pulse
I_2	current intensity before pulse application
IAA	indole-3-acetic acid
I_{AP}	anode peak current intensity
I_{CP}	cathode peak current intensity
Id2	inhibitor of DNA-bind-2

IDLV	integrase-defective lentivirus vector
IE	indicator electrode
IEAPs	ionic electroactive polymers
IFNα-2b	interferon alpha-2b
IFN-γ	interferon gamma
I_{fwd}	forward mode peak current intensity
IGF	insulin-like growth factor
IL	interleukin
I_P	peak´s maximum intensity current
IPNs	interpenetrating polymeric networks
iPSC	induced pluripotent stem cell
IPTG	isopropyl β-D-1-thiogalactopyranoside
IR	infrared
I_{rev}	reverse mode peak current intensity
ISE	ion selective electrodes
IVD	in vitro diagnostic
k	global constant in Eq. (13.3)
Kij	selectivity coefficient of the indicator electrode for the interfering ion *j*
KRAB	Krüppel associated box
KRAS	Kirsten rat sarcoma viral oncogene homolog
KSP	kinesin spindle protein
LAPC	locally advanced pancreatic cancer
LbL	layer-by-layer
LC-MS	liquid chromatography-MS
LCST	lower critical solution temperature
LDA	linear discriminant analysis
LDL	low density lipoprotein
LHR	luteinizing hormone receptor
LLV	leukolike vector
LODER	local drug eluter
LPS	lipopolysaccharides
Lys	lysine
LYS	lysozyme
M1	proinflammatory, classically activated macrophage
M2	prohealing, alternatively activated macrophage
MAGE	multiplex automated genome engineering
MALDI-ToF-MS	matrix-assisted laser desorption/ionization-time of flight-MS
MB	methylene blue
MCP	monocyte chemotactic protein
MEMS	microelectromechanical systems
MFA	metabolic flux analysis
MHC-I	major histocompatibility complex 1
MHC-II	major histocompatibility complex 2
MIP	molecularly imprinted polymers
MIP-1α	macrophage inflammatory protein 1 alpha
MIP-1β	macrophage inflammatory protein 1 beta
miRNA	micro-RNA
MLP	melittin-like peptide
MMP	matrixmetalloproteinases

MNPs	magnetic nanoparticles
MO-MAGE	microarray-oligonucleotide MAGE
MPS	mononuclear phagocyte system
MRI	magnetic resonance imaging
mRNA	messenger RNA
MS	mass spectrometry
MSC	mesenchymal stem cells
MTX	methotrexate
MUC1	mucin 1
MudPIT	multidimensional protein identification technology
MVL5	*N*1-[2-((1*S*)-1-[(3-aminopropyl)amino]-4-[di(3-amino-propyl)amino] butylcarboxamido)ethyl]-3,4-di[oleyloxy]-benzamide
MWCNTs	multiwalled carbon nanotubes
MYC	myelocytomatosis oncogene cellular homolog
n	number of electrons
NAE	*N*-acylethanolamide
NAG	*N*-acetylgalactosamine
NAPE	*N*-acylphosphatidylethanolamine
NAs	nucleic acids
NDi	naphthalene diimide
NHEJ	non-homologous end joining
NHS	*N*-hydroxysuccinimidyl; *N*-hydroxysuccinimide
NLC	nanostructured lipid carriers
NMR	nuclear magnetic resonance
NPs	nanoparticles
NT-3	neurotrophin-3
ON	oligonucleotides
OPN	osteopontin
ORF	open reading frame
P	polar
P	proline
PAA	polyacrylamide; polyacrylic acid
PAF	platelet-activating factor
PAMAM	poly(amido amine)
PAR-1	protease-activated receptor-1
PAs	peptide amphiphiles
PbAE	poly(β-amino esters)
PBAE	poly(β-amino esters)
PBAVE	polybutylamino vinyl ether polymer
PBS	phosphate buffered saline
PCL	poly-e-caprolactone
PCSK9	protein convertase subtilisin/kexin type 9
PDA	polydopamine
PDGF	platelet-derived growth factor
PDITC	*p*-phenylene diisothiocyanate
PDMAEMA	poly(2-dimethylaminoethyl methacrylate)
PDMS	poly(dimethylsiloxane)
PDX-1	pancreatic and duodenal homeobox gene 1
PEG	polyethylene glycol

PEI	polyethylenimine
PEO	polyethylene oxide
PET	positron emission tomography
pFN	plasma fibronectin
PGA	polyglycolic acid
PKN3	protein kinase N3
PKs	pharmacokinetics
PLA	polylactic acid; polylactide
PLGA	poly-lactic-*co*-glycolic acid; poly(lactide-*co*-glycolide)
PlGF-2	placenta growth factor-2
PLK1	polo-like kinase 1
PLL	poly(lysine)-based dendrimers
PLS	partial least squares
PMAA	poly(methacrylic acid)
PMMA	poly(methyl methacrylate)
PNH	paroxysmal nocturnal hemoglobinuria
PNIPAAm	poly(*N*-isopropylacrylamide)
PNS	peripheral nervous system
PoPD	poly(*o*-phenylenediamine)
PPARα	peroxisome proliferator-associated receptor alpha
PPI	poly(propylene imine
pre-miRNA	precursor micro-RNA
pri-miRNA	primary micro-RNA
PRRs	pattern recognition receptors
PtNPs	platinum nanoparticles
γ-PVA	poly-γ-glutamic acid
PVA	poly(vinyl alcohol)
PVC	polyvinyl chloride
PVDF	poly(vinylidene fluoride)
PVX	potato virus X
PZT	lead zirconate titanate
QCM	quartz crystal microbalance
QSI	quorum sensing inhibitor
R	ideal gas constant
R	arginine
RASSL	receptors activated solely by synthetic ligands
RBC	red blood cell
RBS	ribosome-binding site
RE	reference electrode
Re	Reynolds number
RGD	arginine-glycine-aspartate
rGS	reduced graphene oxide sheet
RHCC	right-handed coiled coil
RIDL	dominant lethal genetic system
RISC	RNA-induced silencing complex
RNA	ribonucleic acid
RNAi	RNA interference
ROS	reactive oxygen species
RRM2	ribonuclease reductase

SA	simulated annealing
SAH	*Staphylococcus aureus* α-hemolysin
SAM	self-assembled monolayers
SAVE	synthetic attenuated virus engineering
SAWs	surface acoustic waves
SCRIBE	synthetic cellular recorders integrating biological events
SCs	Schwann cells
SEDDS	self-emulsifying drug-delivery systems
SELEX	systematic evolution of ligands by exponential enrichment
SHED	stem cells from human exfoliated deciduous teeth
shRNA	short hairpin RNA
SH-SAW	shear horizontal SAW
SiO2@MWCNTs	functionalized silica/multiwalled carbon nanotubes core-shell nanocomposites
siRNA	small-interfering RNA
SIS	small intestinal submucosa
SLN	solid lipid nanoparticles
SNALP	stable nucleic acid lipid particles
SPE	screen-printed electrodes
SPIONs	superparamagnetic iron oxide nanoparticles
SPR	surface plasmon resonance
SRM	selected reaction monitoring
ss	single strand
ssAON	single-stranded antisense oligonucleotides
ssDNA	single-stranded DNA
SSI	site-specific incorporation
SSTs	single-stranded tiles
strep	streptavidin
S-Tube	straight nanotube structure
STV	streptavidin
SWCNT	single-walled carbon nanotubes
SWV	square wave voltammetry
T	absolute temperature
t	time
T	threonine
TALEN	transcription activator-like effector nucleases
Tb	toluidine blue
TCPs	tissue culture polystyrene
TCR	T-cell receptor
TENGs	tissue engineered nerve grafts
TET	tetracycline
TG2	tissue transglutaminase
TGF-α	transforming growth factor-alpha
TGF-β	transforming growth factor beta
Thi	thionine
THR	thrombin
Ti	titanium
TIE-2	tyrosine kinase receptor 2
TIR	translation initiation rate

TISAB	total ionic strength adjustment buffer solution
TLR	toll-like receptors
TMPRSS2/EGR	transmembrane protease, serine 2/erythroblast transformation-specific related gene
TMV	tobacco mosaic virus
TNF	Tumor necrosis factor
TNF-α	tumour necrosis factor alpha
TRAIL	TNF-related apoptosis-inducing ligand
tTA	transactivator
TTR	transthyretin
T-VEC	talimogene laherparepvec
Tyr	tyrosine
uAAs	unnatural amino acids
UBM	urinary bladder matrix
UCST	upper critical solution temperature
URAT1	uric acid transporter
UTR	untranslated regions
v	scan rate
V^D	D-form of valine
VEGF	vascular endothelial growth factor
VLPs	virus-like particles
VNPs	virus nanoparticles
WE	working electrode
Y	complex conductance
YAP/TAZ	Yes-associated protein/transcriptional coactivator with PDZ binding motif
Z	electrical impedance
ZFN	zinc-finger nuclease.
zi	ionic charge of species i
Zr	zirconium
αSMA	alpha smooth muscle actin
β-CDs	β-cyclodextrins
γ	activity coefficient
ΔI	difference between two current intensities
φ	phase shift between the voltage-time and current-time functions
2D	two-dimensional
3D	three-dimensional

Index

Note: Page numbers followed by *f* indicates figures and *t* indicates tables.

T